Neurodegeneration and Alzheimer's Disease

Neurodegeneration and Alzheimer's Disease

The Role of Diabetes, Genetics, Hormones, and Lifestyle

Edited by

Editors:
Ralph N. Martins
Edith Cowan University
Joondalup
Australia

Macquarie University
Sydney
Australia

Charles S. Brennan
Lincoln University
Christchurch
New Zealand

Associate Editors:
W.M.A.D. Binosha Fernando
Edith Cowan University
Joondalup
Australia

Margaret A. Brennan
Lincoln University
Christchurch
New Zealand

Stephanie J. Fuller
Edith Cowan University
Joondalup
Australia

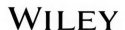

This edition first published 2019
© 2019 John Wiley & Sons Ltd

All rights reserved. No part of this publication may be reproduced, stored in a retrieval system, or transmitted, in any form or by any means, electronic, mechanical, photocopying, recording or otherwise, except as permitted by law. Advice on how to obtain permission to reuse material from this title is available at http://www.wiley.com/go/permissions.

The right of Ralph N. Martins, Charles S. Brennan, W.M.A.D. Binosha Fernando, Margaret A. Brennan and Stephanie J. Fuller to be identified as the authors of this editorial material has been asserted in accordance with law.

Registered Office(s)
John Wiley & Sons, Inc., 111 River Street, Hoboken, NJ 07030,USA
John Wiley & Sons Ltd, The Atrium, Southern Gate, Chichester, West Sussex, PO19 8SQ,UK

Editorial Office
The Atrium, Southern Gate, Chichester, West Sussex, PO19 8SQ,UK

For details of our global editorial offices, customer services, and more information about Wiley products visit us at www.wiley.com.

Wiley also publishes its books in a variety of electronic formats and by print-on-demand. Some content that appears in standard print versions of this book may not be available in other formats.

Limit of Liability/Disclaimer of Warranty
While the publisher and authors have used their best efforts in preparing this work, they make no representations or warranties with respect to the accuracy or completeness of the contents of this work and specifically disclaim all warranties, including without limitation any implied warranties of merchantability or fitness for a particular purpose. No warranty may be created or extended by sales representatives, written sales materials or promotional statements for this work. The fact that an organization, website, or product is referred to in this work as a citation and/or potential source of further information does not mean that the publisher and authors endorse the information or services the organization, website, or product may provide or recommendations it may make. This work is sold with the understanding that the publisher is not engaged in rendering professional services. The advice and strategies contained herein may not be suitable for your situation. You should consult with a specialist where appropriate. Further, readers should be aware that websites listed in this work may have changed or disappeared between when this work was written and when it is read. Neither the publisher nor authors shall be liable for any loss of profit or any other commercial damages, including but not limited to special, incidental, consequential, or other damages.

Library of Congress Cataloging-in-Publication data has been applied for

ISBN: 9781119356783

Cover Design: Wiley
Cover Images: © Irina Shatilova/Shutterstock, © Henrik5000/iStock.com, © corgarashu/Shutterstock, © Andrey Prokhorov/iStock.com

Set in 10/12pt WarnockPro by SPi Global, Chennai, India

Printed and bound in Singapore by Markono Print Media Pte Ltd

10 9 8 7 6 5 4 3 2 1

Contents

List of Contributors *xv*

1   Current Understanding of Alzheimer's Disease and Other Neurodegenerative Diseases, and the Potential Role of Diet and Lifestyle in Reducing the Risks of Alzheimer's Disease and Cognitive Decline *1*
Charles S. Brennan, Margaret A. Brennan, W.M.A.D. Binosha Fernando and Ralph N. Martins
References *7*

2   Alzheimer's Disease and Other Neurodegenerative Diseases *9*
Stephanie J. Fuller, Hamid R. Sohrabi, Kathryn G. Goozee, Anoop Sankaranarayanan and Ralph N. Martins

2.1   Introduction *9*
2.2   Alzheimer's Disease *9*
2.2.1   Pathology *9*
2.2.2   Symptoms *10*
2.2.3   Incidence *11*
2.2.4   Onset and Risk Factors *12*
2.2.5   Treatment *12*
2.2.6   Potential for AD Prevention *13*
2.3   Frontotemporal Lobe Dementia *13*
2.3.1   Neuropathology and Causes *14*
2.3.2   Treatment *15*
2.3.3   Diagnosis and Clinical Overlap with Other Diseases *15*
2.4   Vascular Dementia *16*
2.4.1   Symptoms and Diagnosis *16*
2.4.2   Causes and Risk Factors *16*
2.4.3   Prevention and Treatment *17*
2.4.4   Dementia with Lewy Bodies *18*
2.4.5   Causes *18*
2.4.6   Symptoms *18*
2.4.7   Diagnosis of DLB *18*
2.4.7.1   Clinical Approach to Dementias *19*

2.5	Parkinson's Disease	*19*
2.5.1	Onset	*22*
2.5.2	Causes and Risk Factors	*22*
2.5.3	Incidence	*22*
2.5.4	Pathology	*22*
2.5.5	Treatment	*23*
2.6	Huntington's Disease	*24*
2.6.1	Genetics of the Disease	*24*
2.6.2	Incidence and Prevalence	*25*
2.6.3	Pathology	*25*
2.6.4	Treatment	*26*
2.7	Motor Neuron Diseases	*27*
2.7.1	Amyotrophic Lateral Sclerosis	*27*
2.7.2	Spinal Muscular Atrophy	*27*
2.7.3	Hereditary Spastic Paraplegia	*27*
2.7.4	Onset of MND and Differential Diagnosis	*28*
2.7.5	Incidence, Causes, and Risk Factors	*28*
2.7.6	Pathology	*29*
2.7.7	Treatment	*30*
2.8	Prion Diseases	*30*
2.8.1	Causes	*31*
2.8.2	Symptoms and Diagnosis	*31*
2.8.3	Treatment	*32*
2.8.4	Differential Diagnosis of the Various Types of Dementia	*32*
2.8.5	DLB Treatment	*33*
2.9	Summary	*33*
	References	*34*
3	**Current and Developing Methods for Diagnosing Alzheimer's Disease** *43*	
	Stephanie J. Fuller, Nicholas Carrigan, Hamid R. Sohrabi and Ralph N. Martins	
3.1	Introduction	*43*
3.2	Classical Post-Mortem Diagnosis	*43*
3.2.1	Plaques	*44*
3.2.2	Neurofibrillary Tangles (NFT)	*44*
3.2.3	Cerebral Amyloid Angiopathy (CAA)	*44*
3.2.4	Glial Responses	*45*
3.2.5	Brain Shrinkage	*45*
3.2.6	Loss of Synapses and Neurons	*45*
3.3	Clinical Diagnosis	*45*
3.3.1	Initial Assessment/Screening Tools	*47*
3.3.1.1	Mini-Mental State Examination (MMSE)	*47*
3.3.1.2	Montreal Cognitive Assessment (MoCA)	*47*
3.3.1.3	Clinical Dementia Rating (CDR)	*47*
3.3.1.4	Clock Drawing	*48*
3.3.1.5	Seven-Minute Screen	*48*
3.3.1.6	Alzheimer's Disease Assessment Scale (ADAS-Cog)	*48*
3.3.1.7	Psychogeriatric Assessment Scales (PAS)	*48*

3.3.1.8	Dementia Rating Scale (DRS)	49
3.3.1.9	Mini-Cog	49
3.3.1.10	Rowland Universal Dementia Assessment Scale (RUDAS)	49
3.3.1.11	The Consortium to Establish a Registry for Alzheimer's Disease (CERAD) Neuropsychological Battery (nb) and Other Tests	49
3.4	Brain Imaging in the Diagnosis of Alzheimer's Disease and Other Dementias	51
3.4.1	Imaging Tests in AD Diagnosis: Established Tests	51
3.4.1.1	Computed Tomography (CT)	51
3.4.1.2	Electroencephalography (EEG)	51
3.4.1.3	Magnetic Resonance Imaging (MRI), for the Assessment of Morphological Changes, and the Detection of Stroke	52
3.4.1.4	Positron Emission Tomography (PET)	52
3.4.1.5	FDG-PET	52
3.4.2	Imaging Tests in AD Diagnosis: More Recently Developed Tests	52
3.4.2.1	MRI for Measuring Regional Blood Flow	53
3.4.2.2	Single Photon Emission Computed Tomography (SPECT) Scan	54
3.4.2.3	PiB-PET	54
3.4.3	The Rapidly Evolving Diagnostic Criteria	55
3.4.4	CSF Biomarkers of AD	56
3.4.4.1	Aβ, Tau, and AβPP-Related Biomarkers	56
3.4.4.2	Other Potential CSF Protein Biomarkers	57
3.4.4.3	Potential Lipid Biomarkers in the CSF	58
3.4.5	Blood Biomarkers of AD	60
3.4.5.1	Aβ Peptides in Plasma	60
3.4.5.2	Other Potential Blood Biomarkers	62
3.4.5.3	Blood Proteins	62
3.4.6	Blood Lipids	64
3.4.7	Metabolites	65
3.4.8	Blood Platelets	66
3.4.9	Genetic Risk Factors	67
3.4.10	The Eye as a Window to the Brain	68
3.4.11	miRNA Tests	69
3.5	Conclusions	71
	References	72
4	**The Link Between Diabetes, Glucose Control, and Alzheimer's Disease and Neurodegenerative Diseases**	**89**
	Giuseppe Verdile, Paul E. Fraser and Ralph N. Martins	
4.1	Introduction	89
4.2	The Impact of Type 2 Diabetes on the Brain	90
4.3	Evidence from Cell Culture, Animal, and Clinical Studies	93
4.3.1	CNS Insulin Signalling and Disruptions in AD	93
4.3.2	The Accumulation of Aβ Is Associated with Impaired Insulin Signalling	94
4.3.3	Insulin Resistance Promotes the Accumulation of Aβ	95
4.3.4	Impairments in Insulin Signalling Can Induce Hyperphosphorylation of Tau	96
4.3.5	Type 2 Diabetes and Neuroinflammation	96

4.3.6	Oxidative Stress and Mitochondrial Dysfunction in T2D and AD *97*
4.3.7	Targeting Type 2 Diabetes to Slow Down Progression/Prevent Neurodegeneration and Cognitive Decline *99*
4.4	Conclusions *103*
	References *103*

5 Diet and Nutrition, and their Influence on Alzheimer's Disease and other Neurodegenerative Diseases *117*
Stephanie R. Rainey-Smith, Rhona Creegan, Stephanie J. Fuller, Michele L. Callisaya and Velandai Srikanth

5.1	Introduction *117*
5.2	Dietary Patterns *118*
5.3	Key Macronutrients *119*
5.3.1	Dietary Fatty Acids *119*
5.3.2	Cholesterol *120*
5.3.3	Polyunsaturated Fatty Acids *121*
5.3.4	Dietary Carbohydrates *122*
5.4	Key Micronutrients *124*
5.4.1	Water Soluble Vitamins *125*
5.4.1.1	B Vitamins *125*
5.4.2	Fat Soluble Vitamins *128*
5.4.2.1	Vitamin A (Retinol, Retinal, and Retinoic Acid) *128*
5.4.2.2	Vitamin D *129*
5.4.2.3	Vitamin E *130*
5.4.3	Dietary Minerals *131*
5.4.3.1	Selenium *131*
5.4.3.2	Manganese *132*
5.4.3.3	Zinc, Iron, Copper, and Calcium *132*
5.5	Conclusion *134*
	References *135*

6 Carbohydrate and Protein Metabolism: Influences on Cognition and Alzheimer's Disease *149*
W.M.A.D. Binosha Fernando, Veer B. Gupta, Vijay Jayasena, Charles S. Brennan and Ralph N. Martins

6.1	Carbohydrates *149*
6.1.1	Carbohydrate Digestion *149*
6.1.2	Glucose Ingestion and Use *151*
6.1.3	Glucose and Insulin, Insulin Resistance, and Type 2 Diabetes (Short Summary) *151*
6.1.4	Relative Intake of Carbohydrate and Its Impacts on Neurodegenerative Disease Risk *152*
6.1.5	Ketogenic Diets *154*
6.1.6	Glucose and Its Effects on Cognition *154*
6.1.7	Possible Mechanisms Related to Memory Enhancement with Glucose *157*
6.1.7.1	Glucose and the Hippocampus *158*
6.1.7.2	Glucose Availability in Brain Cells *158*

6.1.7.3	Glucose and the Central Cholinergic System	*159*
6.1.7.4	ATP-Regulated Potassium (K-ATP) Channels and Brain Control of Glucose Homeostasis *159*	
6.1.7.5	Effects of High Fructose Diets *160*	
6.1.7.6	Sucrose *161*	
6.2	Proteins *161*	
6.2.1	Protein Metabolism in General *162*	
6.2.2	Links Between Specific Amino Acids and Brain Function *163*	
6.2.2.1	Tryptophan *163*	
6.2.2.2	Tyrosine *164*	
6.2.3	Clinical Studies of Protein Supplementation *165*	
6.2.4	Links Between Loss of Protein Function and Neurodegeneration *167*	
6.2.5	Clearance Mechanisms Associated with Proteinopathies Involved in Neurodegeneration *168*	
6.2.6	Role of Protein Crosslinking and Inflammation in Neurodegeneration and AD *170*	
6.3	Conclusion *171*	
	References *171*	

7   Fat and Lipid Metabolism and the Involvement of Apolipoprotein E in Alzheimer's Disease *189*
   Eugene Hone, Florence Lim and Ian J. Martins

7.1	Introduction *189*	
7.2	Alzheimer's Disease *189*	
7.3	Cholesterol and Lipid Metabolism *190*	
7.3.1	Cholesterol Synthesis and Metabolism *190*	
7.3.2	Oxysterols *191*	
7.3.2.1	Oxysterols in AD *191*	
7.3.3	Pathways of Dietary (Exogenous) Lipid Homeostasis *192*	
7.3.4	Pathways of Endogenous Lipid Homeostasis *193*	
7.3.5	Peripheral Clearance of Lipoproteins and Reverse Cholesterol Transport *195*	
7.3.5.1	Lipoproteins in the CNS *197*	
7.4	Apolipoprotein E Alleles and Isoforms *197*	
7.4.1	ApoE in the Brain *198*	
7.4.2	Apolipoprotein E and Alzheimer's Disease *198*	
7.4.2.1	ApoE Binding to Aβ *199*	
7.4.2.2	ApoE in the Cellular Clearance of Aβ *200*	
7.4.2.3	ApoE and Antioxidant Properties *201*	
7.4.2.4	ApoE and Tissue Transglutaminase *201*	
7.4.2.5	Apolipoprotein J (Clusterin, CLU) *202*	
7.5	LRP-1 in the Brain and Its Role in Aβ Clearance *203*	
7.5.1	LDL, HDL, and AD *203*	
7.5.2	Statins, Cholesterol, and AD *204*	
7.6	The Role of Lipid Rafts in Neurodegenerative Diseases *205*	
7.7	Changes to Glycerophospholipids in Alzheimer's Disease *206*	
7.7.1	Omega-3 and Omega-6 Fatty Acids *207*	

7.7.1.1	Omega-3 Fatty Acids, Modern Diets, and Health Implications	208
7.8	Sphingolipids	208
7.8.1	Ceramides	208
7.8.2	Sulfatides	209
7.8.3	Gangliosides	209
7.9	Conclusions	210
	References	210
8	**Inflammation in Alzheimer's Disease, and Prevention with Antioxidants and Phenolic Compounds – What Are the Most Promising Candidates?**	**233**
	Matthew J. Sharman, Giuseppe Verdile, Shanmugam Kirubakaran and Gerald Münch	
8.1	Introduction	233
8.2	Inflammation and the Immune Response in AD	233
8.2.1	The Role of Microglia and Astrocytes in Chronic Inflammation in AD	233
8.3	Oxidative Stress	236
8.3.1	Advanced Glycation End Products	237
8.3.2	Involvement of the Complement System in AD	238
8.3.3	Involvement of Cytokines and Chemokines in Inflammation	239
8.3.4	Inflammation – Susceptibility to Aβ Deposition or Aggregation	240
8.3.5	Inflammation Can Influence AβPP Metabolism and Aβ Clearance Directly	241
8.4	Current Medications for AD	242
8.4.1	Current Medications – Acetylcholinesterase Inhibitors and Memantine	242
8.5	Disease Modification and Treatment Approaches	243
8.5.1	Non-Steroidal Anti-Inflammatory Drugs (NSAID)	243
8.6	Some Anti-inflammatory Foods, Supplements, and Newly Developed Drugs for the Treatment of AD	244
8.6.1	Cinnamon/Cinnamaldehyde	244
8.6.2	(−)Epigallocatechin-3-Gallate (EGCG) and Other Green Tea Polyphenols	245
8.6.3	Curcumin	247
8.6.4	Other Polyphenolic Antioxidants	248
8.6.5	Omega-3 (n-3) Essential Fatty Acids	249
8.6.6	Lipoic Acid	250
8.7	Conclusion	253
	References	253
9	**Cognitive Impairments in Alzheimer's Disease and Other Neurodegenerative Diseases**	**267**
	Hamid R. Sohrabi and Michael Weinborn	
9.1	Introduction	267
9.2	Dementia due to Alzheimer's Disease	268
9.2.1	Subjective Cognitive Decline [4] and Mild Cognitive Impairment (MCI)	268

9.2.2	Memory Impairments in AD	*271*
9.2.2.1	Episodic Memory	*271*
9.2.2.2	Semantic Memory	*272*
9.2.2.3	Prospective Memory (PM)	*272*
9.2.3	Attention and Executive Dysfunction in AD	*273*
9.2.4	Language	*274*
9.2.5	Visuospatial Abilities	*276*
9.2.6	Dementia with Lewy Bodies and Parkinson's Disease with Dementia	*276*
9.2.7	Vascular Dementia	*277*
9.2.8	Frontotemporal Dementia	*279*
9.3	Conclusions	*281*
	References	*282*

10	**Animal Models of Alzheimer's Disease**	*291*
	Prashant Bharadwaj	
10.1	Introduction	*291*
10.2	Transgenic Mouse Models	*292*
10.3	Knock-in AD Mice Models	*296*
10.4	Non-Transgenic and Other Mammalian Animal Models	*297*
10.5	Drug Development and Translational Issues	*298*
10.6	Correlations Between Animal Models of AD and Human AD	*300*
10.7	Experimental Design and Reporting	*301*
10.8	The Future of Animal Models in AD	*302*
	References	*303*

11	**The Products of Fermentation and Their Effects on Metabolism, Alzheimer's Disease, and Other Neurodegenerative Diseases: Role of Short-Chain Fatty Acids (SCFA)**	*311*
	W.M.A.D Binosha Fernando, Charles S. Brennan and Ralph N. Martins	
11.1	Introduction	*311*
11.2	Fermentable Substrates and Short-Chain Fatty Acids	*312*
11.2.1	Colonic Microflora and Fermentation	*313*
11.2.1.1	Probiotics and Prebiotics	*313*
11.2.2	Propionic Acid (PPA)	*315*
11.2.3	Acetic Acid	*315*
11.2.4	Butyric Acid	*315*
11.2.5	Short-Chain Fatty Acids and Free Fatty-Acid Receptor Signalling	*316*
11.2.6	Short-Chain Fatty Acids and Energy Intake	*316*
11.2.7	Short-Chain Fatty Acids and Energy Expenditure	*319*
11.2.8	Regulation of Fatty-Acid Metabolism by SCFA	*320*
11.2.9	Effect of Short-Chain Fatty Acids on Glucose Regulation	*320*
11.2.10	Regulation of Cholesterol Metabolism by Short-Chain Fatty Acids	*321*
11.2.11	Regulation of Inflammation by Short-Chain Fatty Acids	*322*
11.2.12	Short-Chain Fatty Acids and Neuroprotection	*324*
11.3	Conclusions	*325*
	References	*326*

12	**Hormonal Expression Associated with Alzheimer's Disease and Neurodegenerative Diseases** *335*
	Giuseppe Verdile, Anna M. Barron and Ralph N. Martins
12.1	The Hypothalamic–Pituitary–Gonadal (HPG) Axis *335*
12.1.1	Dysregulation of the HPG Axis During Ageing *336*
12.2	Roles for Sex Steroids and Gonadotropins in the Neurodegenerative Process in AD *339*
12.2.1	Sex Steroids Modulate Aβ Accumulation *340*
12.2.2	Sex Steroids and Oxidative Stress *342*
12.2.3	Sex Steroids and Inflammation *344*
12.2.4	Testosterone and Diabetes *346*
12.2.5	A Role for Gonadotropins in AD Pathogenesis *347*
12.3	Hormone-based Therapies *349*
12.3.1	The Oestrogens *349*
12.3.2	Testosterone Therapy *350*
12.3.3	Selective Oestrogen or Androgen Receptor Modulators (SERM or SARM) *352*
12.3.4	Gonadotropin-Lowering Agents *354*
12.4	Conclusions *355*
	References *355*
13	**The Link Between Exercise and Mediation of Alzheimer's Disease and Neurodegenerative Diseases** *371*
	Belinda Brown and Tejal M. Shah
13.1	Introduction *371*
13.2	Physical Activity Promotes Health and Well-being *372*
13.3	Neuroplasticity *372*
13.4	The Link Between Physical Activity and Cognition Across the Human Lifespan *373*
13.4.1	Childhood *373*
13.4.2	Adulthood and Midlife *374*
13.4.3	Older Adults *375*
13.5	Physical Activity Reduces the Risk of Dementia and AD *376*
13.6	Mechanisms Underlying the Relationship Between Exercise and Brain Health *376*
13.6.1	Evidence from Molecular and Cellular Research *377*
13.6.2	Neurotrophins *378*
13.6.3	Hormonal Pathways *379*
13.6.4	Cardiovascular and Metabolic Mechanisms *380*
13.6.5	Evidence from Neuroimaging Studies *380*
13.7	The Effect of Genetics on the Relationship Between Exercise and Brain Health *381*
13.8	Future Directions *382*
	References *382*

14		**Current and Prospective Treatments for Alzheimer's Disease (and Other Neurodegenerative Diseases)** *391*
		Steve Pedrini, Mike Morici and Ralph N. Martins
14.1		Introduction *391*
14.2		Current and Potential Medical Treatments *391*
14.2.1		Treatments That Influence Neurotransmission *391*
14.2.1.1		Cholinergic System *391*
14.2.1.2		Other Neurotransmitters *396*
14.2.2		Cholesterol-Lowering Medications *399*
14.2.3		Immunotherapy *400*
14.2.3.1		Active Immunotherapy (Aβ) *401*
14.2.3.2		Active Immunotherapy (tau) *402*
14.2.3.3		Passive Immunotherapy (Aβ) *402*
14.2.3.4		Passive Immunotherapy (tau) *404*
14.2.4		Targeting the Aβ-Producing Pathway *405*
14.2.4.1		α-Secretase *406*
14.2.4.2		β-Secretase *406*
14.2.4.3		γ-Secretase *407*
14.2.5		Other Compounds Affecting Aβ *408*
14.2.6		Other Compounds Affecting Tau *410*
14.2.7		Inflammatory Targets *411*
14.3		Conclusions *412*
		References *412*
15		**The Role of Genetics in Alzheimer's Disease and Parkinson's Disease** *443*
		Tenielle Porter, Aleksandra K. Gozt, Francis L. Mastaglia and Simon M. Laws
15.1		Introduction *443*
15.2		Genetics of Alzheimer's Disease *444*
15.3		Autosomal Dominant AD (ADAD) *445*
15.3.1		Understanding the Importance of APP and the Presenilins in AD *445*
15.4		Amyloid Precursor Protein (*APP*) *447*
15.5		Presenilin 1 (*PSEN1*) *447*
15.6		Presenilin 2 (*PSEN2*) *448*
15.7		Genetic Contributions to Sporadic Late-Onset AD (LOAD) *449*
15.8		Cholesterol Metabolism *449*
15.8.1		Apolipoprotein E (*APOE*) *449*
15.8.2		Clusterin (*CLU*) *452*
15.8.3		ATP-Binding Cassette Transporter A7 (*ABCA7*) *453*
15.9		Immune Response *454*
15.9.1		Complement Receptor 1 (*CR1*) *454*
15.9.2		CD33 (Myeloid Cell Surface Antigen *CD33*; Sialic Acid-Binding Immunoglobulin-Like Lectin 3) *455*
15.9.3		Membrane Spanning 4 Domains, Subfamily A (*MS4A*) *456*
15.9.4		Triggering Receptor Expressed on Myeloid Cells 2 (*TREM2*) *456*

15.9.5	Further Genetic Associations Implicating the Immune Response *457*
15.10	Endocytosis *458*
15.10.1	Bridging Integrator 1 (*BIN1*) *459*
15.10.2	Phosphatidylinositol Binding Clathrin Assembly Lymphoid Myeloid Protein (*PICALM*) *460*
15.10.3	CD2-Associated Protein (*CD2AP*) *461*
15.10.4	Further Genetic Associations Implicating Endocytosis *462*
15.10.5	Variants in *APP* and Genes for APP-Metabolising Proteins *463*
15.10.6	Further Mechanisms Implicated Through Genetic Associations *464*
15.11	Genetics of Parkinson's Disease *465*
15.12	Monogenic forms of PD *466*
15.12.1	Autosomal Dominant Forms *466*
15.12.1.1	PARK 1 (*SNCA*) *466*
15.12.1.2	PARK 8 (*LRRK2*) *467*
15.12.1.3	PARK 11 (*GIGYF2*) *468*
15.12.1.4	PARK 17 (*VPS35*) *468*
15.12.1.5	PARK 18 (*EIF4G1*) *468*
15.12.2	Autosomal Recessive Forms *469*
15.12.2.1	PARK 2 (*PRKN*) *469*
15.12.2.2	PARK 6 (*PINK 1*) *469*
15.12.2.3	PARK 7 (*DJ-1*) *470*
15.12.2.4	PARK 9 (*ATP13A2*) *470*
15.12.2.5	PARK 14 (*PLA2G6*) *470*
15.12.2.6	PARK 15 (*FBXO7*) *471*
15.12.3	Genetic Contributions to Late-Onset Sporadic PD (LOPD) *471*
15.12.4	Common Variants in PD Genes *471*
15.12.5	Glucocerebrosidase (*GBA*) *472*
15.12.6	Immune-Inflammatory Genes *472*
15.12.7	Mitochondrial DNA Variants *473*
15.13	Conclusion *473*
	References *474*

Final Thoughts Regarding Alzheimer's Disease, Diet, and Health *499*
Charles S. Brennan, Margaret A. Brennan, W.M.A.D. Binosha Fernando, Stephanie J. Fuller and Ralph N. Martins

List of Abbreviations *503*

Index *511*

List of Contributors

Anna M. Barron
School of Psychiatry and Clinical Neurosciences
University of Western Australia
Perth, WA, Australia

and

Lee Kong Chian School of Medicine
Nanyang Technological University
Singapore

Prashant Bharadwaj
Centre of Excellence for Alzheimer's Disease Research and Care
School of Medical Sciences
Edith Cowan University
Joondalup, WA, Australia

and

School of Pharmacy and Biomedical Sciences
Curtin Health and Innovation Research Institute (CHIRI)
Faculty of Health Sciences
Curtin University
Perth, WA, Australia

and

Australian Alzheimer's Research Foundation
Ralph and Patricia Sarich Neuroscience Research Institute
Nedlands, WA, Australia

Charles S. Brennan
Department of Wine, Food and Molecular Biosciences
Centre for Food Research and Innovation
Lincoln University
Christchurch, New Zealand

and

School of Food Science
South China University of Technology
Guangzhou, China

and

School of Food Science
Tianjin University of Commerce
Tianjin, China

and

Riddett Institute Palmerston North
New Zealand

Margaret A. Brennan
Department of Wine, Food and Molecular Biosciences
Centre for Food Research and Innovation
Lincoln University
Christchurch, New Zealand

and

College of Food Science
South China University of Technology
Guangzhou, China

and

School of Food Science
Tianjin University of Commerce
Tianjin, China

Belinda Brown
School of Psychology and Exercise Science
Murdoch University
Perth, WA, Australia

and

Australian Alzheimer's Research Foundation
Ralph and Patricia Sarich Neuroscience Research Institute
Nedlands, Australia

Michele L. Callisaya
Menzies Institute for Medical Research, University of Tasmania
Hobart, TAS, Australia

and

Peninsula Clinical School
Central Clinical School Monash University
Melbourne, Vic, Australia

Nicholas Carrigan
Older Adult Mental Health Service
Western Australia Country Health Service (SouthWest)
Bunbury, WA, Australia

and

School of Medical and Health Sciences
Centre of Excellence for Alzheimer's Disease Research and Care
Edith Cowan University
Joondalup, WA, Australia

and

Australian Alzheimer's Research Foundation Ralph and Patricia Sarich Neuroscience Research Institute
Nedlands, WA, Australia

Rhona Creegan
Omega Nutrition Health
Perth, WA, Australia

W.M.A.D. Binosha Fernando
Centre of Excellence for Alzheimer's Disease Research and Care
School of Medical and Health Sciences
Edith Cowan University
Joondalup, WA, Australia

and

Australian Alzheimer's Research Foundation
Ralph and Patricia Sarich Neuroscience Research Institute
Nedlands, WA, Australia

Paul E. Fraser
Tanz Centre for Research in Neurodegenerative Diseases
University of Toronto
Canada

Stephanie J. Fuller
School of Medical and Health Sciences
Centre of Excellence for Alzheimer's Disease Research and Care
Edith Cowan University
Joondalup, WA, Australia

Kathryn G. Goozee
Department of Biomedical Sciences
Macquarie University
Sydney, NSW, Australia

and

School of Psychiatry and Clinical Neurosciences
University of Western Australia
Perth, WA, Australia

and

Cooperative Research Centre for Mental Health
Carlton, Vic, Australia

and

Kara Institute of Neurological Diseases
Sydney, NSW, Australia

and

Anglicare
Sydney, NSW, Australia

Aleksandra K. Gozt
Collaborative Genomic Group
Centre of Excellence for Alzheimer's Disease Research and Care
School of Medical Sciences
Edith Cowan University
Joondalup, WA, Australia

Veer B. Gupta
School of Medicine
Deakin University
Geelong, Vic, Australia

Eugene Hone
Centre of Excellence for Alzheimer's Disease Research and Care
School of Medical and Health Sciences
Edith Cowan University
Joondalup, WA, Australia

and

Cooperative Research Centre for Mental Health
Carlton, Vic, Australia

Vijay Jayasena
School of Science and Health
Western Sydney University
Sydney, NSW, Australia

Shanmugam Kirubakaran
Department of Pharmacology and Molecular Medicine Research Group
School of Medicine
Western Sydney University
Sydney, NSW, Australia

Simon M. Laws
Collaborative Genomic Group
Centre of Excellence for Alzheimer's Disease Research and Care
School of Medical Sciences
Edith Cowan University
Joondalup, WA, Australia

and

Cooperative Research Centre for Mental Health
Carlton, Vic, Australia

and

School of Pharmacy and Biomedical Sciences
Faculty of Health Sciences
Curtin Health Innovation Research Institute
Curtin University
Bentley, WA, Australia

Florence Lim
Centre of Excellence for Alzheimer's Disease Research and Care
School of Medical and Health Sciences
Edith Cowan University
Joondalup, WA, Australia

and

Cooperative Research Centre for Mental Health
Carlton, Vic, Australia

Ian J. Martins
Centre of Excellence for Alzheimer's Disease Research and Care
School of Medical and Health Sciences
Edith Cowan University
Joondalup, WA, Australia

and

Cooperative Research Centre for Mental Health
Carlton, Vic, Australia

Ralph N. Martins
School of Medical and Health Sciences
Centre of Excellence for Alzheimer's
Disease Research and Care
Edith Cowan University
Joondalup, WA, Australia

and

Department of Biomedical Sciences
Macquarie University
Sydney, NSW, Australia

and

School of Psychiatry and Clinical
Neurosciences
University of Western Australia
Perth, WA, Australia

and

KaRa Institute of Neurological Diseases
Sydney, NSW, Australia

and

Australian Alzheimer's Research
Foundation
Ralph and Patricia Sarich Neuroscience
Research Institute
Nedlands, WA, Australia

Francis L. Mastaglia
Institute for Immunology and Infectious
Diseases
Murdoch University
Murdoch, WA, Australia

Mike Morici
Centre of Excellence for Alzheimer's
Disease Research and Care
School of Medical and Health Sciences
Edith Cowan University
Joondalup, WA, Australia

Gerald Münch
Department of Pharmacology and
Molecular Medicine Research Group
School of Medicine
Western Sydney University
Sydney, NSW, Australia

Steve Pedrini
Centre of Excellence for Alzheimer's
Disease Research and Care
School of Medical and Health Sciences
Edith Cowan University
Joondalup, WA, Australia

and

Australian Alzheimer's Research
Foundation
Ralph and Patricia Sarich Neuroscience
Research Institute
Nedlands, WA, Australia

Tenielle Porter
Collaborative Genomic Group
Centre of Excellence for Alzheimer's
Disease Research and Care
School of Medical Sciences
Edith Cowan University
Joondalup, WA, Australia

and

Cooperative Research Centre for Mental
Health
Carlton, Vic, Australia

Stephanie R. Rainey-Smith
Centre of Excellence for Alzheimer's
Disease Research and Care
School of Medical and Health Sciences
Edith Cowan University
Joondalup, WA, Australia

and

Australia Alzheimer's Research
Foundation
Ralph and Patricia Sarich Neuroscience
Research Institute
Nedlands, WA, Australia

Anoop Sankaranarayanan
Department of Psychiatry
School of Medicine
Western Sydney University
Sydney, NSW, Australia

Tejal M. Shah
Department of Biomedical Sciences
Macquarie University
Sydney, NSW, Australia

and

Centre of Excellence for Alzheimer's
Disease Research and Care
School of Medical and Health Sciences
Edith Cowan University
Joondalup, WA, Australia

Matthew J. Sharman
School of Health Sciences
University of Tasmania
Launceston, TAS, Australia

Hamid R. Sohrabi
School of Medical and Health Sciences
Centre of Excellence for Alzheimer's
Disease Research and Care
Edith Cowan University
Joondalup, WA, Australia

and

Department of Biomedical Sciences
Macquarie University
Sydney, NSW, Australia

and

School of Psychiatry and Clinical
Neurosciences
University of Western Australia
Perth, WA, Australia

and

Cooperative Research Centre for Mental
Health
Carlton, Vic, Australia

and

KaRa Institute of Neurological Diseases
Sydney, NSW, Australia

and

Australian Alzheimer's Research
Foundation
Ralph and Patricia Sarich Neuroscience
Research Institute
Nedlands, WA, Australia

Velandai Srikanth
Department of Medicine, Peninsula
Health
Melbourne, Vic, Australia

and

Peninsula Clinical School, Central
Clinical School
Monash University
Melbourne, Vic, Australia

Giuseppe Verdile
School of Pharmacy and Biomedical
Sciences
Faculty of Health Sciences
Curtin Health Innovation Research
Institute
Curtin University of Technology
Bentley, WA, Australia

and

Centre of Excellence for Alzheimer's
Disease Research and Care
School of Medical and Health Sciences
Edith Cowan University
Joondalup, WA, Australia

and

Australian Alzheimer's Research
Foundation
Ralph and Patricia Sarich Neuroscience
Research Institute
Nedlands, WA, Australia

Michael Weinborn
School of Psychology
University of Western Australia
Crawley, WA, Australia

and

Centre of Excellence for Alzheimer's Disease Research and Care
School of Medical and Health Sciences
Edith Cowan University
Joondalup, WA, Australia

and

Australian Alzheimer's Research Foundation
Ralph and Patricia Sarich Neuroscience Research Institute
Nedlands, WA, Australia

1

Current Understanding of Alzheimer's Disease and Other Neurodegenerative Diseases, and the Potential Role of Diet and Lifestyle in Reducing the Risks of Alzheimer's Disease and Cognitive Decline

Charles S. Brennan[1,2,3,4], *Margaret A. Brennan*[1,2,4], *W.M.A.D. Binosha Fernando*[5,9] *and Ralph N. Martins*[5,6,7,8,9]

[1] *Department of Wine, Food and Molecular Biosciences, Centre for Food Research and Innovation, Lincoln University, PO Box 85084, Lincoln, Christchurch, New Zealand*
[2] *School of Food Science, South China University of Technology, Guangzhou, China*
[3] *Riddet Institute, Palmerston North, New Zealand*
[4] *School of Food Science, Tianjin University of Commerce, Tianjin, China*
[5] *School of Medical and Health Sciences, Centre of Excellence for Alzheimer's Disease Research and Care, Edith Cowan University, Joondalup, WA, Australia*
[6] *Department of Biomedical Sciences, Macquarie University, Sydney, NSW, Australia*
[7] *School of Psychiatry and Clinical Neurosciences, University of Western Australia, Perth, WA, Australia*
[8] *KaRa Institute of Neurological Diseases, Sydney, NSW, Australia*
[9] *Australian Alzheimer's Research Foundation, Ralph and Patricia Sarich Neuroscience Research Institute, Nedlands, WA, Australia*

This book is intended to give an up-to-date overview of what is currently known about neurodegenerative diseases, focusing particularly on Alzheimer's disease (AD). Current and developing diagnostic tests are described, and the pathological relationships between AD and other conditions now believed to be risk factors for AD are also described. In particular, we discuss cardiovascular disease, obesity, insulin resistance and type 2 diabetes, focusing on abnormal lipid and sugar metabolism linked to these conditions, and how this is related to AD risk. We provide evidence that improved diet and exercise may reduce AD risk, not just the risk of the other conditions mentioned above. Hopefully this book will provide some food for thought concerning easily adoptable non-pharmacological methods to reduce AD risk, which would need to be adopted at early pre-clinical stages of the disease.

Diet and health are intrinsically linked, and the effect of dietary intakes on our health has been researched and documented for millennia. The consumption of protein, fat, carbohydrates, vitamins and minerals is required for our physiological function. Certain food-based chemicals – bioactive compounds – yield health benefits beyond their mere chemical constituents, and can modify the biological functionality and health of our cells. These bioactive compounds may help enhance repair of our bodies from injuries, mediate the risk of certain diseases (cancer, coronary heart disease) through altering the physiological functions of our cells and organs. There is strong public awareness in terms of the old adage 'you are what you eat', however the information available to the public ranges from scientifically based research, to traditional dietary remedies, to dangerous fad diets. There is also a plethora of food products that have been designed by the food

---

Neurodegeneration and Alzheimer's Disease: The Role of Diabetes, Genetics, Hormones, and Lifestyle,
First Edition. Edited by Ralph N. Martins, Charles S. Brennan, W.M.A.D. Binosha Fernando, Margaret A. Brennan and Stephanie J. Fuller.
© 2019 John Wiley & Sons Ltd. Published 2019 by John Wiley & Sons Ltd.

industry to provide consumers with foods or supplements designed to combat all sorts of illnesses and disorders.

We have long known that there is a connection between the over-consumption of calories and weight gain, particularly fats and carbohydrates. For example, an excess of refined carbohydrates has been associated with overweight, obesity, type 2 diabetes and a number of metabolic disorders and now also, as described in this book, neurodegenerative diseases such as AD and cerebrovascular disease. However, despite this knowledge, and despite the introduction of numerous public health intervention programmes by governments and medical bodies, the percentage of the population which can be classified as overweight or obese continues to rise. Though there is research evidence that some genetic traits predispose certain people to easier weight gain, leading to obesity, this rise in obesity is believed by most to be mainly a result of increased calorie intake and reduced calorie expenditure.

Recently there has been an increased interest in the role the food industry has played in the production of modern food materials. Researchers and popular writers alike are keen to blame the food industry for today's nutritional problems by suggesting that modern food processing techniques produce what some people call high-calorie, energy-dense, nutrient-poor foods, and it would be foolish to ignore the fact that the food industry has played a part in the situation we find ourselves in. If we are consuming more calories as a population than we were 20 or 50 or 70 years ago, and if many of the foods consumed are highly processed, then this has a double impact on our nutritional status. Combine this with the fact that most of us are becoming more sedentary in our work and social lives, then the balance would be that we will be prone to storing excess calories. As described in this book, overweight and obesity as well as high consumption of refined carbohydrates lead to insulin resistance, type 2 diabetes and cardiovascular disease, which are in epidemic proportions in western countries. There is a train of thought that suggests that this overconsumption of calories is a 'western' problem; however, the situation is manifesting itself to be a global problem, with dramatic increases in Asian countries in recent years (for instance, rapid rises in obesity and diabetes levels in China, Malaysia, Singapore and Taiwan, to name a few).

Fat and lipid metabolism has been studied at length in relation to cardiovascular health, and more recently this topic has become important in AD studies. A few decades ago, all fats were regarded as unhealthy, and a high fat intake, particularly cholesterol, was considered to be the main dietary problem when taking into account the increasing rate of obesity, hypertension and cardiovascular disease in western countries. This led to the food industry generating products that were low in fat. However, to compensate on flavour, these foods often contained higher sugar and salt levels than previously. More recent research indicates that cholesterol is not the main problem, that long-chain saturated fat is a greater problem than cholesterol, and that high sugar intake from carbonated drinks, confectionery and processed foods has only exacerbated the increasing obesity level. Furthermore, lifestyle changes [1] have created a demand for more convenience foods, and foods with a long shelf life. These foods are generally more highly processed than those which were available 30–70 years ago. There is also scientific research which indicates that food processing affects the structure of the protein, fat and carbohydrate components (including sugar in the carbohydrate fraction) in foods. These changes may have led to longer shelf-life, or made the foods more desirable, however many have a high salt or high sugar content, and may contain undesirable fats such as trans-fatty acids. In addition, our intake of essential fatty acids has changed with the advent of processed foods and other western dietary changes. The intake of essential polyunsaturated fatty acids, in particular the omega-3 and omega-6 fatty acids, has considerable influence on our brain health, levels of inflammation and brain function, yet our intake, and the ratio of omega-6 : omega-3 fatty acids has changed over the millennia. There is evidence that we evolved on a diet with a ratio of omega-6 : omega-3 fats of approximately 1 : 1, yet a western diet has a ratio of approximately 15 : 1, and omega-6 fatty acids are linked to increased brain inflammation, as discussed in this book.

Several chapters in this book describe how excess refined carbohydrate intake disrupts the metabolic functions of the body. Once these are compromised, the body is subjected to stress. This stress is in the form of chronic inflammation and oxidative stress [2], which then negatively influences cellular functionality, cellular signalling and in the brain – neurological function. These are some of the findings of studies illustrating that obesity and type 2 diabetes are significant risk factors for the development of neurological disorders including AD [3].

Two chapters of the book discuss the various common causes and symptoms of dementia, differential diagnosis, AD diagnostic tests, and current treatments. AD is characterised by gradual cognitive impairment, and the risk of developing this condition increases with age, such that, past the age of 65, the risk doubles every five years. Pathologically, the disease is characterised by the death of neurons in the cerebral cortex, hippocampus and forebrain, which is associated with the formation of extracellular amyloid deposits, intracellular neurofibrillary tangles consisting of hyper-phosphorylated tau protein, as well as inflammation [4]. Although medications are available for the treatment of AD, these medications only serve to reduce the cognitive symptoms of some people with AD and then only for a relatively short period. There are also medications that can reduce other symptoms of Alzheimer's, such as anxiety and sleeplessness, and these are all discussed in this book. However, there are currently no medications that can stop the eventual continuing neurological degeneration and resultant cognitive degeneration of Alzheimer's. As mentioned earlier, one of the main messages of this book is that, if we can manipulate our diet and lifestyle at mid-life, and reduce our risks associated with excess calorie intake, overweight, obesity and type 2 diabetes, we may be able to achieve long-term prevention or delay of the disorder.

We should be concerned about food consumption and obesity. This could be discussed in terms of a change in lifestyle opportunities, or self-esteem or peer perception. The way weight issues contribute to psychological and personal well-being has been studied extensively in the past. More importantly, there is a health cost associated with these issues. Increased weight and obesity have been documented to be associated with a reduction in life expectancy through greater risk factors associated with type 2 diabetes, coronary heart disease, metabolic complications and more recently AD and other neurodegenerative diseases.

Epidemiological studies have investigated the effect of certain diets on longevity and health, particularly the Mediterranean diet and Okinawan diets. Laboratory studies have also investigated the relationship between certain food components and the manipulation of physiological effects either through whole animal studies, or through *in vitro* experiments using cell culture. Many epidemiological and longitudinal studies have illustrated that there is an increased risk for AD and cognitive impairment in future years, in those individuals exhibiting obesity and diabetes. Several chapters of this book discuss glucose metabolism [5], insulin resistance, carbohydrate metabolism, and how a high intake of refined carbohydrate and sugar can lead to dysregulated brain glucose metabolism, inflammation and oxidative stress, and how all of the above are linked to AD.

Many studies have reported a correlation between diets rich in saturated fatty acids and increased low-density lipoprotein, decreased high-density lipoprotein and what is now regarded as high blood cholesterol levels; this in turn has been associated with the development of neurological impairment through cerebral inflammation, and increased development of Aβ deposition in the brain. Other studies have indicated that as people age, the content of docosahexaenoic acid (DHA) in the brain decreases. Furthermore, animal studies have shown that DHA supplementation improves cognitive functions through the regulation of cell lipids and Aβ production. These are some of the findings that support the change from a diet rich in saturated fats to one rich in polyunsaturated fats, particularly the omega-3 fatty acids. Lipids in the diet and how they relate to the risk of AD are discussed in a chapter of this book.

Mounting scientific data indicates that antioxidants contribute to the neutralisation of oxidative reactions occurring in the body [6], and increased intake of dietary fibre can aid weight control, glucose metabolism and the gut–brain axis. For instance, research has suggested that there is a strong link between the consumption of fruits and vegetables in adults, and the diminishing of the risks associated with the onset of cognitive decline, possibly due to the reduction in incidence or severity of the associated conditions of cardiovascular disease, obesity and type 2 diabetes. However, it is fair to mention that neurodegeneration can arise for a number of reasons which are not solely diet-related (such as genetic predisposition to neurodegenerative diseases, environmental stimuli, hormonal imbalances, stress situations), and interestingly mitochondrial dysfunction, or cell energy impairment, apoptosis, and overproduction of reactive oxygen species is the final common pathogenic mechanism in neurodegenerative diseases [2].

Our own natural antioxidant system, which consists of enzymes as well as biochemical compounds, is crucial in balancing the oxidative stress within our bodies and minimising any damage caused by free radicals [7]. These mechanisms are discussed in this book, as well as changes to this system which have been observed in type 2 diabetes, obesity, ageing and AD.

It is known now that AD develops in the brain for around 20 years before cognitive symptoms emerge. Eventually the cognitive impairment reaches a level where a diagnosis of possible/probable AD is made, using the diagnostic criteria described in detail in a chapter in this book. Again, there is somewhat of a chicken and egg situation regarding dietary imbalances – a bad diet may increase risk of AD and accelerate its development in the brain, then once a person has some level of cognitive impairment, either as self-reported memory loss or as diagnosed, measured mild-cognitive impairment (but not yet clinical AD), there is the risk of withdrawal from normal social life, and the development of depression and anxiety, and these can increase the likelihood of developing dietary problems such as a lower quality of nutrition. In turn this can lead to weight loss, lack of mobility and a further reduction in the quality of life. Intervention studies using rat models as well as clinical studies have indicated that there is a potential to slow the progression of neurological impairment using dietary and lifestyle interventions. This could be in the form of improving the overall diet, promoting the consumption of bioactive ingredients from certain foods, a reduction in energy consumption, improved mineral uptake and/or maintenance/increased levels of physical activity to improve physiological function and cardiovascular health. The important message here is that if we know a person is in the early preclinical stages of Alzheimer's, there may be sufficient time (at least 10 years) in which preventative treatments or diets can be applied, with the aim of delaying cognitive decline.

Good vitamin and antioxidant [6] intake has been associated with resistance to cognitive decline, and vitamins are discussed in this book, in relation to oxidative stress and AD. For instance folic acid, vitamin B6, and vitamin B12 have been reported to be related to the maintenance of cognitive function [3, 8]. Part of the mechanisms behind this could relate to the fact that these vitamins are physiologically important for the development and repair of neuronal networks, and this may also be associated with the links between vitamins and minerals in cell signalling and development. Individuals who have low levels of vitamin B12 appear to be more prone to the development of neurological impairments. Similarly, it has been suggested that avoiding vitamin C deficiencies can help maintain cognitive function through immunomodulation and protection of neurons [9]. The form in which these vitamins and minerals are ingested is of importance, most likely due to their bioavailability, so that it has been suggested that ingestion of foods rich in antioxidant vitamins (rather than supplements), or combinations of vitamins (such as C and E) may help delay the onset of AD [10], and in fact it has been shown that dietary supplementation using individual vitamins has little effect. Furthermore, studies which investigate the potential use of single refined compounds on neurodegenerative diseases may be hard to translate to normal dietary situations, and it is most likely that a combination of healthy foods is likely to be most effective.

Within this book you will find a variety of tests for determining cognitive impairment, and tests to distinguish between several different types of neurodegenerative conditions, including AD, dementia with Lewy bodies, and fronto-temporal dementia, for example. You will also discover many novel potential methods for the diagnosis of AD. Diagnosis at preclinical stages is the aim now, as the prevention or the slowing of the onset of AD, when the disease is in the very early stages of development, is emerging as the most likely avenue for an effective reduction in AD incidence. Therefore, intervention studies need to be carried out on people with very early stages of AD, preferably well before the onset of symptoms, to determine how dietary change and particular food components may affect the development of AD as well as other neurological disorders. However, a diagnosis of Alzheimer's is clearly not necessary to adopt a healthier diet and lifestyle.

One area of research that has proven of considerable interest in recent years is the antioxidant and medicinal value of plant-based foods, with the aim of providing treatments, including preventative treatments for many conditions. Harnessing these ingredients is not new: traditional European, western or Chinese medicine practices are rich in examples of such uses of common plant species. For instance, Chinese medicinal practices utilise mushroom materials to combat a number of metabolic disorders. This has been a particular research focus of our laboratories. Whilst the consumer in the UK, USA or NZ may be accustomed to 4–5 different types of mushroom species which are commonly available in the supermarkets, there are over 900 different species of mushroom in China. We have shown that mushrooms are a rich source of bioactive compounds such as β-glucans, peptides, chitinous substances, terpenes, sterols and phenolic compounds [11, 12]. In addition, we and other researchers have illustrated that these bioactive compounds are useful in terms of anti-inflammatory, antioxidant, anti-cancer, anti-virus, anti-microbial, anti-diabetic and immune modulating ingredients, and some have the potential to stimulate axon generation during brain development [11–13]. With respect to AD, the capacity of several medicinal mushroom species to inhibit the enzyme BACE-1 (one of the enzymes required to produce Aβ amyloid peptide of AD from its precursor, amyloid precursor protein [APP]) was investigated *in vitro*, and it was discovered that extracts of *Auricularia polytricha* (wood ear mushroom) can reduce the activity of the enzyme [14]. When scopolamine-stressed mice were fed mushroom extracts rich in phenolic compounds (for instance from *Inonotus obliquus*), their performance in memory tests improved; whereas in cell culture experiments involving 6-hydroxydopamine-induced stress, a mushroom compound dihydroxybenzalacetone led to protection against neurodegeneration [15, 16].

Chinese tea, green tea, and even black teas have been investigated for the effects of tea phenolic compounds on obesity, oxidative stress, diabetes and neurological functionality [17]. Arguably, tea is the most widely consumed beverage in the world, and tea is a rich source of bioactive ingredients, of which catechins and theanine are the two most studied. These components have been shown to have a neuroprotective effect by inhibiting Aβ formation through inhibiting fibrillar aggregation, and via inhibition of acetylcholinesterase [18, 19]. Catechins can make up between 12% and 24% of the dry weight of tea leaves, and mainly include epigallocatechin (EGC), epicatechin (EC), catechin, epicatechin-3-gallate (ECG) and epigallocatechin-3-gallate (EGCG); whereas theanine commonly makes up 1–2% of tea. The process of making tea naturally extracts these compounds into the liquid which we then consume. Both catechins and theanine have been shown to cross the blood–brain barrier and enter brain tissue [17, 20]. The catechins in both green and black tea have been shown to be potent antioxidant compounds. For instance, the antioxidant activity of tea polyphenols has been shown to inhibit the release free radicals and to limit cellular damage [21]. The polyphenol antioxidants in tea are discussed in greater detail in the chapter on inflammation.

The consumption of caffeine has also been shown to protect against cognitive impairment. Finnish researchers evaluated data over a number of years relating to a cohort of over 1000 people, and illustrated that the consumption of three cups of coffee a day can delay the progression of AD. These effects have been suggested to be due to the caffeine content of coffee. Research has indicated that the consumption of 300 micrograms of caffeine daily may reduce the risk of AD, slow cognitive impairment and reduce Aβ levels in the brain and blood [22]. There is also evidence caffeine may inhibit the rate of Aβ production and hence the formation of toxic Aβ fibrils which have been linked with neurodegeneration. Caffeine can act as an antioxidant, however coffee is rich in many other antioxidants, and the combination of these may be providing the benefits of coffee.

The study of the genetics of AD has also revealed that particular forms of many genes are linked to increased risk of the disease. The main risk factor gene is apolipoprotein E, for which possession of the e4 allele increases several-fold the risk of developing AD. However, particular forms of many other genes and genetic mutations have been shown to influence Alzheimer's risk, and the study of these other genes is revealing considerable information about the metabolic and biochemical pathways involved in disease pathogenesis, as described in detail in the chapter on genetics.

Another chapter of the book describes the importance of fermentation in our digestive process. Fermentation in our gut produces short-chain fatty acids which have been shown to have a myriad of beneficial effects, including reducing the risk of type 2 diabetes and inflammation. The importance of prebiotics and probiotics in our diet has become a popular topic in health food conversations, yet more clinical research is needed to gain a better understanding of the gut–brain axis and how it influences our health. Having said this, animal studies have provided a huge amount of valuable information concerning AD, especially the studies of AD-model transgenic mice. The major animal models which have been studied over the years are reviewed in one of the book's chapters, including their uses and limitations.

Epidemiological experiments, as well as the *in vivo* and *in vitro* trials conducted on numerous food items, have given rise to a prolific nutraceutical industry endeavouring to provide consumers with a range of supplements to enhance lifestyles and reduce the incidence of many conditions. However, these nutraceuticals should only be regarded as a supplementation to an enhanced lifestyle which includes physical fitness, reduction of stress and healthy eating. The whole issue of diet and human nutrition is a complex relationship of factors which interact to exert effects on physiological function and health. A key message of this book concerns the deficiencies of the western diet, and how overall dietary changes to mimic the Mediterranean diet or Okinawan diet (both linked to health and longevity) are advisable. Such changes are recommended due to the health promoting properties of antioxidants and anti-inflammatory compounds as well as essential fats and vitamins to be found in fresh foods, coupled with reductions in the intake of meat, processed foods, and especially refined carbohydrates. We hope that the chapters of this book explain the background knowledge of AD and some other neurological conditions, and help illustrate the potential new ways in which we can utilise new knowledge that is being obtained in scientific research, to benefit our health and well-being.

References

1. Pasinetti, G.M. and Eberstein, J.A. (2008). Metabolic syndrome and the role of dietary lifestyles in alzheimer's disease. *J. Neurochem.* 106: 1503–1514.
2. Emerit, J., Edeas, M., and Bricaire, F. (2004). Neurodegenerative diseases and oxidative stress. *Biomed. Pharmacother.* 58: 39–46.
3. Cukierman, T., Gerstein, H.C., and Williamson, J.D. (2005). Cognitive decline and dementia in diabetes – systematic overview of prospective observational studies. *Diabetologia* 48: 2460–2469.
4. Claeysen, S., Cochet, M., Donneger, R. et al. (2012). Alzheimer culprits: cellular crossroads and interplay. *Cell. Signalling* 24: 1831–1840.
5. Shorr, R.I., de Rekeneire, N., Resnick, H.E. et al. (2006). Glycemia and cognitive function in older adults using glucose-lowering drugs. *J. Nutr. Health Aging* 10: 297–301.
6. Luchsinger, J.A., Tang, M.X., Shea, S., and Mayeux, R. (2003). Antioxidant vitamin intake and risk of Alzheimer disease. *Arch. Neurol.* 60: 203–208.
7. Halliwell, B. (2001). Role of free radicals in the neurodegenerative diseases: therapeutic implications for antioxidant treatment. *Drugs Aging* 18: 685–716.

8 Clarke, R., Smith, A.D., Jobst, K.A. et al. (1998). Folate, vitamin B12, and serum total homocysteine levels in confirmed Alzheimer disease. *Arch. Neurol.* 55: 1449–1455.

9 Harrison, F.E. (2012). A critical review of vitamin C for the prevention of age-related cognitive decline and Alzheimer's disease. *J. Alzheimer's Dis. JAD* 29: 711–726.

10 Zandi, P.P., Anthony, J.C., Khachaturian, A.S. et al. (2004). Reduced risk of Alzheimer disease in users of antioxidant vitamin supplements: the Cache County Study. *Arch. Neurol.* 61: 82–88.

11 Xikun, L., BM, A., Luca, S. et al. (2016). How the inclusion of mushroom powder can affect the physicochemical characteristics of pasta. *Int. J. Food Sci. Technol.* 51: 2433–2439.

12 Vallee, M., Lu, X., Narciso, J.O. et al. (2017). Physical, predictive glycaemic response and antioxidative properties of black ear mushroom (Auricularia auricula) extrudates. *Plant Foods Hum. Nutr.* 72: 301–307.

13 Wasser, S.P. (2002). Medicinal mushrooms as a source of antitumor and immunomodulating polysaccharides. *Appl. Microbiol. Biotechnol.* 60: 258–274.

14 Bennett, L., Sheean, P., Zabaras, D., and Head, R. (2013). Heat-stable components of wood ear mushroom, Auricularia polytricha (higher Basidiomycetes), inhibit in vitro activity of beta secretase (BACE1). *Int. J. Med. Mushrooms* 15: 233–249.

15 Giridharan, V.V., Thandavarayan, R.A., and Konishi, T. (2011). Amelioration of scopolamine induced cognitive dysfunction and oxidative stress by Inonotus obliquus – a medicinal mushroom. *Food Funct.* 2: 320–327.

16 Gunjima, K., Tomiyama, R., Takakura, K. et al. (2014). 3, 4-dihydroxybenzalacetone protects against Parkinson's disease-related neurotoxin 6-OHDA through Akt/Nrf2/glutathione pathway. *J. Cell. Biochem.* 115: 151–160.

17 Trevisanato, S.I. and Kim, Y.I. (2000). Tea and health. *Nutr. Rev.* 58: 1–10.

18 Grelle, G., Otto, A., Lorenz, M. et al. (2011). Black tea theaflavins inhibit formation of toxic amyloid-beta and alpha-synuclein fibrils. *Biochemistry* 50: 10624–10636.

19 Harvey, B.S., Musgrave, I.F., Ohlsson, K.S. et al. (2011). The green tea polyphenol (−)-epigallocatechin-3-gallate inhibits amyloid-β evoked fibril formation and neuronal cell death in vitro. *Food Chem.* 129: 1729–1736.

20 Mandel, S.A., Amit, T., Weinreb, O., and Youdim, M.B. (2011). Understanding the broad-spectrum neuroprotective action profile of green tea polyphenols in aging and neurodegenerative diseases. *J. Alzheimers Dis.* 25: 187–208.

21 Koh, S.H., Kim, S.H., Kwon, H. et al. (2003). Epigallocatechin gallate protects nerve growth factor differentiated PC12 cells from oxidative-radical-stress-induced apoptosis through its effect on phosphoinositide 3-kinase/Akt and glycogen synthase kinase-3. *Brain Res. Mol. Brain Res.* 118: 72–81.

22 Arendash, G.W. and Cao, C. (2010). Caffeine and coffee as therapeutics against Alzheimer's disease. *J. Alzheimers Dis.* 20 (Suppl 1): S117–S126.

2

Alzheimer's Disease and Other Neurodegenerative Diseases

Stephanie J. Fuller[1], Hamid R. Sohrabi[1,2,3,4,5,8], Kathryn G. Goozee[2,3,4,5,6], Anoop Sankaranarayanan[7] and Ralph N. Martins[1,2,3,5,8]

[1] School of Medical and Health Sciences, Centre of Excellence for Alzheimer's Disease Research and Care, Edith Cowan University, Joondalup, WA, Australia
[2] Department of Biomedical Sciences, Macquarie University, Sydney, NSW, Australia
[3] School of Psychiatry and Clinical Neurosciences, University of Western Australia, Perth, WA, Australia
[4] Cooperative Research Centre for Mental Health, Carlton, VIC, Australia
[5] KaRa Institute of Neurological Diseases, Sydney, NSW, Australia
[6] Anglicare, Sydney, NSW, Australia
[7] Department of Psychiatry, School of Medicine, Western Sydney University, Australia
[8] Australian Alzheimer's Research Foundation, Ralph and Patricia Sarich Neuroscience Research Institute, Nedlands, WA, Australia

2.1 Introduction

Worldwide there are over 50 million people living with dementia, and this number is expected to double every 20 years to reach 150 million by 2050. The cost to the community and government health systems, as well as the stress on families and carers will also increase markedly. Dementia can be caused by several conditions, most of which afflict the elderly, and a few are genetic in origin. This chapter will discuss the most common causes of Alzheimer's disease (AD) as well as the major other forms of neurodegeneration that can lead to dementia. The aspects of the conditions that are discussed in this chapter include disease pathology, incidence, symptoms, diagnosis, risk factors, and treatment. With respect to AD, other chapters of this book cover some of these topics in much greater detail.

2.2 Alzheimer's Disease

2.2.1 Pathology

AD is characterised pathologically by the loss of synapses and neurons in the cerebral cortex, particularly the temporal lobe and parietal lobe, and parts of the frontal cortex, also the hippocampus and other subcortical regions. There is associated brain shrinkage, intracellular neurofibrillary tangles (NFT) and extracellular amyloid deposits known as plaques. These plaques consist mostly of aggregates of a 4 kDa 39–43 amino

---

Neurodegeneration and Alzheimer's Disease: The Role of Diabetes, Genetics, Hormones, and Lifestyle,
First Edition. Edited by Ralph N. Martins, Charles S. Brennan, W.M.A.D. Binosha Fernando, Margaret A. Brennan and Stephanie J. Fuller.
© 2019 John Wiley & Sons Ltd. Published 2019 by John Wiley & Sons Ltd.

acid peptide known as amyloid-beta or Aβ. Aβ peptides aggregate readily, especially the longer Aβ42 peptides, with small soluble oligomers believed to be toxic, whereas larger aggregates are thought to be relatively benign. The NFT are made up of hyperphosphorylated tau protein, and are not unique to AD: they are found in other neurodegenerative conditions (other tauopathies) such as chronic traumatic encephalopathy, progressive supranuclear palsy (PSP), subacute sclerosing panencephalitis and Huntington's disease [1–3].

2.2.2 Symptoms

AD has a long pre-clinical period of around 20 years, during which time synaptic, neuronal and brain matter loss occur gradually. Eventually the brain pathology gives rise to early symptoms which include short-term memory loss, word finding problems, difficulties when making decisions and carrying out complex or multi-step tasks, confusion, delusions, anxiety and withdrawal from society. This gradual decline in cognition and behaviour becomes severe enough to impair one's independent daily living activities, job-related tasks and daily functions (e.g. leisure activities) [4]. Symptoms that usually appear later include hallucinations, loss of recognition of close relatives and friends, changes in personality and behaviour, needing help with daily living activities, and wandering. Late symptoms include losing the ability to communicate, and requiring help for most daily activities including dressing, eating, and bathroom use. The order of presentation of symptoms is highly variable; and also dependent on the person's pre-existing lifestyle patterns and personality traits. In addition, the pathology locus adds variability. It is also important to note that many of these signs and symptoms can occur as a result of other neurodegenerative conditions, and that often a person may have symptoms arising from multiple conditions, for example Alzheimer's disease occurring together with vascular dementia (VaD).

As the AD neuropathological changes progress, the patient becomes unable to walk without help, muscles become quite rigid, and the patient loses the ability to eat and swallow, and to control bladder and bowel functions. In 2011, the National Institute on Aging (NIA) and the Alzheimer's Association (AA) published the criteria on diagnosis of dementia due to AD, incorporating a framework previously published by McKhann et al. [4, 5]. Using the 1984 framework, the current criteria distinguish between probable and possible AD based on the strength of the clinical evidence. Of note, the diagnosis of AD dementia can currently be confirmed only after an autopsy with supporting clinical diagnosis prior to death. Table 2.1 provides the main diagnostic criteria for dementia due to AD, using the National Institute on Aging–Alzheimer's Association (NIA-AA) criteria [4].

The disease is life-limiting, thus a patient will typically survive 8–10 years after diagnosis, although some survive up to 20 years. Common causes of death are pneumonia (due to impaired swallowing causing the accidental intake of food or beverages into the lungs) and other infections, dehydration and malnutrition [6].

Less than 1% of AD cases are due to the inheritance of genetic mutations; these usually result in an early onset form of the disease. The genes affected include the amyloid beta precursor protein (*APP*) gene, and the presenilin-1 (*PSEN1*) and presenilin-2 (*PSEN2*) genes. The discovery of these genes and studies of their protein products led to the finding that the AD-related mutations all cause an increase in the production of the longer Aβ peptides (Aβ42) or an increase in ratio of the longer Aβ peptides (Aβ42/Aβ40),

Table 2.1 Primary diagnostic criteria for dementia due to Alzheimer's disease (AD).[a]

Probable AD dementia	Possible AD dementia

1) Symptoms have a gradual onset over months to years (Insidious onset).
2) Clear-cut history of worsening of cognition by report or observation.
3) The initial and most prominent cognitive deficits are evident on history and examination in one of the following categories.
   a) Amnestic presentation: Impairment in learning and recall of recently learned information.
   b) Non-amnestic presentations [b]:
   Language presentation: manifested by word-finding.
   Visuospatial presentation manifested by spatial cognition, including object agnosia, impaired face recognition, simultanagnosia, and alexia.
   Executive dysfunction manifested by impaired reasoning, judgement, and problem solving.
4) The diagnosis of probable AD dementia should not be applied when there is evidence of (i) substantial concomitant cerebrovascular disease (e.g. stroke associated with current clinical presentation; multiple or extensive infarcts or severe white matter hyperintensity burden); or (ii) presence of the core features of other dementias (e.g. features of dementia with Lewy bodies; behavioural variant frontotemporal dementia; semantic variant primary progressive aphasia or non-fluent/agrammatic variant primary progressive aphasia); or (iii) evidence for another concurrent neurological disease or medical comorbidity; or use of medication with significant impact on cognition.
	This diagnostic category is used when the core clinical criteria for AD dementia is met but one of the following two circumstances is also present:
	
	1) Atypical course is diagnosed in the presence of cognitive deficits for AD dementia, but either has a sudden onset of cognitive impairment or lack of evidence for progressive cognitive decline.
	2) Etiologically mixed presentation is diagnosed when one of the following conditions is present: (i) substantial concomitant cerebrovascular disease (e.g. stroke, multiple or extensive infarcts, or severe white matter hyperintensity); or (ii) presence of the core features of other dementias (e.g. dementia with Lewy bodies; behavioural variant frontotemporal dementia; semantic variant primary progressive aphasia or non-fluent/agrammatic variant primary progressive aphasia); or (iii) evidence for another concurrent neurological disease, or a non-neurological medical comorbidity or use of medication with significant impact on cognition.

a) This table is based on the criteria published by McKhan et al. [4]. Aphasia: impaired ability to produce or understand speech; alexia: reduction in understanding of written language; simultanagnosia: inability to perceive more than one object at a time.
b) In the non-amnestic presentations, in addition to the presenting deficits, impairment in other cognitive domains is also noticeable.

supporting the hypothesis that overproduction of Aβ peptides (Aβ42 peptides in particular) which aggregate in the brain in AD is central to disease pathogenesis [7].

2.2.3 Incidence

In 2016, it was estimated that nearly 44 million people had AD or a related dementia around the world. In the USA in 2016, one in nine people over 65 had AD, one in three over 85 had AD, and about 16 million people will have AD by 2050, unless a cure or preventative treatment is found (http://www.alzheimers.net/resources/alzheimers-statistics). In Australia, over 425,416 people currently have dementia (www.dementia.org.au/statistics, 2018), and this is expected to increase to over 1,100,000 by 2050 (http://www.natsem.canberra.edu.au/publications/?publication=economic-cost-of-dementia-in-australia-2016-2056). It is a leading cause of death in older adults in western countries. In Australia it is the second leading cause of death of older adults, and the primary cause of death in older women.

The single biggest risk factor for AD is increasing age, with the incidence approximately doubling with every five years over the age of 65.

2.2.4 Onset and Risk Factors

Some AD cases (1%) are caused by inheritance of a dominant pathogenic mutation as mentioned above. In families that are affected, mutation-carrying family members usually develop symptoms between the ages of 35 and 65 years, and the disease progression is faster than progression in late-onset (mostly sporadic) cases. For the more common sporadic form of AD, there are no clear causes, though many risk factors have been identified. Genetic risk factors exist, with the strongest being possession of apolipoprotein E ε4 (*APOE* ε4) alleles: each *APOE* ε4 allele lowers the average age of onset by about eight years, compared to people with no *APOE* ε4 alleles [8]. People with one *APOE* ε4 allele have a fivefold increased risk of developing AD, and those with two *APOE* ε4 alleles have a 20-fold increased risk of developing the disease [9, 10]

More recent sequencing technologies have enabled the identification of rare disease variants, and have unmasked mutations which lead to an intermediate risk of AD in the genes *PLD3*, *TREM2*, *UNC5C*, *AKAP9* and *ADAM10* [11]. It is hoped that characterising the links to these genes may help develop novel treatments for the disease, and the genetics of AD is discussed in greater detail in Chapter 15.

The discovery of a link between *APOE* and AD dementia has triggered 25 years of research concerning ApoE and its physiological role in AD. In addition, the link between *APOE* ε4 alleles and cardiovascular diseases led to studies of the risk of AD due to other conditions. For example, genome-wide association studies have found linkages between late-onset AD and various genes involved in cholesterol and lipid metabolism such as clusterin (*CLU*), sortilin related receptor-1 (*SORL1*, involved in intracellular transport and processing of AβPP) and ATP binding cassette subfamily A member 7 (*ABCA7*), highlighting the important link that must exist between AD and the dysregulation of lipid metabolism [11]. It is now known that cardiovascular problems, type 2 diabetes, metabolic syndrome, mid-life hypertension, smoking, hyperlipidaemia and obesity all increase the risk of AD [12, 13].

2.2.5 Treatment

There is currently no effective treatment or cure for AD. There are treatments that can potentially ameliorate symptoms and stave off cognitive decline for up to 6–12 months. For example, due to synaptic damage in AD, acetylcholine levels are low, therefore cholinesterase inhibitors (such as donepezil, galantamine, and rivastigmine) can be given to slow the clearance of this important neurotransmitter, therefore increasing the levels of acetylcholine available to support neural connectivity. However, as the disease progresses, these medications are unable to sustain their effectiveness. Memantine is another class of AD medication used often as a second line of intervention. It targets the abnormally high glutamate levels which occur in AD: memantine partially blocks the N-Methyl-D-aspartate (NMDA) receptors, achieving a reduction in glutamate levels, slowing the influx of toxic levels of calcium into cells. This has the potential of slowing the disease progression to some extent, as high intracellular calcium leads to faster cellular damage. Conditions that frequently coexist with AD may also be treated, such as depression, sleep disturbances, anxiety, hallucinations and delusions. However, the side effects of medications can be significant, and can contribute to other health problems [14, 15].

2.2.6 Potential for AD Prevention

It is known that chronic inflammation, oxidative stress, mitochondrial dysfunction, and disruptions to glucose and lipid metabolism occur early in AD, and it is thought these may be AD pathology-initiating events [16, 17]. There is accumulating evidence that minimising these metabolic changes can help reduce the development of these and other AD risk factors. For example, diet modification and increases in exercise are known to reduce the risk of insulin resistance, inflammation and oxidative stress, and to improve blood lipid profiles. The Australian Imaging Biomarker and Lifestyle (AIBL) research cohort has enabled a longitudinal investigation into the effect of diet and exercise on AD risk [18] and results of these studies support the concept that dietary improvements [19–21] and regular exercise [22, 23] may reduce AD risk and/or AD symptom development. Dietary changes that would be recommended would include decreasing intake of processed foods, sugar and saturated fats, whilst increasing intake of fresh fruit and vegetables, fish, whole grains and seeds, and healthy fats, to reflect a traditional Mediterranean diet. Further longitudinal studies will hopefully consolidate these findings.

2.3 Frontotemporal Lobe Dementia

Frontotemporal lobe dementia, or frontotemporal dementia (FTD or FTLD), also known as Pick's disease, is one of the most common forms of dementia in people under 65 years of age, with onset usually between 40 and 60 years of age. Due to the younger onset age, the prominent behavioural symptoms are sometimes confused with those of psychiatric disorders [24]. The three types of FTD include behavioural variant FTD, progressive non-fluent aphasia, and semantic dementia. The behavioural variant is the most commonly diagnosed, with symptoms including a loss of inhibitions, which can result in socially inappropriate behaviour, loss of empathetic and sympathetic capacity, repetitive or compulsive behaviours, and the development of a craving for sweet or fatty foods, junk food, and alcohol. Unlike AD, memory is not affected, whereas both AD and behavioural FTD patients have problems with planning, decision-making, and managing finances.

The other two FTD types are known as the language variants, and initial symptoms involve slowly-developing speech problems. In non-fluent aphasia, speech is slow and hesitant, errors in grammar occur, for example minor words or conjunctions such as 'the' and 'to' may be missing. In semantic dementia, names of familiar objects are forgotten, and there may be difficulty recognising familiar people and objects. Unlike behavioural FTD and AD, planning, organising, and memory are relatively unchanged in the early stages.

In later stages, the three forms of FTD eventually progress such that advanced FTD patients develop symptoms of all three types. There may also be aggression, agitation, and other symptoms commonly found in AD. The disease progression is between 2 and 10 years from the time of diagnosis, demonstrating a high fatality rate [25, 26].

2.3.1 Neuropathology and Causes

All FTD cases show atrophy and neuronal loss in the frontal and temporal lobes of the brain, as well as gliosis and spongy change, however there can be considerable histological differences, such that FTD can be said to have different pathological subtypes [27]. One subtype (Pick's disease), named after the physician who first documented FTD, is characterised by the presence of hyperphosphorylated tau-filled structures (Pick bodies) in neurons and glial cells [28], and accounts for about 45% of cases (FTD-tau). Over 50% of FTD patients have ubiquitin +ve inclusions with no tau present, yet the inclusions have TDP- 43 present (FTD-TDP). Two much rarer forms of FTD have been detected, one which is characterised by having ubiquitin and fused in-sarcoma protein (FUS) detected in the inclusions (FTD-FUS), and the other has ubiquitin together with other as yet unknown proteins (FTD-UPS) [29–33]. The proteins present in the inclusions to a greater or lesser extent determine the clinical phenotypes, for example, FTD-FUS is always associated with behavioural variant FTD, non-fluent aphasia is commonly associated with the presence of tau pathology, and semantic aphasia is more often linked with TDP-43 presence in inclusions, although tau is sometimes seen. There is often considerable overlap with AD and FTD, particularly in the case of logopenic aphasia (a newly identified subtype of aphasia that involves impairments in naming and sentence repetition), both in clinical symptom development and underlying neuropathology, suggesting common pathological mechanisms [34].

Mutations in several genes have been linked to specific subtypes of FTD. However, most people who develop FTD have no family history, and the cause is unknown. In the study of FTD genetics, an early finding was that tau +ve frontotemporal dementia with parkinsonism (FTDP-17) is linked to mutations in the microtubule associated protein tau (*MAPT*) gene on chromosome 17, which encodes the tau protein. Disturbances in tau metabolism and structure are clearly relevant to the disease pathogenesis, as the neuropathology caused by the mutations is influenced by the position of the *MAPT* mutation [35]. Mutations in the *TDP-43* gene, transactive response DNA binding protein (*TARDBP*), also have been found in FTD, though they are very rare, whereas the main gene linked to FTD-TDP is the gene for progranulin protein (*GRN*, also on chromosome 17). Another gene linked to familial FTD that is characterised by ubiquitin +ve inclusions (but no tau and rarely TDP-43) is *VCP*, which codes for a structural protein Valosin-Containing Protein. Cases with this form of FTD also usually have signs of amyotrophic lateral sclerosis (ALS), inclusion body myopathy, and Paget's disease of bone. Recent genome-wide screening studies have indicated other potential loci are linked to FTD, that have genes that influence neuronal genesis, differentiation and axonal outgrowth, elements of the immune system, and possibly lysosomal and autophagy pathways [36, 37]. Other genome-wide screening studies have identified risk loci (C9orf72 and UNC13A) that are common to both FTD and ALS, also indicating that pathogenic changes to neurotransmitter release and synaptic function are common to both ALS and FTD-TDP [38].

2.3.2 Treatment

There is no cure or treatment that will stop the disease process, therefore the treatments available involve managing difficult behaviours such as aggression and loss of sexual inhibition. Pharmacological interventions for the management of these behaviours, as well as repetitive behaviours, include SSRI (selective serotonin reuptake inhibitors) or an atypical antipsychotic drug. Many such treatments are still being tested in clinical trials; trials so far have been limited to small case series or open label trials, and not all studies have reported improvements. Behavioural strategies and patient management are important over the course of this disease, and it is also important to provide support for carers [25, 39] as most patients eventually need full-time care. The AD medications donepezil and memantine have been tested in clinical trials with limited success and many side effects. Non-pharmacological interventions include physical therapy for gait, speech therapy, and exercise; as well as socialisation when apathy and depression become evident [40]. Potential therapies currently in clinical trials include anti-tau antibodies; therapies to reduce tau phosphorylation and aggregation; the non-steroidal anti-inflammatory medication salsalate which inhibits tau acetylation; and TPI-287 which is a chemotherapy treatment that mimics paclitaxel in promoting microtubule stability [39].

2.3.3 Diagnosis and Clinical Overlap with Other Diseases

Early symptoms help to indicate the type of FTD, however the clinical heterogeneity in familial and sporadic forms of FTD is considerable. Furthermore, FTD frequently overlaps clinically with three other neurodegenerative diseases that result in profound motor deficits: corticobasal degeneration (CBD), PSP, and ALS [24].

Magnetic resonance imaging (MRI) scans can detect clear localised brain atrophy, and there is reliably detectable hypometabolism in the frontal cortex by $[^{18}F]$-fluorodeoxyglucose (FDG)-positron emission tomography (PET) for example [29]. The development of β-amyloid PET imaging with ligands such as ^{11}C-Pittsburgh Compound B has transformed the detection and understanding of pre-clinical AD, the diagnosis of AD for clinical trials, and the ability to determine efficacy of potential therapies. The use of similar imaging using recently developed tau-specific ligands such as ^{18}F THK5351 and ^{18}F-T807 to measure tau deposits in patients will help considerably with differential diagnosis and the understanding of pathogenesis of AD and FTD, while detecting any overlap between these and other tauopathies [41, 42]. There are currently no cerebrospinal fluid (CSF) or blood biomarkers specific for FTD.

Behavioural assessments are the most important in assessments of patients who potentially have the behavioural variant FTD, and seem to be more sensitive in distinguishing this form of FTD from AD, than standard cognitive testing. A combination of behavioural and motor symptom evaluations, cognitive assessments, MRI, and other more specialised brain scans if available (FDG-PET and PiB-PET for example) are sometimes necessary to reach an accurate diagnosis – necessary for appropriate management of these different conditions, and for clinical trials [29].

2.4 Vascular Dementia

Vascular dementia (VaD) [38], also known as multi-infarct dementia [37], is the second most common type of dementia. There are different types, with the most common being cortical dementia (the main one known as multi-infarct dementia) and subcortical vascular dementia (or Binswanger's disease). Hereditary forms of VaD are rare, and the sporadic forms are mostly caused by degenerative blood vessel disorders such as atherosclerosis, small vessel disease, and cerebral amyloid angiopathy (CAA) [43]. VaD rarely occurs on its own, it often overlaps with AD, and both conditions have increasing incidence with increasing age. Overall, dementia affects about 10% of those aged over 65 years with 20% of those over 80 years exhibiting severe dementia.

2.4.1 Symptoms and Diagnosis

Patients typically present with a history of one or more transient neurological events, which may spontaneously resolve over 24–48 hours with no noticeable lasting effect. However, a history of multiple episodes often compound to result in cognitive deterioration, with one or more disturbing changes. Apart from cognitive changes, there may also be reports of headaches, visual disturbances, weakness in an arm or leg, loss of speech, or confusion – all of which may be transient, yet full recovery of function is rare. Depending on the pathology locus, cognitive changes can include loss of memory, difficulties with problem solving, orientation, perception, and concentration. Differentiating between VaD and AD is often difficult, the presence of physical symptoms strongly suggests VaD, yet the mental deterioration that occurs in AD is very similar, although rarely reported to be stepwise in progression as seen in VaD.

Diagnosis will involve obtaining a detailed history of cognitive problems, blood tests to rule out chemical or hormone imbalances, and brain imaging with computed tomography (CT) or MRI. These can help exclude other causes of dementia such as brain tumours, and will often show up both current and significant past strokes. The degree, location, and spread of white matter/foci seen on MRI can also assist in diagnosis [44]. Diagnosis will often reveal the presence of AD as well – estimated to co-exist with VaD in 25–50% of cases, depending on each reported study [45–47]. For example, neuropathology studies have shown that signs of cerebrovascular disease such as stroke, small vessel disease, microinfarction, and CAA are found in the majority of cases of older onset dementia [46, 48]. The cognitive decline in VaD is very similar to that of AD, however it can be modulated by reducing the risk factors such as managing cholesterol levels, exercise, and lowering blood pressure for example, with the aim of preventing strokes. Untreated vascular dementia usually ends in a patient requiring care around the clock, and eventually death from stroke, heart disease, or infection.

2.4.2 Causes and Risk Factors

The evidence suggests that vascular dementia is caused by chronic reduced blood flow to the brain, usually as a result of a series of strokes, though occasionally due to a single stroke. The loss of blood flow causes localised neuropathology and tissue death.

Often the strokes can be so mild as to go unnoticed, or be dismissed as just headaches, yet the neurological damage accumulates over time. Risk factors for VaD include:

- Hypertension
- High cholesterol levels
- Diabetes mellitus
- Obesity
- Dyslipidaemia
- Smoking
- High homocysteine levels
- Atrial fibrillation

Large cohort studies have shown that cardiovascular diseases, possibly due to embolic stroke or chronic cerebral hypoperfusion can lead to an increased risk of cognitive impairment and dementia, to such an extent that the cognitive impairment and dementia can be seen to be an extension of the cardiovascular illness [47, 49]. This link is well established in VaD, and is becoming a lot more evident in also contributing to AD. All the risk factors listed above are also risk factors for AD, which may explain the high percentage of patients with both pathologies. Having more than one pathology also appears to increase the rate of cognitive decline.

2.4.3 Prevention and Treatment

An infarct is the damaged or dead tissue caused by a thrombus or embolus blocking blood flow to a part of the brain, thus damaging or killing the cells in the affected region. There is no treatment that can reverse the damage done by infarcts. However, emergency treatment within a couple of hours of a stroke or transient ischaemic attack (TIA – or mini stroke) can reduce the level of damage and help prevent a recurrence. Such treatments include oxygen therapy to support brain perfusion, aspirin to prevent blood clotting, and tissue plasminogen activator given intravenously to help break blood clots. Later treatment can involve surgical blood vessel repair. A TIA is a warning signal that a patient should take preventative medication and adopt some preventative measures. Lifestyle changes including changing one's diet, increasing exercise, improving quality of sleep, and losing weight are key to reducing risk factors such as diabetes and cardiovascular disease. Similarly, following a stroke, diet improvements, cognitive rehabilitation, and physical activity are recommended, and statin therapy is often recommended following stroke or TIA to prevent further vascular events, though this is more effective against cardiovascular events rather than stroke [50].

Other pharmacological treatments include anticholinergic medications and antihypertensive medications [47]. AD treatments have been trialled on vascular dementia patients, with little success, though donepezil has shown some benefits [51]. Other treatments that have shown promise are cerebrolysin, which has demonstrated some beneficial effects on global outcome, though cognition was not assessed [52]; and SSRI, which have also been shown to be beneficial on global outcome [53], and many more are currently being trialled [54].

2.4.4 Dementia with Lewy Bodies

This form of dementia, Lewy body Dementia (DLB), is one of the Lewy body diseases along with Parkinson's disease (PD), PD dementia, and multiple system atrophy [55]. It is a neurodegenerative disease characterised principally by widespread neuronal loss as well as the build-up of intracellular α-synuclein protein deposits (Lewy bodies) in the remaining neurons in the brain stem and neocortex of a patient. In multiple system atrophy, these deposits are predominantly be found in the glial cells [56]. As with the Aβ amyloid peptide aggregates in AD, it is thought that the oligomers/protofibrils of the α-synuclein protein, and not the large aggregates, have toxic effects on cell membranes and at synapses, and negatively influence mitochondrial function and protein degradation [57]. DLB is the most common form of dementia after AD and VaD, with onset usually after the age of 50, and an increasing prevalence with increasing age. The prevalence of DLB is around 4% of all dementias, though reports have varied widely, possibly due to missed diagnoses [58, 59]. Similarly, in a systematic review, DLB accounted for 3–7% of all dementia cases in incidence studies [59].

2.4.5 Causes

Most cases are sporadic with no obvious cause. However, the finding of point mutations as well as duplications and triplications of the α-synuclein gene being linked to early onset forms of familial α-synucleinopathy supports the concept that aggregated α-synuclein species which disrupt synaptic function and cause neuronal death, lead to neuropathology and symptoms of the synucleinopathies [60]. DLB linkage to chromosome 2q35-q36 has also been reported, but comprehensive genetic and mutation analysis has not revealed any specific gene or pathogenic mutation [61].

2.4.6 Symptoms

The first symptoms of DLB usually include impaired attention, visuospatial function, and executive function. These can vary in a person, even from hour to hour. Other early symptoms include motor problems usually seen in PD, depression, and visual hallucinations. Unlike AD, memory problems only occur much later [62]. Tremors are less common than in Parkinson's, yet a shuffling gait, blank facial expression, constipation, sleeping problems including rapid eye movement sleep behaviour disorder (SBD), and difficulties swallowing food often occur. Postural hypotension can also occur, resulting in fainting episodes, which can obviously result in injury [63]. The symptoms are believed to result from loss of both cholinergic (cognitive degeneration) and dopaminergic (loss of motor control) neurons.

2.4.7 Diagnosis of DLB

It is difficult to discuss this without mentioning the problems of differential diagnosis – clinical symptoms of DLB and AD overlap considerably [64]. Furthermore, many subjects presenting with symptoms may be developing more than one form of dementia – for example AD and DLB combined, and it is important to establish if Lewy body diseases are involved in a dementia diagnosis due to the sensitivity of DLB patients to many pharmaceuticals [63]. For example, LB patients have a hypersensitivity to neuroleptic and antiemetic medications that affect dopaminergic or cholinergic systems, such as chlorpromazine, haloperidol, trifluoperazine, risperidone, or thioridazine [65, 66]. Furthermore, benzodiazepines, anaesthetics, and some antidepressants may lead to delusions and hallucinations [66]. Pre-clinical diagnosis of this condition is being studied extensively, and promising early markers for DLB include the presence of sleep disturbances (SBD), autonomic dysfunction or hyposmia, 123I-metaiodobenzylguanidine cardiac scintigraphy to detect cardiac sympathetic denervation, measures of substantia nigra pathology, and skin biopsy for α-synuclein in peripheral autonomic nerves. Although there are currently no effective treatments or preventative therapies for DLB, preclinical diagnosis enables clinical trials at very early stages, and reduces the risk of dangerous side effects from inappropriate prescription of some of the above-mentioned medications [63].

In DLB, physical problems usually appear early, which would be very rare in AD or VaD. It has been suggested that a combination of clinical tests and imaging tests is the best option currently, with the symptoms of REM sleep behaviour disorder, severe neuroleptic sensitivity, and the 'gold standard' detection of reduced striatal dopamine transporter activity by functional imaging together strongly suggesting a DLB diagnosis [65]. However, despite the development of consensus diagnostic criteria, the sensitivity of differential diagnosis of DLB is still low. Other imaging techniques that have been proven useful include PET scans showing the characteristic nigrostriatal degeneration in DLB (as mentioned above), regional cerebral blood flow, FDG-PET, the use of single-photon emission computed tomography (SPECT) tracers, and MRI scans to show alterations in structure and white matter integrity [67].

2.4.7.1 Clinical Approach to Dementias

Early diagnosis is critical to instituting appropriate treatment strategies to delay progression of these illnesses. Table 2.2 explains some basic information and steps needed to differentiate the different types of dementias clinically (focusing on the main four types, Alzheimer's disease, Vascular Dementia, Lewy Body Dementia and Behavioural variant of Frontotemporal Dementia).

2.5 Parkinson's Disease

Similar to AD, PD is another neurodegenerative disease that affects the central nervous system and takes many years to develop. However, it mainly affects the motor system, with early symptoms including shaking (tremor), slowness of movements, rigidity, balance problems, and especially difficulty walking. Sleep disorders are common in PD, and it is likely that they exacerbate cognitive decline in PD [68]. Behavioural changes as well as depression are also common in PD. As the disease advances, patients experience further deterioration in gait, a reduced speed of walking, and a progressively greater requirement for physical assistance with daily living activities. Visual hallucinations and delusions can occur, and dementia is also a common in the late stages of PD [69].

Table 2.2 Clinical differentiation between Alzheimer's disease, vascular dementia, Lewy body dementia, and fronto-temporal dementia.

Characteristic	Alzheimer's dementia (AD)	Vascular dementia (VaD)	Lewy body dementia (DLB)	Frontotemporal dementia (FTD)
Age of onset	Typical onset after 65 yr of age, with increasing prevalence as age advances. Nearly 5% have an earlier age of onset, by 60 yr of age	Typical onset is after 65 yr of age, with increasing risk corresponding to age	Typical onset is between 50 and 55 yr of age	Typically manifests between 45 and 65 yr of age
Type	Cortical dementia	Subcortical dementia	Cortico-subcortical dementia	Cortical dementia
Progression of illness	Insidious onset	Typically described as having an acute onset with stepwise decline	Characterised by a fluctuating course and earlier admission to residential care due to behavioural symptoms	Rapid progress
Memory	Severe amnesia with impairments in immediate and delayed recall	Variable; patients have deficits in short-term or immediate memory abilities due to dysfunction in retrieval	Variable; although immediate recall is affected, patients with DLB can often recall a much greater proportion of this information after a delay. One possible explanation for this may be related to compromised attentional deficit in DLB	Preserved episodic memory especially in the behavioural variant

Visuospatial function	Impaired and can be impaired early in 20–43% patients	Generally preserved	Early impairments can be a hallmark	Preserved
Executive functions	Affected, but less severe compared to VaD	Severe impairment in attention, and problem solving	Impaired	Impaired social cognition and multitasking early; as disease progresses other abnormalities reflecting advanced involvement of prefrontal areas
Speech	Usually word-finding deficits (anomia). Verbal fluency impaired (semantic or category more than phonemic)	Depends on areas affected	Slowed dysarthric speech, with impaired prosody and occasional rush of speech	Semantic variant display empty, circumlocutory speech reflecting loss of semantic knowledge. Progressive non-fluent aphasia is characterised by progressive decline in language output. Speech is non-fluent, effortful and lacking in prosody

Aphasia: impaired ability to produce or understand speech; prosody: patterns of stress and intonation in language; semantic: understanding meaning in language; dysarthric: slurred or slow speech; phonemic: relating to the sound of words or letters; circumlocutory: unnecessarily using too many words when fewer would do.

2.5.1 Onset

There is no clear test for PD; the diagnosis is based on the presence of several of the following early symptoms – resting tremor of a hand or limb, slowness of movement (bradykinesia), reduced arm swing, physical rigidity, and slowed cognition. There may also be balance problems, a change in handwriting to smaller letters and words, loss of smell, sleep disorders, long-term constipation, a change in voice, and face 'masking' – an uncharacteristic blank or serious facial expression.

2.5.2 Causes and Risk Factors

Like Alzheimer's, PD is believed to have a long pre-clinical phase, such that about 50% of dopaminergic neurons in the substantia nigra have been lost by the time PD symptoms appear [70]. There is no specific known cause of PD, although a small proportion are known to be caused by genetic factors. Environmental factors have been associated with an increased risk of PD, including pesticide exposure, head injuries, and possibly heavy metal exposure [71, 72]. While smoking is contraindicated for most health conditions, a higher incidence of PD is reported in non-smokers [73]. With respect to dementia in PD, advanced age, being male, hallucinations, smoking, hypertension, and especially REM sleep behaviour disorders increase the risk of dementia in PD, whereas higher education is mildly protective [74].

2.5.3 Incidence

The proportion of the population at any given time in industrialised countries is about 0.3%, yet is age-related, such that 1% of people over 60 are affected, yet 4% of people over 80 are affected [71]. Some (but not all) studies suggest it is more common in men than women.

2.5.4 Pathology

PD is considered a synucleinopathy due to the abnormal accumulation of α-synuclein protein in the brain in the form of Lewy bodies. The accumulated aberrant soluble oligomeric protofibrils of α-synuclein are the pathological hallmark of PD, and these protofibrils are thought to be toxic as they disrupt neuronal cell function [75]. There are three main synucleinopathies: PD, dementia with Lewy bodies, and multiple system atrophy, with the differences being the cell types and brain structures affected [55]. Alpha-synuclein pathology is found in both sporadic and inherited forms of AD. The death of the dopaminergic neurons in the substantia nigra leads to the major symptoms of PD, due to a lack of dopamine, yet symptoms don't appear until 50–80% of these specific neurons die.

Alpha-synuclein is encoded by the *SNCA* gene, and is expressed mostly in neurons in the neocortex, substantia nigra, hippocampus, thalamus, and cerebellum. The protein is mostly found in presynaptic termini. Interestingly, α-synuclein is expressed strongly in the neuronal mitochondria of the hippocampus, olfactory bulb, striatum, and thalamus, and mitochondria are often damaged early in the process of neuronal degeneration [76]. Inherited forms of the disease manifest in people from 20 to 60 years of age, and several genes have now been linked to PD. These have been labelled *Park1*, *Park2* and so on, in order of discovery, with *Park1* being *SNCA*, *Park2* being *Parkin*, for example [77]. PD-linked Parkin mutations mostly cause disease onset before the age of 30 years, whereas mutations in *Park8* (the *LRRK2* gene, of unknown function) are the most frequent causes of familial PD, causing 2–40% of early onset PD cases in certain populations [77]. It has also been shown that gene dosage can influence risk of PD, most likely by increasing total α-synuclein levels. This is supported by the finding that point mutations in *SNCA* that cause inefficient lysosomal degradation of α-synuclein also lead to PD [78]. Genetic studies have shown that other *SNCA* mutations can be linked to an increased risk of sporadic PD [75, 79].

2.5.5 Treatment

There is no cure for PD; however, there are several medications and treatments that can reduce symptoms and improve quality of life considerably. Firstly, a good exercise program is recommended, to help minimise involuntary movements and improve coordination and balance. There is also evidence that exercise may protect the residual dopamine-producing neurons, and/or restore the dysfunctional cortico-basal ganglia motor control circuit in people with PD [80], and it may also reduce the incidence of Parkinson's in vulnerable populations. Occupational and speech therapists as well as physiotherapists can provide specific supportive therapies [69].

Anti-cholinergic medications were the first group of medications to treat PD. They block the effect of acetylcholine to re-balance its levels with the diminishing dopamine. These medications include benztropine, biperidine, and benzhexol. Such medications are now rarely used as they have been replaced mostly by dopamine agonists, and levodopa [81].

Dopamine agonists such as bromocriptone and pergolide mimic the action of dopamine, and are often given at early PD stages. At later stages of PD, dopamine agonists can still be used, but often the loss of dopamine in the brain in PD can be treated by giving levodopa, a precursor of dopamine which is converted to dopamine in the brain. This treatment can work for many years, yet as the disease progresses, the response is weaker, or unpredictable, and other treatments are needed.

Other medications include amantadine, which has both anti-cholinergic and dopamine agonist properties, as it can reduce drug-induced involuntary movements (dyskinesia), catechol-o-methyl transferase inhibitors such as entacapone to reduce levodopa breakdown in the intestines and the brain, and monoamine oxidase type B inhibitors such as selegiline, to prevent breakdown of available dopamine, thus prolonging the action of levodopa [81, 82].

In some cases where patients are relatively young and otherwise healthy, and who have problems with fluctuations in responses to drug treatments, subthalamic deep brain stimulation can be performed. This does have some side-effects though, as semantic and verbal fluency can be affected, and other speech disturbances can also occur, particularly when left-sided or bilateral procedures are carried out [83].

In later stages when cognitive function is significantly affected, cholinesterase inhibitors such as rivastigmine can improve global cognition. Other medications that have been shown to be beneficial include clozapine, an inhibitor of serotonin and dopamine receptors (reduces psychosis), the tricyclic antidepressants nortriptyline and pramipexole (reduce depression), and atomoxetine, a noradrenergic reuptake inhibitor (improves attention) [69].

In people treated with levodopa, it may take about 15 years to reach a stage of high dependency, depending on age and other conditions. PD eventually becomes highly debilitating, and life expectancy can be significantly reduced.

For three decades, cell therapy has been tested as potential treatment for PD. Such cell transplants can involve either autologous (from the same individual) cells or non-autologous cells, each with their own advantages and drawbacks – for example, the ethical issues surrounding the use of non-autologous cells need to be considered, as well as immune rejection. Nevertheless, recent research suggests such therapy will provide a realistic treatment option, as a result of advances in pluripotent stem cell biotechnology [84]. For example, the potential of inducible pluripotent stem cells (iPSC) has improved recently with new techniques such as the removal of c-Myc-containing cells minimising the risk of tumour formation [85]. The first approved clinical trial using iPSCs to treat PD patients was started in 2016 in Melbourne, Australia, by the International Stem Cell Corporation [86] and other clinical trials are being planned.

Alternative cell therapy methods have also been investigated, including the conversion of fibroblasts into neurons without going through an inducible PSC stage. These exciting innovations will hopefully provide the step forward needed in PD treatment [84, 87, 88].

2.6 Huntington's Disease

Huntington's disease (HD), also known as Huntington's chorea, is a progressive disorder of motor, cognitive, and psychiatric disturbances. HD is a genetic disease that is inherited in an autosomal dominant manner [89] in about 90% of cases, with the remaining 10% being due to a new mutation. The diagnosis of suspected HD involves the presence of progressive motor disability featuring chorea (involuntary jerky movements), including reduced manual dexterity, slurred speech, swallowing problems, and balance problems [89]. Psychological and cognitive symptoms can also appear early, and may include cognitive decline, changes in personality and depression, whereas later psychiatric symptoms can include anxiety, aggression, depression leading to suicidal tendencies, and worsened addictions such as alcoholism and gambling [90]. Other symptoms include apathy, hallucinations, olfactory dysfunction, general weight loss, rigidity and, in later stages, an inability to walk, speak or swallow properly, leading to high levels of care being required [89].

2.6.1 Genetics of the Disease

The mutant protein in HD – huntingtin – originates from the Huntingtin gene (*HTT*), which has a trinucleotide (CAG) repeat of variable length. This CAG repeat translates to a polyglutamine strand of variable length at the N-terminus of the protein – 28 repeats or less are considered normal – whereas over 36 repeats leads to the production of huntingtin with abnormal characteristics, which are believed to result in a toxic gain of function [89, 91]. During reproduction, CAG repeats over 28 are unstable, with this lack of stability increasing as the number of repeats increases. With 28–35 repeats, parents are unaffected, yet with 36–40 repeats, 'reduced penetrance' of the disease can develop into fully penetrant HD by the next generation [91]. Disease onset age can be predicted approximately by measuring an individual's CAG repeat length, with longer repeats usually indicating a younger age of onset [92].

2.6.2 Incidence and Prevalence

The average of onset is from 35 to 44 years, with the disease developing earlier with each successive generation if the father is the origin of the mutation, as the CAG repeats are reproduced with greater instability in spermatogenesis than in oogenesis [91]. A 2012 review found that, on average, the yearly worldwide incidence of HD was 0.38/100 000, with incidence being lower in Asian countries compared to Australia, Europe, and North America, as the latter countries have a greater number of huntingtin gene haplotypes. Similarly, the average prevalence was 5.70/100 000 in European, North American, and Australian populations, yet was only 0.40/100 000 in Asia [93]. Although some might argue that this variation could be attributed, at least in part, to differences in case-ascertainment and/or diagnostic criteria, there is consistent evidence of a lower incidence in Asian populations [94].

2.6.3 Pathology

On a macroscopic level, certain areas of the brain are clearly more vulnerable to HD damage than others. The striatum is the most affected brain region, with considerable atrophy occurring, followed by cortical atrophy, firstly in the posterior frontal and then occipital, parietal, and other cortical regions. In late stages there can be up to 25% brain atrophy [95]. Some striatal and early cortical atrophy can be detected prior to onset of symptoms, by which stage there is also widespread neuronal loss in the caudate nucleus (30–40%) [96]. In fact, at a cellular level, HD is primarily characterised by considerable neuronal loss in the striatum and cortex, and again, many other brain regions are similarly affected, such as the thalamus, substantia nigra, and cerebellum. In the striatum, GABAergic medium-size spiny neurons are most affected and degeneration of these neurons occurs progressively. There is also often white matter pathology, even at pre-symptomatic stages [97]. Early synaptic dysfunction is manifested by disrupted glutamate release in the striatum, followed by progressive disconnection between the cortex and striatum.

Huntingtin is a 348 kDa protein expressed ubiquitously, and it is also found in many different subcellular compartments, possibly as a result of the many huntingtin gene splice forms, the protein's numerous caspase and calpain cleavage sites, and the post-translational modifications that are possible [98]. The recent discovery of human-specific isoforms of the protein, including one with a novel exon, may help shed some light on the human-specific pathogenesis of the disease [99]. The function of huntingtin has still not been properly characterised, but there is evidence huntingtin plays a role in endocytosis, axonal and vesicular transport, cell signalling, mitochondrial function, and cell survival pathways [100].

In HD, the huntingtin extra CAG repeats translate to a longer glutamine stretch at the protein's N-terminus. This irregularity is not unique to HD, an abnormal increase in CAG repeats is found in several inherited neurodegenerative 'trinucleotide repeat disorders', often referred to as Polyglutamine diseases. These disorders have different proteins involved with no sequence similarity, and quite unique patterns of neurodegeneration, such that the only common factor is the increase in number of CAG repeats. HD brains and other polyglutamine diseases are also characterised by the presence of intracellular aggregates (inclusions). In HD, these inclusions are found in neuronal nuclei and neuronal processes in the striatal and cortical neurons. They consist of a mixture of granules, straight and tortuous filaments, as well as fibrils, and comprise mostly of truncated forms of the mutant huntingtin protein [101].

Several possible means for HD neurodegeneration of the striatum and the cortex have been suggested – including proteosomal dysfunction, induction of autophagy or apoptosis, mitochondrial failure, disrupted transcription, defective glutamate biology, disruption in provision of brain-derived neurotrophic factor (BDNF) to the striatum, and excitotoxicity at extrasynaptic NMDA receptors [97, 102, 103]. HD neurodegeneration is most likely due to a combination of the above, due to defective huntingtin protein, and/or due to the cellular and functional disruption caused by the aggregated protein fragments [101]. Changes in cortical blood flow are also evident in HD, and a few reports suggest that in pre-clinical HD, cortical blood flow may be an important influence on the rate of neurodegeneration, disease onset, and the rate of progression [104].

2.6.4 Treatment

There are currently no effective pharmacological treatments that stop or prevent the progression of HD pathology. Most treatments that have been trialled have been antichoreic, and tetrabenazine – a monoamine-depleting agent which reduces the amount of dopamine reaching neurons, to modulate both GABA and glutamate transmission – is currently the most effective medication for this purpose, according to Cochrane database reviews [105]. Other medications that reduce the chorea include benzodiazepines such as clonazepam and diazepam, or antipsychotic medication such as olanzapine, risperidone, and quetiapine, which also reduce delusions and violent outbursts, yet have considerable side effects including stiffness, sedation and tremor [89, 106].

Many therapies are under investigation, including inhibitors of apoptosis, huntingtin aggregation, inflammation, oxidative damage and excitotoxicity, as well as modulators of mitochondrial function and transcription [89, 107]. Gene silencing therapies are being developed, including RNAi and antisense oligonucleotides [108, 109]. Other gene silencing therapy being trialled is aiming at personalised therapy, to target only the pathogenic allele [110]. Neural transplantation studies for HD have also been carried out in a small number of people, with variable results [111].

Donepezil (an AD medication) has been trialled to see if it can reduce cognitive and motor impairments in HD, however without success. The AD medication memantine, which influences the NMDA pathway, is currently being trialled for HD [89]. Mood stabilisers such as carbamazepine help reduce irritability; others include sodium valproate and olanzapine.

Depression can be severe in HD, and antidepressants that have been used include selective serotonin reuptake inhibitors (SSRI) such as fluoxetine and citalopram, tricyclic antidepressants such as amitriptyline, and others such as mirtazapine, clozapine and duloxetine [89, 112]. Suicide attempts are twice as common in HD as in the general population, and significant psychological support, tailored regular exercise, and occupational therapy is needed to help HD patients.

2.7 Motor Neuron Diseases

This is a group of neurological conditions that principally affect motor neurons, which control voluntary muscles of the body. Motor neuron diseases (MND) are characterised by progressive loss of motor neurons of the spinal cord (lower motor neurons) or motor neurons of the brain (upper motor neurons), or a combination of both, leading to atrophy and/or spasticity of the associated muscles. Thus, although the MND-related conditions have distinct names, MND can be described as existing on a spectrum: from a pure lower motor neuron; to mixed upper and lower motor neuron; to a pure upper motor neuron variant in addition to regional variants restricted to the arms, legs, or bulbar region [113, 114]. Spinal muscular atrophy (SMA), ALS, and hereditary spastic paraplegia (HSP) are the most common; others include primary lateral sclerosis (PLS), progressive muscular atrophy, progressive bulbar palsy and pseudobulbar palsy.

2.7.1 Amyotrophic Lateral Sclerosis

The main form of MND, amyotrophic lateral sclerosis (ALS), is also known as Lou Gehrig's disease. Like most other MND, ALS is characterised by muscle stiffness, muscle twitching, and gradual worsening weakness due to muscles decreasing in size. It is a progressive mixed upper and lower MND, mostly sporadic (85%), and invariably fatal, approximately 3–5 years after diagnosis [113, 115]. Approximately 5% of cases with ALS develop dementia of the frontotemporal type (FTD), and this ALS-FTD is characterised by behaviour changes, and sometimes language dysfunction. ALS and ALS-FTD are discussed in greater detail below.

2.7.2 Spinal Muscular Atrophy

SMA is a neurodegenerative disease caused by progressive degeneration of lower motor neurons in the anterior horn of the spinal cord, resulting in hypotonia, muscle atrophy, and paralysis. Spine deformities can develop, as well as contractures of major joints. Due to the high variability in age of onset and clinical types, SMA is divided into five types. Type 0 has a prenatal onset, with early respiratory failure, severe neonatal hypotonia, and severe weakness detected at birth, and survival from this most severe form is rarely past six months. Type I (severe SMA, Werdnig-Hoffmann disease) has an onset usually before six months, bulbar and respiratory muscles are affected early, and symptoms usually start with muscle weakness, poor muscle tone, lack of motor development, and feeding problems. Type I patients rarely reach two years of age. At the other end of the spectrum, Type IV has an adult age of onset, with initial symptoms involving pronounced proximal weakness. Both Type III and IV SMA patients usually have a normal life expectancy [116].

2.7.3 Hereditary Spastic Paraplegia

This is usually divided into pure and complicated forms, with the pure forms often split into two groups, Type 1 with onset before 35 years, and Type 2 with onset after 35 years. Type 1 patients usually have a slow and variable course of disease, whereas Type 2 cases evolve more rapidly, and in these cases muscle weakness, sensory loss, and urinary symptoms are more severe. Overall, HSP patients present initially with gait disturbance or walking difficulties, leg stiffness, and urinary problems. The age of onset for HSP can be from infancy to the eighth decade, and unlike most inherited conditions, the age of onset within an affected family can vary widely, possibly because some symptoms are mild and not reported for many years. HSP hallmark characteristics include spasticity and hyperreflexia of lower limbs, progressive gait disturbance, and extensor plantar responses. Despite muscle problems, there is usually little or no muscle weakness [117]. In complicated HSP, clinical features which may be seen in addition to spastic paraparesis include amyotrophy (particularly in the hand), dementia, epilepsy, cardiac defects, sensory neuropathy, deafness, and retinal changes, amongst others [117]. This condition is compatible with a normal life expectancy, such that most patients die in old age of coincidental illnesses.

2.7.4 Onset of MND and Differential Diagnosis

Patients initially present with walking, tripping, or falling problems, weakness in legs and feet, and sometimes hand weakness or clumsiness. There may also be muscle twitching (fasciculations) especially in the arms and shoulders, slurred speech, and trouble swallowing. Eventually symptoms worsen, muscle wastage occurs leading to weight loss, and breathing problems can lead to the need for devices to help breathe at night. At later stages symptoms worsen, some patients will opt for a tracheotomy to enable the use of a respirator, a gastrostomy tube can be used to maintain caloric intake and hydration, and frontotemporal dementia can occur [115].

There is considerable overlap in symptoms of the various MND, and ALS is often confused with primary lateral sclerosis (PLS). It has been suggested that patients presenting with spasticity who do not develop wasting within three years most likely have PLS [118]. Patients with ALS are also more likely to have hyporeflexia [119]. PLS is a disease of the upper motor neurons, whereas progressive muscular atrophy only involves the lower motor neurons in the spinal cord. In progressive bulbar palsy, the lowest motor neurons of the brain stem are affected the most, causing slurred speech and difficulty chewing and swallowing. However, there are almost always mildly abnormal signs in the arms and legs [115].

2.7.5 Incidence, Causes, and Risk Factors

Some forms of MND are inherited, but the causes of most MND are not known. A person is considered to be suffering from familial ALS if there is a history of at least one other blood relative with the disease, and many families have been investigated to determine the potential genetic link. As a result, over 30 genetic mutations or variants have been shown to account for familial ALS. The most common ones include a *C9ORF72* hexanucleotide repeat (GGGGCC) expansion which accounts for approximately 40% of familial ALS in North America and Europe, yet, for the moment, little is known about the protein linked to this gene. Superoxide dismutase (*SOD1*) variants have been linked to the disease in about 12% of familial cases, and variations in 'transactive response DNA binding protein 43' (*TARDBP*) and the 'fused in sarcoma' (*FUS*) genes are each responsible for a small percentage of cases [120]. These percentages are averages, and figures vary depending on the population being examined. Over 160 pathogenic *SOD1* variants are now known, and there is evidence that *SOD1* variants result in a toxic gain of function. The pathological hallmarks found post-mortem in the brain and spinal cord of *SOD1* ALS as well as other ALS cases include intracellular neuronal and astrocytic ubiquitinated proteins and protein aggregates in inclusions (though mostly not involving TDP-43; see below) [120–122]. TDP-43 is a transcription factor usually found in the nucleus, yet which is abnormally found in the cytoplasm in MND, where it may be phosphorylated (pho-TDP-43), and often ubiquitinated, and also found intracellularly in inclusions [122, 123]. Variants of the *TARDBP* gene, which codes for TDP-43, appear to cause dysregulation of gene expression including RNA splicing, as well as a toxic gain of function of mutant TDP-43 protein. As in wild-type TDP-43 proteinopathy, mutant TDP-43 in *TARDBP*-linked ALS brain tissue is characterised by its cytoplasmic accumulation as aggregated and insoluble deposits.

Interestingly, studies of the *SOD1*G93A ALS mutation in a mouse model have shown a close interaction at hippocampal synapses between SOD1 and APP, the protein precursor of the Aβ peptide which is thought to be toxic in AD, such that there are SOD1-APP conformational changes and APP processing changes [124]. More recent analysis has shown that patients with ALS have increased APP and Aβ expression, with the latter correlating with cytoplasmic pho-TDP-43 expression. There was also higher phosphorylated tau expression in the hippocampus, though no significant deposition of Aβ aggregates in the brain [123]. Interestingly, deposition of TDP-43 is also the major feature of tau-negative frontotemporal dementia (FTD) which is clinically very similar to ALS. In fact, abnormally hyper-phosphorylated and ubiquitinated TDP-43 is found in several conditions which are sometimes collectively known as the TDP-43 proteinopathies. Other TDP-43 proteinopathies include chronic traumatic encephalopathy and a subset of AD [125]. The finding that pathogenic mutations in the *TARDBP* gene is linked to ALS implicates TDP-43 as a key mediator of pathogenesis in both ALS and a subgroup of FTD which is characterised by ubiquitinated protein inclusions (known as FTD-U or ALS-FTD) [126].

It has been suggested that sporadic ALS and other MND are caused by environmental (heavy metals, electromagnetic fields, sport, herbicides, fertilisers, and insecticides), viral, or as yet unknown genetic factors [127]. Rates of MND in most of the world are also mostly unknown. ALS is the most common MND, and in the USA approximately 2/100 000 people develop it each year, thus it is a rare disease. Similarly, ALS affects about 2.2 people/100 000 in Europe [128]. Other reports indicate ALS cases occur at a rate of around 1.2–4.0/100 000 in Caucasian populations, and at a lower rate in other ethnic populations [129, 130]. MND appear to affect men more than women, for example sporadic ALS affects men : women in a ratio of 1.3 : 1. Onset of the condition is usually between the ages of 40 and 60, although familial forms have an average age of onset of 46 years.

2.7.6 Pathology

On a macroscopic level, there is widespread muscle atrophy, affecting the proximal and distal extremities, the tongue, intercostal muscles, and the diaphragm. The brain often shows little gross change, though the precentral gyrus may be atrophied, and, in cases with accompanying dementia, the frontal and temporal lobes may also show some atrophy. Brain histological features will include a loss of motor neurons, for example in ALS there is a loss of both upper and lower motor neurons, with associated astrogliosis. In the relevant brain or spinal cord sections, immunohistochemical staining with ubiquitin antibodies will reveal neuronal cytoplasmic inclusions, especially in ALS. Staining for TDP-43 will colocalise with ubiquitin staining in ALS (as well as ALS-FTD), though not in ALS cases linked to an *SOD1* mutation [32, 131].

2.7.7 Treatment

There are no cures for any of the MND. The only medication that is approved for treatment of MND in Australia is riluzole, which acts by blocking glutamatergic transmission and, if prescribed early in the disease, can prolong lifespan for up to two to three months. Other treatments involve multidisciplinary teams that provide physiotherapy, speech therapy, district nurse help, psychological help, orthotic help, neurologist help and advice, and palliative care. These deal with issues that occur at various stages of the disease, such as self-care (assistive equipment); communication difficulties (alternative communication devices); disease progression; mobility (specialised equipment); breathing difficulties (assisted ventilation); and eating and drinking difficulties (gastrostomy) [132]. Genetic testing of family members of familial MND families can also be carried out, with the help of neurologists and disease-specific genetic counsellors.

Promising results from studies of potential new therapies are providing some hope for the future though. MicroRNA studies have shown that certain miRNA are altered in the early stages of SMA for example, miR-9, miR-206, and miR-132 in spinal cord, skeletal muscle, and serum from SMA transgenic mice, as well as in serum from SMA patients; furthermore it has been shown that antisense RNA therapy can alter levels of these miRNA [133]. This supports the concept that antisense RNA may provide potential anti-MND therapy in the future. There is also evidence from pre-clinical models that stem cell therapy, particularly from studies of ALS, may provide effective treatment. For example, spinal cord neural progenitor cells are being investigated as potentially useful cells for intraspinal transplantation in phase I and phase IIa trials, with the aim of replacing motor neurons and modulating toxicity [134, 135]. Transcranial magnetic stimulation has been tested for both diagnosis and treatment of MND, with most research having been carried out with respect to ALS [136]; however, results have been variable.

2.8 Prion Diseases

Also known as transmissible spongiform encephalopathies (TSE), prion diseases are a group of neurodegenerative diseases which include Creutzfeldt-Jakob disease (CJD), Gerstmann-Sträussler-Scheinker syndrome (GSS), kuru and fatal familial insomnia in humans; scrapie in sheep, goats and mufflons; transmissible mink encephalopathy in ranch-reared mink; chronic wasting disease of mule deer and elk; bovine spongiform encephalopathy (BSE) or 'mad cow disease' in cattle and its analogues in several exotic species of antelopes and wild felids in zoological gardens, and feline spongiform encephalopathy in domestic cats [137]. These invariably fatal diseases all involve modification of the prion proteins (PrP), which then become infectious pathogens that are devoid of nucleic acid. Transmission of the condition from one animal to another was first shown by Gajdusek and Morris in the 1960s, for example see [138], yet prion diseases were thought to be caused by a slow virus at the time. It has since been shown, with some controversy, that modified forms of PrP (Prp^{sc} named after scrapie in sheep, versus the normal cellular form PrP^c) with β-sheet structure and associated modified physical and biochemical properties, can act as infective agents in other sheep or in humans, for example. Other interesting findings were that scrapie, like kuru and CJD, produced death of the host without any sign of an immune response to a foreign infectious agent, and that the Prp^{sc} is highly resistant to heat, radiation, and formalin treatment [139].

2.8.1 Causes

There are some rare familial forms of CJD which cause about 10% of cases, and more than 20 mutations in the PrP gene have been documented to cause the human form. Prion diseases can also occur sporadically at a rate of 1/1,000,000. Between 1986 and 1998, there was an alarming rise in cases of CJD, and all evidence suggests it was caused by the consumption of animals that had been infected with the bovine form of the disease. These are referred to as vCJD cases ("v" for variant), and they occurred in the UK and Canada. To date, over 170 people have died of vCJD, and a British and Irish inquiry into BSE concluded the transmission was caused by cattle being fed the remains of other cattle in the form of meat and bone meal (MBM), a protein supplement in concentrated feeds [140].

2.8.2 Symptoms and Diagnosis

Typical symptoms include rapidly progressing dementia, visual and cerebellum function abnormalities, personality changes, hallucinations, anxiety, depression, paranoia, obsessive-compulsive symptoms, and psychosis. Physical problems that develop include myoclonia, speech problems, ataxia, changes in gait, and seizures. The duration of the disease is variable, and can be from just a few weeks to six months, though some patients have been known to survive for more than two years following diagnosis [141].

A diagnosis of CJD is not very simple as the symptoms overlap those of many other forms of dementia. First symptoms usually include cognitive, cerebellar, behavioural, constitutional, sensory, motor, and visual changes, in descending order of frequency. To meet WHO criteria for probable CJD, patients should undergo an electroencephalogram to detect periodic epileptiform discharges, or should be tested for elevated 14-3-3 protein, tau and neuron-specific enolase in the CSF, and also have evidence of at least two of the following – myoclonus, pyramidal/extrapyramidal findings, visual or cerebellar deficits, and akinetic mutism. However, many of these changes overlap with changes seen in DLB and Hashimoto's encephalopathy (another rapidly progressive dementia), so will not provide an accurate diagnosis [142]. Brain MRI sequences obtained using one or more of fluid attenuated inversion recovery (FLAIR), diffusion weighted imaging (DWI), and apparent diffusion coefficient (ADC) studies will help with diagnosis, providing over 90% sensitivity and specificity in the detection of sporadic CJD [142, 143]. In particular, high signal changes in the basal ganglia and cerebral cortex on FLAIR and DWI are useful in the diagnosis of sporadic CJD [144].

2.8.3 Treatment

There is no cure for CJD, and although some treatments such as quinacrine, doxycycline, and pentosane polysulfate have been trialled, none have been proven to be effective [145].

2.8.4 Differential Diagnosis of the Various Types of Dementia

As mentioned previously, AD usually presents with memory problems, unlike DLB, and the physical problems of DLB are not usually found in AD or VaD, thus helping diagnosis. However, the diagnosis of DLB is difficult, due to the overlap with the symptoms of AD, VaD, and PD, as discussed above, and due to the often concurrent development of other forms of dementia, especially AD. Furthermore, within the synucleinopathies, cognitive impairment and depression associated with hippocampal dysfunction are common to all the disorders.

There is a more rapid cognitive and physical decline in the first few months of DLB [63, 146]. Thus to some extent, DLB and Parkinson's disease dementia (PDD), both synucleinopathies, are differentiated by the difference in onset time of dementia symptoms relative to Parkinsonian symptoms. PDD is the diagnosis when dementia symptoms arise more than a year after the onset of Parkinsonian symptoms, whereas DLB is diagnosed when cognitive symptoms begin at the same time or within a year of Parkinsonian symptoms [65]. However, it would be preferable to detect these conditions well before symptoms have been present for a while, and many studies have researched the underlying pathology and are continuing to refine the many imaging techniques mentioned in the section above in order to differentiate between AD, DLB, and PD.

Research into CSF biomarkers has determined that changes seen in AD are often also seen in DLB and FTD for example, with some subtle differences now emerging that may make differential diagnosis possible. For instance, phosphorylated tau (P-tau) is one of the core CSF biomarkers for AD, yet P-tau is also found in DLB and FTD. Nevertheless, the phosphorylation of tau protein appears to be different in DLB compared to AD, such that levels of tau phosphorylated at threonine 231 (Thr231-phosphorylated tau) may differentiate between AD and FTD, and there is also evidence tau phosphorylated at threonine 181 (Thr181-phosphorylated tau) can enhance classification between AD and DLB [147, 148]. CSF levels of α-synuclein have been proposed as a biomarker for the synucleinopathies – PD, DLB, and multiple system atrophy – however one study found a higher level of α-synuclein in the CSF, when comparing DLB with AD or healthy controls [149, 150]. As it currently stands, it appears that diagnosis will have to rely on imaging studies, CSF samples in some cases, and neuropsychological evaluation. Ideally peripheral biomarkers, such as blood biomarkers, will become available. In fact, recent research suggests blood biomarker panels are showing considerable promise, particularly in the case of AD [151–153], where comparisons to PiB-PET imaging results have been made, as well as cross-validation in autosomal dominant AD cohorts [154]. Importantly, these diagnostic tools have been shown to detect AD at preclinical stages, which is essential for treatments to be successful, if aiming to prevent disease progression and symptom onset. Eventually it is hoped that disease-specific biomarker panels are developed for all these conditions, or at least a series of panels that will be able to differentiate between the different conditions.

2.8.5 DLB Treatment

When considering appropriate treatment, it is useful to divide the array of symptoms into five categories: cognitive, neuropsychiatric, movement, autonomic, and sleep. Unfortunately, as already alluded to above, the management of one symptom of DLB often leads to unwanted side-effects in another symptom. For example, DLB-associated problems with attention, executive function, and visuospatial ability respond well to anti-cholinesterase treatment, yet there are potential adverse effects including cardiac and gastrointestinal dysautonomia [155]. Certain symptoms can be diminished using specific treatments, for example daytime sleepiness (which can be treated with caffeine in those without restless leg syndrome), and constipation or diarrhoea (which can be treated with fibre, exercise, or misoprostol, for example), genito-urinary symptoms and postural hypotension [155].

2.9 Summary

From the descriptions of the neurodegenerative conditions above, it can be seen that there are many different pathologies, symptoms, and disease time courses, yet none of these conditions have a cure. At best, some have treatments that reduce the severity of symptoms, to a greater or lesser extent. The symptoms of the various neurodegenerative conditions show much overlap in the initial clinical presentations, often requiring several specialist assessments, neuroimaging tests, and sometimes genetic tests before differential diagnosis is given, and even then, sometimes only a 'probable' diagnosis is possible.

The most common neurodegenerative condition that leads to dementia in the elderly is AD, an illness that reveals symptoms only once considerable and irreversible synaptic and neuronal loss has already occurred. With no cure or effective treatment available despite considerable research, the therapeutic research focus is now aiming at prevention and slowing down the disease progress, and, as can be seen in the rest of this book, AD preventative and disease-slowing therapies are being researched extensively.

Being able to determine that a patient is in the pre-clinical or early symptomatic stages of AD, either as the only pathology, or in combination with another neurodegenerative condition, is essential to provide disease-specific treatments. The Australian Imaging, Biomarker and Lifestyle [151] study of ageing that is mentioned repeatedly in this book is one of a few highly characterised longitudinal studies of large cohorts around the world that has provided invaluable information concerning lifestyle aspects that influence risk of AD, as well as supportive information concerning which other conditions increase the risk of developing AD. Mid-life obesity, cardiovascular disease, hypertension, type 2 diabetes, insulin resistance, and dyslipidaemia are all conditions that are linked to chronic inflammation, oxidative stress, and an increased risk of AD. All of these conditions can be ameliorated by lifestyle changes, particularly dietary modifications and increases in levels of physical activity and management of cardiovascular risk factors. These lifestyle changes are discussed with relevance to reducing risk of AD, but have a greater applicability, as they would also reduce the risk or symptom level of some of the other neurodegenerative conditions too, such as VaD and PD, quite apart from reducing cardiovascular disease, type 2 diabetes, and all the other related conditions listed above.

References

1 Kovacs, G.G. (2016). Molecular pathological classification of neurodegenerative diseases: turning towards precision medicine. *Int. J. Mol. Sci.* 17 (2): 189. https://doi.org/10.3390/ijms17020189.
2 Jellinger, K.A. and Bancher, C. (1998). Neuropathology of Alzheimer's disease: a critical update. *J. Neural Transm. Suppl.* 54: 77–95.
3 Fernandez-Nogales, M., Cabrera, J.R., Santos-Galindo, M. et al. (2014). Huntington's disease is a four-repeat tauopathy with tau nuclear rods. *Nat. Med.* 20: 881–885.
4 McKhann, G.M., Knopman, D.S., Chertkow, H. et al. (2011). The diagnosis of dementia due to Alzheimer's disease: recommendations from the National Institute on Aging-Alzheimer's Association workgroups on diagnostic guidelines for Alzheimer's disease. *Alzheimers Dement.* 7: 263–269.
5 McKhann, G., Drachman, D., Folstein, M. et al. (1984). Clinical diagnosis of Alzheimer's disease: report of the NINCDS-ADRDA Work Group under the auspices of Department of Health and Human Services Task Force on Alzheimer's Disease. *Neurology* 34: 939–944.
6 Tarawneh, R. and Holtzman, D.M. (2012). The clinical problem of symptomatic Alzheimer disease and mild cognitive impairment. *Cold Spring Harbor Perspect. Med.* 2: a006148.
7 Selkoe, D.J. and Hardy, J. (2016). The amyloid hypothesis of Alzheimer's disease at 25 years. *EMBO Mol. Med.* 8: 595–608.
8 Corder, E.H., Saunders, A.M., Strittmatter, W.J. et al. (1993). Gene dose of apolipoprotein E type 4 allele and the risk of Alzheimer's disease in late onset families. *Science* 261: 921–923.
9 Strittmatter, W.J. (2012). Medicine: old drug, new hope for Alzheimer's disease. *Science* 335: 1447–1448.
10 Hauser, P.S. and Ryan, R.O. (2013). Impact of apolipoprotein E on Alzheimer's disease. *Curr. Alzheimer Res.* 10: 809–817.
11 Giri, M., Zhang, M., and Lu, Y. (2016). Genes associated with Alzheimer's disease: an overview and current status. *Clin. Interv. Aging* 11: 665–681.
12 de Toledo Ferraz Alves, T.C., Ferreira, L.K., Wajngarten, M., and Busatto, G.F. (2010). Cardiac disorders as risk factors for Alzheimer's disease. *J. Alzheimers Dis.* 20: 749–763.
13 Luchsinger, J.A. and Mayeux, R. (2004). Cardiovascular risk factors and Alzheimer's disease. *Curr. Atheroscler. Rep.* 6: 261–266.
14 Birks, J. (2006). Cholinesterase inhibitors for Alzheimer's disease. *Cochrane Database Syst. Rev.* CD005593. https://doi.org/10.1002/14651858.CD005593.
15 Szeto, J.Y. and Lewis, S.J. (2016). Current treatment options for Alzheimer's disease and Parkinson's disease dementia. *Curr. Neuropharmacol.* 14: 326–338.
16 Verdile, G., Keane, K.N., Cruzat, V.F. et al. (2015). Inflammation and oxidative stress: the molecular connectivity between insulin resistance, obesity, and Alzheimer's disease. *Mediators Inflamm.* 2015: 105828.
17 Veurink, G., Fuller, S.J., Atwood, C.S., and Martins, R.N. (2003). Genetics, lifestyle and the roles of amyloid beta and oxidative stress in Alzheimer's disease. *Ann. Hum. Biol.* 30: 639–667.

18 Ellis, K.A., Bush, A.I., Darby, D. et al., and Group AR (2009). The Australian Imaging, Biomarkers and Lifestyle (AIBL) study of aging: methodology and baseline characteristics of 1112 individuals recruited for a longitudinal study of Alzheimer's disease. *Int. Psychogeriatr.* 21: 672–687.

19 Gardener, S., Gu, Y., Rainey-Smith, S.R. et al., and Group AR (2012). Adherence to a Mediterranean diet and Alzheimer's disease risk in an Australian population. *Transl. Psychiatry* 2: e164.

20 Gardener, S.L., Rainey-Smith, S.R., Barnes, M.B. et al. (2015). Dietary patterns and cognitive decline in an Australian study of ageing. *Mol. Psychiatry* 20: 860–866.

21 Gardener, S.L., Rainey-Smith, S.R., Sohrabi, H.R. et al., and Group AR (2017). Increased carbohydrate intake is associated with poorer performance in verbal memory and attention in an APOE genotype-dependent manner. *J. Alzheimers Dis.* 58: 193–201.

22 Brown, B.M., Peiffer, J.J., and Martins, R.N. (2013). Multiple effects of physical activity on molecular and cognitive signs of brain aging: can exercise slow neurodegeneration and delay Alzheimer's disease? *Mol. Psychiatry* 18: 864–874.

23 Brown, B.M., Sohrabi, H.R., Taddei, K. et al., and Dominantly Inherited Alzheimer N (2017). Habitual exercise levels are associated with cerebral amyloid load in presymptomatic autosomal dominant Alzheimer's disease. *Alzheimers Dement.* 13: 1197–1206.

24 Bang, J., Spina, S., and Miller, B.L. (2015). Frontotemporal dementia. *Lancet* 386: 1672–1682.

25 Chan, D.K., Reutens, S., Liu, D.K., and Chan, R.O. (2011). Frontotemporal dementia – features, diagnosis and management. *Aust. Fam. Physician* 40: 968–972.

26 Cardarelli, R., Kertesz, A., and Knebl, J.A. (2010). Frontotemporal dementia: a review for primary care physicians. *Am. Fam. Physician* 82: 1372–1377.

27 Mackenzie, I.R. and Neumann, M. (2016). Molecular neuropathology of frontotemporal dementia: insights into disease mechanisms from postmortem studies. *J. Neurochem.* 138 (Suppl 1): 54–70.

28 Dickson, D.W. (2001). Neuropathology of Pick's disease. *Neurology* 56: S16–S20.

29 Pan, X.D. and Chen, X.C. (2013). Clinic, neuropathology and molecular genetics of frontotemporal dementia: a mini-review. *Transl. Neurodegener.* 2: 8.

30 Roeber, S., Mackenzie, I.R., Kretzschmar, H.A., and Neumann, M. (2008). TDP-43-negative FTLD-U is a significant new clinico-pathological subtype of FTLD. *Acta Neuropathol.* 116: 147–157.

31 Mackenzie, I.R., Neumann, M., Bigio, E.H. et al. (2009). Nomenclature for neuropathologic subtypes of frontotemporal lobar degeneration: consensus recommendations. *Acta Neuropathol.* 117: 15–18.

32 Cairns, N.J., Bigio, E.H., Mackenzie, I.R. et al., and Consortium for Frontotemporal Lobar D (2007). Neuropathologic diagnostic and nosologic criteria for frontotemporal lobar degeneration: consensus of the Consortium for Frontotemporal Lobar Degeneration. *Acta Neuropathol.* 114: 5–22.

33 Neumann, M., Kwong, L.K., Sampathu, D.M. et al. (2007). TDP-43 proteinopathy in frontotemporal lobar degeneration and amyotrophic lateral sclerosis: protein misfolding diseases without amyloidosis. *Arch. Neurol.* 64: 1388–1394.

34 Henry, M.L. and Gorno-Tempini, M.L. (2010). The logopenic variant of primary progressive aphasia. *Curr. Opin. Neurol.* 23: 633–637.

35 Hardy, J., Momeni, P., and Traynor, B.J. (2006). Frontal temporal dementia: dissecting the aetiology and pathogenesis. *Brain* 129: 830–831.

36 Ferrari, R., Grassi, M., Salvi, E. et al. (2015). A genome-wide screening and SNPs-to-genes approach to identify novel genetic risk factors associated with frontotemporal dementia. *Neurobiol. Aging* 36 (2904): e2913–e2926.

37 Ferrari, R., Hernandez, D.G., Nalls, M.A. et al. (2014). Frontotemporal dementia and its subtypes: a genome-wide association study. *Lancet Neurol.* 13: 686–699.

38 Diekstra, F.P., Van Deerlin, V.M., van Swieten, J.C. et al. (2014). C9orf72 and UNC13A are shared risk loci for amyotrophic lateral sclerosis and frontotemporal dementia: a genome-wide meta-analysis. *Ann. Neurol.* 76: 120–133.

39 Tsai, R.M. and Boxer, A.L. (2016). Therapy and clinical trials in frontotemporal dementia: past, present, and future. *J. Neurochem.* 138 (Suppl 1): 211–221.

40 Merrilees, J. (2007). A model for management of behavioral symptoms in frontotemporal lobar degeneration. *Alzheimer Dis. Assoc. Disord.* 21: S64–S69.

41 Harada, R., Okamura, N., Furumoto, S. et al. (2016). 18F-THK5351: a novel PET radiotracer for imaging neurofibrillary pathology in Alzheimer disease. *J. Nucl. Med.* 57: 208–214.

42 Johnson, K.A., Schultz, A., Betensky, R.A. et al. (2016). Tau positron emission tomographic imaging in aging and early Alzheimer disease. *Ann. Neurol.* 79: 110–119.

43 Thal, D.R., Grinberg, L.T., and Attems, J. (2012). Vascular dementia: different forms of vessel disorders contribute to the development of dementia in the elderly brain. *Exp. Gerontol.* 47: 816–824.

44 Kim, K.W., MacFall, J.R., and Payne, M.E. (2008). Classification of white matter lesions on magnetic resonance imaging in elderly persons. *Biol. Psychiatry* 64: 273–280.

45 Jellinger, K.A. (2007). The enigma of vascular cognitive disorder and vascular dementia. *Acta Neuropathol.* 113: 349–388.

46 Schneider, J.A., Arvanitakis, Z., Bang, W., and Bennett, D.A. (2007). Mixed brain pathologies account for most dementia cases in community-dwelling older persons. *Neurology* 69: 2197–2204.

47 Lo Coco, D., Lopez, G., and Corrao, S. (2016). Cognitive impairment and stroke in elderly patients. *Vasc. Health Risk Manag.* 12: 105–116.

48 Sonnen, J.A., Larson, E.B., Crane, P.K. et al. (2007). Pathological correlates of dementia in a longitudinal, population-based sample of aging. *Ann. Neurol.* 62: 406–413.

49 Abete, P., Della-Morte, D., Gargiulo, G. et al. (2014). Cognitive impairment and cardiovascular diseases in the elderly. A heart-brain continuum hypothesis. *Ageing Res. Rev.* 18: 41–52.

50 Manktelow, B.N. and Potter, J.F. (2009). Interventions in the management of serum lipids for preventing stroke recurrence. *Cochrane Database Syst. Rev.* CD002091. https://doi.org/10.1002/14651858.CD002091.pub2.

51 Gorelick, P.B., Scuteri, A., Black, S.E. et al., and American Heart Association Stroke Council CoE, Prevention CoCNCoCR, Intervention, Council on Cardiovascular S, Anesthesia (2011). Vascular contributions to cognitive impairment and dementia: a statement for healthcare professionals from the American Heart Association/American Stroke Association. *Stroke* 42: 2672–2713.

52 Muresanu, D.F., Heiss, W.D., Hoemberg, V. et al. (2016). Cerebrolysin and Recovery After Stroke (CARS): a randomized, placebo-controlled, double-blind, multicenter trial. *Stroke* 47: 151–159.

53 Mead, G.E., Hsieh, C.F., Lee, R. et al. (2013). Selective serotonin reuptake inhibitors for stroke recovery: a systematic review and meta-analysis. *Stroke* 44: 844–850.

54 Mijajlovic, M.D., Pavlovic, A., Brainin, M. et al. (2017). Post-stroke dementia – a comprehensive review. *BMC Med.* 15: 11.

55 Yang, W. and Yu, S. (2017). Synucleinopathies: common features and hippocampal manifestations. *Cell. Mol. Life Sci.* 74 (8): 1485–1501. https://doi.org/10.1007/s00018-016-2411-y.

56 Braak, H. and Braak, E. (2000). Pathoanatomy of Parkinson's disease. *J. Neurol.* 247 (Suppl 2): II3–II10.

57 Ingelsson, M. (2016). Alpha-Synuclein oligomers-neurotoxic molecules in Parkinson's disease and other Lewy body disorders. *Front Neurosci.* 10: 408.

58 Vann Jones, S.A. and O'Brien, J.T. (2014). The prevalence and incidence of dementia with Lewy bodies: a systematic review of population and clinical studies. *Psychol. Med.* 44: 673–683.

59 Hogan, D.B., Fiest, K.M., Roberts, J.I. et al. (2016). The prevalence and incidence of dementia with Lewy bodies: a systematic review. *Can. J. Neurol. Sci.* 43 (Suppl 1): S83–S95.

60 Schulz-Schaeffer, W.J. (2010). The synaptic pathology of alpha-synuclein aggregation in dementia with Lewy bodies, Parkinson's disease and Parkinson's disease dementia. *Acta Neuropathol.* 120: 131–143.

61 Meeus, B., Nuytemans, K., Crosiers, D. et al. (2010). Comprehensive genetic and mutation analysis of familial dementia with Lewy bodies linked to 2q35-q36. *J. Alzheimers Dis.* 20: 197–205.

62 Simard, M., van Reekum, R., and Cohen, T. (2000). A review of the cognitive and behavioral symptoms in dementia with Lewy bodies. *J. Neuropsychiatry Clin. Neurosci.* 12: 425–450.

63 Donaghy, P.C. and McKeith, I.G. (2014). The clinical characteristics of dementia with Lewy bodies and a consideration of prodromal diagnosis. *Alzheimers Res. Ther.* 6: 46.

64 Gurnani, A.S. and Gavett, B.E. (2016). The differential effects of Alzheimer's disease and Lewy body pathology on cognitive performance: a meta-analysis. *Neuropsychol. Rev.* 27 (1): 1–17. https://doi.org/10.1007/s11065-016-9334-0.

65 McKeith, I.G., Dickson, D.W., Lowe, J. et al., and Consortium on DLB (2005). Diagnosis and management of dementia with Lewy bodies: third report of the DLB Consortium. *Neurology* 65: 1863–1872.

66 Wang, F., Feng, T.Y., Yang, S. et al. (2016). Drug therapy for behavioral and psychological symptoms of dementia. *Curr. Neuropharmacol.* 14: 307–313.

67 Mak, E., Su, L., Williams, G.B., and O'Brien, J.T. (2014). Neuroimaging characteristics of dementia with Lewy bodies. *Alzheimers Res. Ther.* 6: 18.

68 Huang, J., Zhuo, W., Zhang, Y. et al. (2017). Cognitive function characteristics of Parkinson's disease with sleep disorders. *Parkinsons Dis.* 2017: 4267353.

69 Yang, Y., Tang, B.S., and Guo, J.F. (2016). Parkinson's disease and cognitive impairment. *Parkinsons Dis.* 2016: 6734678.

70 Noyce, A.J., Lees, A.J., and Schrag, A.E. (2016). The prediagnostic phase of Parkinson's disease. *J. Neurol. Neurosurg. Psychiatry* 87: 871–878.

71 de Lau, L.M. and Breteler, M.M. (2006). Epidemiology of Parkinson's disease. *Lancet Neurol.* 5: 525–535.

72 Noyce, A.J., Bestwick, J.P., Silveira-Moriyama, L. et al. (2012). Meta-analysis of early nonmotor features and risk factors for Parkinson disease. *Ann. Neurol.* 72: 893–901.

73 Checkoway, H., Powers, K., Smith-Weller, T. et al. (2002). Parkinson's disease risks associated with cigarette smoking, alcohol consumption, and caffeine intake. *Am. J. Epidemiol.* 155: 732–738.

74 Xu, Y., Yang, J., and Shang, H. (2016). Meta-analysis of risk factors for Parkinson's disease dementia. *Transl. Neurodegener.* 5: 11.

75 Stefanis, L. (2012). Alpha-Synuclein in Parkinson's disease. *Cold Spring Harbor Perspect. Med.* 2: a009399.

76 Liu, G., Zhang, C., Yin, J. et al. (2009). Alpha-Synuclein is differentially expressed in mitochondria from different rat brain regions and dose-dependently down-regulates complex I activity. *Neurosci. Lett.* 454: 187–192.

77 Klein, C. and Westenberger, A. (2012). Genetics of Parkinson's disease. *Cold Spring Harbor Perspect. Med.* 2: a008888.

78 Eriksen, J.L., Przedborski, S., and Petrucelli, L. (2005). Gene dosage and pathogenesis of Parkinson's disease. *Trends Mol. Med.* 11: 91–96.

79 Winkler, S., Hagenah, J., Lincoln, S. et al. (2007). Alpha-Synuclein and Parkinson disease susceptibility. *Neurology* 69: 1745–1750.

80 Hou, L., Chen, W., Liu, X. et al. (2017). Exercise-induced neuroprotection of the nigrostriatal dopamine system in Parkinson's disease. *Front. Aging Neurosci.* 9: 358.

81 Kitamura, Y., Kakimura, J., and Taniguchi, T. (2002). Antiparkinsonian drugs and their neuroprotective effects. *Biol. Pharm. Bull.* 25: 284–290.

82 Radad, K., Gille, G., and Rausch, W.D. (2005). Short review on dopamine agonists: insight into clinical and research studies relevant to Parkinson's disease. *Pharmacol. Rep.* 57: 701–712.

83 Alomar, S., King, N.K., Tam, J. et al. (2017). Speech and language adverse effects after thalamotomy and deep brain stimulation in patients with movement disorders: a meta-analysis. *Mov. Disord.* 32: 53–63.

84 Yasuhara, T., Kameda, M., Sasaki, T. et al. (2017). Cell therapy for Parkinson's disease. *Cell Transplant.* 26: 1551–1559.

85 Nakagawa, M., Koyanagi, M., Tanabe, K. et al. (2008). Generation of induced pluripotent stem cells without Myc from mouse and human fibroblasts. *Nat. Biotechnol.* 26: 101–106.

86 Barker, R.A., Parmar, M., Kirkeby, A. et al. (2016). Are stem cell-based therapies for Parkinson's disease ready for the clinic in 2016? *J. Parkinsons Dis.* 6: 57–63.

87 Vierbuchen, T., Ostermeier, A., Pang, Z.P. et al. (2010). Direct conversion of fibroblasts to functional neurons by defined factors. *Nature* 463: 1035–1041.

88 Jiang, H., Xu, Z., Zhong, P. et al. (2015). Cell cycle and p53 gate the direct conversion of human fibroblasts to dopaminergic neurons. *Nat. Commun.* 6: 10100.

89 Warby, S.C., Graham, R.K., and Hayden, M.R. (1993). Huntington disease. In: *GeneReviews(R)* (ed. R.A. Pagon, M.P. Adam, H.H. Ardinger, et al.). Seattle (WA): University of Washington.

90 van Duijn, E., Kingma, E.M., and van der Mast, R.C. (2007). Psychopathology in verified Huntington's disease gene carriers. *J. Neuropsychiatry Clin. Neurosci.* 19: 441–448.

91 Walker, F.O. (2007). Huntington's disease. *Lancet* 369: 218–228.

92 Langbehn, D.R., Brinkman, R.R., Falush, D. et al., and International Huntington's Disease Collaborative G (2004). A new model for prediction of the age of onset and penetrance for Huntington's disease based on CAG length. *Clin. Genet.* 65: 267–277.

93 Pringsheim, T., Wiltshire, K., Day, L. et al. (2012). The incidence and prevalence of Huntington's disease: a systematic review and meta-analysis. *Mov. Disord.* 27: 1083–1091.

94 Rawlins, M.D., Wexler, N.S., Wexler, A.R. et al. (2016). The prevalence of Huntington's disease. *Neuroepidemiology* 46: 144–153.

95 Halliday, G.M., McRitchie, D.A., Macdonald, V. et al. (1998). Regional specificity of brain atrophy in Huntington's disease. *Exp. Neurol.* 154: 663–672.

96 Vonsattel, J.P., Myers, R.H., Stevens, T.J. et al. (1985). Neuropathological classification of Huntington's disease. *J. Neuropathol. Exp. Neurol.* 44: 559–577.

97 Raymond, L.A., Andre, V.M., Cepeda, C. et al. (2011). Pathophysiology of Huntington's disease: time-dependent alterations in synaptic and receptor function. *Neuroscience* 198: 252–273.

98 Mort, M., Carlisle, F.A., Waite, A.J. et al. (2015). Huntingtin exists as multiple splice forms in human brain. *J. Huntingtons Dis.* 4: 161–171.

99 Ruzo, A., Ismailoglu, I., Popowski, M. et al. (2015). Discovery of novel isoforms of huntingtin reveals a new hominid-specific exon. *PLoS One* 10: e0127687.

100 Zuccato, C., Valenza, M., and Cattaneo, E. (2010). Molecular mechanisms and potential therapeutic targets in Huntington's disease. *Physiol. Rev.* 90: 905–981.

101 Rubinsztein, D.C. and Carmichael, J. (2003). Huntington's disease: molecular basis of neurodegeneration. *Expert Rev. Mol. Med.* 5: 1–21.

102 Nopoulos, P.C. (2016). Huntington disease: a single-gene degenerative disorder of the striatum. *Dialogues Clin. Neurosci.* 18: 91–98.

103 Reiner, A., Dragatsis, I., and Dietrich, P. (2011). Genetics and neuropathology of Huntington's disease. *Int. Rev. Neurobiol.* 98: 325–372.

104 Chen, J.J., Salat, D.H., and Rosas, H.D. (2012). Complex relationships between cerebral blood flow and brain atrophy in early Huntington's disease. *Neuroimage* 59: 1043–1051.

105 Mestre, T., Ferreira, J., Coelho, M.M. et al. (2009). Therapeutic interventions for symptomatic treatment in Huntington's disease. *Cochrane Database Syst. Rev.* CD006456. https://doi.org/10.1002/14651858.CD006456.pub2.

106 Coppen, E.M. and Roos, R.A. (2017). Current pharmacological approaches to reduce chorea in Huntington's disease. *Drugs* 77: 29–46.

107 Frank, S. (2014). Treatment of Huntington's disease. *Neurotherapeutics* 11: 153–160.

108 Pfister, E.L. and Zamore, P.D. (2009). Huntington's disease: silencing a brutal killer. *Exp. Neurol.* 220: 226–229.

109 Aronin, N. and DiFiglia, M. (2014). Huntingtin-lowering strategies in Huntington's disease: antisense oligonucleotides, small RNAs, and gene editing. *Mov. Disord.* 29: 1455–1461.

110 Kay, C., Skotte, N.H., Southwell, A.L., and Hayden, M.R. (2014). Personalized gene silencing therapeutics for Huntington disease. *Clin. Genet.* 86: 29–36.

111 Barker, R.A., Mason, S.L., Harrower, T.P. et al., and collaboration N-U (2013)). The long-term safety and efficacy of bilateral transplantation of human fetal striatal tissue in patients with mild to moderate Huntington's disease. *J. Neurol. Neurosurg. Psychiatry* 84: 657–665.

112 Videnovic, A. (2013). Treatment of Huntington disease. *Curr. Treat. Options Neurol.* 15: 424–438.

113 Statland, J.M., Barohn, R.J., McVey, A.L. et al. (2015). Patterns of weakness, classification of motor neuron disease, and clinical diagnosis of sporadic amyotrophic lateral sclerosis. *Neurol. Clin.* 33: 735–748.

114 Patten, S.A., Armstrong, G.A., Lissouba, A. et al. (2014). Fishing for causes and cures of motor neuron disorders. *Dis. Model Mech.* 7: 799–809.

115 Kinsley, L. and Siddique, T. (1993). Amyotrophic lateral sclerosis overview. In: *GeneReviews(R)* (ed. R.A. Pagon, M.P. Adam, H.H. Ardinger, et al.). Seattle (WA): University of Washington.

116 Prior, T.W. and Finanger, E. (1993). Spinal muscular atrophy. In: *GeneReviews(R)* (ed. R.A. Pagon, M.P. Adam, H.H. Ardinger, et al.). Seattle (WA).

117 McDermott, C., White, K., Bushby, K., and Shaw, P. (2000). Hereditary spastic paraparesis: a review of new developments. *J. Neurol. Neurosurg. Psychiatry* 69: 150–160.

118 Tartaglia, M.C., Rowe, A., Findlater, K. et al. (2007). Differentiation between primary lateral sclerosis and amyotrophic lateral sclerosis: examination of symptoms and signs at disease onset and during follow-up. *Arch. Neurol.* 64: 232–236.

119 Gordon, P.H., Cheng, B., Katz, I.B. et al. (2009). Clinical features that distinguish PLS, upper motor neuron-dominant ALS, and typical ALS. *Neurology* 72: 1948–1952.

120 Boylan, K. (2015). Familial amyotrophic lateral sclerosis. *Neurol. Clin.* 33: 807–830.

121 Andersen, P.M. (2006). Amyotrophic lateral sclerosis associated with mutations in the CuZn superoxide dismutase gene. *Curr. Neurol. Neurosci. Rep.* 6: 37–46.

122 Scotter, E.L., Chen, H.J., and Shaw, C.E. (2015). TDP-43 proteinopathy and ALS: insights into disease mechanisms and therapeutic targets. *Neurotherapeutics* 12: 352–363.

123 Gomez-Pinedo, U., Villar-Quiles, R.N., Galan, L. et al. (2016). Immununochemical markers of the amyloid cascade in the hippocampus in motor neuron diseases. *Front. Neurol.* 7: 195.

124 Rabinovich-Toidman, P., Rabinovich-Nikitin, I., Ezra, A. et al. (2015). Mutant SOD1 increases APP expression and phosphorylation in cellular and animal models of ALS. *PLoS One* 10: e0143420.

125 Tremblay, C., St-Amour, I., Schneider, J. et al. (2011). Accumulation of transactive response DNA binding protein 43 in mild cognitive impairment and Alzheimer disease. *J. Neuropathol. Exp. Neurol.* 70: 788–798.

126 Van Deerlin, V.M., Leverenz, J.B., Bekris, L.M. et al. (2008). TARDBP mutations in amyotrophic lateral sclerosis with TDP-43 neuropathology: a genetic and histopathological analysis. *Lancet Neurol.* 7: 409–416.

127 Bozzoni, V., Pansarasa, O., Diamanti, L. et al. (2016). Amyotrophic lateral sclerosis and environmental factors. *Funct. Neurol.* 31: 7–19.

128 Kiernan, M.C., Vucic, S., Cheah, B.C. et al. (2011). Amyotrophic lateral sclerosis. *Lancet* 377: 942–955.
129 Walling, A.D. (1999). Amyotrophic lateral sclerosis: Lou Gehrig's disease. *Am. Fam. Physician* 59: 1489–1496.
130 Roberts, A.L., Johnson, N.J., Chen, J.T. et al. (2016). Race/ethnicity, socioeconomic status, and ALS mortality in the United States. *Neurology* 87: 2300–2308.
131 Saberi, S., Stauffer, J.E., Schulte, D.J., and Ravits, J. (2015). Neuropathology of amyotrophic lateral sclerosis and its variants. *Neurol. Clin.* 33: 855–876.
132 Hogden, A., Foley, G., Henderson, R.D. et al. (2017). Amyotrophic lateral sclerosis: improving care with a multidisciplinary approach. *J. Multidiscip. Healthc.* 10: 205–215.
133 Catapano, F., Zaharieva, I., Scoto, M. et al. (2016). Altered levels of MicroRNA-9, -206, and -132 in spinal muscular atrophy and their response to antisense oligonucleotide therapy. *Mol. Ther. Nucleic. Acids* 5: e331.
134 Haidet-Phillips, A.M. and Maragakis, N.J. (2015). Neural and glial progenitor transplantation as a neuroprotective strategy for Amyotrophic Lateral Sclerosis (ALS). *Brain Res.* 1628: 343–350.
135 Faravelli, I., Riboldi, G., Nizzardo, M. et al. (2014). Stem cell transplantation for amyotrophic lateral sclerosis: therapeutic potential and perspectives on clinical translation. *Cell. Mol. Life Sci.* 71: 3257–3268.
136 Ni, Z. and Chen, R. (2015). Transcranial magnetic stimulation to understand pathophysiology and as potential treatment for neurodegenerative diseases. *Transl. Neurodegener.* 4: 22.
137 Liberski, P.P. (2012). Historical overview of prion diseases: a view from afar. *Folia Neuropathol.* 50: 1–12.
138 Gibbs, C.J. Jr., Gajdusek, D.C., Asher, D.M. et al. (1968). Creutzfeldt-Jakob disease (spongiform encephalopathy): transmission to the chimpanzee. *Science* 161: 388–389.
139 Prusiner, S.B. (1998). Prions. *Proc. Natl. Acad Sci. U.S.A.* 95: 13363–13383.
140 Kimberlin, R.H. and Wilesmith, J.W. (1994). Bovine spongiform encephalopathy: epidemiology, low dose exposure and risks. *Ann. N.Y. Acad. Sci.* 724: 210–220.
141 Chen, C. and Dong, X.P. (2016). Epidemiological characteristics of human prion diseases. *Infect. Dis. Poverty* 5: 47.
142 Rosenbloom, M.H. and Atri, A. (2011). The evaluation of rapidly progressive dementia. *Neurologist* 17: 67–74.
143 Shiga, Y., Miyazawa, K., Sato, S. et al. (2004). Diffusion-weighted MRI abnormalities as an early diagnostic marker for Creutzfeldt-Jakob disease. *Neurology* 63: 443–449.
144 Tian, H.J., Zhang, J.T., Lang, S.Y., and Wang, X.Q. (2010). MRI sequence findings in sporadic Creutzfeldt-Jakob disease. *J. Clin. Neurosci.* 17: 1378–1380.
145 Diack, A.B., Head, M.W., McCutcheon, S. et al. (2014). Variant CJD. 18 years of research and surveillance. *Prion* 8: 286–295.
146 Metzler-Baddeley, C. (2007). A review of cognitive impairments in dementia with Lewy bodies relative to Alzheimer's disease and Parkinson's disease with dementia. *Cortex* 43: 583–600.
147 Hampel, H., Blennow, K., Shaw, L.M. et al. (2010). Total and phosphorylated tau protein as biological markers of Alzheimer's disease. *Exp. Gerontol.* 45: 30–40.

148 Spiegel, J., Pirraglia, E., Osorio, R.S. et al. (2016). Greater specificity for cerebrospinal fluid P-tau231 over P-tau181 in the differentiation of healthy controls from Alzheimer's disease. *J. Alzheimers Dis.* 49: 93–100.

149 Schade, S. and Mollenhauer, B. (2014). Biomarkers in biological fluids for dementia with Lewy bodies. *Alzheimers Res. Ther.* 6: 72.

150 Shi, M., Bradner, J., Hancock, A.M. et al. (2011). Cerebrospinal fluid biomarkers for Parkinson disease diagnosis and progression. *Ann. Neurol.* 69: 570–580.

151 Pedrini, S., Gupta, V.B., Hone, E. et al., and Group AR (2017). A blood-based biomarker panel indicates IL-10 and IL-12/23p40 are jointly associated as predictors of beta-amyloid load in an AD cohort. *Sci. Rep.* 7: 14057.

152 Doecke, J.D., Laws, S.M., Faux, N.G. et al., and Alzheimer's Disease Neuroimaging I, Australian Imaging B, Lifestyle Research G (2012). Blood-based protein biomarkers for diagnosis of Alzheimer disease. *Arch. Neurol.* 69: 1318–1325.

153 O'Bryant, S.E., Xiao, G., Barber, R. et al., Texas Alzheimer's R, Care C, and Alzheimer's Disease Neuroimaging I (2011). A blood-based screening tool for Alzheimer's disease that spans serum and plasma: findings from TARC and ADNI. *PLoS One* 6: e28092.

154 Johnstone, D., Milward, E.A., Berretta, R., and Moscato, P., and Alzheimer's Disease Neuroimaging I(2012). Multivariate protein signatures of pre-clinical Alzheimer's disease in the Alzheimer's disease neuroimaging initiative (ADNI) plasma proteome dataset. *PLoS One* 7: e34341.

155 Boot, B.P. (2015). Comprehensive treatment of dementia with Lewy bodies. *Alzheimers Res. Ther.* 7: 45.

3

Current and Developing Methods for Diagnosing Alzheimer's Disease

Stephanie J. Fuller[1], Nicholas Carrigan[1,2,3], Hamid R. Sohrabi[1,3,4,5,6,7] and Ralph N. Martins[1,3,4,5,6]

[1] *Centre of Excellence for Alzheimer's Disease Research and Care, School of Medical and Health Sciences, Edith Cowan University, Joondalup, WA, Australia*
[2] *Older Adult Mental Health Service, Western Australia Country Health Service (South West), Bunbury, WA, Australia*
[3] *Australian Alzheimer's Research Foundation, Ralph and Patricia Sarich Neuroscience Research Institute, Nedlands, WA, Australia*
[4] *Department of Biomedical Sciences, Macquarie University, Sydney, NSW, Australia*
[5] *School of Psychiatry and Clinical Neurosciences, University of Western Australia, Perth, WA, Australia*
[6] *KaRa Institute of Neurological Diseases, Sydney, NSW, Australia*
[7] *Cooperative Research Centre for Mental Health, Carlton, VIC, Australia*

3.1 Introduction

It is of the utmost importance to develop techniques to diagnose Alzheimer's disease (AD) as early as possible in the pre-clinical stages. This fact has been revealed in recent years by specialised brain imaging techniques which have confirmed a long-held theory that considerable and irreversible synaptic and neuronal cell loss has been developing for many years in the brain prior to detectable clinical signs and symptoms. It is therefore crucial that better pre-clinical diagnostic methods are developed to aid in monitoring, testing, as well as eventually applying disease-modifying treatments, to slow or prevent the onset of dementia. A delay of even a couple of years can make a huge difference to the person affected, their family and the community at large, both from the personal and financial points of view.

3.2 Classical Post-Mortem Diagnosis

Confirming an AD diagnosis has traditionally required the post-mortem examination of the brain, to demonstrate the presence of extracellular amyloid plaques and fibrils, and intracellular neurofibrillary tangles (NFT). Other brain pathological changes that can be observed include microglial infiltration, widespread loss of synapses and neurons, and brain shrinkage.

3.2.1 Plaques

Amyloid plaques consist mostly of aggregated A-beta (Aβ) 4 kDa peptides, and are considered the hallmark pathology seen in an AD brain. Also known as senile or neuritic plaques, these usually contain other proteins, especially proteins related to inflammatory processes, and the central plaque core is usually found surrounded by a corona of abnormal neurites, microglial cells, and sometimes reactive astrocytes [1]. Aβ peptides (ranging from 39 to 43 amino acids) are normal breakdown products of a widely expressed transmembrane protein, the amyloid-β protein precursor protein (AβPP or sometimes abbreviated to APP). In AD however, the peptide is most likely produced in excess, and the longer forms are produced to a greater extent – this is of importance, as the longer forms (Aβ1-42 in particular) aggregate much more readily into oligomers, and then amyloid fibrils. Plaque deposition usually starts in the isocortex – the frontal, temporal and occipital lobes of the grey matter of the cortex, then can be detected in the entorhinal cortex, hippocampal formation, amygdala, insular, and cingulated cortices, although the topographical distribution is not as predictable as that of NFT (see below) [2]. Post-mortem examination of brains of elderly people who had been cognitively normal can often reveal plaques (and other AD-related brain neuropathology), and it is most likely that these plaques represent pre-clinical stages of the disease.

3.2.2 Neurofibrillary Tangles (NFT)

The other major pathological hallmark of AD is the presence of NFT in specific regions of the brain, though NFT are not AD-specific as they can be found in other neuropathological conditions as well. NFT are abnormal fibrils that are wound together in a helical fashion, consisting mostly of aggregates (paired helical filaments) of the microtubule-associated protein tau. In AD, this tau is abnormally hyper-phosphorylated, with phosphate groups attached at specific sites on the protein. As with plaques, other proteins are often associated with NFT, but are not believed to be of primary importance to the structure. NFT are found intra-neuronally, and have the microscopic appearance of swirls or strands of fibres when stained. The development of NFT in the AD brain follows a much more specific pattern than plaques, and the severity of AD cognitive symptoms also mirrors more closely the extent of NFT deposition [2, 3]. The pattern of NFT deposition has been described by Braak and Braak as having six stages, as follows: the first NFT appear in the trans-entorhinal region (stage I) along with the entorhinal cortex itself, followed by the hippocampal CA1 region (stage II). NFT then accumulate in limbic structures such as the subiculum of the hippocampal formation (stage III) and the amygdala, thalamus, and claustrum (stage IV). Eventually, NFT spread to all isocortical areas, with the associative areas being affected earlier (stage V) than the primary sensory, motor, and visual areas (stage VI) [4]. These different stages are well defined, and often used for the pathological diagnosis and staging of AD.

3.2.3 Cerebral Amyloid Angiopathy (CAA)

Most AD patients will show some degree of amyloid deposition in the walls of blood vessels; this is known as cerebral amyloid angiopathy (CAA). This amyloid deposition occurs in cortical capillaries, small arterioles, and larger arteries as well as leptomeningeal arteries. Veins are rarely involved. As with brain amyloid plaques, this amyloid consists mostly of aggregated Aβ peptides, although there are a lot more of the shorter (Aβ1-40) forms present. If severe, there is the risk of leakage from blood vessel walls, causing life-threatening lobar haemorrhages.

3.2.4 Glial Responses

Dense (older) amyloid plaques often have activated microglial cells and reactive astrocytes associated with them, suggesting Aβ is a major trigger of the glial response. However, there is also a strong association between the level of astrocytosis and microgliosis and the amount of NFT in the brain, indicating the glial response is also linked to neurofibrillary degeneration and associated neuropathology [5].

3.2.5 Brain Shrinkage

Brain atrophy is typically found in AD, with a pattern of symmetrical cortical atrophy, mainly in the medial temporal lobes. In contrast, the sensory, visual, and primary motor areas are spared. As a result of the brain atrophy, the lateral ventricles can appear quite dilated (hydrocephalus *ex vacuo*), and this can be visualised quite early in the course of the disease using magnetic resonance imaging (MRI). Such imaging techniques are often used in diagnosis to rule out other conditions such as stroke, and can also indicate whether severe CAA is present. Brain shrinkage is discussed again later in the section on imaging tests in clinical diagnosis.

3.2.6 Loss of Synapses and Neurons

The loss of neurons and synapses is one of the main reasons for cortical atrophy of the AD brain. Synaptic loss occurs early in the disease, which is understandable, as a loss of synaptic communication would lead to cognitive decline. In fact, many studies have determined synaptic density to be the best correlate of cognitive decline in AD [2, 6, 7]. Synaptic loss also precedes neuronal loss, and as there are many synapses per neuron, synaptic loss is a more sensitive indicator of developing neuropathology.

Post-mortem studies of AD brains have shown that neuron loss occurs in a regional and laminar pattern that matches that of NFT development; studies have also shown that the neuronal loss in any particular region exceeds the number of NFT present. Thus, although not as good a correlate as synaptic density, neuronal loss does correlate better with cognitive decline than the number of NFT. It has been shown that there is a reduction in neuron numbers in the hippocampus and cerebral cortex of symptomatic AD subjects, whereas in asymptomatic subjects with the histopathology (plaques and NFT) of AD, yet who display no cognitive decline, a significant reduction in neurons is not detected in these AD-sensitive brain regions [8]. This supports the concept that amyloid plaques and NFT can be present in a cognitively healthy person, and do not cause cognitive decline on their own: significant neuronal (and synaptic) loss must occur for symptoms to appear.

3.3 Clinical Diagnosis

The first step in the diagnosis of dementia in a patient usually involves a visit to a general practitioner, either by the affected person due to the development of memory problems, or by a family member or close friend who is concerned about memory or behavioural changes in their relative or friend. Sometimes a general practitioner will notice signs of dementia whilst treating a patient's other conditions. Other common conditions which can present with a similar cognitive picture include delirium, depression, and pain syndromes; and these conditions need to be excluded before a diagnosis of dementia can be made. Dementia is a syndrome which is associated with many diseases, and involves impairment in several brain functions including memory, perception, personality, and cognitive skills. In the case of AD, early symptoms include memory problems, particularly short-term memory; changes in behaviour and mood; loss of ability to perform routine daily living tasks; confusion, for example about time of day or familiar places; problems with language (aphasia), as well as object misplacement and the storage of objects in inappropriate places (https://fightdementia.org.au/about-dementia-and-memory-loss/how-can-i-find-out-more/warning-signs-of-dementia). A collateral history from family or carers is an important part of the clinical diagnostic process. This can also identify risks associated with the impaired individual wandering, using natural gas appliances, or driving motor vehicles or farm machinery for instance. Sometimes, the presence of risky behaviour can facilitate the diagnosis and prompt strategies to ensure safety.

Later symptoms include more severe memory problems, an inability to perform core living activities such as eating and dressing, and greater communication problems. Behavioural and Psychological Symptoms of Dementia (BPSD) refer to the non-cognitive presentations of dementia, which include depression, agitation, sundowning, delusions, aggression, and apathy. These symptoms present more commonly in the later stages of the disease, but can occur at any stage.

A general practitioner's initial tests are usually to rule out other possible causes of dementia symptoms [9]. Such other causes include:

- acute infection
- metabolic disorders
- electrolyte imbalances
- anaemia
- thyroid/thyroid stimulating hormone imbalance
- vitamin deficiency (e.g. vitamin B12 deficiency)
- drug side-effects, drug interaction, and dosing problems.

Most of the above-mentioned causes can be ruled out quickly by urine and blood tests. Furthermore, brief cognitive tests may also be performed, for example the Mini-Mental State Examination (MMSE) [10] to screen for the presence and level of cognitive impairment, however once other likely causes are ruled out, a general practitioner usually refers a patient to a geriatrician, neurologist, and/or psychiatrist, for further testing. These specialists will conduct lengthy clinical examination and may ask for a more comprehensive combination of neuropsychological assessments, focusing on specific domains of cognition. Functional and behavioural assessments may also be carried out, although these are usually of greater use in more severe stages of dementia. Behavioural assessment investigates the non-cognitive aspects of dementia, which include personality, mood, psychotic symptoms, and unusual behaviours, as well as sleep, eating, and sexual disorders. Assessment of non-cognitive characteristics improves the clinical diagnostic accuracy, and aids in assessing care requirements and distinguishing different causes of dementia.

Other tests that can be requested or carried out by specialists include one or more brain scans, the most commonly used of these are detailed below. However, such scans are expensive, time-consuming, and some are only available in major cities, as part of certain research programs.

3.3.1 Initial Assessment/Screening Tools

3.3.1.1 Mini-Mental State Examination (MMSE)

The MMSE is the most commonly administered cognitive test for dementia screening [11] in English-speaking countries. The test is scored out of a possible maximum of 30, and includes questions concerning time and place orientation (10 points), word registration (3 points), attention (5 points), delayed word recall (3 points), various verbal tasks (8 points), and visuo-construction (1 point) [10, 12]. A score greater than or equal to 25 points indicates normal cognition. Below this, scores can indicate severe (≤ 9 points), moderate (10–18 points), or mild (19–24 points) cognitive impairment [13].

The test only takes about 10 minutes to administer, useful for busy general practitioners. However, this test has certain disadvantages, as it is affected by level of education, age, practice effect, and ceiling effect (i.e. high scores above the cut-off score for dementia can be achieved by impaired individuals increasing the false negative rates). Despite these limitations, the MMSE has been shown to help differentiate between different types of dementia. For example, AD patients score significantly lower on orientation to time and place, and recall, compared to patients with dementia with Lewy bodies (DLB) [14, 15], vascular dementia, or dementia due to Parkinson's disease (PD) [16].

3.3.1.2 Montreal Cognitive Assessment (MoCA)

The Montreal Cognitive Assessment (MoCA) has been a more recently developed measure for screening of mild cognitive impairment (MCI) and cognitive impairment [17]. The MoCA has some advantages as compared to the MMSE, including having more comprehensive assessment of cognition, a lower ceiling effect, the ability to detect MCI, and so on. It assesses different cognitive domains including executive functioning, visuo-constructional skills, memory, attention, language, verbal fluency, abstract thinking, and orientation and takes only 10 minutes to administer. It gives a total score of 30 and has a cut-off score of 26 or above for normal cognitive functioning [17]. As the MoCA is not copyrighted, it has been recently more commonly used in various large observational and clinical trials and, over time, more data will clarify its utility and accuracy. However, it has been argued that the cut-off score of 26 is too high and may increase the potential for false positive diagnosis [18]. Clinicians should consider education, age, social, and ethno-racial groups as they interpret the performance of patients on this measure.

3.3.1.3 Clinical Dementia Rating (CDR)

The Clinical Dementia Rating (CDR) is one of the most commonly used semi-structured global rating measures for diagnosis and for determining the severity of dementia [19]. The CDR incorporates information obtained from both an informant and the patient to determine the presence and stage of dementia syndrome. It allows assessment of a patient's cognitive functioning on six different domains including memory, orientation, judgement and problem solving, community affairs, home and hobbies, and personal care [20]. The CDR provides a Global Score range of 0–3, where a score of

0, 0.5, 1, 2, and 3 indicates no dementia, questionable, mild, moderate, and severe dementia, respectively [20]. More recently a Clinical Dementia Rating Sum of Boxes Score (CDR-SOB) has been developed that provides a wider range of scores, as well as allowing to determine the changes within each of the CDR Global Scores [21]. The Standardised Outcome Measure (SOM) Score range for each of the Global scores include the following: Global Score 0.5 = 0.5–4.0; Global Score 1 = 4.5–9.0; Global score 2 = 9.5–15.5; and Global score 3 = 16.0–18.0 [21].

3.3.1.4 Clock Drawing

The clock drawing test can be administered using a blank piece of paper, but sometimes the patient is given a page with a large circle already present. Patients are instructed to draw a clock face (if not already there) and all the numbers, and to place hands on the face to show a specific time, usually 10 minutes past 11 (or sometimes 20 past 8). This is a short test, originally devised to investigate constructional apraxia, but is now often used in conjunction with the MMSE in dementia screening tests, or as part of the seven-minute screen and Mini-Cog test and MoCA.

Limitations of this test include the fact that scoring is to some degree subjective, and although scoring standardisation has been put forward [22], several different scoring protocols have been devised [23]. For example, the Watson method is based on dividing the clock into quadrants and the score is determined by the number of digits in each quadrant, however the positioning of the hands on the clock is ignored [24], whereas the Sunderland method takes into account number and hand positions [25].

3.3.1.5 Seven-Minute Screen

This is a short cognitive assessment test used in general practice as a screening assessment tool. It includes the Clock Drawing test, Verbal fluency test, Temporal Orientation test, and Enhanced Cued Recall test. This test requires a minimum of training to administer, hence it is a quick screening tool often used in primary care to determine the presence of dementia [26]. However, it should be noted that the greater the dementia, the longer the test takes to administer.

3.3.1.6 Alzheimer's Disease Assessment Scale (ADAS-Cog)

The Alzheimer's Disease Assessment Scale (ADAS) was originally designed to measure the severity of the most important symptoms of AD, whereas the ADAS-Cog is a combination of tests often used to measure primary outcome in clinical trials of anti-dementia drugs. The ADAS-Cog consists of 11 tasks which measure disturbances in memory, language, attention, praxis and other cognitive abilities considered to be core symptoms of AD. The scoring is not difficult, although the test requires greater training to administer and score than the MMSE for example. The test is more thorough than the MMSE, and AD severity (staging) is possible to a degree, though this test is not a substitute for extensive neuropsychological testing [27].

One disadvantage is that the test takes approximately 30 minutes to administer and is prone to practice effect, and thus is not practical as a screening tool for general practitioner use in a standard consultation.

3.3.1.7 Psychogeriatric Assessment Scales (PAS)

The Psychogeriatric Assessment Scales (PAS) provide assessments of the clinical changes seen in dementia and depression. Six independent scales are obtained:

three scales are derived from an interview with the subject (Cognitive Impairment, Depression, Stroke) and three from an interview with an informant (Cognitive Decline, Behaviour Change, Stroke). The interviews are relatively easy to score, and they can be carried out with minimal training [28]. Longitudinal studies have found the cognitive decline scale to be particularly useful, as it allows a valid retrospective assessment of change, and has predictive validity for subsequent cognitive deterioration [29].

The limitations of this testing format include the fact that the patients need to be fluent in English, the informant needs to be as objective as possible, and the level of cognitive decline measured in the cognitive impairment scale may be influenced by pre-morbid intelligence and level of education.

3.3.1.8 Dementia Rating Scale (DRS)
This cognitive assessment scale is intended for patients who are not able to complete standard neurological tests, as they already have quite severe symptoms of dementia. Such patients are often institutionalised due to the stage of their dementia. The testing therefore provides increased discrimination and sensitivity to differentiate individuals with substantial cognitive deficits [30]. Testing using the dementia rating scale (DRS) needs to be done by a clinician, and covers attention, preservation, construction, conceptualisation, as well as verbal and non-verbal memory.

A second edition of the Mattis Dementia Rating Scale 2 (MDRS-2) [31], as well as an alternate MDRS-2 test (MDRS-2 AF) [32] for serial assessments have been developed, and one study evaluating the MDRS-2 found that the test is quite reliable in differentiating less severe dementia subgroups from healthy elderly controls. The test could detect MCI in subjects, though couldn't differentiate amnestic MCI from MCI due to PD [31].

3.3.1.9 Mini-Cog
This brief test consists of three parts, and can be administered in less than five minutes by any individual. It includes the clock drawing test, and the learning and recall of three unrelated words, to determine verbal recall. This test takes less time to administer than the MMSE and is about as accurate in diagnosing dementia, if the MMSE cut-off score is 25 [33]. It is also less susceptible to language problems and educational level than the MMSE. However, the Mini-Cog is not useful if the subject is visually impaired, or has motor impairments that make writing or drawing difficult.

3.3.1.10 Rowland Universal Dementia Assessment Scale (RUDAS)
This assessment scale was developed in Australia to overcome the cultural, educational level and language problems sometimes encountered in other tests such as the MMSE. It is valid across cultures, and is easily administered by primary health care clinicians [34]. The test consists of 6 items, takes less than 10 minutes to administer, and a recent systematic review of the test found that it performs as well as the MMSE. It is more widely applicable as it can be used to test people from culturally and linguistically diverse populations [35].

3.3.1.11 The Consortium to Establish a Registry for Alzheimer's Disease (CERAD) Neuropsychological Battery (nb) and Other Tests
The Consortium to establish a registry for Alzheimer's disease (CERAD) was funded in 1986 by the National Institute on Aging [36] to develop standardised assessments

for patients with AD. The consortium developed comprehensive and reliable batteries of neuropsychological and clinical tests at various clinical sites, with a cohort of approximately 1500 subjects in total, evaluated for up to seven years. Post-mortem neuropathology was also investigated when possible, to obtain neuropathologic confirmation of clinical diagnoses. The assessment combinations covered the areas of clinical, neuropsychological and behavioural assessments for dementia, family history interviews, and assessments of care needs. Thus these assessments were quite comprehensive, included several other individual tests mentioned here (such as the MMSE), and were originally used to differentiate AD from healthy controls, as they were found to discriminate between healthy controls, mild and moderate dementia [37]. The information now collected as part of the CERAD-nb includes measures of verbal fluency, confrontational naming (15-item Boston Naming Test), the MMSE, a patient's clinical history, a physical examination, laboratory and neuroimaging tests, and informant reports. Investigations into possible systemic disorders are also included, as are investigations into depression, parkinsonism, and cerebrovascular disease. Other tests include the Blessed DRS, the CDR scale, Short Blessed Test, calculation, clock and language tests, constructional praxis performance and recall tests. Ultimately the tests can give a good indication of a differential diagnosis of either AD alone, AD associated with other disorders, or non-AD dementia (see Table 3.1).

One benefit of these tests is that they can be carried out in languages other than English, such as Chinese, Japanese, Italian, Spanish and German. This battery of tests has been found to be useful in distinguishing early AD from normal elderly controls, particularly the verbal memory subtests [38]. More importantly, a more recent study has found that CERAD total scores are a practical way of screening for prodromal AD and

Table 3.1 List of tests used in CERAD clinical and neuropsychological assessment.

Assessment type	Test or source
Demographic data	Obtained from subject and/or informant
Clinical history	Obtaining details of cognitive impairment, history of medication use, family history, determining presence/absence of depression, PD, cerebrovascular disease and other systemic illnesses
Clinical examinations	Physical examination and neurological examination
Laboratory and imaging studies	Blood tests to investigate deficiencies such as vitamin B12 or iron deficiency, and other laboratory studies, as well as neuroimaging studies such as MRI
Neuropsychological tests	Mini-Mental State Examination
	Boston Naming Test
	Verbal fluency
	Word list memory
	Word list recall
	Word list recognition
	Recall of Constructional Praxis
Clinical diagnosis	Clinical Dementia Rating scale for staging level of dementia
	Evaluations to determine presence/absence or coexistence of other illnesses that are also likely to cause cognitive impairment or dementia

assessing cognitive progression in MCI. Furthermore, the CERAD compound scores have been found to be more accurate than the MMSE in discriminating progressing MCI subjects from controls [39], but this may not be surprising considering the range and number of tests included in the CERAD tests.

The main disadvantage of the CERAD tests is that they are time-consuming, and although they can be used for research purposes as well as for patient care, they are too time-consuming for screening purposes. However, for the purpose of monitoring disease progression, a shorter combination of the CERAD subtests has been put together (that includes the MMSE, clock drawing test, verbal fluency, and constructional praxis) and has been shown to provide a promising and time-efficient method for measuring cognitive deterioration during AD follow-up [40].

3.4 Brain Imaging in the Diagnosis of Alzheimer's Disease and Other Dementias

Neuroimaging is widely believed to be highly useful for excluding other (sometimes reversible) causes of dementia, such as normal-pressure hydrocephalus, brain tumours, and subdural haematoma, and for excluding other likely causes such as strokes and ischaemia due to cerebrovascular disease. In fact, imaging has been used in AD studies for over four decades, starting with computed tomography (CT), then MRI to rule out some other causes of dementia. With the development of structural and functional magnetic resonance imaging (fMRI), and more recently positron emission tomography (PET) which have made use of tracers of various kinds, imaging can now help to a greater extent in the diagnosis, as well as the differential diagnosis of AD.

The greatest advances in imaging involve the new PET techniques and specific tracers which are making the diagnosis of AD possible at pre-clinical stages, making it feasible to monitor disease development, and to test potential disease-modifying therapies that may slow or even stop the progress of the disease. The aim is obviously to prevent the manifestation of symptoms if possible, or at least to delay the onset of symptoms for as long as possible. It is probably safe to assume that the earlier disease detection is possible, the better the chances of preserving cognitive function.

3.4.1 Imaging Tests in AD Diagnosis: Established Tests

3.4.1.1 Computed Tomography (CT)
CT scans to aid in the diagnosis of AD were developed before structural MRI techniques were adopted, and are still used regularly to help rule out tumours, to detect damage from small or large strokes or head trauma, to detect fluid build-up in the brain, and to investigate brain atrophy. Although CT scans can show loss of brain tissue, for example in the temporal lobe, CT scans are proving to be not as good as scans from new MRI techniques, when used for the detection of AD at earlier stages.

3.4.1.2 Electroencephalography (EEG)
An electroencephalograph (EEG) is a non-invasive procedure that can be used repeatedly at any age, with virtually no risks or limitations, and is helpful in the diagnosis of brain disorders. It is often helpful in identifying some disorders that can mimic AD in specific clinical contexts.

3.4.1.3 Magnetic Resonance Imaging (MRI), for the Assessment of Morphological Changes, and the Detection of Stroke

This form of imaging is very helpful for imaging soft tissues like the brain. An MRI is beneficial in ruling out other causes of dementia, such as tumours or strokes. It also helps to show physical changes in the brain that are associated with AD.

3.4.1.4 Positron Emission Tomography (PET)

PET scanning is a three-dimensional imaging technique, which utilises the injection of a radioactive tracer, to enable the examination of specific aspects of the brain or other internal organs. PET imaging can reveal, for example, a region of the brain causing a patient to have seizures, is useful in evaluating degenerative brain diseases such as AD, Huntington's, PD, frontotemporal lobe dementia (FTLD), and DLB, and can also differentiate between them to some extent.

3.4.1.5 FDG-PET

Using particular tracers, PET scans can show the difference in brain activity between a normal brain and one affected by AD. For example, 18F-2-fluoro-2-deoxy-D-glucose (FDG)-PET is a powerful method for detection of disease-related impairment of cerebral glucose metabolism in neurodegenerative diseases, and it has gained popularity in the early and differential diagnosis of AD. AD causes hypometabolism of mainly the temporoparietal areas including the angular gyrus, precuneus, and the posterior cingulate cortex, especially its retrosplenial part [41]. The hypometabolism in the posterior cingulate cortex is an early and sensitive marker of AD, mild reductions have been observed even in asymptomatic subjects who have a higher genetic risk of developing AD (carriers of the apolipoprotein E, APOE ε4 gene), and these reductions in glucose metabolism appear to precede reductions in hippocampal volume or metabolism [42]. Metabolic activity in the temporal cortex is often lower in AD, and as the disease worsens, frontal metabolism also declines. Changes are usually bilateral, although some asymmetry may be observed [41]. Other neurodegenerative diseases also show regional reductions in brain glucose metabolism, including FTLD (which has several subtypes) and DLB. Furthermore, depression and other psychiatric diseases can also cause metabolic changes in the brain. However, unlike AD, some of these other conditions result in more asymmetrical changes in brain glucose metabolism, or alternatively, the brain regions most affected are different to those affected in AD [41]. Therefore together with cognitive symptoms and other medical history, FDG-PET analysis can help considerably towards a differential diagnosis.

3.4.2 Imaging Tests in AD Diagnosis: More Recently Developed Tests

No cure or effective treatment exists for AD once symptoms have developed, despite decades of extensive research. As a result, the focus has shifted towards prevention, or slowing down of the disease process, to delay onset of symptoms for as long as possible. It is known that the disease develops over at least two decades, therefore detecting brain pathological changes as early as possible is of the utmost importance, for the dual purposes of understanding early pathology, and developing effective early treatments. Many recent studies have made advances towards this aim, as can be seen below.

3.4.2.1 MRI for Measuring Regional Blood Flow

In brain tissue, regional blood flow is tightly coupled to regional glucose consumption, and MRI technologies that have been recently developed to measure brain regional blood flow are proving to be just as sensitive to brain metabolic changes as FDG-PET, and sometimes less invasive and less expensive. The most common methods for measuring cerebral blood flow are based on dynamic susceptibility contrast (DSC) imaging, blood oxygen level dependent fMRI (BOLD), and arterial spin labelling (ASL) fMRI. Unlike CT or PET tracers, MRI contrast agents and their concentration in tissue/blood cannot be measured in absolute concentrations, but rather in relation to their interaction with neighbouring hydrogen protons [43]. DSC involves the use of an intravascular contrast agent such as gadolinium chelate, making it similar to PET. BOLD fMRI uses an endogenous tracer, it indirectly measures brain regional cognitive activity in subjects carrying out specific tasks by exploiting local differences in the magnetic field due to changes in the relative concentrations of oxygenated and de-oxygenated haemoglobin following brain activation [44]. It has been found that the elderly display a greater magnitude and extent of activation of the BOLD signal when compared to younger adults, possibly reflecting a compensatory recruitment due to functional and structural deterioration of synaptic and neural health [45]. Although variance in BOLD signals, particularly with relation to ageing, is still being characterised [46], this fMRI technique has shown a lot of promise, and recent studies have shown that the fMRI BOLD signal is reliable across scanning sessions of an elderly population with amnestic Mild Cognitive Impairment (aMCI), and thus could be used for tracking longitudinal change in observational and interventional studies in aMCI [47]. Interestingly, increased activation has been associated with several risk factors for AD, including possession of the *APOE* ε4 allele [45], and type 2 diabetes [48]. Furthermore, BOLD fMRI has been used to determine cerebrovascular reactivity for anatomic regions underlying the default-mode network (implicated in AD and other brain disorders) in subjects at mid-life with a high risk of cardiovascular disease, or with diabetes and dyslipidemia, and revealed a non-significant reduction in cerebrovascular reactivity, suggesting reduced vascular function [49]. Such studies provide further evidence that such changes in the brain may function as a pre-clinical marker of neurodegeneration, a higher risk of stroke [50] and cognitive dysfunction later in life [49]. A recent AD-transgenic (Tg2576) mouse study showed that resting state fMRI using BOLD to investigate functional connectivity (FC) could be capable of revealing hyper-synchronised FC before deposition of Aβ and hypo-synchronised FC at later stages, providing further evidence this non-invasive imaging technique has pre-clinical diagnostic potential [51].

ASL uses endogenous arterial blood water – this water is labelled magnetically by applying a 180° radiofrequency inversion pulse in layers just beneath the brain slice about to be imaged [52]. As with BOLD, no injection of tracer or radioactivity is necessary for ASL, and for the purpose of AD diagnosis, the technique could be carried out just after initial structural MRI, for example if the structural MRI results reveal neurodegeneration indicative of AD. Many recent advances in ASL techniques have been made, and ASL perfusion and perfusion-based fMRI methods have been applied in many clinical studies, involving investigations of acute and chronic cerebrovascular disease [50], neurodegenerative disorders for example in comparisons of AD and Parkinson's disease [53], in differentiating presenile AD and frontotemporal dementia [54], for detecting pre-clinical AD [55], as well as for investigations of brain development, central nervous system (CNS) neoplasms and epilepsy [52]. One recent study demonstrated that, with the use of automated methods, age- and sex-adjusted ASL perfusion maps could be used to classify and predict diagnosis of AD, stable MCI as well as the conversion of MCI to AD, with good to excellent accuracy, supporting the concept that this method will be used more widely in the coming years [56]. However, one other recent ASL MRI study found that higher cerebral blood flow in cognitively normal *APOE* ε3 carriers was associated with better verbal memory functions, whereas *APOE* ε4 carriers showed the opposite, suggesting dysregulation or differences within the neurovascular unit, when compared to *APOE* ε3 carriers. This demonstrates that *APOE* genotype may need to be considered when evaluating results of ASL MRI, and supports the vascular theory of AD risk [57].

3.4.2.2 Single Photon Emission Computed Tomography (SPECT) Scan

Single photon emission computed tomography (SPECT) is a non-invasive technique for creating very clear, three-dimensional pictures of a major organ, such as the brain or heart. SPECT scans use radionuclide imaging – thus involving the injection of a very small amount of a radioactive tracer. A SPECT scan can map blood flow in certain regions of the brain, and is useful in evaluating specific brain functions. This might reveal abnormalities that are characteristic of AD. In one study, brain perfusion using 99mTc-HMPAO-SPECT and Brodmann areas mapping in mild AD showed that such scans may be useful as an ancillary tool, revealing perfusion impairments in early AD [58]. Dopamine transporter SPECT is a special type of SPECT used in Parkinson's disease and Lewy body dementia. Recent studies have found that SPECT followed by statistical analysis that involves three-dimensional stereotactic surface projection can help distinguish between depression and early stages of AD [59]. Furthermore, a recent French study suggests that hypoperfusion in the inferior parietal cortex, as measured by hexamethylpropyleneamine oxime-SPECT, is associated with a negative predictive value of 90%, thus discriminating well between AD and other cognitive disorders [60].

3.4.2.3 PiB-PET

PET using the amyloid-specific tracer ^{11}C Pittsburgh compound B (PiB) has facilitated the *in vivo* detection and quantitation of Aβ deposition in the brain [61]. This radioactive analogue of the Thioflavin T dye, binds specifically to fibrillar Aβ. A major contributor to this research has been the Australian Imaging Biomarker and Lifestyle (AIBL) study of ageing. AIBL recruited 1166 people aged over 60, and monitored them for over 10 years, taking blood samples every 18 months. A large number of the participants (n = 423) also underwent amyloid PET imaging using PiB-PET, as well as MRI brain imaging [62]. It has been shown that PiB-PET imaging allows the detection of amyloid deposition more than a decade prior to manifestation of symptoms, and can help determine people with MCI who are likely to progress to AD [63]. Early cross-sectional analysis of the baseline data revealed links between cognition, brain amyloid burden, structural brain changes, biomarkers, and lifestyle factors [64]. It was also evident early on that there was a strong relationship between Aβ deposition and brain atrophy very early in the disease process [65]. One meta-analysis of PiB-PET studies indicates that this technology provides 83–100% sensitivity and 41–100% specificity in identifying the conversion of MCI to AD, with pooled estimates for the long-term follow-up subgroup providing 95% sensitivity and

57% specificity [66]. Similarly, a recent Cochrane database systematic review of nine PiB-PET studies of MCI patients, which were aimed at detecting who would convert to AD, found 83–100% sensitivity and 46–88% specificity. However the studies showed a heterogeneity in methodology and interpretation that made it difficult to compare the studies. Due to high cost, the review also could not recommend this screening method for routine clinical practice [67]. Nevertheless, in clinical studies of pre-clinical AD, such diagnostic methods are of the utmost importance as they help us to determine and characterise earlier stages of the disease, and can help to monitor effects of potential preventative treatments.

A more recent study has shown that PET imaging in transgenic mice using a different amyloid plaque tracer, ^{11}C-AZD2184, and the astroglial tracer ^{11}C-deuterium-L-deprenyl (^{11}C-DED), detects astrocytosis before amyloid deposition occurs in these mice [68]. These results are promising as they suggest ^{11}C-DED may detect AD-related neuropathology which occurs prior to amyloid deposition; however, the AD-specificity of these changes needs to be determined. Recent AIBL studies have helped determine the extent and nature to which carriage of *APOE* ε4 alleles increases the risk for clinical disease progression from cognitively normal status. For example, being *APOE* ε4 +ve (compared to *APOE* ε4 −ve) increased the risk 2.66-fold over a 72-month period [69]. Furthermore, a recent cross-sectional study involving most of the AIBL cohort (including a subset, all of whom had undergone Aβ PiB-PET imaging as well as MRI hippocampal volume measurement) investigated the relationship between *APOE* ε4 allele status and Aβ levels, hippocampal volume, as well as memory [70]. It was found that *APOE* ε4 alleles influence Aβ levels, episodic memory and hippocampal volume in a dose-dependent manner. Such studies increase our understanding of AD, and add to the evidence that determining a person's *APOE* ε4 allele status is important when assessing a person's risk of AD.

3.4.3 The Rapidly Evolving Diagnostic Criteria

In 2011, the criteria and guidelines for diagnosing AD in the USA were changed. The National Institute on Aging/Alzheimer's Association Diagnostic Guidelines for Alzheimer's Disease expanded the definition of AD to include two earlier phases of the disease: (i) presymptomatic and (ii) mildly symptomatic pre-dementia, along with (iii) dementia caused by AD. This reflects the rapidly increasing amount of evidence (as mentioned in sections above) that AD brain pathology begins years, perhaps decades, before cognitive symptoms are noticeable [71]. Furthermore, since the mid-1990s, the literature on MCI has mushroomed, describing the gradual cognitive impairments that occur in patients preceding the threshold point where the level of impairments in cognitive function and daily living activities results in a dementia diagnosis [72].

More recently, as a result of the vast increase in information concerning pre-clinical biomarkers of AD, the National Institute on Aging–Alzheimer's Association (NIA-AA) Preclinical Workgroup developed AD staging criteria, for the purposes of dividing the pre-clinical phase of AD into three pathogenic stages: a significant help in clinical studies of pre-clinical AD [73]. The stages include:

- *Stage 0*. No biomarker abnormalities
- *Stage 1*. Significant amyloid deposition, as detected by PET amyloid tracer retention and low cerebrospinal fluid (CSF) Aβ1-42.

- *Stage 2.* Stage 1 observations, as well as neurodegeneration indicators, including cortical thinning/hippocampal atrophy as detected by structural MRI, high CSF tau/phospho-tau, and abnormal brain glucose metabolism, as measured by FDG-PET for example.
- *Stage 3.* Stage 2 observations as well as subtle cognitive changes that are greater impairments than would be expected for the age, though not as severe as MCI impairments.
- Using this classification method, there is also a 'SNAP' (suspected non-AD pathology) category, which includes those subjects with neurodegeneration indicators, yet no amyloid deposition.

The value of such pre-clinical classification is evident when one considers how important it is to know such stages when assessing potential treatments and/or preventative measures.

3.4.4 CSF Biomarkers of AD

The CSF is in direct contact with the brain, thus is a medium likely to reflect pathological biochemical changes developing in the brain. A lumbar puncture to obtain CSF can be carried out, to investigate biomarkers of AD and/or several other disorders of the CNS. CSF analysis is also useful when an inflammatory or infectious aetiology is suspected. Furthermore, lumbar punctures have been used to distinguish atypical presentations of AD from other neurodegenerative dementias [9].

3.4.4.1 Aβ, Tau, and AβPP-Related Biomarkers

As Aβ peptides and tau metabolism are known to be perturbed in AD, levels of various forms of these proteins/peptides have been investigated extensively. A pattern of protein changes, namely lower than normal Aβ1-42 levels, as well as increased levels of Thr181-phosphorylated tau and increased total tau levels, is considered to be most consistent with AD, and assays for these can be performed by specialised laboratories [74–77]. In certain clinical settings and for clinical trials, such tests have been performed, and with new ultrasensitive technologies, may significantly increase the diagnostic accuracy [78]. However, the aim is now to determine whether these CSF changes can be predictive. In support of this potential, increased levels of total tau and phosphorylated tau have been observed up to 10 years prior to the onset of clinical symptoms in familial AD cases [79, 80]. Lower CSF levels of Aβ1-42 have also been detected prior to symptom onset in familial AD [80, 81]. MCI patients have been investigated, and some studies do suggest CSF levels of Aβ1-42, total tau and Thr181-phosphorylated tau may be useful when trying to predict MCI progression to AD [82, 83]. However, other studies have indicated that these markers are not reliable enough on their own [84]. In one comparative study with a six-year follow-up, the ability of the MMSE, the clock drawing test, and CSF Thr181-phosphorylated tau and Aβ1-42 levels were evaluated to determine how well these tests could predict conversion from MCI to AD. The MMSE results and clock drawing test were found to classify 81% of cases correctly, whereas the CSF biomarkers were slightly better, at 83% correct. When combined, the three tests were more accurate than the individual tests in predicting MCI conversion to AD, underscoring the value of using more than one diagnostic method [12]. The changes in CSF total tau and Thr181-phosphorylated tau have been shown to correlate to some extent with NFT load at autopsy, and regional brain atrophy as determined by MRI, whereas CSF levels of Aβ1-42 have been shown to correlate inversely (to a degree) with brain amyloid load, as determined by PET [80].

CSF levels of secreted forms of the amyloid precursor, APP, have also been investigated. The α-secretase and β-secretase that initially cleave APP produce the soluble forms sAPPα and sAPPβ, respectively. Some studies of AD CSF have shown increased sAPPβ levels occur together with decreased Aβ42 and increased tau [85, 86]. Other have shown higher sAPPα and sAPPβ levels in MCI compared to AD [87], whereas some have shown no change in sAPPα levels in AD CSF [85, 86, 88]. Interestingly, one recent study has shown diurnal dynamics of APP metabolism: a diurnal pattern in Aβ levels has been recognised for a while, and it now appears the soluble APP forms follow the same pattern in healthy people, with the lowest levels occurring in the morning, and highest in the evening. This pattern diminishes with age, and is lost in people who have cerebral amyloid, as is the correlation between soluble APP levels and Aβ levels, supporting the concept that normal Aβ/APP metabolism and clearance mechanisms are disturbed in AD [88]. These recent findings also show the importance of standardising CSF collection methods and times, when considering utilising APP metabolites as biomarkers.

A 2014 Cochrane database systematic review of 14 studies of CSF Aβ levels, when used for diagnosis of AD and other forms of dementia in people with MCI, found that low CSF Aβ levels provided little benefit when used to try to diagnose prodromal AD. The review concluded that CSF Aβ levels alone did not provide an accurate test for AD [89]. In contrast, a 2014 meta-analysis of 50 studies determined that CSF Aβ levels could discriminate AD from other dementias, as it found that CSF Aβ1-42 levels were significantly lower in AD compared to frontotemporal dementia ($p < 0.001$), Parkinson's dementia ($p < 0.023$), and vascular dementia ($p < 0.001$), and could also differentiate from MCI ($p < 0.001$) [90]. This review included more recent studies and a greater number (50) of studies. A 2015 systematic review of 17 studies suggested lower CSF Aβ1-42 levels were potentially useful in differential diagnosis of AD versus non-AD dementias (and controls), yet not useful in the differential diagnosis of MCI [91]. A recent review of CSF studies has shown that the combined measurement of CSF Aβ1-42, total tau, and Thr181-phosphorylated tau levels can diagnose AD with a sensitivity and specificity reaching 92% and 89%, respectively [92, 93]. The 2017 Cochrane Database systematic review which evaluated 15 studies came to the conclusion that there is considerable variability between study methodology and cohorts and that the above CSF biomarkers may be more useful for ruling out AD, rather than for definite diagnosis [94]. Further reviews, standardisation of study methods, as well as more longitudinal studies will clarify the value of CSF Aβ and tau levels in AD diagnosis.

3.4.4.2 Other Potential CSF Protein Biomarkers

Many other CSF protein biomarkers have been investigated through extensive proteomic studies. Most of the potential biomarkers found can be linked to various aspects of AD neuropathology, such as inflammation, oxidative stress, synapse loss, and neuronal dysfunction. Early studies of candidate CSF biomarkers found clusterin, kininogen, transthyretin, β2-microglobulin, zinc-α2-glycoprotein, α(1)β-glycoprotein, retinol binding protein, and the apolipoproteins E, A1, and A4, as all of these proteins were found to be altered in AD compared to controls [95, 96]. More recently, studies have found changes in neprilysin which is involved in Aβ metabolism [97], changes to neurofilament proteins and visinin-like protein 1 (a neuronal calcium sensor protein) [98, 99], and increases in YKL-40, a potential biomarker of inflammation, in early stages of AD [100, 101]. Other protein inflammatory factors, such as interleukins-1 and -6, α1-antichymotrypsin, and tumour necrosis factor alpha (TNFα), have been found to be altered in AD, though the results have been inconsistent [102, 103]. A study of proteomic changes in CSF in pre-symptomatic familial early onset familial Alzheimer's disease (EOAD) mutation carriers has found some of the same CSF protein changes previously reported in late-onset (sporadic) Alzheimer's disease (LOAD), including changes to APP, transferrin, α(1)β-glycoprotein, complement components, afamin precursor, spondin 1, plasminogen, haemopexin, and neuronal pentraxin receptor levels [104]. Other proteins which were discovered for the first time in this study include calsyntenin 3, di-N-acetyl-chitobiase, AMPA (α-amino-3-hydroxy-5-methyl-4-isoxazolepropionic acid) 4 glutamate receptor, CD99 antigen, and secreted phosphoprotein 1. Further studies are needed to validate these results, and to determine if levels of these proteins also change in pre-clinical stages in LOAD subjects. A recent systematic review of CSF biomarkers of AD found that apart from the three core biomarkers (Aβ1-42, total tau, and Thr181-phosphorylated tau), neurofilament light chain (NFL) could probably be considered similarly consistent as a biomarker, whereas the proteins neuron-specific enolase, visinin-like protein 1, heart fatty acid binding protein, and YKL-40 (also known as chitinase 3-like protein 1, or human cartilage glycoprotein-39) were found to be moderately associated with AD [74].

Other longitudinal CSF studies have found elevated levels of the synaptic marker neurogranin in MCI and AD [105], as well as changes to neuronal cell adhesion molecule (NrCAM) and chromogranin A [106]. More recent studies have found that CSF neurogranin levels correlate with the progression of MCI [107], and that an increase in the level of another synaptic protein SNAP25 might indicate AD [108]. Comparisons of different conditions is helping to determine whether CSF biomarkers can help differentiate between different neurodegenerative disorders; for example, idiopathic normal-pressure hydrocephalus may be associated with significantly reduced levels of CSF Aβ42, t-tau, and p-tau compared to healthy controls; whereas compared to AD, both t-tau and p-tau were significantly decreased in idiopathic normal-pressure hydrocephalus, and CSF Aβ42 was slightly increased [109].

3.4.4.3 Potential Lipid Biomarkers in the CSF

There is strong evidence that brain lipid composition is altered in AD pathology, including at pre-clinical stages [110–112]. For example, levels of certain phospholipids, such as choline and ethanolamine phospholipids and their metabolites, are reduced in AD, and these changes have been reported to correlate with AD severity, tau pathology, and loss of neuronal signalling [113]. Studies have indicated inositol, serine, and glycerol-containing phospholipids are involved in AD pathology, sometimes detectable at early stages of AD [114–116], and levels of sphingolipids and particularly the ceramide precursors of sphingolipids have been reported to be altered, and to be associated with early AD pathology [117–119].

CSF levels of lipids have been investigated in AD, and the levels of phospholipids, cholesterol, and fatty acids have all been observed to decrease in AD when compared to controls [120, 121]. CSF sulfatide levels are also lower in AD [120, 122]. In a recent study of nanoparticle and supernatant fractions of CSF, it was found that levels of certain sphingomyelins were lower in AD compared to control, and that levels of three sphingomyelin species were also lower in MCI CSF. Acid sphingomyelinase activity correlated with Aβ1-42 levels in cognitively normal individuals, but once MCI was present, this correlation was lost [123]. Another study of sphingomyelins in brain tissue in AD found that carrying *APOE* ε4 alleles led to an increase in ceramide (22:0) and sulfatide levels and lower ceramide (C24:0) levels, but only once the disease was present, suggesting that *APOE* ε4-carriers develop the disease differently to non-carriers, and indicating *APOE* ε4 status may be important when investigating CSF lipid levels [124]. The importance of sphingolipid metabolism in AD pathogenesis has also been highlighted by other recent findings that Aβ1-42 oligomers inhibit sphingosine kinase (SphK1) expression and activity, thus disturbing sphingolipid metabolism and causing oxidative stress. Upregulation of the p53 protein has also been implicated in the Aβ1-42-induced cell death mechanism and is generally believed to play an important role in neurodegeneration in AD [125, 126]. Pro-survival mechanisms are also activated following Aβ1-42 treatment, such as the upregulation of the mitochondrial sirtuins Sirt 3, 4, and 5. These are important in the regulation of mitochondrial energy dynamics and anti-oxidative pathways, but despite upregulation of these proteins and other pro-survival mechanisms, Aβ1-42 treatment still kills many neuronal cells in *in vitro* systems [125]. These *in vitro* systems, with the use of specific inhibitors, have highlighted the importance of increased p53 levels and reduced SphK1 activity in early AD pathogenesis. These may act as potential CSF biomarkers of early stages of AD, however such changes also occur in other neurodegenerative conditions such as Parkinson's disease [127]. Perhaps more importantly, such studies have provided new avenues for therapeutic strategy [125].

AD CSF has also been reported to have higher levels of the phosphatidylcholine metabolite glycerophosphocholine (GPCh) than control CSF [128], a lower ratio of lysophosphatidylcholine/phosphatidylcholine compared to controls [129], alterations to glycerophospholipids and phospholipase A2 activity compared to controls [130], and elevated sphingomyelin levels compared to controls [131].

The ability of the CSF biomarkers total tau, Thr181-phosphorylated tau, and Aβ1-42 to predict AD in people with MCI has been found to be as accurate as the MMSE and clock drawing cognitive tests, after a six-year follow-up [12]. Furthermore, the combination of the two sets of tests was found to be significantly more accurate in predicting AD. A recent review has found CSF biomarkers to be more accurate in the short term in ruling out progression to AD, rather than demonstrating progression. The predictive value of the CSF biomarkers was also found to increase with longer term follow-up and yet to decline with age [132]. Another review found that the CSF biomarkers can be used to discriminate AD from healthy ageing (including psychiatric disorders like depression), to diagnose AD in its pre-clinical phase or in atypical forms with prominent non-memory impairment [133]. It is also claimed that CSF biomarkers can identify AD in patients with mixed pathologies and clarify ambiguous (AD versus non-AD) dementia diagnoses [133]. As mentioned earlier, a recent meta-analysis of 50 studies supports these claims, as it found that CSF Aβ1-42 levels were significantly lower in AD compared to frontotemporal dementia, Parkinson's dementia, and vascular dementia, and could also differentiate from MCI [90]. Despite such claims, there is still considerable between-laboratory variability in absolute levels of the biomarkers, due to differences in CSF collection methods, storage, and analytical protocols. Ideally research and clinical groups will reach consensus concerning analytical methods, and eventually cut-off values for the CSF biomarkers of AD will be determined [134].

Cholesterol metabolism is known to be disturbed in AD, including at early stages of the disease. Studies have shown that CSF levels of the cholesterol metabolites 24OH-cholesterol and 27OH-cholesterol are higher in both MCI and AD [135], when compared to controls. The metabolite 27OH-cholesterol is produced in the periphery, whereas 24OH-cholesterol is the main brain cholesterol metabolite.

Biomarker studies such as those described above indicate that there is enormous scope for further AD CSF biomarker investigation. However, obtaining CSF from patients is invasive and uncomfortable, and although may be very informative in clinical trials, CSF testing is unlikely to be used routinely for diagnosis. With so many promising potential blood biomarkers, it is hoped that a reliable blood biomarker panel will soon be available to help with AD diagnosis, particularly pre-clinical AD diagnosis.

3.4.5 Blood Biomarkers of AD

As we have just mentioned above, obtaining CSF is invasive, uncomfortable, and thus CSF biomarkers are not likely to be used for general screening. Neuropsychiatric tests are clearly safer and less invasive, however they are time-consuming, and only detect disease once dementia symptoms have appeared. Therefore, these are of little use if wishing to apply potential preventative treatments at the earliest (pre-clinical) stages possible. Imaging tests such as PiB-PET may detect disease early in the pathogenic process, yet are expensive, time-consuming, and not applicable for population screening.

A blood test for AD would be preferable, and blood biomarkers have been investigated in earnest for many years by many research groups. However, there are many potential problems with blood screening. Firstly, AD may be a systemic disease to some extent, yet the pathology is seen primarily in the brain, early stages of the disease process are still not properly understood and, for the moment, changes that may be detected in the general circulation are also not well understood. Nevertheless, these stages are being characterised rapidly, partly by such blood biomarker studies, which will allow researchers to determine AD-specific blood changes. Secondly, there are numerous other age-associated conditions, and medications to treat them, that may also cause changes to the blood proteome. These include cardiovascular diseases, diabetes-related changes, inflammatory conditions such as rheumatoid arthritis and osteoarthritis, chronic kidney disease, liver problems, obesity, and various cancers, quite apart from other brain conditions that may occur concurrently with AD, such as cerebrovascular disease, Lewy body disease, Parkinson's disease, and fronto-temporal dementia [136]. Age- and disease-associated damage to the integrity of the blood–brain barrier will also influence the proteins found in blood plasma/serum. However, blood–brain barrier leakage may be useful as brain-specific disease-related proteins may leak into the periphery, adding valuable biomarkers to the circulation.

3.4.5.1 Aβ Peptides in Plasma

Changes to Aβ metabolism are clearly central and early events in AD pathogenesis. Changes in CSF levels of Aβ1-42, Aβ1-40, and phosphorylated tau have been characterised to an extent that they can be used as part of AD diagnosis, therefore it is not surprising that plasma levels of the peptides have also been investigated to see if plasma Aβ peptide levels can be used as biomarkers. However, investigations into blood levels of the Aβ peptides have produced contradictory results.

Initial studies investigated familial AD families, and showed that people carrying AD-associated mutations had higher plasma levels of Aβ1-42 [137], however such findings may not apply to sporadic AD. Later studies found no change between sporadic AD, other dementias and healthy controls, although it was found that plasma levels of Aβ do increase with age [138, 139]. On the other hand, in one study of over 800 people, high baseline plasma Aβ1-42 and Aβ1-40 levels were associated with faster declines in multiple cognitive domains, over approximately 4.5 years [140] and another study found that plasma Aβ1-42 levels were higher in women with MCI, compared to healthy control women, yet this association was not found in men [141]. Some studies have found lower Aβ1-42/Aβ1-40 ratios to be associated with increased AD risk [142], and overall, the findings in a 2012 review found inconsistent results [143]. More recent studies are suggesting lower plasma Aβ1-42 levels, and plasma Aβ1-42/Aβ1-40 ratios are relevant: a report from the AIBL study, where plasma Aβ1-42, Aβ1-40, and N-terminal cleaved fragments were measured using both a commercial multiplex assay and a well-documented ELISA (enzyme-linked immunosorbent assay), found that plasma Aβ1-42 levels correlated inversely with brain PiB-PET-determined plaque load [144]. This result is supported by a more recent similar study of MCI subjects [145], and another longitudinal study of MCI conversion to AD, which demonstrated lower plasma Aβ1-42 levels, and lower plasma Aβ1-42/Aβ1-40 ratios were linked to later conversion to AD [146]. The results agrees with the concept of conversion to AD correlating with a decline in plasma Aβ1-42 levels, and a decline in plasma Aβ1-42/Aβ1-40 ratios. More recent results from the AIBL study support the results, as they showed that lower baseline plasma Aβ1-42 and the Aβ1-42/Aβ1-40 ratio were significant putative biomarkers of cognitive decline, following a 36-month update [147]. Blood exosomes have also been investigated, and the exosomal levels of total tau, Thr181-phosphorylated tau, Ser396-phosphorylated tau, and Aβ1-42 were significantly higher in patients with AD than in matched controls, a change that could be detected in some cognitively normal individuals who later developed AD, up to 10 years before clinical diagnosis [148]. These are encouraging results, yet they need to be replicated.

A more recent study has found that plasma levels of Aβ oligomers, as measured by a multimer detection system, are higher in patients with AD than in normal control individuals, and that they correlate well with conventional AD biomarkers [149]; whereas another study has found that chemically treated (protease inhibitors and phosphatase inhibitors) plasma prior to Aβ measurement results in Aβ1-40 levels and the Aβ1-42/Aβ1-40 ratio being significantly different between subjects considered PiB+ve and those who are PiB−ve for amyloid deposition. There was also good correlation with global PiB-measured deposition. Another study has found red blood cell-associated Aβ1-42 to increase with increasing levels of cognitive decline [150], and yet another recent study has also suggested plasma Aβ may be useful as a brain amyloidosis biomarker, though in a different way. The turnover of Aβ1-38, Aβ1-40, and Aβ1-42 in human plasma was investigated, and the study found faster fractional turnover of Aβ1-42 relative to Aβ1-40, as well as lower Aβ1-42 and Aβ1-42/Aβ1-40 concentrations in amyloid-positive participants, suggesting blood Aβ1-42 shows similar concentration changes to those seen in CSF [151]. Longitudinal studies will help determine the value of all the above findings, and whether plasma Aβ1-40 and Aβ1-42 levels (or erythrocyte-associated Aβ) will be of value as part of a panel of AD biomarkers [144, 152].

3.4.5.2 Other Potential Blood Biomarkers

Extensive research into blood serum or plasma biomarkers has revealed a huge range of potential biomarkers aside from the Aβ peptides, including proteins, peptides, lipids, as well as mRNA (discussed in a later section).

The development of several highly sensitive and sophisticated techniques has led to extensive proteomics and lipidomics studies of plasma, in the search for biomarkers of AD. With the knowledge that AD is accompanied by inflammation and oxidative stress, it is no surprise that many of the biomarkers that have been found are linked to such factors. Metabolic dysregulation, including changes to lipid metabolism, has also been recorded in AD, and markers of these changes have also been found in biomarker searches. For the moment, none of the individual biomarkers or panels of biomarkers provide conclusive clear diagnosis of AD, although the sensitivity and specificity of some of the biomarker panels are now reaching similar levels to neuropsychological tests in some studies [136, 153, 154]. For example, Burnham et al. investigated 176 analytes in plasma from over 800 subjects and reported that 5 of these analytes showed significant differences between subjects with high compared to low levels of PiB-PET-determined amyloid deposits [155]. A model based on nine markers achieved a sensitivity and specificity of 80% and 82%, respectively, for predicting amyloid burden. Validation using a different cohort, the Alzheimer's Disease Neuroimaging Initiative (ADNI) yielded similar results (sensitivity 79% and specificity 76%). An important complicating factor is these studies, which will reduce as longitudinal biomarker studies gain more data, is the fact that the elderly 'control' subjects in these studies may have undetected early AD, or pathology from other conditions, and in turn, the AD subjects may be affected by multiple medical comorbidities. Furthermore, many of the biomarkers found are common to other neuropathological conditions, thus not providing specificity [136, 153].

3.4.5.3 Blood Proteins

Some of the important studies on AD biomarkers include one by Ray et al. which investigated 120 signalling proteins in 259 plasma samples. The study produced a panel of 18 signalling proteins, linked to haematopoiesis, immune responses, apoptosis, and neuronal support (including epidermal growth factor, interleukin-1a, -3, and -11, TNFα, and angiopoietin), for which changes could reportedly distinguish AD from control subjects with a 90% accuracy rate. Possibly more importantly, the panel appeared to identify MCI subjects who would progress to AD in two to six years [156]. Unfortunately, a later evaluation of this panel of biomarkers could only find epidermal growth factor, platelet derived growth factor-BB, and chemokine ligand-15 to be different between AD and controls, and that these biomarkers could not distinguish from other dementias [157]. Hu et al. found alterations in levels of 17 analytes to be associated with MCI/very early AD or AD, and of these, four were found to be altered in three independent cohorts, providing supportive evidence for this data. The four potential biomarkers are apoE (protein), B-type natriuretic peptide, C-reactive protein and pancreatic polypeptide (PP) [158]. Some of these biomarker studies are helping to elucidate potential disease mechanisms and reasons for genetic variability – for example, high levels of PP have been quite consistently associated with AD as well as with MCI, however they have also been found in non-AD dementias. Despite the fact that changes in PP are proving to be not specific to AD, it is likely to be useful in a panel of biomarkers, and interestingly, studies of PP have shown associations with AD vary according to *APOE* ε4 status and the presence of type 2 diabetes, providing information that may help elucidate the links between weight loss and AD, glycaemic control and AD, as well as age-related lower somatostatin levels, *APOE* ε4 status and AD [159]. Similarly, plasma levels of NFL, as measured via the Single-Molecule Array (Simoa) method, show a marked increase in AD and MCI patients compared with controls, with a diagnostic performance similar to CSF biomarkers [160]. However, high plasma NFL is also found in other neurodegenerative disorders, therefore NFL would only be useful on a panel of biomarkers. In other biomarker-linked studies, investigating correlations between the different biomarker groups, analysis has shown that β-2 microglobulin, the light chain of the major histocompatibility complex (MHC)-class I, may be a master regulator of many seemingly unrelated biomarker proteins, implying a central role for the immune system in AD [161].

The ε4 allele of *APOE* is the major genetic risk factor for the development of sporadic and familial late-onset AD [162, 163]. Lower CSF apoE levels in AD relative to controls have been recorded consistently [164, 165]. However, studies of plasma apoE levels carried out around the same time did not provide consistent results. More recently, in studies with more sensitive techniques, reports have suggested that plasma levels of apoE are lower in AD. For example, the AIBL study has found that total apoE levels in plasma, as well as plasma apoE ε4 levels, were significantly lower in AD compared to controls, and correlated with increasing amyloid deposition in the brain, as determined by PiB-PET [166]. Later results from the same AIBL study confirmed previous reports that apoE levels are influenced by genotype, with ε2/ε2 carriers having the highest plasma apoE protein levels and ε4/ε4 carriers having the lowest [167]. In another recent study which involved over 75 000 participants, low plasma levels of apoE were found to be associated with increased risk of AD and other dementias in the general population, independent of ε2/ε3/ε4 *APOE* genotype [168]. Low plasma apoE has also been found to correlate with smaller hippocampal size in MCI and normal control subjects, especially in people with *APOE* ε4 alleles [169], supporting the concept that plasma apoE may represent a peripheral marker for developing AD. At this stage it is not known why lower levels of apoE occur in APOE ε4 allele carriers (both in the brain and plasma), however it is likely that these lower apoE levels may contribute to AD pathogenesis and progression by not being sufficient to carry out normal physiological apoE functions as part of the regulation of lipid metabolism in the periphery and brain. This would apply especially if the body is stressed by obesity, cardiovascular problems, insulin resistance, and type 2 diabetes – all risk factors for AD. For example, it is known that apoE promotes Aβ degradation, suggesting that reduced brain apoE levels lower the brain's Aβ clearance capacity [170]. Overall, plasma apolipoprotein levels have been linked to cognitive status and cognitive decline in elderly individuals [171], and in a recent study of very old individuals, the levels of most apolipoproteins were found to decrease with age, apoE levels were found to be at their highest, and the elderly were found to have the lowest frequency of *APOE* ε4 alleles [172].

Clusterin has been suggested as a potential biomarker, as some studies have shown plasma levels to be associated with longitudinal brain atrophy and disease stage. However, clusterin is being investigated as a diagnostic marker for colorectal cancer [173] and obesity-associated systemic inflammation [174], suggesting clusterin may have limited value due to lack of specificity, though may be useful as part of a biomarker panel. In fact, a recent study of AD, MCI and elderly control plasma samples from three independent cohorts has found clusterin to be highly useful as part of a panel of 10 proteins (transthyretin, clusterin, cystatin C, α1-acid-glycoprotein, intercellular adhesion molecule, complement C4, pigment epithelium derived factor, α1-antitrypsin, Regulated on Activation Normal T Cell Expressed and Secreted [RANTES], and ApoC3). This panel has been strongly associated with disease severity in MCI subjects, predicting progression to AD (accuracy 87%, sensitivity 85%, and specificity 88%) [175]. Other studies by the same group have discovered that plasma levels of several cytokines were associated with clinical and/or imaging evidence of disease severity. Interleukin-10, in particular, was associated with both forms of evidence, indicating strong potential as a biomarker of disease progression [176]. More recent studies of clusterin in the AIBL cohort have found plasma clusterin could predict both MCI and AD from healthy controls with greater than 80% accuracy for AD and greater than 75% accuracy for MCI at both baseline and 18-month time points [177], correlated well with PiB-measured brain Aβ levels; and plasma levels of clusterin were found to be higher in AD compared to healthy controls at baseline and 18 months ($p = 0.0003$) [178]. Another research group has also found higher plasma clusterin to correlate with lower MMSE scores [179]. All of these results support the use of clusterin as part of a biomarker panel.

3.4.6 Blood Lipids

The involvement of the lipid transporter apoE in AD pathology, and the *APOE* allele-dependent variation in AD risk, suggest strongly that lipids and disruptions to lipid metabolism are important in AD pathogenesis. Lipidomics studies have searched for blood-based changes to lipid profiles, both for biomarker searches as well as for the purpose of further characterisation of disease pathology.

Levels of the brain-specific cholesterol metabolite 24-hydroxycholesterol have been found to be higher in the blood of AD patients, however this metabolite is now known to be a marker for several other neurodegenerative diseases [180], indicating this could be a useful biomarker, though only as part of a panel of biomarkers. In other lipidomics studies, results have indicated that levels of certain blood phospholipids are altered in AD, such as phosphatidylethanolamine and phosphatidylcholine [148, 181]. In particular, the lipidomics study by Mapstone et al. assembled and validated a set of 10 lipids (including one lyso-phosphatidylcholine (18:2) and seven phosphatidylcholine species) from peripheral blood that predicted conversion from cognitively normal to either aMCI or AD within a two to three year time-frame with over 90% accuracy [148]. This impressive result provides optimism concerning the development of a reliable pre-clinical diagnostic tool, and highlights the concept that disturbances in lipid and cholesterol metabolism, in concert with oxidative stress, are involved early in AD pathogenesis. Lower serum levels of lyso-phosphatidylcholine (18:2) have been observed in AD patients in other studies too [182], and more recently the ratio of plasma phosphatidylcholines to lysophosphatidylcholines was found to differentiate AD and MCI patients from healthy controls [183]. However, an attempt at replicating the results above of Mapstone et al. using two larger independent cohorts failed, underscoring the importance of validation [184].

In other studies, presenilin-1 mutation carriers have been found to demonstrate altered phospholipid and sphingolipid metabolism in AD, and this needs further investigation in sporadic AD [185]. On the other hand, serum plasmalogen ethanolamines, thought to help protect against reactive oxygen species, have been reported to be lower in AD, and levels have been observed to correlate with dementia severity as determined by ADAS-Cog scoring [186].

Ceramides are central molecules of sphingolipid biosynthesis and catabolism. Several lines of evidence have suggested that the generation of free radicals by ceramides and Aβ contributes to the neurotoxicity seen in AD, in particular in the mitochondria [187]. Mielke et al. investigated sphingolipids in detail, and determined that over a one-year follow-up, high plasma ceramide levels, particularly d18:1–C22:0 and d18:1–C24:0, predicted cognitive decline and hippocampal volume loss among amnestic MCI patients, suggesting the predictive value of peripheral ceramides [188]. In other studies of 33 sphingomyelin species in plasma, higher levels of ceramide species and lower sphingomyelin levels were detected in AD compared to age-matched controls [189], results supported by further studies by Mielke et al., who also showed high plasma ceramide and low sphingomyelin levels were associated with a faster rate of cognitive decline [190]. Plasma ceramide studies suggest that, although these lipids may be useful in determining disease progression, for the moment, the overlap in levels of these lipids between groups prevent these lipids from being disease biomarkers [191]. Nevertheless, the many studies of this lipid group have helped to show that ceramides are linked to tau phosphorylation, apoptosis, oxidative stress, and Aβ-linked neurodegeneration, and although the mechanisms involved are still under debate, these studies are providing further characterisation of early AD pathogenesis as well as avenues for potential preventative therapy.

A more recent study of a potential lipid biomarker panel found several significant differences between controls, MCI and/or AD, yet not enough to produce an AD-specific biomarker panel [192]; another study investigated serum lipid peroxidation markers as AD biomarkers, yet found these were more indicative of subcortical small vessel disease [193]. More promising, however, is a recent lipidomics analysis which found a combination of 24 molecules could classify AD with greater than 70% accuracy [194]; hopefully further studies will improve this potential panel of biomarkers. Furthermore, a recent targeted brain and blood metabolomics study has shown that perturbations in sphingolipid metabolism appear to be biologically relevant biomarkers for the early detection of AD [195]. Blood platelet lipids have also shown changes in AD, and general blood metabolite investigations have also shown lipid changes in AD – see sections below.

3.4.7 Metabolites

Potential metabolite biomarkers have been investigated by some groups. Metabolomics profiling of plasma samples has been carried out using various mass spectrometry (MS)-based platforms, to find differences between control, MCI, and AD samples. In one study, Ultra-Performance Liquid Chromatography (UPLC)/Mass Spectrometry (MS) was used to show that MCI and AD plasma levels of progesterone, lysophosphatidylcholines, tryptophan, L-phenylalanine, dihydrosphingosine, and phytosphingosine were significantly different from the levels found in control subjects, indicating promise for such metabolites being biomarkers of pre-clinical AD stages [196]. Another metabolomics study found that the combination of differences in thymine, arachidonic acid, 2-aminoadipic acid, N,N-dimethylglycine, and 5,8-tetradecadienoic acid in plasma could differentiate amnestic MCI from control subjects [197]. Yet another study carried out non-targeted metabolomics research and found 23 altered canonical pathways when comparing MCI and control plasma. Lysine metabolism was significantly altered in MCI versus controls, and other pathways found to be altered include amino acid metabolism, the Krebs cycle, mitochondrial function, neurotransmitter metabolism, and lipid biosynthesis [198]. These studies may provide a selection of valuable biomarkers for a diagnostic panel, and are advancing our understanding of early AD pathogenic mechanisms.

3.4.8 Blood Platelets

Blood platelets are another potential source of peripheral AD biomarkers. Early studies reported altered membrane fluidity, whereas more recent studies have found significantly lower levels of phospholipase A(2) activity in AD compared to controls, and somewhat lower activity in MCI subjects [199]. Platelet proteome analysis has discovered AD-related changes in many protein levels, particularly secretory granule proteins, as well as proteins in the lipid homeostasis and glycoprotein synthesis pathways [200]. One recent study used platelet levels of monoamine oxidase B, apoE and tropomyosin 1 to differentiate AD from control subjects, and achieved a sensitivity of 94% and specificity of 89%. A biochip incorporating tests for these biomarkers was developed, and was shown to identify AD patients with an accuracy of 92% [201]. A recent review found that most platelet AD biomarkers are indicators of either oxidative stress or changes to membrane integrity [202], and from recent studies which have discovered that lower platelet serotonin (5 HT) levels [203] and lower platelet ADAM10 levels [204] are associated with AD, it can be concluded that platelets continue to show promise as a source of AD biomarkers. In support of this, another recent study of soluble platelet lysates found the lipid known as phosphatidylcholine aeC40:4 could differentiate AD from controls, whereas four other lipids could differentiate MCI from controls [205].

Overall, the blood biomarkers that have been found mostly fit into AD-related pathological cascades which occur in various pathways such as the inflammatory/immune system, endocrine system, oxidative stress, blood coagulation, cytokine, growth factor, and lipid metabolism and transport pathways. The various cross-sectional and longitudinal studies have found a myriad of potential biomarkers, and have put together several reasonably successful biomarker panels that can match current diagnostic sensitivity and specificity. To improve on these results, it is likely that some standardisation will be necessary. The time of collection, fasting status of the subjects, sample handling, preparation and storage, and eventually assay methods can all be controlled and optimised. There are many other variables and confounding elements that can influence the results of these particular assays. We have already mentioned several, such as the numerous age-associated conditions, and medications to treat them, including cardiovascular diseases, diabetes-related changes, inflammatory conditions such as rheumatoid arthritis and osteoarthritis, chronic kidney disease, liver problems, obesity, and many cancers, quite apart from other brain conditions that may occur concurrently with AD, such as cerebrovascular disease, Lewy body disease, Parkinson's disease, and fronto-temporal dementia [136]. The cohorts of the different studies have also been classified as elderly controls, MCI and AD using different criteria, which provides another source of variability. The control groups in particular are of concern, as they may include people with undetected developing AD, and/or may have any number of other conditions, depending on study exclusion criteria. Any biomarker panel would eventually need to be applicable to any person in the population, however for the purposes of biomarker panel development, cohort selection needs to be very clearly defined, and perhaps standardised to some extent [206].

3.4.9 Genetic Risk Factors

A family history of late-life cognitive impairment is a well-recognised risk factor for the development of MCI and AD. Twin studies support this concept, as AD heritability in that context has been measured to be between 58% and 79% [207]. As mentioned earlier, the primary genetic risk factor for late-onset AD is the ε4 allele of the *APOE* gene, an allele far more common amongst AD sufferers than in the general population. On average, *APOE* ε4 alleles are also known to cause a younger age of onset of AD, a greater accumulation of brain amyloid, and a more precipitous cognitive decline, particularly in the early stages, and in a dose-dependent manner [208]. Many other genetic variants have been identified as minor risk factors for cognitive decline and AD, and the genes for some of these have known roles in neuronal and memory functions, such as brain-derived neurotrophic factor (*BDNF*) and catechol-o-methyltransferase (*COMT*). The *BDNF* Val66Met polymorphism, for example, has been shown to cause faster declines in episodic memory and hippocampal volume in individuals who already have amnestic MCI and high PiB-PET-determined levels of brain Aβ, compared to people lacking that polymorphism [209]. Like many other genetic variants though, polymorphisms in *BDNF* and *COMT* do not contribute as much on their own to AD risk when compared to *APOE* alleles; however, when combined, and added to *APOE* allelic effects, the increased genetic risk score has been found to be associated with a nearly fourfold increased risk of cognitive impairment [210]. Similarly, another study also constructed a genetic risk score to predict progression from MCI to AD using genotype information concerning 8 genetic variants (16 total alleles, not including *APOE*) which had been identified by genome-wide association studies (GWAS), with each allele weighted by its AD risk odds ratio. Although the weighted genetic risk score was not significant, the authors found that subjects who possessed a total of six or more risk alleles progressed from MCI to AD twice as quickly (over an average of 26.3 months follow-up) as those who possessed fewer than six risk alleles [211]. In other studies, GWAS have associated the C allele of CD33 with an increased risk of AD and a more severe decline, and a recent study has found that in people with *APOE* ε4 alleles, carrying the C allele of CD33 leads to an even greater risk of AD dementia than the *APOE* ε4 alleles alone [212].

A more recent review of GWAS found associations with AD or AD-biomarkers only at 17 single nucleotide polymorphisms, located in 11 positions, which were either in genes, small nuclear RNA, or non-coding RNA regions [213]; and most of the protein-coding genes were expressed in human brain and correlated with *APOE* expression, showing again the strong link with lipid metabolism. Studies of polymorphisms in interleukin-1 (IL-1), IL-6, TNFα, IL-4, and particularly IL-10, however, are also showing the importance of inflammation in the context of AD [36, 214]. Future genetic risk studies will be needed to verify all these results, and to expand the studies to include more AD-associated gene polymorphisms as they are discovered. For the moment though, testing for *APOE* allele status would contribute significantly to the value of any AD biomarker panel.

3.4.10 The Eye as a Window to the Brain

People in the early stages of AD, sometimes at pre-clinical stages, may complain of visual disturbances such as problems reading and bumping into things. Examination of visual problems can reveal anomalies of colour vision, spatial contrast sensitivity, fundus examination, backward masking, and eye motility [215, 216]. Pathological examination of an AD subject's eye will reveal abnormalities from the cellular level to the functional level of the visual cortex.

The eye is an easily accessible mostly transparent tissue that is linked to the brain via the optic nerve, thus making it an attractive tissue to investigate the potential for clinical AD diagnosis. Several sensitive non-invasive investigative techniques are already established for the examination of the eye, such as slit lamp examination and optical coherence tomography; these may potentially serve in the diagnosis of AD. Furthermore, the deposition of amyloid has been investigated in tissues aside from the brain, and has been found in ocular structures such as the lens. The presence of cataracts, in particular age-related cataracts such as supranuclear cataracts, has been linked to AD risk; and post-mortem studies have shown these cataracts to be colocalised with enhanced Aβ immunoreactivity in the lenses of AD subjects [217]. Another study identified amyloid plaques in AD retinas at post-mortem as well as *in vivo* in AD-model transgenic mice, using a curcumin-based fluorochrome [218], and other studies of AD-model transgenic mice support these findings [219, 220]. One study using an Aβ-specific fluorescent ligand and laser scanning device could detect a higher average signal in probable AD cases compared to controls [221]. All these results suggest some promise for this method as a diagnostic tool. Some other studies which have also investigated Aβ immunoreactivity in the eyes of AD patients have not confirmed the original findings [222]; however, more recently, Kerbage et al. [223] provided evidence that the Aβ-specific fluorescent ligand could be used *in vivo* to differentiate between AD and control patients, to a better extent than a PET marker. Further studies are needed to replicate findings, and to investigate whether inconsistencies in study results are due to methodological and/or sensitivity problems, yet there is now considerable evidence ocular Aβ may be useful as a biomarker [224].

Some AD-associated changes to the retinal vasculature have also been reported via optical coherence tomography and laser Doppler techniques, including vascular narrowing, reduced branching, and non-optimal branching geometry [225, 226]. In addition, a reduced pupil light-response has been recorded in AD [227, 228]. This change in response to bright light together with the changes to the retinal vasculature have been recorded in pre-clinical disease stages – in asymptomatic people with brain amyloid deposits – indicating these changes may be useful in pre-clinical diagnosis. Furthermore, the changes seen in AD are not the same as those seen in vascular dementia, which centre around retinal venular widening, thus helping in differential diagnosis too [229].

Recent studies have found a significant correlation between increased pupillary size and CSF levels of Aβ and tau [230]. Furthermore, retinal oxygen saturation in arterioles and venules has also been found to be elevated in AD patients compared to controls

[231], and a recent meta-analysis of 11 optical coherence tomography studies has found that the mean peri-papillary retina nerve fibre layer thickness is significantly reduced in MCI (p = 0.03) and AD (p < 0.0001) compared to healthy controls [232]. In support of this, other recent studies have found that retinal nerve fibre thinning as well as reduced total macular and macular ganglion cell volumes are each associated with atrophy of the medial temporal lobe – a neuropathological hallmark of AD – in neurologically normal older adults [233], and that retinal vascular changes such as the amplitude of retinal venous pulsations correlate (in this case negatively) with Aβ deposition levels as measured by PET amyloid imaging [234]. Another recent review has shown that the type of retinal ganglion cells showing neurodegeneration appears to be disease specific, with AD changes being different to those seen in Parkinson's and Huntington's diseases [235]. Therefore there is now promising evidence that ocular changes in early stages of AD may provide biomarkers that may aid pre-clinical diagnosis and treatment [236].

3.4.11   miRNA Tests

The microRNA (miRNA) are a novel class of small (18–25 nucleotides), single-stranded non-coding RNA involved in the post-transcriptional regulation of gene expression. Their mechanism of action is mediated by complementary binding to the 3′ untranslated region (3′-UTR) of mRNA, leading to degradation or translational repression of the target mRNA. Extracellular miRNA seem to derive mainly from three sources: (i) passive leakage from damaged cells; (ii) active secretion via microvesicles, released by most cell types; and (iii) active secretion in complexes of miRNA-associated proteins, such as Argonaute2. Microvesicles can be isolated from most bodily fluids including blood, urine and CSF, and provide a rich source of biomarkers for disease diagnosis. Exosomes in particular, 80–100 nm vesicles originating in the endosomal pathway, have been shown to contain protein and RNA, including miRNA. Interestingly, miRNA have also been found to be very stable in CSF and blood, possibly partly due to the fact that they can be transported by liposomes or lipoproteins which protect them from degradation [237].

Altered expression of miRNA is now recognised as a feature of many disease states, including in the neurodegeneration of AD, Parkinson's disease, amyotrophic lateral sclerosis, and Huntington's disease pathogenesis [238]. The diversity of miRNA, and their potential to target multiple pathways, offers novel clinical applications for miRNA as biomarkers and therapeutic agents in neurodegenerative diseases. AD-specific changes in miRNA have been recorded, for example miRNA linked to BACE1, the enzyme that cleaves the N-terminus of Aβ. The first such changes recorded were lower brain levels of the miR-29a/b-1 cluster [239]; lower brain tissue levels of miR-29c [240] and miRNA-339-5p [241] have also been noted. These miRNA were found to upregulate BACE1 expression in culture, and the miRNA were either predicted or found to bind to the BACE1-3′-UTR.

More recently, other AD-specific miRNA changes have been detected in body fluids such as CSF and plasma, and publications are indicating such body fluids to be very promising sources of AD biomarkers [242]. For example, miRNA related to the immune system, often linked to many disease pathways, have been found to be altered in AD CSF [243]. More recently, CSF investigations by OpenArray technology discovered the differential expression of many miRNA in AD (including miR-103, miR-375, miR-505, miR-708, miR-4467, miR-219, miR-296, miR-766, and miR-3622b-3p) [244]. Confirmatory analysis (MANCOVA – multivariate analysis of covariance) in the same study revealed miR-100, miR-146a, and miR-1274a to be differentially expressed in AD, reaching Bonferroni corrected significance. Furthermore, a combination of miR-100, miR-375, and miR-103 was found to classify AD and controls subjects with ~95% accuracy. Other studies have found pro-inflammatory miRNA-9, miRNA-125b, miRNA 146a, and miRNA-155 are increased in extracellular fluid and CSF in AD patients, regulating innate immune and inflammatory responses in the AD brain [245]. Interestingly, the same research group has shown *in vitro* that anti-miRNA strategies may be useful in preventing the miRNA-induced inflammatory signalling that occurs in AD, thus providing avenues for anti-AD therapy [246].

Studies are indicating plasma may be a source of AD miRNA biomarkers [242]. Early studies found higher plasma levels of miR-34a and 181b in AD, with miR-181b being higher in *APOE* e4 carrying individuals [247]. Other studies of miRNA levels as diagnostic markers in blood serum have detected that the miRNAs miR-137, -181c, -9, and -29a/b, which have all been linked to ceramide regulation, were downregulated in both probable AD and amnestic MCI/probable early AD subjects compared to healthy controls, as well as in mouse risk factor models (mice fed high-fat diets) [248]. These findings are particularly interesting as they consolidate the theory that cardiovascular disease/obesity/dyslipidemia are linked to AD pathogenesis, however, from the point of view of disease biomarkers, it is important to note that it has not yet been determined whether these other conditions have similar miRNA profiles to AD, and these miRNA changes have also not been investigated in other neuropathological diseases. Other biomarker investigations have found that miR-125b and miR-181c are down-regulated while miR-9 is up-regulated in serum of AD patients compared with normal controls, with miR125b results correlating well with the MMSE results amongst AD patients [249]. Furthermore, quantitative reverse transcriptase-polymerase chain reaction (qRT-PCR) was used to show that plasma miRNA-34a and miRNA-29b levels are lower in AD when compared to healthy controls [250]. Some studies have investigated serum/plasma miRNA levels in other neurodegenerative disorders as well as AD, and so far these studies have indicated that serum miRNA-125b, miRNA-23a, and miRNA-26b are downregulated in AD, compared with non-inflammatory and inflammatory neurological controls, and frontotemporal dementia [251]. QRT-PCR has also shown that serum miRNA-31, -93, -143, and -146a are markedly decreased in AD compared with controls. Furthermore, the study showed miRNA-93, and -146a are significantly elevated in MCI compared with controls, and that the panel of miRNA-31, -93, and -146a can be used to discriminate AD from vascular dementia [252]. Other studies comparing MCI and controls found that the levels of miRNA-206 and -132 are significantly higher in MCI than in controls, and the combination of these two miRNAs could achieve the AUC (area under the curve) of 0.98 [253].

This is a relatively new field that has gained considerable focus very quickly, and the encouraging recent results above suggest that a selection of miRNAs, either alone or in combination with other blood biomarkers of protein or lipid origin for example, will be developed into a biomarker panel that can detect pre-clinical AD, and differentiate between AD and other neurodegenerative diseases. Both 2015 and 2016 reviews concluded that miRNA differences as in the selection of papers mentioned above are not showing much consensus from one laboratory to another, though the results of high-density microarray- and RNA sequencing-based profiles of AD brain and particularly of biological fluid samples are indicating that there are real and significant human population differences in AD onset, incidence, epidemiology, disease course, and progression [254, 255]. Recent studies have confirmed 23 previously reported miRNA, as well as 26 novel biomarkers, appear to be AD biomarkers, and also found that 6 of the most promising miRNA biomarker candidates could differentiate early AD from controls with high specificity and sensitivity [256]. These results support the concept that AD pre-clinical diagnosis using blood miRNA species alone is a distinct possibility.

3.5 Conclusions

Current diagnostic techniques are slow, cumbersome, and require a range of clinical disciplines. The first tests are neuropsychological tests, which of course are only of value once MCI or symptomatic AD is present. Similarly, current treatments are applied once symptoms appear: despite worldwide research for several decades, current treatments for AD at best reduce some of the symptoms for a year or more, by improving neurotransmission. They consist of cholinesterase inhibitors such as rivastigmine; or memantine, which influences NMDA (N-Methyl D-Aspartate) receptor function. Medications can also be used to treat other AD symptoms that can arise such as anxiety, depression, or hallucinations. However, all these medications only treat symptoms, there are no effective drugs that influence the advancing pathology of the disease. With no cure likely, particularly once symptoms are present, preventative or disease-slowing treatments are being pursued, however this avenue requires the identification of people in pre-clinical stages of the disease and/or people at greater risk of developing AD.

Earlier diagnosis via CSF collection (invasive, expensive, and not comfortable for the patient) and/or imaging (limited availability and expensive) is unlikely to be applicable to the general population. Nevertheless, CSF biomarkers are widely used in clinical studies. For example, studies of early onset (autosomal dominant) AD families have increased the understanding of AD pathogenesis, and in spite of known and potential differences to sporadic late-onset AD, current drug trials in such families are benefiting from this unique resource. Comparing and characterising CSF biomarkers from AD mutation-carrying members of these families many years before expected age of disease onset, and observing changes caused by potential treatments, is helping to accelerate therapy development, and is providing some hope for these families as well as the general population [80].

The developments in blood-based biomarkers over the last 10 years give much hope that a reliable blood-based panel of biomarkers will soon be available. Longitudinal studies by groups around the world now have valuable 'banks' of plasma samples that can be used between groups for assay validation in the search for pre-clinical biomarkers. A large body of data from previous studies is available to be used to characterise the metabolic and pathological changes in early AD, both in the brain and the periphery, especially in the pre-clinical years of the disease. However, many recent studies suggest that other less common avenues for diagnosis may win the race for providing reliable pre-clinical diagnosis. In particular, studies of miRNA have been particularly fruitful in the last few years, as have studies of non-invasive eye scans. Most recently, Aβ levels in saliva have been investigated and shown promise in distinguishing AD from healthy controls.

Whichever test, or more likely combination of pre-clinical tests is eventually adopted, it is clear that early diagnosis will facilitate research into the earlier stages of AD, improve our knowledge concerning aetiology and risk factors, and improve our chances of effective preventative intervention. Studies of treatment options have shifted focus onto preventative therapies, medications, and lifestyle changes. This explains the increased interest in pre-clinical diagnosis, and diagnosis as early as possible. Considerable evidence points to the importance of diabetes, dyslipidemia, inflammation, and cardiovascular health in increasing AD risk, as discussed in detail in the rest of this book. Genetic studies are also helping to determine populations at greater risk, and to reveal biochemical pathways involved in pathogenesis. It is clear that a pre-clinical diagnostic test or battery of tests will be a huge step forward in AD treatment development, and cannot come soon enough.

References

1 Perl, D.P. (2010). Neuropathology of Alzheimer's disease. *Mt. Sinai J. Med.* 77: 32–42.
2 Serrano-Pozo, A., Frosch, M.P., Masliah, E., and Hyman, B.T. (2011). Neuropathological alterations in Alzheimer disease. *Cold Spring Harb. Perspect. Med.* 1: a006189.
3 Arriagada, P.V., Growdon, J.H., Hedley-Whyte, E.T., and Hyman, B.T. (1992). Neurofibrillary tangles but not senile plaques parallel duration and severity of Alzheimer's disease. *Neurology* 42: 631–639.
4 Braak, H. and Braak, E. (1991). Neuropathological stageing of Alzheimer-related changes. *Acta Neuropathol.* 82: 239–259.
5 Serrano-Pozo, A., Mielke, M.L., Gomez-Isla, T. et al. (2011). Reactive glia not only associates with plaques but also parallels tangles in Alzheimer's disease. *Am. J. Pathol.* 179: 1373–1384.
6 DeKosky, S.T. and Scheff, S.W. (1990). Synapse loss in frontal cortex biopsies in Alzheimer's disease: correlation with cognitive severity. *Ann. Neurol.* 27: 457–464.
7 Terry, R.D., Masliah, E., Salmon, D.P. et al. (1991). Physical basis of cognitive alterations in Alzheimer's disease: synapse loss is the major correlate of cognitive impairment. *Ann. Neurol.* 30: 572–580.
8 Andrade-Moraes, C.H., Oliveira-Pinto, A.V., Castro-Fonseca, E. et al. (2013). Cell number changes in Alzheimer's disease relate to dementia, not to plaques and tangles. *Brain* 136: 3738–3752.
9 Maalouf, M., Ringman, J.M., and Shi, J. (2011). An update on the diagnosis and management of dementing conditions. *Rev. Neurol. Dis.* 8: e68–e87.
10 Folstein, M.F., Folstein, S.E., and McHugh, P.R. (1975). "Mini-mental state": a practical method for grading the cognitive state of patients for the clinician. *J. Psychiatr. Res.* 12: 189–198.
11 Ismail, Z., Rajji, T.K., and Shulman, K.I. (2010). Brief cognitive screening instruments: an update. *Int. J. Geriatr. Psychiatry* 25: 111–120.
12 Palmqvist, S., Hertze, J., Minthon, L. et al. (2012). Comparison of brief cognitive tests and CSF biomarkers in predicting Alzheimer's disease in mild cognitive impairment: six-year follow-up study. *PLoS One* 7: e38639.

13 Mungas, D. (1991). In-office mental status testing: a practical guide. *Geriatrics* 46: 54–58, 63, 66.
14 Palmqvist, S., Hansson, O., Minthon, L., and Londos, E. (2009). Practical suggestions on how to differentiate dementia with Lewy bodies from Alzheimer's disease with common cognitive tests. *Int. J. Geriatr. Psychiatry* 24: 1405–1412.
15 Ala, T.A., Hughes, L.F., Kyrouac, G.A. et al. (2002). The Mini-Mental State exam may help in the differentiation of dementia with Lewy bodies and Alzheimer's disease. *Int. J. Geriatr. Psychiatry* 17: 503–509.
16 Jefferson, A.L., Cosentino, S.A., Ball, S.K. et al. (2002). Errors produced on the mini-mental state examination and neuropsychological test performance in Alzheimer's disease, ischemic vascular dementia, and Parkinson's disease. *J. Neuropsychiatry Clin. Neurosci.* 14: 311–320.
17 Nasreddine, Z.S., Phillips, N.A., Bédirian, V. et al. (2005). The Montreal Cognitive Assessment, MoCA: a brief screening tool for mild cognitive impairment. *J. Am. Geriatr. Soc.* 53: 695–699.
18 Rossetti, H.C., Lacritz, L.H., Cullum, C.M., and Weiner, M.F. (2011). Normative data for the Montreal Cognitive Assessment (MoCA) in a population-based sample. *Neurology* 77: 1272–1275.
19 Hughes, C.P., Berg, L., Danziger, W. et al. (1982). A new clinical scale for the staging of dementia. *Br. J. Psychiatry* 140: 566–572.
20 Morris, J.C. (1997). Clinical dementia rating: a reliable and valid diagnostic and staging measure for dementia of the Alzheimer type. *Int. Psychogeriatr.* 9: 173–176.
21 O'Bryant, S.E., Waring, S.C., Cullum, C.M. et al. (2008). Staging dementia using clinical dementia rating scale sum of boxes scores: a Texas Alzheimer's research consortium study. *Arch. Neurol.* 65: 1091–1095.
22 Shulman, K.I. (2000). Clock-drawing: is it the ideal cognitive screening test? *Int. J. Geriatr. Psychiatry* 15: 548–561.
23 Richardson, H.E. and Glass, J.N. (2002). A comparison of scoring protocols on the Clock Drawing Test in relation to ease of use, diagnostic group, and correlations with Mini-Mental State Examination. *J. Am. Geriatr. Soc.* 50: 169–173.
24 Watson, Y.I., Arfken, C.L., and Birge, S.J. (1993). Clock completion: an objective screening test for dementia. *J. Am. Geriatr. Soc.* 41: 1235–1240.
25 Sunderland, T., Hill, J.L., Mellow, A.M. et al. (1989). Clock drawing in Alzheimer's disease: a novel measure of dementia severity. *J. Am. Geriatr. Soc.* 37: 725–729.
26 Meulen, E.F., Schmand, B., van Campen, J.P. et al. (2004). The seven minute screen: a neurocognitive screening test highly sensitive to various types of dementia. *J. Neurol. Neurosurg. Psychiatry* 75: 700–705.
27 Pena-Casanova, J. (1997). Alzheimer's disease assessment scale – cognitive in clinical practice. *Int. Psychogeriatr.* 9 (Suppl 1): 105–114.
28 Jorm, A.F., Mackinnon, A.J., Henderson, A.S. et al. (1995). The psychogeriatric assessment scales: a multi-dimensional alternative to categorical diagnoses of dementia and depression in the elderly. *Psychol. Med.* 25: 447–460.
29 Jorm, A.F., Christensen, H., Jacomb, P.A. et al. (2001). The cognitive decline scale of the psychogeriatric assessment scales (PAS): longitudinal data on its validity. *Int. J. Geriatr. Psychiatry* 16: 261–265.

30 Marson, D.C., Dymek, M.P., Duke, L.W., and Harrell, L.E. (1997). Subscale validity of the Mattis Dementia Rating Scale. *Arch. Clin. Neuropsychol.* 12: 269–275.

31 Matteau, E., Dupre, N., Langlois, M. et al. (2011). Mattis Dementia Rating Scale 2: screening for MCI and dementia. *Am. J. Alzheimers Dis. Other Demen.* 26: 389–398.

32 Schmidt, K.S., Lieto, J.M., Kiryankova, E., and Salvucci, A. (2006). Construct and concurrent validity of the Dementia Rating Scale-2 alternate form. *J. Clin. Exp. Neuropsychol.* 28: 646–654.

33 Borson, S., Scanlan, J.M., Chen, P., and Ganguli, M. (2003). The Mini-Cog as a screen for dementia: validation in a population-based sample. *J. Am. Geriatr. Soc.* 51: 1451–1454.

34 Storey, J.E., Rowland, J.T., Basic, D. et al. (2004). The Rowland Universal Dementia Assessment Scale (RUDAS): a multicultural cognitive assessment scale. *Int. Psychogeriatr.* 16: 13–31.

35 Naqvi, R.M., Haider, S., Tomlinson, G., and Alibhai, S. (2015). Cognitive assessments in multicultural populations using the Rowland Universal Dementia Assessment Scale: a systematic review and meta-analysis. *CMAJ* 187: E169–E175.

36 Magalhaes, C.A., Carvalho, M.D.G., Sousa, L.P. et al. (2017). Alzheimer's disease and cytokine IL-10 gene polymorphisms: is there an association? *Arq. Neuropsiquiatr.* 75: 649–656.

37 Morris, J.C., Heyman, A., Mohs, R.C. et al. (1989). The Consortium to Establish a Registry for Alzheimer's Disease (CERAD): Part I. Clinical and neuropsychological assessment of Alzheimer's disease. *Neurology* 39: 1159–1165.

38 Sotaniemi, M., Pulliainen, V., Hokkanen, L. et al. (2012). CERAD-neuropsychological battery in screening mild Alzheimer's disease. *Acta Neurol. Scand.* 125: 16–23.

39 Paajanen, T., Hanninen, T., Tunnard, C. et al. (2014). CERAD neuropsychological compound scores are accurate in detecting prodromal Alzheimer's disease: a prospective AddNeuroMed study. *J. Alzheimers Dis.* 39: 679–690.

40 Hallikainen, I., Martikainen, J., Lin, P.J. et al. (2014). The progression of Alzheimer's disease can be assessed with a short version of the CERAD neuropsychological battery: the Kuopio ALSOVA study. *Dement. Geriatr. Cogn. Dis. Extra* 4: 494–508.

41 Herholz, K. (2014). Guidance for reading FDG PET scans in dementia patients. *Q. J. Nucl. Med. Mol. Imaging* 58: 332–343.

42 Protas, H.D., Chen, K., Langbaum, J.B. et al. (2013). Posterior cingulate glucose metabolism, hippocampal glucose metabolism, and hippocampal volume in cognitively normal, late-middle-aged persons at 3 levels of genetic risk for Alzheimer disease. *JAMA Neurol.* 70: 320–325.

43 Bammer, R., Skare, S., Newbould, R. et al. (2005). Foundations of advanced magnetic resonance imaging. *NeuroRx* 2: 167–196.

44 Borogovac, A. and Asllani, I. (2012). Arterial spin labeling (ASL) fMRI: advantages, theoretical constrains, and experimental challenges in neurosciences. *Int. J. Biomed. Imaging* 2012: 818456.

45 Woodard, J.L. and Sugarman, M.A. (2012). Functional magnetic resonance imaging in aging and dementia: detection of age-related cognitive changes and prediction of cognitive decline. *Curr. Top Behav. Neurosci.* 10: 113–136.

46 Grady, C.L. and Garrett, D.D. (2014). Understanding variability in the BOLD signal and why it matters for aging. *Brain Imaging Behav.* 8: 274–283.

47 Zanto, T.P., Pa, J., and Gazzaley, A. (2014). Reliability measures of functional magnetic resonance imaging in a longitudinal evaluation of mild cognitive impairment. *Neuroimage* 84: 443–452.

48 Huang, R.R., Jia, B.H., Xie, L. et al. (2016). Spatial working memory impairment in primary onset middle-age type 2 diabetes mellitus: an ethology and BOLD-fMRI study. *J. Magn. Reson. Imaging* 43: 75–87.

49 Haight, T.J., Bryan, R.N., Erus, G. et al. (2015). Vascular risk factors, cerebrovascular reactivity, and the default-mode brain network. *Neuroimage* 115: 7–16.

50 Leoni, R.F., Mazzetto-Betti, K.C., Silva, A.C. et al. (2012). Assessing cerebrovascular reactivity in carotid steno-occlusive disease using MRI BOLD and ASL techniques. *Radiol. Res. Pract.* 2012: 268483.

51 Shah, D., Praet, J., Latif Hernandez, A. et al. (2016). Early pathologic amyloid induces hypersynchrony of BOLD resting-state networks in transgenic mice and provides an early therapeutic window before amyloid plaque deposition. *Alzheimers Dement.* 12: 964–976.

52 Wolf, R.L. and Detre, J.A. (2007). Clinical neuroimaging using arterial spin-labeled perfusion magnetic resonance imaging. *Neurotherapeutics* 4: 346–359.

53 Le Heron, C.J., Wright, S.L., Melzer, T.R. et al. (2014). Comparing cerebral perfusion in Alzheimer's disease and Parkinson's disease dementia: an ASL-MRI study. *J. Cereb. Blood Flow Metab.* 34: 964–970.

54 Steketee, R.M., Bron, E.E., Meijboom, R. et al. (2016). Early-stage differentiation between presenile Alzheimer's disease and frontotemporal dementia using arterial spin labeling MRI. *Eur. Radiol.* 26: 244–253.

55 Wierenga, C.E., Hays, C.C., and Zlatar, Z.Z. (2014). Cerebral blood flow measured by arterial spin labeling MRI as a preclinical marker of Alzheimer's disease. *J. Alzheimers Dis.* 42 (Suppl 4): S411–S419.

56 Collij, L.E., Heeman, F., Kuijer, J.P. et al. (2016). Application of machine learning to arterial spin labeling in mild cognitive impairment and Alzheimer disease. *Radiology* 281: 865–875.

57 Zlatar, Z.Z., Bischoff-Grethe, A., Hays, C.C. et al. (2016). Higher brain perfusion may not support memory functions in cognitively normal carriers of the ApoE epsilon4 allele compared to non-carriers. *Front. Aging Neurosci.* 8: 151.

58 Valotassiou, V., Papatriantafyllou, J., Sifakis, N. et al. (2015). Clinical evaluation of brain perfusion SPECT with Brodmann areas mapping in early diagnosis of Alzheimer's disease. *J. Alzheimers Dis.* 47: 773–785.

59 Kirino, E. (2017). Three-dimensional stereotactic surface projection in the statistical analysis of single photon emission computed tomography data for distinguishing between Alzheimer's disease and depression. *World J. Psychiatry* 7: 121–127.

60 Andriuta, D., Moullart, V., Schraen, S. et al. (2017). Inferior parietal cortex hypoperfusion is the most specific imaging marker for AD patients with positive CSF biomarker assays in a memory clinic in France. *Alzheimer Dis. Assoc. Disord.* 32: 89–93.

61 Mathis, C.A., Mason, N.S., Lopresti, B.J., and Klunk, W.E. (2012). Development of positron emission tomography beta-amyloid plaque imaging agents. *Semin. Nucl. Med.* 42: 423–432.

62 Klunk, W.E., Engler, H., Nordberg, A. et al. (2004). Imaging brain amyloid in Alzheimer's disease with Pittsburgh compound-B. *Ann. Neurol.* 55: 306–319.

63 Rowe, C.C., Bourgeat, P., Ellis, K.A. et al. (2013). Predicting Alzheimer disease with beta-amyloid imaging: results from the Australian imaging, biomarkers, and lifestyle study of ageing. *Ann. Neurol.* 74: 905–913.

64 Ellis, K.A., Rowe, C.C., Villemagne, V.L. et al., Group Ar (2010). Addressing population aging and Alzheimer's disease through the Australian imaging biomarkers and lifestyle study: collaboration with the Alzheimer's disease neuroimaging initiative. *Alzheimers Dement.* 6: 291–296.

65 Chetelat, G., Villemagne, V.L., Bourgeat, P. et al., Australian Imaging B, Lifestyle Research G (2010). Relationship between atrophy and beta-amyloid deposition in Alzheimer disease. *Ann. Neurol.* 67: 317–324.

66 Ma, Y., Zhang, S., Li, J. et al. (2014). Predictive accuracy of amyloid imaging for progression from mild cognitive impairment to Alzheimer disease with different lengths of follow-up: a meta-analysis. [Corrected]. *Medicine (Baltimore)* 93: e150.

67 Zhang, S., Smailagic, N., Hyde, C. et al. (2014). (11)C-PiB-PET for the early diagnosis of Alzheimer's disease dementia and other dementias in people with mild cognitive impairment (MCI). *Cochrane Database Syst. Rev.* (7): CD010386. https://doi.org/10.1002/14651858.CD010386.pub2.

68 Rodriguez-Vieitez, E., Ni, R., Gulyas, B. et al. (2015). Astrocytosis precedes amyloid plaque deposition in Alzheimer APPswe transgenic mouse brain: a correlative positron emission tomography and in vitro imaging study. *Eur. J. Nucl. Med. Mol. Imaging* 42: 1119–1132.

69 Hollands, S., Lim, Y.Y., Laws, S.M. et al., Group AR (2017). APOEvarepsilon4 genotype, amyloid, and clinical disease progression in cognitively normal older adults. *J. Alzheimers Dis.* 57: 411–422.

70 Lim, Y.Y., Williamson, R., Laws, S.M. et al., Group AR (2017). Effect of APOE genotype on amyloid deposition, brain volume, and memory in cognitively normal older individuals. *J. Alzheimers Dis.* 58: 1293–1302.

71 McKhann, G.M., Knopman, D.S., Chertkow, H. et al. (2011). The diagnosis of dementia due to Alzheimer's disease: recommendations from the National Institute on Aging-Alzheimer's Association workgroups on diagnostic guidelines for Alzheimer's disease. *Alzheimers Dement.* 7: 263–269.

72 Jack, C.R. Jr., Albert, M.S., Knopman, D.S. et al. (2011). Introduction to the recommendations from the National Institute on Aging-Alzheimer's Association workgroups on diagnostic guidelines for Alzheimer's disease. *Alzheimers Dement.* 7: 257–262.

73 Jack, C.R. Jr., Knopman, D.S., Weigand, S.D. et al. (2012). An operational approach to National Institute on Aging-Alzheimer's Association criteria for preclinical Alzheimer disease. *Ann. Neurol.* 71: 765–775.

74 Olsson, B., Lautner, R., Andreasson, U. et al. (2016). CSF and blood biomarkers for the diagnosis of Alzheimer's disease: a systematic review and meta-analysis. *Lancet Neurol.* 15: 673–684.

75 Iqbal, K., Wang, X., Blanchard, J. et al. (2010). Alzheimer's disease neurofibrillary degeneration: pivotal and multifactorial. *Biochem. Soc. Trans.* 38: 962–966.

76 Blennow, K. and Hampel, H. (2003). CSF markers for incipient Alzheimer's disease. *Lancet Neurol.* 2: 605–613.

77 Mattsson, N., Zetterberg, H., Hansson, O. et al. (2009). CSF biomarkers and incipient Alzheimer disease in patients with mild cognitive impairment. *JAMA* 302: 385–393.

78 Andreasson, U., Blennow, K., and Zetterberg, H. (2016). Update on ultrasensitive technologies to facilitate research on blood biomarkers for central nervous system disorders. *Alzheimers Dement. (Amst)* 3: 98–102.

79 Bateman, R.J., Xiong, C., Benzinger, T.L. et al. (2012). Clinical and biomarker changes in dominantly inherited Alzheimer's disease. *N. Engl. J. Med.* 367: 795–804.

80 Schindler, S.E. and Fagan, A.M. (2015). Autosomal dominant Alzheimer disease: a unique resource to study CSF biomarker changes in preclinical AD. *Front. Neurol.* 6: 142.

81 Moonis, M., Swearer, J.M., Dayaw, M.P. et al. (2005). Familial Alzheimer disease: decreases in CSF Abeta42 levels precede cognitive decline. *Neurology* 65: 323–325.

82 Parnetti, L., Chiasserini, D., Eusebi, P. et al. (2012). Performance of abeta1-40, abeta1-42, total tau, and phosphorylated tau as predictors of dementia in a cohort of patients with mild cognitive impairment. *J. Alzheimers Dis.* 29: 229–238.

83 Trojanowski, J.Q., Vandeerstichele, H., Korecka, M. et al., Alzheimer's Disease Neuroimaging I (2010). Update on the biomarker core of the Alzheimer's disease neuroimaging initiative subjects. *Alzheimers Dement.* 6: 230–238.

84 Parnetti, L. and Chiasserini, D. (2011). Role of CSF biomarkers in the diagnosis of prodromal Alzheimer's disease. *Biomark. Med.* 5: 479–484.

85 Lewczuk, P., Kamrowski-Kruck, H., Peters, O. et al. (2010). Soluble amyloid precursor proteins in the cerebrospinal fluid as novel potential biomarkers of Alzheimer's disease: a multicenter study. *Mol. Psychiatry* 15: 138–145.

86 Gabelle, A., Roche, S., Geny, C. et al. (2010). Correlations between soluble alpha/beta forms of amyloid precursor protein and Abeta38, 40, and 42 in human cerebrospinal fluid. *Brain Res.* 1357: 175–183.

87 Alexopoulos, P., Tsolakidou, A., Roselli, F. et al. (2012). Clinical and neurobiological correlates of soluble amyloid precursor proteins in the cerebrospinal fluid. *Alzheimers Dement.* 8: 304–311.

88 Dobrowolska, J.A., Kasten, T., Huang, Y. et al. (2014). Diurnal patterns of soluble amyloid precursor protein metabolites in the human central nervous system. *PLoS One* 9: e89998.

89 Ritchie, C., Smailagic, N., Noel-Storr, A.H. et al. (2014). Plasma and cerebrospinal fluid amyloid beta for the diagnosis of Alzheimer's disease dementia and other dementias in people with mild cognitive impairment (MCI). *Cochrane Database Syst. Rev.* (6): CD008782. https://doi.org/10.1002/14651858.CD008782.pub4.

90 Tang, W., Huang, Q., Wang, Y. et al. (2014). Assessment of CSF Abeta42 as an aid to discriminating Alzheimer's disease from other dementias and mild cognitive impairment: a meta-analysis of 50 studies. *J. Neurol. Sci.* 345: 26–36.

91 Mo, J.A., Lim, J.H., Sul, A.R. et al. (2015). Cerebrospinal fluid beta-amyloid1-42 levels in the differential diagnosis of Alzheimer's disease – systematic review and meta-analysis. *PLoS One* 10: e0116802.

92 Niemantsverdriet, E., Valckx, S., Bjerke, M., and Engelborghs, S. (2017). Alzheimer's disease CSF biomarkers: clinical indications and rational use. *Acta Neurol. Belg.* 117: 591–602.

93 Sunderland, T., Linker, G., Mirza, N. et al. (2003). Decreased beta-amyloid1-42 and increased tau levels in cerebrospinal fluid of patients with Alzheimer disease. *JAMA* 289: 2094–2103.

94 Ritchie, C., Smailagic, N., Noel-Storr, A.H. et al. (2017). CSF tau and the CSF tau/ABeta ratio for the diagnosis of Alzheimer's disease dementia and other dementias in people with mild cognitive impairment (MCI). *Cochrane Database Syst. Rev.* (3): CD010803. https://doi.org/10.1002/14651858.CD010803.pub2.

95 Puchades, M., Hansson, S.F., Nilsson, C.L. et al. (2003). Proteomic studies of potential cerebrospinal fluid protein markers for Alzheimer's disease. *Brain Res. Mol. Brain Res.* 118: 140–146.

96 Davidsson, P., Westman-Brinkmalm, A., Nilsson, C.L. et al. (2002). Proteome analysis of cerebrospinal fluid proteins in Alzheimer patients. *Neuroreport* 13: 611–615.

97 Maruyama, M., Higuchi, M., Takaki, Y. et al. (2005). Cerebrospinal fluid neprilysin is reduced in prodromal Alzheimer's disease. *Ann. Neurol.* 57: 832–842.

98 de Jong, D., Jansen, R.W., Pijnenburg, Y.A. et al. (2007). CSF neurofilament proteins in the differential diagnosis of dementia. *J. Neurol. Neurosurg. Psychiatry* 78: 936–938.

99 Tarawneh, R., Lee, J.M., Ladenson, J.H. et al. (2012). CSF VILIP-1 predicts rates of cognitive decline in early Alzheimer disease. *Neurology* 78: 709–719.

100 Perrin, R.J., Craig-Schapiro, R., Malone, J.P. et al. (2011). Identification and validation of novel cerebrospinal fluid biomarkers for staging early Alzheimer's disease. *PLoS One* 6: e16032.

101 Craig-Schapiro, R., Perrin, R.J., Roe, C.M. et al. (2010). YKL-40: a novel prognostic fluid biomarker for preclinical Alzheimer's disease. *Biol. Psychiatry* 68: 903–912.

102 Craig-Schapiro, R., Fagan, A.M., and Holtzman, D.M. (2009). Biomarkers of Alzheimer's disease. *Neurobiol. Dis.* 35: 128–140.

103 Babic, M., Svob Strac, D., Muck-Seler, D. et al. (2014). Update on the core and developing cerebrospinal fluid biomarkers for Alzheimer disease. *Croat. Med. J.* 55: 347–365.

104 Ringman, J.M., Schulman, H., Becker, C. et al. (2012). Proteomic changes in cerebrospinal fluid of presymptomatic and affected persons carrying familial Alzheimer disease mutations. *Arch. Neurol.* 69: 96–104.

105 Thorsell, A., Bjerke, M., Gobom, J. et al. (2010). Neurogranin in cerebrospinal fluid as a marker of synaptic degeneration in Alzheimer's disease. *Brain Res.* 1362: 13–22.

106 Wildsmith, K.R., Schauer, S.P., Smith, A.M. et al. (2014). Identification of longitudinally dynamic biomarkers in Alzheimer's disease cerebrospinal fluid by targeted proteomics. *Mol. Neurodegener.* 9: 22.

107 Kvartsberg, H., Duits, F.H., Ingelsson, M. et al. (2015). Cerebrospinal fluid levels of the synaptic protein neurogranin correlates with cognitive decline in prodromal Alzheimer's disease. *Alzheimers Dement.* 11: 1180–1190.

108 Brinkmalm, A., Brinkmalm, G., Honer, W.G. et al. (2014). SNAP-25 is a promising novel cerebrospinal fluid biomarker for synapse degeneration in Alzheimer's disease. *Mol. Neurodegener.* 9: 53.

109 Chen, Z., Liu, C., Zhang, J. et al. (2017). Cerebrospinal fluid Abeta42, t-tau, and p-tau levels in the differential diagnosis of idiopathic normal-pressure hydrocephalus: a systematic review and meta-analysis. *Fluids Barriers CNS* 14: 13.

110 Nitsch, R.M., Blusztajn, J.K., Pittas, A.G. et al. (1992). Evidence for a membrane defect in Alzheimer disease brain. *Proc. Natl. Acad. Sci. U. S. A.* 89: 1671–1675.

111 Soderberg, M., Edlund, C., Alafuzoff, I. et al. (1992). Lipid composition in different regions of the brain in Alzheimer's disease/senile dementia of Alzheimer's type. *J. Neurochem.* 59: 1646–1653.

112 Han, X. (2010). Multi-dimensional mass spectrometry-based shotgun lipidomics and the altered lipids at the mild cognitive impairment stage of Alzheimer's disease. *Biochim. Biophys. Acta* 1801: 774–783.

113 Bennett, S.A., Valenzuela, N., Xu, H. et al. (2013). Using neurolipidomics to identify phospholipid mediators of synaptic (dys)function in Alzheimer's disease. *Front. Physiol.* 4: 168.

114 Bader Lange, M.L., Cenini, G., Piroddi, M. et al. (2008). Loss of phospholipid asymmetry and elevated brain apoptotic protein levels in subjects with amnestic mild cognitive impairment and Alzheimer disease. *Neurobiol. Dis.* 29: 456–464.

115 Morel, E., Chamoun, Z., Lasiecka, Z.M. et al. (2013). Phosphatidylinositol-3-phosphate regulates sorting and processing of amyloid precursor protein through the endosomal system. *Nat. Commun.* 4: 2250.

116 Chan, R.B., Oliveira, T.G., Cortes, E.P. et al. (2012). Comparative lipidomic analysis of mouse and human brain with Alzheimer disease. *J. Biol. Chem.* 287: 2678–2688.

117 Han, X., MH, D., DW, M.K. Jr. et al. (2002). Substantial sulfatide deficiency and ceramide elevation in very early Alzheimer's disease: potential role in disease pathogenesis. *J. Neurochem.* 82: 809–818.

118 Han, X. (2010). The pathogenic implication of abnormal interaction between apolipoprotein E isoforms, amyloid-beta peptides, and sulfatides in Alzheimer's disease. *Mol. Neurobiol.* 41: 97–106.

119 Grimm, M.O., Grimm, H.S., Patzold, A.J. et al. (2005). Regulation of cholesterol and sphingomyelin metabolism by amyloid-beta and presenilin. *Nat. Cell Biol.* 7: 1118–1123.

120 Mulder, M., Ravid, R., Swaab, D.F. et al. (1998). Reduced levels of cholesterol, phospholipids, and fatty acids in cerebrospinal fluid of Alzheimer disease patients are not related to apolipoprotein E4. *Alzheimer Dis. Assoc. Disord.* 12: 198–203.

121 Fonteh, A.N., Cipolla, M., Chiang, J. et al. (2014). Human cerebrospinal fluid fatty acid levels differ between supernatant fluid and brain-derived nanoparticle fractions, and are altered in Alzheimer's disease. *PLoS One* 9: e100519.

122 Han, X., Fagan, A.M., Cheng, H. et al. (2003). Cerebrospinal fluid sulfatide is decreased in subjects with incipient dementia. *Ann. Neurol.* 54: 115–119.

123 Fonteh, A.N., Ormseth, C., Chiang, J. et al. (2015). Sphingolipid metabolism correlates with cerebrospinal fluid Beta amyloid levels in Alzheimer's disease. *PLoS One* 10: e0125597.

124 Bandaru, V.V., Troncoso, J., Wheeler, D. et al. (2009). ApoE4 disrupts sterol and sphingolipid metabolism in Alzheimer's but not normal brain. *Neurobiol. Aging* 30: 591–599.

125 Cieslik, M., Czapski, G.A., and Strosznajder, J.B. (2015). The molecular mechanism of amyloid beta42 peptide toxicity: the role of sphingosine kinase-1 and mitochondrial sirtuins. *PLoS One* 10: e0137193.

126 Aubry, S., Shin, W., Crary, J.F. et al. (2015). Assembly and interrogation of Alzheimer's disease genetic networks reveal novel regulators of progression. *PLoS One* 10: e0120352.

127 Pyszko, J.A. and Strosznajder, J.B. (2014). The key role of sphingosine kinases in the molecular mechanism of neuronal cell survival and death in an experimental model of Parkinson's disease. *Folia Neuropathol.* 52: 260–269.

128 Walter, A., Korth, U., Hilgert, M. et al. (2004). Glycerophosphocholine is elevated in cerebrospinal fluid of Alzheimer patients. *Neurobiol. Aging* 25: 1299–1303.

129 Mulder, C., Wahlund, L.O., Teerlink, T. et al. (2003). Decreased lysophosphatidylcholine/phosphatidylcholine ratio in cerebrospinal fluid in Alzheimer's disease. *J. Neural Transm. (Vienna)* 110: 949–955.

130 Fonteh, A.N., Chiang, J., Cipolla, M. et al. (2013). Alterations in cerebrospinal fluid glycerophospholipids and phospholipase A2 activity in Alzheimer's disease. *J. Lipid Res.* 54: 2884–2897.

131 Kosicek, M., Zetterberg, H., Andreasen, N. et al. (2012). Elevated cerebrospinal fluid sphingomyelin levels in prodromal Alzheimer's disease. *Neurosci. Lett.* 516: 302–305.

132 Verhey, F.R. and Visser, P.J. (2013). Use of cerebrospinal fluid (CSF) biomarkers for Alzheimer's type dementia: diagnosis in mild cognitive impairment. *Ned. Tijdschr. Geneeskd.* 157: A5596.

133 Engelborghs, S. (2013). Clinical indications for analysis of Alzheimer's disease CSF biomarkers. *Rev. Neurol. (Paris)* 169: 709–714.

134 Fourier, A., Portelius, E., Zetterberg, H. et al. (2015). Pre-analytical and analytical factors influencing Alzheimer's disease cerebrospinal fluid biomarker variability. *Clin. Chim. Acta* 449: 9–15.

135 Wang, H.L., Wang, Y.Y., Liu, X.G. et al. (2016). Cholesterol, 24-hydroxycholesterol, and 27-hydroxycholesterol as surrogate biomarkers in cerebrospinal fluid in mild cognitive impairment and Alzheimer's disease: a meta-analysis. *J. Alzheimers Dis.* 51: 45–55.

136 Henriksen, K., O'Bryant, S.E., Hampel, H. et al. (2014). The future of blood-based biomarkers for Alzheimer's disease. *Alzheimers Dement.* 10: 115–131.

137 Scheuner, D., Eckman, C., Jensen, M. et al. (1996). Secreted amyloid beta-protein similar to that in the senile plaques of Alzheimer's disease is increased in vivo by the presenilin 1 and 2 and APP mutations linked to familial Alzheimer's disease. *Nat. Med.* 2: 864–870.

138 Tamaoka, A., Fukushima, T., Sawamura, N. et al. (1996). Amyloid beta protein in plasma from patients with sporadic Alzheimer's disease. *J. Neurol. Sci.* 141: 65–68.

139 Fukumoto, H., Tennis, M., Locascio, J.J. et al. (2003). Age but not diagnosis is the main predictor of plasma amyloid beta-protein levels. *Arch. Neurol.* 60: 958–964.

140 Cosentino, S.A., Stern, Y., Sokolov, E. et al. (2010). Plasma ss-amyloid and cognitive decline. *Arch. Neurol.* 67: 1485–1490.

141 Assini, A., Cammarata, S., Vitali, A. et al. (2004). Plasma levels of amyloid beta-protein 42 are increased in women with mild cognitive impairment. *Neurology* 63: 828–831.

142 Graff-Radford, N.R., Crook, J.E., Lucas, J. et al. (2007). Association of low plasma Abeta42/Abeta40 ratios with increased imminent risk for mild cognitive impairment and Alzheimer disease. *Arch. Neurol.* 64: 354–362.

143 Koyama, A., Okereke, O.I., Yang, T. et al. (2012). Plasma amyloid-beta as a predictor of dementia and cognitive decline: a systematic review and meta-analysis. *Arch. Neurol.* 69: 824–831.

144 Lui, J.K., Laws, S.M., Li, Q.X. et al., Group AR (2010). Plasma amyloid-beta as a biomarker in Alzheimer's disease: the AIBL study of aging. *J. Alzheimers Dis.* 20: 1233–1242.

145 Devanand, D.P., Schupf, N., Stern, Y. et al. (2011). Plasma Abeta and PET PiB binding are inversely related in mild cognitive impairment. *Neurology* 77: 125–131.

146 Fei, M., Jianghua, W., Rujuan, M. et al. (2011). The relationship of plasma Abeta levels to dementia in aging individuals with mild cognitive impairment. *J. Neurol. Sci.* 305: 92–96.

147 Rembach, A., Watt, A.D., Wilson, W.J. et al., Group AR (2014). Plasma amyloid-beta levels are significantly associated with a transition toward Alzheimer's disease as measured by cognitive decline and change in neocortical amyloid burden. *J. Alzheimers Dis.* 40: 95–104.

148 Mapstone, M., Cheema, A.K., Fiandaca, M.S. et al. (2014). Plasma phospholipids identify antecedent memory impairment in older adults. *Nat. Med.* 20: 415–418.

149 Wang, M.J., Yi, S., Han, J.Y. et al. (2017). Oligomeric forms of amyloid-beta protein in plasma as a potential blood-based biomarker for Alzheimer's disease. *Alzheimers Res. Ther.* 9: 98.

150 Lauriola, M., Paroni, G., Ciccone, F. et al. (2017). Erythrocyte associated Amyloid-beta as potential biomarker to diagnose dementia. *Curr. Alzheimer Res.* 15: 381–385.

151 Ovod, V., Ramsey, K.N., Mawuenyega, K.G. et al. (2017). Amyloid beta concentrations and stable isotope labeling kinetics of human plasma specific to central nervous system amyloidosis. *Alzheimers Dement.* 13: 841–849.

152 Toledo, J.B., Shaw, L.M., and Trojanowski, J.Q. (2013). Plasma amyloid beta measurements - a desired but elusive Alzheimer's disease biomarker. *Alzheimers Res. Ther.* 5: 8.

153 Sutphen, C.L., Fagan, A.M., and Holtzman, D.M. (2014). Progress update: fluid and imaging biomarkers in Alzheimer's disease. *Biol. Psychiatry* 75: 520–526.

154 Forlenza, O.V., Diniz, B.S., Teixeira, A.L. et al. (2013). Mild cognitive impairment: Part 2: biological markers for diagnosis and prediction of dementia in Alzheimer's disease. *Rev. Bras. Psiquiatr.* 35: 284–294.

155 Burnham, S.C., Faux, N.G., Wilson, W. et al., Alzheimer's Disease Neuroimaging I, Australian Imaging B, Lifestyle Study Research G (2014). A blood-based predictor for neocortical Abeta burden in Alzheimer's disease: results from the AIBL study. *Mol. Psychiatry* 19: 519–526.

156 Ray, S., Britschgi, M., Herbert, C. et al. (2007). Classification and prediction of clinical Alzheimer's diagnosis based on plasma signaling proteins. *Nat. Med.* 13: 1359–1362.

157 Bjorkqvist, M., Ohlsson, M., Minthon, L., and Hansson, O. (2012). Evaluation of a previously suggested plasma biomarker panel to identify Alzheimer's disease. *PLoS One* 7: e29868.

158 Hu, W.T., Holtzman, D.M., Fagan, A.M. et al., Alzheimer's Disease Neuroimaging I (2012). Plasma multianalyte profiling in mild cognitive impairment and Alzheimer disease. *Neurology* 79: 897–905.

159 Roberts, R.O., Aakre, J.A., Cha, R.H. et al. (2015). Association of pancreatic polypeptide with mild cognitive impairment varies by APOE epsilon4 allele. *Front. Aging Neurosci.* 7: 172.

160 Mattsson, N., Andreasson, U., Zetterberg, H., and Blennow, K., Alzheimer's Disease Neuroimaging I (2017). Association of plasma neurofilament light with neurodegeneration in patients with Alzheimer disease. *JAMA Neurol.* 74: 557–566.

161 Rembach, A., Stingo, F.C., Peterson, C. et al., Group AR (2015). Bayesian graphical network analyses reveal complex biological interactions specific to Alzheimer's disease. *J. Alzheimers Dis.* 44: 917–925.

162 Saunders, A.M., Strittmatter, W.J., Schmechel, D. et al. (1993). Association of apolipoprotein E allele epsilon 4 with late-onset familial and sporadic Alzheimer's disease. *Neurology* 43: 1467–1472.

163 Hyman, B.T., Gomez-Isla, T., Rebeck, G.W. et al. (1996). Epidemiological, clinical, and neuropathological study of apolipoprotein E genotype in Alzheimer's disease. *Ann. N. Y. Acad. Sci.* 802: 1–5.

164 Lehtimaki, T., Pirttila, T., Mehta, P.D. et al. (1995). Apolipoprotein E (apoE) polymorphism and its influence on ApoE concentrations in the cerebrospinal fluid in Finnish patients with Alzheimer's disease. *Hum. Genet.* 95: 39–42.

165 Demeester, N., Castro, G., Desrumaux, C. et al. (2000). Characterization and functional studies of lipoproteins, lipid transfer proteins, and lecithin:cholesterol acyltransferase in CSF of normal individuals and patients with Alzheimer's disease. *J. Lipid Res.* 41: 963–974.

166 Gupta, V.B., Laws, S.M., Villemagne, V.L. et al., Group AR (2011). Plasma apolipoprotein E and Alzheimer disease risk: the AIBL study of aging. *Neurology* 76: 1091–1098.

167 Gupta, V.B., Wilson, A.C., Burnham, S. et al., Group AR (2015). Follow-up plasma apolipoprotein E levels in the Australian imaging, biomarkers and lifestyle flagship study of ageing (AIBL) cohort. *Alzheimers Res. Ther.* 7: 16.

168 Rasmussen, K.L., Tybjaerg-Hansen, A., Nordestgaard, B.G., and Frikke-Schmidt, R. (2015). Plasma levels of apolipoprotein E and risk of dementia in the general population. *Ann. Neurol.* 77: 301–311.

169 Teng, E., Chow, N., Hwang, K.S. et al., Alzheimer's Disease Neuroimaging I (2015). Low plasma ApoE levels are associated with smaller hippocampal size in the Alzheimer's disease neuroimaging initiative cohort. *Dement. Geriatr. Cogn. Disord.* 39: 154–166.

170 Jiang, Q., Lee, C.Y., Mandrekar, S. et al. (2008). ApoE promotes the proteolytic degradation of Abeta. *Neuron* 58: 681–693.

171 Song, F., Poljak, A., Crawford, J. et al. (2012). Plasma apolipoprotein levels are associated with cognitive status and decline in a community cohort of older individuals. *PLoS One* 7: e34078.

172 Muenchhoff, J., Song, F., Poljak, A. et al. (2017). Plasma apolipoproteins and physical and cognitive health in very old individuals. *Neurobiol. Aging* 55: 49–60.

173 Bertuzzi, M., Marelli, C., Bagnati, R. et al. (2015). Plasma clusterin as a candidate pre-diagnosis marker of colorectal cancer risk in the Florence cohort of the European Prospective Investigation into Cancer and Nutrition: a pilot study. *BMC Cancer* 15: 56.

174 Won, J.C., Park, C.Y., Oh, S.W. et al. (2014). Plasma clusterin (ApoJ) levels are associated with adiposity and systemic inflammation. *PLoS One* 9: e103351.

175 Hye, A., Riddoch-Contreras, J., Baird, A.L. et al. (2014). Plasma proteins predict conversion to dementia from prodromal disease. *Alzheimers Dement.* 10: 799–807e.2.

176 Leung, R., Proitsi, P., Simmons, A. et al. (2013). Inflammatory proteins in plasma are associated with severity of Alzheimer's disease. *PLoS One* 8: e64971.

177 Gupta, V.B., Doecke, J.D., Hone, E. et al., Group AR (2016). Plasma apolipoprotein J as a potential biomarker for Alzheimer's disease: Australian imaging, biomarkers and lifestyle study of aging. *Alzheimers Dement. (Amst)* 3: 18–26.

178 Gupta, V.B., Hone, E., Pedrini, S. et al., Group AR (2017). Altered levels of blood proteins in Alzheimer's disease longitudinal study: results from Australian imaging biomarkers lifestyle study of ageing cohort. *Alzheimers Dement. (Amst)* 8: 60–72.

179 Hsu, J.L., Lee, W.J., Liao, Y.C. et al. (2017). The clinical significance of plasma clusterin and Abeta in the longitudinal follow-up of patients with Alzheimer's disease. *Alzheimers Res. Ther.* 9: 91.

180 Bandaru, V.V. and Haughey, N.J. (2014). Quantitative detection of free 24S-hydroxycholesterol, and 27-hydroxycholesterol from human serum. *BMC Neurosci.* 15: 137.

181 Gonzalez-Dominguez, R., Garcia-Barrera, T., and Gomez-Ariza, J.L. (2014). Metabolomic study of lipids in serum for biomarker discovery in Alzheimer's disease using direct infusion mass spectrometry. *J. Pharm. Biomed. Anal.* 98: 321–326.

182 Cui, Y., Liu, X., Wang, M. et al. (2014). Lysophosphatidylcholine and amide as metabolites for detecting Alzheimer disease using ultrahigh-performance liquid chromatography-quadrupole time-of-flight mass spectrometry-based metabonomics. *J. Neuropathol. Exp. Neurol.* 73: 954–963.

183 Klavins, K., Koal, T., Dallmann, G. et al. (2015). The ratio of phosphatidylcholines to lysophosphatidylcholines in plasma differentiates healthy controls from patients with Alzheimer's disease and mild cognitive impairment. *Alzheimers Dement. (Amst)* 1: 295–302.

184 Casanova, R., Varma, S., Simpson, B. et al. (2016). Blood metabolite markers of preclinical Alzheimer's disease in two longitudinally followed cohorts of older individuals. *Alzheimers Dement.* 12: 815–822.

185 Chatterjee, P., Lim, W.L., Shui, G. et al. (2016). Plasma phospholipid and sphingolipid alterations in Presenilin1 mutation carriers: a pilot study. *J. Alzheimers Dis.* 50: 887–894.

186 Wood, P.L., Mankidy, R., Ritchie, S. et al. (2010). Circulating plasmalogen levels and Alzheimer disease assessment scale-cognitive scores in Alzheimer patients. *J. Psychiatry Neurosci.* 35: 59–62.

187 Jazvinscak Jembrek, M., Hof, P.R., and Simic, G. (2015). Ceramides in Alzheimer's disease: key mediators of neuronal apoptosis induced by oxidative stress and Abeta accumulation. *Oxid. Med. Cell. Longev.* 2015: 346783.

188 Mielke, M.M., Haughey, N.J., Bandaru, V.V. et al. (2010). Plasma ceramides are altered in mild cognitive impairment and predict cognitive decline and hippocampal volume loss. *Alzheimers Dement.* 6: 378–385.

189 Han, X., Rozen, S., Boyle, S.H. et al. (2011). Metabolomics in early Alzheimer's disease: identification of altered plasma sphingolipidome using shotgun lipidomics. *PLoS One* 6: e21643.

190 Mielke, M.M., Haughey, N.J., Bandaru, V.V. et al. (2011). Plasma sphingomyelins are associated with cognitive progression in Alzheimer's disease. *J. Alzheimers Dis.* 27: 259–269.

191 Mielke, M.M. and Haughey, N.J. (2012). Could plasma sphingolipids be diagnostic or prognostic biomarkers for Alzheimer's disease? *Clin. Lipidol.* 7: 525–536.

192 Costa, A.C., Joaquim, H.P.G., Forlenza, O. et al. (2017). Plasma lipids metabolism in mild cognitive impairment and Alzheimer's disease. *World J. Biol. Psychiatry* 1–7.

193 Swardfager, W., Yu, D., Scola, G. et al. (2017). Peripheral lipid oxidative stress markers are related to vascular risk factors and subcortical small vessel disease. *Neurobiol. Aging* 59: 91–97.

194 Proitsi, P., Kim, M., Whiley, L. et al. (2017). Association of blood lipids with Alzheimer's disease: a comprehensive lipidomics analysis. *Alzheimers Dement.* 13: 140–151.

195 Varma, V.R., Oommen, A.M., Varma, S. et al. (2018). Brain and blood metabolite signatures of pathology and progression in Alzheimer disease: a targeted metabolomics study. *PLoS Med* 15: e1002482.

196 Liu, Y., Li, N., Zhou, L. et al. (2014). Plasma metabolic profiling of mild cognitive impairment and Alzheimer's disease using liquid chromatography/mass spectrometry. *Cent. Nerv. Syst. Agents Med. Chem.* 14: 113–120.

197 Wang, G., Zhou, Y., Huang, F.J. et al. (2014). Plasma metabolite profiles of Alzheimer's disease and mild cognitive impairment. *J. Proteome Res.* 13: 2649–2658.

198 Trushina, E., Dutta, T., Persson, X.M. et al. (2013). Identification of altered metabolic pathways in plasma and CSF in mild cognitive impairment and Alzheimer's disease using metabolomics. *PLoS One* 8: e63644.

199 Gattaz, W.F., Forlenza, O.V., Talib, L.L. et al. (2004). Platelet phospholipase a(2) activity in Alzheimer's disease and mild cognitive impairment. *J. Neural Transm. (Vienna)* 111: 591–601.

200 Donovan, L.E., Dammer, E.B., Duong, D.M. et al. (2013). Exploring the potential of the platelet membrane proteome as a source of peripheral biomarkers for Alzheimer's disease. *Alzheimers Res. Ther.* 5: 32.

201 Veitinger, M., Oehler, R., Umlauf, E. et al. (2014). A platelet protein biochip rapidly detects an Alzheimer's disease-specific phenotype. *Acta Neuropathol.* 128: 665–677.

202 Veitinger, M., Varga, B., Guterres, S.B., and Zellner, M. (2014). Platelets, a reliable source for peripheral Alzheimer's disease biomarkers? *Acta Neuropathol. Commun.* 2: 65.

203 Tajeddinn, W., Fereshtehnejad, S.M., Seed Ahmed, M. et al. (2016). Association of platelet serotonin levels in Alzheimer's disease with clinical and cerebrospinal fluid markers. *J. Alzheimers Dis.* 53: 621–630.

204 Manzine, P.R., Marcello, E., Borroni, B. et al. (2015). ADAM10 gene expression in the blood cells of Alzheimer's disease patients and mild cognitive impairment subjects. *Biomarkers* 20: 196–201.

205 Oberacher, H., Arnhard, K., Linhart, C. et al. (2017). Targeted metabolomic analysis of soluble lysates from platelets of patients with mild cognitive impairment and Alzheimer's disease compared to healthy controls: is PC aeC40:4 a promising diagnostic tool? *J. Alzheimers Dis.* 57: 493–504.

206 O'Bryant, S.E., Gupta, V., Henriksen, K. et al., Star B, groups Bw (2015). Guidelines for the standardization of preanalytic variables for blood-based biomarker studies in Alzheimer's disease research. *Alzheimers Dement.* 11: 549–560.

207 Gatz, M., Reynolds, C.A., Fratiglioni, L. et al. (2006). Role of genes and environments for explaining Alzheimer disease. *Arch. Gen. Psychiatry* 63: 168–174.

208 Cosentino, S., Scarmeas, N., Helzner, E. et al. (2008). APOE epsilon 4 allele predicts faster cognitive decline in mild Alzheimer disease. *Neurology* 70: 1842–1849.

209 Lim, Y.Y., Villemagne, V.L., Laws, S.M. et al., Group AR (2014). Effect of BDNF Val66Met on memory decline and hippocampal atrophy in prodromal Alzheimer's disease: a preliminary study. *PLoS One* 9: e86498.

210 Wollam, M.E., Weinstein, A.M., Saxton, J.A. et al. (2015). Genetic risk score predicts late-life cognitive impairment. *J. Aging Res.* 2015: 267062.

211 Rodriguez-Rodriguez, E., Sanchez-Juan, P., Vazquez-Higuera, J.L. et al. (2013). Genetic risk score predicting accelerated progression from mild cognitive impairment to Alzheimer's disease. *J. Neural Transm. (Vienna)* 120: 807–812.

212 Hayden, K.M., Lutz, M.W., Kuchibhatla, M. et al. (2015). Effect of APOE and CD33 on cognitive decline. *PLoS One* 10: e0130419.

213 Guo, X., Qiu, W., Garcia-Milian, R. et al. (2017). Genome-wide significant, replicated and functional risk variants for Alzheimer's disease. *J. Neural Transm. (Vienna)* 124: 1455–1471.

214 Su, F., Bai, F., and Zhang, Z. (2016). Inflammatory cytokines and Alzheimer's disease: a review from the perspective of genetic polymorphisms. *Neurosci. Bull.* 32: 469–480.

215 Katz, B. and Rimmer, S. (1989). Ophthalmologic manifestations of Alzheimer's disease. *Surv. Ophthalmol.* 34: 31–43.

216 Laske, C., Sohrabi, H.R., Frost, S.M. et al. (2015). Innovative diagnostic tools for early detection of Alzheimer's disease. *Alzheimers Dement.* 11: 561–578.

217 Goldstein, L.E., Muffat, J.A., Cherny, R.A. et al. (2003). Cytosolic beta-amyloid deposition and supranuclear cataracts in lenses from people with Alzheimer's disease. *Lancet* 361: 1258–1265.

218 Koronyo-Hamaoui, M., Koronyo, Y., Ljubimov, A.V. et al. (2011). Identification of amyloid plaques in retinas from Alzheimer's patients and noninvasive in vivo optical imaging of retinal plaques in a mouse model. *Neuroimage* 54 (Suppl 1): S204–S217.

219 Dutescu, R.M., Li, Q.X., Crowston, J. et al. (2009). Amyloid precursor protein processing and retinal pathology in mouse models of Alzheimer's disease. *Graefes Arch. Clin. Exp. Ophthalmol.* 247: 1213–1221.

220 Melov, S., Wolf, N., Strozyk, D. et al. (2005). Mice transgenic for Alzheimer disease beta-amyloid develop lens cataracts that are rescued by antioxidant treatment. *Free Radic. Biol. Med.* 38: 258–261.

221 Kerbage, C., Sadowsky, C.H., Jennings, D. et al. (2013). Alzheimer's disease diagnosis by detecting exogenous fluorescent signal of ligand bound to Beta amyloid in the lens of human eye: an exploratory study. *Front. Neurol.* 4: 62.

222 Tian, T., Zhang, B., Jia, Y., and Li, Z. (2014). Promise and challenge: the lens model as a biomarker for early diagnosis of Alzheimer's disease. *Dis. Markers* 2014: 826503.

223 Kerbage, C., Sadowsky, C.H., Tariot, P.N. et al. (2015). Detection of amyloid beta signature in the Lens and its correlation in the brain to aid in the diagnosis of Alzheimer's disease. *Am. J. Alzheimers Dis. Other Demen.* 30: 738–745.

224 Shah, T.M., Gupta, S.M., Chatterjee, P. et al. (2017). Beta-amyloid sequelae in the eye: a critical review on its diagnostic significance and clinical relevance in Alzheimer's disease. *Mol. Psychiatry* 22: 353–363.

225 Frost, S., Kanagasingam, Y., Sohrabi, H. et al., Group AR (2013). Retinal vascular biomarkers for early detection and monitoring of Alzheimer's disease. *Transl. Psychiatry* 3: e233.

226 Williams, M.A., McGowan, A.J., Cardwell, C.R. et al. (2015). Retinal microvascular network attenuation in Alzheimer's disease. *Alzheimers Dement. (Amst)* 1: 229–235.

227 Fotiou, D.F., Brozou, C.G., Haidich, A.B. et al. (2007). Pupil reaction to light in Alzheimer's disease: evaluation of pupil size changes and mobility. *Aging Clin. Exp. Res.* 19: 364–371.

228 Frost, S., Kanagasingam, Y., Sohrabi, H. et al., Group AR (2013). Pupil response biomarkers for early detection and monitoring of Alzheimer's disease. *Curr. Alzheimer Res.* 10: 931–939.

229 de Jong, F.J., Schrijvers, E.M., Ikram, M.K. et al. (2011). Retinal vascular caliber and risk of dementia: the Rotterdam study. *Neurology* 76: 816–821.

230 Bittner, D.M., Wieseler, I., Wilhelm, H. et al. (2014). Repetitive pupil light reflex: potential marker in Alzheimer's disease? *J. Alzheimers Dis.* 42: 1469–1477.

231 Einarsdottir, A.B., Hardarson, S.H., Kristjansdottir, J.V. et al. (2016). Retinal oximetry imaging in Alzheimer's disease. *J. Alzheimers Dis.* 49: 79–83.

232 Coppola, G., Di Renzo, A., Ziccardi, L. et al. (2015). Optical coherence tomography in Alzheimer's disease: a meta-analysis. *PLoS One* 10: e0134750.

233 Casaletto, K.B., Ward, M.E., Baker, N.S. et al. (2017). Retinal thinning is uniquely associated with medial temporal lobe atrophy in neurologically normal older adults. *Neurobiol. Aging* 51: 141–147.

234 Golzan, S.M., Goozee, K., Georgevsky, D. et al. (2017). Retinal vascular and structural changes are associated with amyloid burden in the elderly: ophthalmic biomarkers of preclinical Alzheimer's disease. *Alzheimers Res. Ther.* 9: 13.

235 La Morgia, C., Di Vito, L., Carelli, V., and Carbonelli, M. (2017). Patterns of retinal ganglion cell damage in neurodegenerative disorders: parvocellular vs magnocellular degeneration in optical coherence tomography studies. *Front. Neurol.* 8: 710.

236 Javaid, F.Z., Brenton, J., Guo, L., and Cordeiro, M.F. (2016). Visual and ocular manifestations of Alzheimer's disease and their use as biomarkers for diagnosis and progression. *Front. Neurol.* 7: 55.

237 Vickers, K.C., Palmisano, B.T., Shoucri, B.M. et al. (2011). MicroRNAs are transported in plasma and delivered to recipient cells by high-density lipoproteins. *Nat. Cell Biol.* 13: 423–433.

238 Goodall, E.F., Heath, P.R., Bandmann, O. et al. (2013). Neuronal dark matter: the emerging role of microRNAs in neurodegeneration. *Front. Cell. Neurosci.* 7: 178.

239 Hebert, S.S., Horre, K., Nicolai, L. et al. (2008). Loss of microRNA cluster miR-29a/b-1 in sporadic Alzheimer's disease correlates with increased BACE1/beta-secretase expression. *Proc. Natl. Acad. Sci. U. S. A.* 105: 6415–6420.

240 Lei, X., Lei, L., Zhang, Z. et al. (2015). Downregulated miR-29c correlates with increased BACE1 expression in sporadic Alzheimer's disease. *Int. J. Clin. Exp. Pathol.* 8: 1565–1574.

241 Long, J.M., Ray, B., and Lahiri, D.K. (2014). MicroRNA-339-5p down-regulates protein expression of beta-site amyloid precursor protein-cleaving enzyme 1 (BACE1) in human primary brain cultures and is reduced in brain tissue specimens of Alzheimer disease subjects. *J. Biol. Chem.* 289: 5184–5198.

242 Femminella, G.D., Ferrara, N., and Rengo, G. (2015). The emerging role of microRNAs in Alzheimer's disease. *Front. Physiol.* 6: 40.

243 Cogswell, J.P., Ward, J., Taylor, I.A. et al. (2008). Identification of miRNA changes in Alzheimer's disease brain and CSF yields putative biomarkers and insights into disease pathways. *J. Alzheimers Dis.* 14: 27–41.

244 Denk, J., Boelmans, K., Siegismund, C. et al. (2015). MicroRNA profiling of CSF reveals potential biomarkers to detect Alzheimer's disease. *PLoS One* 10: e0126423.

245 Alexandrov, P.N., Dua, P., Hill, J.M. et al. (2012). microRNA (miRNA) speciation in Alzheimer's disease (AD) cerebrospinal fluid (CSF) and extracellular fluid (ECF). *Int. J. Biochem. Mol. Biol.* 3: 365–373.

246 Lukiw, W.J., Alexandrov, P.N., Zhao, Y. et al. (2012). Spreading of Alzheimer's disease inflammatory signaling through soluble micro-RNA. *Neuroreport* 23: 621–626.

247 Schipper, H.M., Maes, O.C., Chertkow, H.M., and Wang, E. (2007). MicroRNA expression in Alzheimer blood mononuclear cells. *Gene Regul. Syst. Bio.* 1: 263–274.

248 Geekiyanage, H., Jicha, G.A., Nelson, P.T., and Chan, C. (2012). Blood serum miRNA: non-invasive biomarkers for Alzheimer's disease. *Exp. Neurol.* 235: 491–496.

249 Tan, L., Yu, J.T., Liu, Q.Y. et al. (2014). Circulating miR-125b as a biomarker of Alzheimer's disease. *J. Neurol. Sci.* 336: 52–56.

250 Kiko, T., Nakagawa, K., Tsuduki, T. et al. (2014). MicroRNAs in plasma and cerebrospinal fluid as potential markers for Alzheimer's disease. *J. Alzheimers Dis.* 39: 253–259.

251 Galimberti, D., Villa, C., Fenoglio, C. et al. (2014). Circulating miRNAs as potential biomarkers in Alzheimer's disease. *J. Alzheimers Dis.* 42: 1261–1267.

252 Dong, H., Li, J., Huang, L. et al. (2015). Serum MicroRNA profiles serve as novel biomarkers for the diagnosis of Alzheimer's disease. *Dis. Markers* 2015: 625659.

253 Xie, B., Zhou, H., Zhang, R. et al. (2015). Serum miR-206 and miR-132 as potential circulating biomarkers for mild cognitive impairment. *J. Alzheimers Dis.* 45: 721–731.

254 Wu, H.Z., Ong, K.L., Seeher, K. et al. (2016). Circulating microRNAs as biomarkers of Alzheimer's disease: a systematic review. *J. Alzheimers Dis.* 49: 755–766.

255 Zhao, Y., Bhattacharjee, S., Dua, P. et al. (2015). microRNA-based biomarkers and the diagnosis of Alzheimer's disease. *Front. Neurol.* 6: 162.

256 Nagaraj, S., Laskowska-Kaszub, K., Debski, K.J. et al. (2017). Profile of 6 microRNA in blood plasma distinguish early stage Alzheimer's disease patients from non-demented subjects. *Oncotarget* 8: 16122–16143.

4

The Link Between Diabetes, Glucose Control, and Alzheimer's Disease and Neurodegenerative Diseases

Giuseppe Verdile[1,2,3], *Paul E. Fraser*[4] *and Ralph N. Martins*[1,2,3,5,6]

[1] School of Pharmacy and Biomedical Sciences, Faculty of Health Sciences, Curtin Health Innovation Research Institute, Curtin University, Bentley, WA, Australia
[2] Centre of Excellence for Alzheimer's Disease Research and Care, School of Medical and Health Sciences, Edith Cowan University, Joondalup, WA, Australia
[3] Australian Alzheimer's Research Foundation, Ralph and Patricia Sarich Neuroscience Research Institute, Nedlands, WA, Australia
[4] Tanz Centre for Research in Neurodegenerative Diseases, University of Toronto, Toronto, ON, Canada
[5] School of Psychiatry and Clinical Neurosciences, University of Western Australia, Perth, WA, Australia
[6] KaRa Institute of Neurological Diseases, Sydney, NSW, Australia

4.1 Introduction

In the last few decades, changes in lifestyle, especially related to over-nutrition and physical inactivity, together with ageing, have increased the global incidence of type 2 diabetes (T2D). According to the International Diabetes Federation (IDF), currently 387 million people around the world have diabetes mellitus, and this number is expected to reach 592 million by 2035. T2D is by far the most common form of diabetes, representing about 90–95% of diabetes cases. In older people (>65 years), the prevalence of T2D is 12–25%, and is characterised by cell and tissue insulin resistance, metabolic dysregulation, and chronic inflammation. Siegfried Hoyers first suggested the concept of disturbances in glucose metabolism and insulin resistance as underlying causes of neurodegeneration and dementia [1, 2], and such clinical abnormalities have been well documented in dementia cases [3, 4]. Epidemiological studies have more recently provided further evidence for this causative link, as T2D has been shown to be associated with accelerated cognitive decline and an increased risk of dementia (by 1.5–2-fold), and it has been suggested that 10% of cases of dementia worldwide may be attributable to the metabolic disturbances associated with T2D [5]. Moreover, cross-sectional and longitudinal studies have indicated that global brain atrophy is strongly associated with T2D, and that the rate of atrophy is greater than that seen in normal ageing [6, 7]. Recently, in the Framingham Heart Study it was reported that diabetes, and in particular the resulting hyperglycaemia, is associated with reduced cognitive performance and reduced brain grey matter volume in young to middle aged adults [8]. Collectively, the evidence indicates that metabolic changes associated with diabetes can potentially drive or exacerbate the early neurodegenerative processes in dementia. However, the molecular underpinnings of this relationship are both complex and poorly understood.

Neurodegeneration and Alzheimer's Disease: The Role of Diabetes, Genetics, Hormones, and Lifestyle,
First Edition. Edited by Ralph N. Martins, Charles S. Brennan, W.M.A.D. Binosha Fernando,
Margaret A. Brennan and Stephanie J. Fuller.
© 2019 John Wiley & Sons Ltd. Published 2019 by John Wiley & Sons Ltd.

In this chapter, we review the evidence of the impact of T2D on the brain that may contribute to cognitive decline and dementia, and discuss potential underlying mechanisms linking T2D with neurodegeneration. We also discuss the potential of therapeutics targeting T2D for preventing or slowing down the progression of AD.

4.2 The Impact of Type 2 Diabetes on the Brain

Following an intake of food, blood glucose levels rise, and insulin is released by pancreatic β-cells in response to this rise. Insulin elicits its anabolic effects via association with the transmembrane insulin receptor (IR) in target tissues. The interaction results in the autophosphorylation of the receptor and the recruitment and phosphorylation of insulin receptor substrate [9] proteins and activation of associated downstream signalling cascades, e.g. phosphatidylinositol-3-kinase (PI3K) and protein kinase B (Akt). Akt is an important regulator of translocation of GLUT4 vesicles to the plasma membrane, which is critical for the intracellular uptake of free glucose in insulin-sensitive tissues.

T2D, which typically develops in middle age (40–50), is characterised at early stages by insulin resistance, which refers to the failure of cells to respond to insulin and to activate signalling – this occurs in insulin-sensitive tissues such as the liver, skeletal muscle, and adipose tissue. Subsequently there is a reduction in uptake and utilisation of glucose in these tissues, resulting in elevated blood glucose concentrations. An increased burden is placed on pancreatic β-cells to produce and secrete more insulin in order to control elevating blood glucose levels. Although initially this compensatory mechanism may reduce glucose levels, persistent insulin resistance and continued exposure of β-cells to excess glucose and lipids promotes β-cell dysfunction, failure, and ultimately cell death, culminating in overt diabetes. In addition to hyperglycaemia, other metabolic disturbances such as hyperinsulinaemia, hypercholesterolaemia, and hyperlipidaemia feature in T2D, and all of these have detrimental effects on the brain.

It is well-known that T2D patients have poorer cognitive function and greater cognitive decline compared to non-T2D controls [5]. Furthermore, studies of the longitudinal impact of T2D on cognitive functioning and neurodegeneration are indicating common metabolic disturbances and causal relationships between T2D and neurodegenerative diseases, particularly AD, yet these relationships remain poorly understood.

Early studies found that AD patients are typically hyperinsulinaemic and that they have concomitant reduced insulin sensitivity, both in fasting states and during glucose tolerance tests [3]. Despite increased plasma insulin levels, cerebrospinal fluid (CSF) insulin levels have been shown to be reduced in AD patients [10]. Initially it was suggested that deficiencies in brain insulin signalling are a consequence of reduced insulin uptake into the brain. However, this is complicated by the evidence that the brain can also produce its own insulin. It is also understood that brain insulin contributes to the control of nutrient homeostasis, reproduction, cognition, and memory; brain insulin also has neurotrophic, neuromodulatory, and neuroprotective effects, indicating that disruptions to insulin levels in the brain may lead to many metabolic and neuronal impairments [11]. Changes to brain insulin uptake may nevertheless be an early event in the disease process, as reduced CSF insulin levels are observed in mild AD and mildly cognitively impaired (MCI) patients [12]. It is well understood that high fat/high sugar diets increase the likelihood of metabolic syndrome, insulin resistance, and T2D; similarly, a high saturated fat and high glycaemic diet also lowers CSF insulin levels in healthy adults [13].

Insulin signalling abnormalities have been implicated in the pathogenesis of AD, as studies have shown that raising plasma insulin to levels found in patients with insulin resistance causes an increase in Aβ levels as well as levels of inflammatory agents in the brain [14]. It is also known that glucose homeostasis is critical for energy generation, neuronal maintenance, neurogenesis, neurotransmitter regulation, cell survival, and synaptic plasticity in the brain [15]. If chronic peripheral hyperinsulinaemia causes lower brain levels of insulin due to lower transport across the blood–brain barrier (BBB), this would disrupt glucose homeostasis, promoting neurodegeneration.

Structural and functional imaging studies have provided evidence that neurodegeneration occurs in diabetic brains. For example, structural magnetic resonance imaging (MRI) studies have shown that T2D is strongly associated with brain atrophy [7]. Longitudinal case control studies have suggested that the rate of global brain atrophy in T2D is up to three times faster than in normal ageing [6, 16], suggesting that T2D accelerates neurodegeneration. Long-term T2D may also be particularly harmful to the brain, as a study showed that individuals who'd had insulin resistance and diabetes longer exhibited smaller brain volumes compared to controls and those at earlier stages of insulin resistance [17]. Both grey and white matter loss have been observed in T2D, indicating loss of brain connectivity [5], most likely contributing to associated cognitive impairment. Grey matter volume changes have also been shown to correlate with insulin resistance in healthy controls as well as AD cases [18]. In other studies, whole-brain connectivity patterns using diffusion tensor imaging have shown reductions in connectivity in type 2 diabetics compared to age-matched controls, and that this was associated with slower processing speeds [19]. Although cerebrovascular lesions and brain atrophy (and thus reduced connectivity) are both thought to mediate the relationship between T2D and cognitive impairment, a cross-sectional study of individuals with and without T2D revealed that, although infarcts were by themselves associated with poorer cognition, brain atrophy was the predominant change linked to cognition at earlier stages of the disease [7]. Whether the combination of vascular and neurodegenerative processes accelerate dementia remains to be determined.

Earlier chapters have described how new brain imaging methods have shown that the Aβ amyloid deposition characteristic of AD develops many years before symptoms appear. Furthermore, it is well known that AD is associated with low brain glucose usage, in a brain region-specific manner. However, some recent imaging studies of cerebral glucose metabolism (^{18}F-deoxyglucose–positron emission tomography: FDG-PET) and amyloid deposition (e.g. ^{11}C-Pittsburg compound B-positron emission tomography: PiB-PET) have produced conflicting results. A recent cross-sectional study using PiB-PET and FDG-PET imaging in the population-based Mayo Clinic Study of Aging [20] showed that, compared to healthy aged controls, aged people with T2D displayed cerebral hypo-metabolism. This result was expected; however, the study showed no differences in neocortical amyloid load, suggesting that the hypo-metabolism in T2D was occurring independent of amyloid deposition. On the other hand, the authors also found that there was a greater association between hypo-metabolism and diabetes in MCI diabetic patients suggesting that this indicator of neuronal injury may be a better determinant (than amyloid deposition) of developing cognitive deficits. This notion was further supported by findings from the Baltimore Longitudinal Study of Aging, where no association was observed between measures of peripheral insulin resistance or glucose homeostasis and neocortical amyloid load [21]. This has been suggested to be due to the fact that the cognitive deficits that can occur in T2D are not always due to developing AD. More recently in the Alzheimer's Disease Neuroimaging Initiative (ADNI) study, no association was shown between T2D and accumulation of neocortical Aβ-amyloid load (PiB-PET) or increases in CSF Aβ42 [22]. Instead, T2D was associated with lower cortical thickness, and an increase in CSF total tau (t-tau) and phosphorylated tau (p-tau). therefore a relationship may occur with other hallmarks of AD. In recent findings from our own studies, we provided further evidence for this relationship in another large well-characterised cohort, the Australian Imaging Biomarker and Lifestyle (AIBL) study [26]. Together, these findings suggest that insulin resistance/T2D is not associated with cerebral accumulation of Aβ-amyloid, but with other hallmarks of the disease.

In related studies, it has been argued that accelerated amyloid deposition may be a feature in type 2 diabetics. For example, in a study undertaken by Wu et al., (2012) amyloid deposition was shown to increase from healthy control levels to early MCI to late MCI, yet glucose utilisation (as measured by FDG-PET) only started to decrease at the late MCI stage, providing evidence that brain metabolism can be normal despite the presence of a significant level of amyloid – a level which usually suggests the presence of significant other AD-related pathogenesis [23]. More recently, higher peripheral insulin resistance (as measured by HOMA-IR) was found to correlate with greater levels of neocortical amyloid load in late-middle-aged, normoglycaemic, non-diabetic, and cognitively normal participants. In the latest study by the same group, cerebral hypometabolism was found to associated with insulin resistance in AD, though hypermetabolism was shown to be associated with insulin resistance in MCI participants [24]. In a more recent study, participants with a parental history of dementia due to AD were recruited from the Wisconsin Alzheimer's Disease Research Center (ADRC), investigating memory in people at risk, causes and treatments (IMPACT) [25]. The study investigated the association between insulin resistance and CSF/AD-related biomarkers including Aβ42, CSF sAPPα/sAPPβ (secreted forms of APP – the amyloid-β precursor protein), and CSF p-tau, and it was shown that increases in HOMA-IR (insulin resistance) were associated with increased CSF levels of sAPPβ (not sAPPα), and there was a modest association with CSF Aβ42. These findings are consistent with insulin resistance promoting amyloidogenic processing of APP. Whether similar associations exist between insulin resistance and PiB-PET load was not assessed, but the findings were consistent with those observed in the group's previous study. However, more recently our own results in the AIBL study have shown that increases in insulin resistance are associated with reductions in cognitive functioning and increases in CSF-tau and CSF-p-tau, and no significant associations with neocortical amyloid load were detected [26]. Our results are more in line with those from ADNI [22]. In our study, we also show that associations appears to be stronger in females. This finding warrants further exploration but is in line with meta-analyses which have suggested that sex mediates T2D associations with dementias and associated co-morbidities, such as stroke, where women are at higher risk [27–29].

From these imaging/biomarker studies, there is yet to be a coherent story on the effects of insulin resistance on indices of neuronal functioning and AD pathology. Sex, age, and family history may all play a role in the different findings observed in the various studies.

One explanation for these results could also be that, in earlier stages of insulin resistance, any developing AD neuropathology is in early pre-clinical stages; then with growing severity of insulin resistance and development of T2D, cerebral hypometabolism and neuronal dysfunction become more prominent. The results are possibly complicated by the age at which insulin resistance develops, with its associated chronic inflammation and oxidative stress, as this may determine whether T2D and AD are co-morbidities or whether T2D may be accelerating AD development. Larger, longitudinal studies of ageing are required to characterise the impact of insulin resistance and T2D on the brain.

Recent evidence suggests that increases in fasting blood glucose are associated with reductions in brain grey matter and hippocampal volume, as well as with impaired attention and memory in young and middle-aged adults [8]. A graded association was observed between fasting blood glucose levels in normal, pre-diabetic and diabetic ranges and measures of brain atrophy. This has clinical relevance as these studies suggest that even at an early stage of diabetes (or pre-diabetes), increases in blood glucose levels have already led to detrimental effects on memory, hippocampal integrity, and regional brain volumes. Unfortunately, results from other studies that have assessed improvements in memory following glycaemic control in the elderly have suggested that such changes may be irreversible. For example, in the ACCORD memory study of elderly patients with T2D, intensive glycaemic control showed a small difference in brain volume, but no evidence of cognitive improvement, and furthermore the targeted treatment was associated with increased mortality [9]. Taken together, these studies demonstrate that age, duration, and severity of pathology impact on the effects of diabetes on the brain and that treatment in late life may not be as effective as preventative strategies that can be implemented at a young age.

4.3 Evidence from Cell Culture, Animal, and Clinical Studies

Cell culture and *in vivo* studies have suggested that the early accumulation of Aβ promotes central nervous system (CNS) insulin resistance, and conversely, insulin resistance has also been shown to promote Aβ accumulation, deposition, and the progression of neurodegeneration in AD. High Aβ levels and insulin resistance both lead to neuronal injury via inflammatory and oxidative stress processes. The interplay between these processes, Aβ deposition, and cerebral insulin resistance is discussed further below.

4.3.1 CNS Insulin Signalling and Disruptions in AD

The brain is now recognised to be a major target for insulin, and insulin signalling is important for neuronal function and survival. Insulin can enter the brain through a receptor-based saturable transporter that is largely saturated by peripheral insulin levels [30–32]. There is evidence that an acute increase in peripheral insulin levels can lead to higher CSF insulin, whereas chronic peripheral hyperinsulinaemia, such as that which occurs in insulin resistance, downregulates IR expression at the BBB, and therefore reduces insulin transport into the brain [33]. As mentioned earlier, insulin can also be produced by neurons, although it has been suggested this may be limited to neuronal progenitor cells [34]. Early studies showed that insulin can act on the hypothalamus, regulating brain metabolism and body energy balance [35–37]; however, more recently, insulin signalling has been recognised to be important for neuronal function in other brain regions, including the hippocampus. Insulin action is also required for neuronal synaptic plasticity, and it facilitates learning and memory [38–40]. Furthermore, insulin has been shown to promote dendritic spine and synapse formation, neuronal stem cell activation, general cell growth and repair, and neuroprotection [41–44]. Due to these widespread effects of insulin, it is clear that disruptions to insulin levels or insulin signalling in the brain will contribute to neuronal dysfunction and degeneration.

Studies of post-mortem brains have shown that neocortical levels of insulin and binding to IR are reduced with age; these changes have also been shown in the AD brain [45]. Subsequent studies comparing AD and healthy control brains have shown reduced gene and protein expression of insulin, IR, insulin signalling molecules, reduced levels of IR insulin binding, and increased phosphorylation of insulin receptor substrate-1 (IRS1) in AD [4, 46–48]. These findings are consistent with the concept that the inhibition of downstream insulin signalling events ultimately results in disruption of neuronal functioning. Importantly, these changes in insulin signalling can be seen in the brains of pre-clinical AD subjects, several years before the onset of clinical symptoms [49], indicating that it is an early event in the disease progression.

4.3.2 The Accumulation of Aβ Is Associated with Impaired Insulin Signalling

It is well known that small Aβ aggregates (oligomers) are major contributors to synaptotoxicity and the neurodegenerative processes in AD (for a recent review see [50]). Evidence over the last decade has suggested that Aβ-induced neurotoxicity may be at least partly mediated through its effects on insulin signalling. Aβ has been shown to interfere directly with insulin receptor signalling by inhibiting autophosphorylation of the receptor [51], and Aβ oligomers have been shown to markedly reduce IR levels and IR activity at the cell surface of hippocampal neuron dendrites [52]. Insulin receptor loss occurs prior to dendritic and synaptic deterioration, and cell culture studies have shown that this IR loss can be completely prevented by administering insulin [53]. This added insulin was also found to protect against Aβ-induced oxidative stress and synaptic spine deterioration, and at submaximal doses of insulin, the diabetes drug rosiglitazone could potentiate the effect. Furthermore, it has been shown that serine phosphorylation of IRS-1 (IRS-1pSer) is common to both AD and T2D, and another anti-diabetes agent, exenatide, has been shown in an AD transgenic mouse model to reduce levels of IRS-1pSer and also reduce c-Jun N-terminal kinase (JNK) activation [54]. Reducing JNK activation is important for reducing AD pathogenesis, as downstream effects of JNK activation include the promotion of tau phosphorylation and inflammatory processes [48, 55–57].

Neurotransmission via the N-methyl-D aspartate receptor (NMDAR) can also be influenced by glucose levels and insulin signalling, in fact there is evidence of cross-talk between insulin receptor signalling and NMDAR signalling. For example, it has been shown that the Aβ oligomeric inhibition of IR is prevented by the NMDAR blocker memantine (used clinically to increase neurotransmission in AD patients, and recent studies have shown that elevated glucose and oligomeric Aβ both disrupt synapses via aberrant protein S-nitrosylation – an effect attenuated by memantine [52]. This followed earlier studies which showed that Aβ-induced NMDAR activation and

Aβ-induced excessive calcium influx [58–61] can stimulate phosphorylation of IRS-1, resulting in the down-regulation of insulin signalling.

4.3.3 Insulin Resistance Promotes the Accumulation of Aβ

The accumulation of Aβ in the brain can result from its overproduction or the impaired removal from the brain. In studies of AD mouse models, high-fat diets that promote obesity and diabetes also promote Aβ accumulation. This can occur through increasing levels of key enzymes that generate Aβ (beta-site APP cleaving enzyme [BACE1] and γ-secretase) [62], through up-regulating autophagosome formation [63] which are known Aβ-generating vesicles, or through hindering the removal of Aβ from the brain.

Impairments in Aβ degradation and/or clearance pathways provide a major mechanism by which Aβ accumulates in the AD brain, particularly in sporadic cases (recently reviewed in [64]). Insulin-degrading enzyme (IDE) can degrade Aβ, and has been shown to be a primary regulator of not only insulin but also Aβ levels [65–67]. The overexpression of IDE in AD mouse models results in a reduction in both amyloid deposition and soluble Aβ levels [68], whilst the depletion of IDE promotes Aβ accumulation [69, 70]. In cell culture studies, the breakdown of Aβ is inhibited by the addition of insulin to media, highlighting the competition between insulin and Aβ for IDE, and showing IDE's preference for insulin [71]. Compared to levels found in brains from control subjects, IDE expression is reduced in AD and MCI brains, providing further support that inadequate IDE expression or activity contributes to promoting AD pathology [65, 72–75]. The study by Zhao et al. showed that levels of IDE continued to reduce during the progression from MCI to AD, and that the IDE levels were inversely correlated with brain Aβ42 levels, supporting the concept that a drop in IDE levels is an early pathological change in AD.

A recent study of AD model mice has provided evidence that T2D may influence Aβ accumulation by both modulating Aβ production and impairing its clearance. The 3xTg-AD mice, which develop peripheral glucose intolerance, were found to have this intolerance enhanced when fed a high-fat diet, the mice also developed pancreatic β-cell degeneration and impaired insulin production. The high-fat diet also caused an increase in brain soluble Aβ levels and memory impairment [62]. The authors found no changes in expression levels of Aβ degrading enzymes (IDE or neprilysin) or low-density lipoprotein (LDL)-receptor-related protein 1 and RAGE (the receptor for advanced glycation end-products), proteins involved in the influx/efflux of Aβ across the BBB. Administering insulin to these mice led to reduced cerebral Aβ levels, reduced levels of BACE1, and increased levels of sAPPα, overall indicating a reduction in Aβ production, possibly due to a shift to the non-amyloidogenic APP breakdown pathway. However, reductions in brain Aβ levels were associated with concomitant increases in blood Aβ levels, leading to the authors concluding that a combination of mechanisms of both reducing Aβ production as well as enhancing clearance into the periphery from the brain underlies insulin's benefits in reversing AD pathology in the mice. Given that the authors found no changes in Aβ degrading enzymes or lipoprotein receptor-related protein-1 (LRP-1)/RAGE, it is unclear how insulin facilitates the transport of Aβ into the blood. It is possible that there is a role for other Aβ transporters including ApoE or ApoJ in this clearance, and future studies could explore this aspect. Although an artificial model of AD, it is interesting that the mouse AD model develops signs of T2D, which are exacerbated by a high–fat diet, as it underscores the strong links between the development of AD and T2D.

4.3.4 Impairments in Insulin Signalling Can Induce Hyperphosphorylation of Tau

There is evidence that deficiencies in insulin signalling can exacerbate neurodegeneration by enhancing the phosphorylation of tau. In AD and other dementias, the hyperphosphorylation of the microtubule associated protein tau to form neurofibrillary tangles (NFT) is an important pathological hallmark, and small aggregates of hyperphosphorylated tau are considered to contribute to neuronal dysfunction and degeneration in AD [76]; in fact NFT levels correlate better with the severity of clinical symptoms than amyloid plaque levels.

Glycogen synthase kinase-3β (GSK-3β) is a key kinase that phosphorylates tau. Its activity is modulated via the serine/threonine kinase Akt. As mentioned earlier, insulin action triggers a complex signalling cascade, leading to the activation of Akt and the downstream inhibition of GSK-3β. Deficiencies or impairments in brain insulin signalling lead to a reduction in Akt activity [56, 57] and Wnt/β-catenin signalling [77], resulting in increases in GSK-3β activity, and promoting the hyperphosphorylation of tau, which eventually results in the misfolding and formation of tau fibrils [78]. Insulin can also regulate tau expression, and a reduction in insulin signalling can result in impaired tau gene expression [56, 57]. This can lead to reduced levels of normal soluble tau whilst levels of hyperphosphorylated tau are rising, exacerbating neuronal cytoskeletal collapse, neurite retraction, and impairments in synapse formation.

The above studies suggest that the onset of insulin resistance and subsequent impaired insulin signalling promote AD pathology. A recent study, however, argues that elevated glucose levels may be the early event that can accelerate AD pathogenesis. To attempt to tease out the effects of elevated blood glucose levels independent of insulin resistance, this recent study combined glucose clamps and *in vivo* microdialysis to assess changes in AD transgenic mice during a hyperglycaemic challenge [79]. The authors found that increased blood glucose levels as a result of the clamp were associated with increased Aβ levels in the interstitial fluid (ISF) in young mice, an effect which persisted after euglycemia was restored. Whilst total Aβ load in the brain did not change, hippocampal metabolism and neuronal activity was reduced. This effect was exacerbated in older mice with established plaque pathology, indicating that age and pathology may influence the brain's response to the metabolic insults. The study also suggests that repeated exposures to acute hyperglycaemia can promote Aβ accumulation, as well as alter hippocampal and neuronal functioning early in the disease process.

4.3.5 Type 2 Diabetes and Neuroinflammation

Chronic inflammation features in the pathogenesis of both T2D and the neurodegeneration seen in AD. For example, in obesity, which is often a precursor to T2D, the secretion of chemo-attractants such as monocyte chemo-attractant protein-1 (MCP-1) and macrophage migration inhibitory factor (MIF); as well as the cytokines interleukin-6 (IL-6), tumour necrosis factor-α (TNFα), and IL-1β, attracts immune cells such as macrophages, dendritic cells, and T-cells to accumulate in adipose tissue. This in turn can increase peripheral lipid, by reducing lipid lipase activity (effectively increasing lipid levels) or by increasing the production of non-esterified free fatty acids. A feedback loop of pro-inflammatory cytokines exacerbates this pathological development, driving further immune cell infiltration and cytokine secretion and disrupting the insulin signalling cascade [80]. In combination with insulin resistance, which reduces the uptake of glucose and fatty acids due to impaired insulin signalling, such changes help promote the T2D phenotype. In fact, TNFα signalling can lead to serine phosphorylation of IRS-1 by kinases, thereby blocking the intracellular actions of insulin [81–83]. In support of this, antibody-mediated blocking of TNFα signalling has been shown to improve insulin sensitivity in peripheral tissues, and help restore glucose homeostasis [84, 85].

Chronic inflammation also appears to be important in early stages of AD [86] and there is much evidence that the metabolic changes seen in T2D can promote CNS inflammation. For example, a number of studies have shown that hyperinsulinaemia can promote inflammatory responses in the CNS [87–89] by increasing the production of the same pro-inflammatory cytokines, IL-1β, TNFα, and IL-6 mentioned above [87, 89–91]. Aβ oligomers can also induce the secretion of pro-inflammatory cytokines through activating microglia, and thus similarly leading to the phosphorylation of IRS-1 and the blocking of insulin signalling [48, 54, 92]. As mentioned above, the cytokine-mediated inhibition of insulin signalling can be blocked by administering TNFα antibodies [84]. Pro-inflammatory cytokines can also cross the BBB and inhibit insulin signalling when cerebral vascular tissue is damaged [93]. Furthermore, inflammation can be mediated by RAGE. In T2D and AD, increased RAGE levels have been proposed to contribute to vascular dysfunction [94, 95]. Aβ can cross the BBB via RAGE, increase the level of cerebrovascular dysfunction, and induce the generation of TNFα and IL-6, contributing further to neurodegeneration [96]. In addition, activated macrophages have been found to be a source of advanced glycation end products (AGE), and AGE-albumin in particular, which is excreted by macrophages, has been implicated in AD and T2D as well as other chronic degenerative diseases. Advanced glycation end-products are not only linked to RAGE signalling and inflammation, but to various hallmarks of the ageing process. Recently, anti-inflammatory molecules that inhibit AGE have been shown to be good candidates for reducing diabetic complications as well as pathogenic changes seen in other degenerative diseases [97, 98].

4.3.6 Oxidative Stress and Mitochondrial Dysfunction in T2D and AD

Numerous studies have shown that oxidative stress plays a major role in neurodegeneration, and is thought to occur early in AD pathogenesis [99–101]. Oxidised lipids, proteins, and DNA are present in AD brains, at levels higher than those found in aged-matched control brains [101]. For example, high levels of lipid peroxidation can be detected in the temporal cortex [102] and it has been shown that levels of lipid peroxidation markers such as 4-hydroxynonenal and malondialdehyde correlate with levels of amyloid deposition in AD brains [103].

Furthermore, proteomic studies of brain tissue have revealed that key enzymes involved in metabolic pathways (i.e. glycolysis) are oxidised in AD, MCI, and pre-clinical AD brains [104–106]. The oxidation of these enzymes, partly caused by excessive generation or reduced removal of reactive oxygen species (ROS), correlates with reductions in cerebral glucose metabolism in AD and MCI [107], thereby impairing neural glucose homeostasis and neuronal functions. Many studies have demonstrated Aβ1-42 induces oxidative stress in the brain, as well as iron-induced oxidative stress in AD; other studies have provided evidence of roles for the superoxide anion, hydroxyl radical, hydrogen peroxide, and nitric oxide in the oxidative stress-mediated neurodegeneration in AD [108]. The fact that increases in Aβ1-42 levels (due to increased production and/or reduced clearance) induce oxidative stress, leading to increased ROS production, and that oxidative stress and ROS production in turn causes greater Aβ1-42 production, leads to a vicious cycle that exacerbates neurodegenerative changes in AD.

Oxidative changes also occur in T2D patients compared to healthy controls, there are increases in protein oxidation and reductions in free radical scavenging capacity, deficits in antioxidant defence enzymes and increases in lipid peroxidation [109]. The oxidative stress processes associated with both pathologies may represent the major underlying link between T2D and AD. Indeed, the progressive worsening of insulin resistance during AD pathogenesis correlates with increased oxidative stress, DNA damage, and protein oxidation [104]. This gives further support to the theory that, in the presence of insulin resistance and reduced glucose utilisation, a vicious cycle involving greater oxidative stress can be established, resulting in the progression of neurodegeneration.

Mitochondria play an important role in energy metabolism and oxidative stress processes since they are major sites for generating ATP (energy), ROS, and endogenous antioxidants. Processes that occur in the mitochondrial matrix leading to energy production include oxidative phosphorylation, fatty acid oxidation, and the citric acid cycle; other processes include haem production and the urea cycle. Functions within a mitochondrial unit clearly need to be tightly regulated and integrated, thus many signalling mechanisms are required to help with such regulation. In an ageing brain as well as in neurodegeneration, a decrease in mitochondrial energy-transducing capacity is often seen, and this is associated with a progressive increase in steady state levels of H_2O_2 and other ROS (i.e. nitric oxide), causing a cell to shift from a reduced state to an oxidised state, where amino acids of susceptible proteins are oxidatively modified (for review see [110]).

With such important roles for mitochondria in energy (ATP) production, ROS homeostasis, and the production of endogenous antioxidants, it is not surprising that mitochondrial dysfunction features, and features early, in a number of degenerative diseases, including AD and T2D. It has been suggested that the impaired mitochondrial oxidative capacity of cells is one of the main underlying causes of insulin resistance and T2D [111]. However, whether mitochondrial dysfunction is a cause or consequence of insulin resistance is still not clear [111]. Interestingly, mitochondrial autophagy itself serves as a major source of ROS production [112].

As approximately 90% of the ATP required for normal neuronal functioning is derived from neuronal mitochondria, impairments in mitochondrial structure or function would be likely to contribute significantly to neurodegeneration. In fact, there is increasing evidence that mitochondrial defects are a key and early feature of several neurodegenerative disorders including AD. Indeed, mitochondrial dysfunction has been detected in AD post-mortem brain, platelets from AD patients, brain tissue from AD mice, and cell culture models (reviewed in [113]). Mitochondrial metabolic dysfunction has been suggested to be an early event in the disease process, as changes in mitochondrial function have been detected prior to significant brain Aβ ('plaque') accumulation; with changes including reductions in mitochondrial enzyme activity (promoting oxidative phosphorylation and ROS generation), increases in oxidative stress, and reduced mitochondrial respiratory efficiency [114]. Indeed, increasing evidence indicates that age-related impairments in mitochondrial function represent a driving force of increased oxidative stress and progression of neurodegeneration in AD [115].

There is also evidence to suggest that insulin resistance and impairments in insulin signalling could be early events which promote mitochondrial dysfunction. Intra-cerebroventricular injection of streptozotocin (STZ, known to be toxic to insulin-producing pancreatic β-cells) into rat brain causes decreases in insulin and IR mRNA levels in frontoparietal cerebral cortex and hippocampal regions, as well as changes in downstream tyrosine kinase activities, inducing an insulin-resistant brain state [116]. More recently, these STZ-induced insulin signalling changes have been shown to be accompanied by mitochondrial abnormalities [117]. Other studies have reported that high-fat diets cause increased mitochondrial ROS production and oxidative stress in skeletal muscle, resulting in peripheral insulin resistance [118]. In a recent study of normal rats and rats with a diabetic phenotype (through pancreatectomy), it was shown that Aβ25-35 administered directly to the hippocampus caused reductions of around 20% in energy intake, and increases in carbohydrate oxidation and energy expenditure of approximately 10%, regardless of the diabetic status of the rats [119]. Furthermore, the Aβ-injected rats with induced diabetes had exacerbated memory impairments. These studies provide evidence that the concurrent development of AD pathology and diabetes-related metabolic changes can be additive with respect to symptoms.

4.3.7 Targeting Type 2 Diabetes to Slow Down Progression/Prevent Neurodegeneration and Cognitive Decline

As discussed in detail in this chapter, insulin resistance, glucose dyshomeostasis and associated impairments in insulin signalling in the brain contribute to AD pathology and neurodegeneration. Thus it stands to reason that improving neuronal insulin sensitivity or restoring glucose homeostasis and targeting insulin signalling are appropriate approaches for developing therapeutics for neurodegenerative diseases such as AD. As discussed in other chapters, this can be achieved through changes in lifestyle (diet and exercise) that can control/slow down the progression of T2D as well as have benefits in protecting against neurodegeneration. However, there is also growing interest in evaluating anti-diabetic medications for potential benefits in slowing down or preventing neurodegeneration. Insulin sensitisers, drugs that stimulate insulin production and improve insulin signalling, and insulin itself, have shown the most promise.

One of the most commonly prescribed drugs for T2D is the insulin sensitiser metformin. This drug can cross the BBB [120, 121]; and its ability to reduce tau phosphorylation [122] and more recently its ability to enhance neurogenesis [123] suggest that it may have neuroprotective actions. Indeed, metformin has been shown to attenuate cognition and AD-like pathology in obese mice. However, evidence for similar benefits of metformin in AD transgenic mouse models is lacking, and there is evidence from clinical studies that metformin usage is associated with a slight increase in risk of AD [124], worsening of cognitive performance in diabetics [125], and worse spatial memory and visual acuity in old male mice [126].

Other insulin sensitisers that have shown more promise than metformin are the thiazolidinediones (TZD), rosiglitazone and pioglitazone. *In vivo* studies have shown efficacy of TZD in attenuating AD pathology by inhibiting inflammatory gene expression, altering Aβ homeostasis, and exhibiting other neuroprotective effects [15, 127, 128]. Rosiglitazone showed promise in small early phase trials, as treatment (4 mg d^{-1} rosiglitazone) for six months of mild AD or amnestic MCI participants resulted in improved memory and the modulation of plasma Aβ levels, compared to placebo [129]. These benefits, however, were not observed in larger phase 3 trials with participants on a lower dose (2 mg d^{-1}) [130]. Compared to other TZD, rosiglitazone has only modest BBB penetration properties, and can be actively transported out of the brain [131], thus using the lower dose in the phase 3 trial may have reduced its insulin-sensitising effect in the brain. This failure in trials and its associated adverse effects, have led to the withdrawal of rosiglitazone as an AD therapeutic.

The other insulin sensitiser is pioglitazone. Although most recent data has suggested that pioglitazone reduces the incidence of dementia [132], trials have produced mixed results. In initial 6-month pilot studies, pioglitazone-treated AD participants showed improved cognition and cerebral blood flow compared to placebo treated participants [133]; whereas in a longer 18-month placebo-controlled, randomised trial, it was found that overall, pioglitazone treatment was well tolerated by participants, yet had no significant benefits on cognition [134]. The authors of this latter study stated that the study was not intended to assess efficacy, and suggested that the severity of AD impacted on beneficial cognitive outcomes. This has been true for most drugs that have been trialled in cohorts of AD patients: most studies have reported no significant benefits after onset of the disease. This has prompted trials on patients at an earlier stage that is widely considered pre-AD: amnestic MCI. However, at this stage, clinical symptoms can nonetheless be considered to have commenced, and brain pathology would already be quite extensive, therefore potential treatments may still not offer significant benefits. This is one of the many reasons for the intensive research to identify biomarkers for pre-clinical diagnosis of the disease, or biomarkers to identify subjects most likely to progress to cognitive decline and AD, as treatment at very early pathogenic stages may be necessary to slow disease progression significantly. One trial implementing such an approach is the TOMMORROW study, a very large (n = 5800) phase III multi-centre trial aimed at assessing the efficacy of pioglitazone at delaying the onset of MCI in those who are cognitively normal but for whom the genetic marker profiles suggest they are at greater risk of MCI. Additional TZD have been evaluated in animal studies, and comparisons have shown pioglitazone to have superior efficacy at improving cognition and attenuating AD pathology [135].

Arguably the most evidence for the benefits of anti-diabetic drugs in AD comes from the use of insulin. Mouse AD model studies have shown insulin to reduce AD pathology and improve cognition AD [62, 136, 137]. Benefits of insulin administration have also consistently been observed in human trials. Acute peripheral insulin administration can enhance cognition [138], and in AD patients it has been found to improve some aspects of cognition, including story recall and attention [139]. The peripheral administration of insulin, however, may not be a suitable approach as most insulin does not enter the CNS and there is a risk in non-diabetics of developing hypoglycaemia, and although this can be mitigated by an infusion of glucose, this would be impractical in a clinical setting. To circumvent these problems, intranasal administration of insulin has been evaluated. Pilot clinical studies have indeed shown benefits. An eight-week trial of daily intranasal delivery improved aspects of cognition (word recall) in cognitively normal individuals, without altering peripheral glucose levels [140]. More recently, in a four-month placebo-controlled randomised trial, intranasal insulin was shown to improve memory in MCI/AD subjects [141], when compared to placebo. Further, these improvements could still be detected two months after treatment cessation, suggesting that insulin has lasting effects on CNS function. Insulin has a short half-life, thus to determine if analogues that have a longer half-life would show benefit, the same group treated AD and MCI patients with the analogue 'insulin determir' [142]. They found that after 21 days' treatment with a daily dose of the analogue, verbal working memory and visuospatial working memory was improved compared to placebo, but there was no treatment effect on daily functioning or executive functioning. This effect was APOE ε4-mediated as improvement was seen in carriers, but not in non-carriers. A very recent treatment comparison of regular insulin treatment with insulin determir showed that the regular insulin-treated group of AD and MCI patients had better memory after two and four months treatment [143]. This was associated with preserved or increased hippocampal volumes, and improved CSF biomarker profile. No significant effects were observed for the insulin determir compared to the placebo group, indicating that efficacy decreased over time.

The findings from these trials indicate that regular insulin treatment may offer benefits over short treatment periods (months), but the effect over longer periods is unknown. To determine the safety of insulin treatment over a prolonged period, and to determine whether benefits are still observed after a longer treatment time, the 18-month Study of Nasal Insulin in the Fight Against Forgetfulness (SNIFF) study is currently underway. This is a phase II/III multi-centre trial that is recruiting MCI and AD subjects, with the aim of evaluating intranasal insulin vs placebo over 18 months, followed by a 6-month open-label extension trial, where all participants will receive insulin.

Although to be addressed in the SNIFF trial, one concern is that the chronic administration of insulin to the CNS may induce hyperinsulinaemic conditions, thereby promoting brain insulin resistance, there may also be off-target effects due to binding to other receptors (for example insulin like-growth factor [IGF] receptors). Indeed, mice cortical neurons or primary neuronal cultures exposed to excessive amounts of insulin raise phosphorylation levels of key molecules (higher basal phosphorylation of Akt and GSK-3β) in the insulin signalling cascade, consistent with insulin resistance [144].

Another way to raise insulin levels or insulin action, yet avoiding potential adverse effects of insulin sensitisers or insulin itself, is to use glucagon-like peptide-1 receptor (GLP-1R) agonists. This group of drugs for diabetics has minor adverse effects compared to thiazolidinediones, and improves glucose homeostasis without the risk of hypoglycaemia [145]. Glucagon-like peptide-1 (GLP-1) is an incretin peptide that is secreted by the intestine in response to food, and in the presence of high glucose, binds its receptor located on pancreatic β-cells, stimulating insulin release. The GLP-1 peptide and its receptors are also present in the brain, where they have been shown to be neuroprotective [146, 147], to promote neurogenesis [147, 148], and to potentiate insulin signalling [149, 150].

As GLP-1 is rapidly degraded (within minutes), more stable analogues have been generated (reviewed in [151]). Of these, exendin-4, exenatide (synthetic exendin-4), and the more stable liraglutide (11–16 hours compared to 2–3 hours) have been approved for use in diabetes. These GLP-1 analogues have also been evaluated in cell culture and animal models, where they have been shown to promote the formation of new synapses, to promote neurogenesis, and to protect against oxidative injury [152–155] and Aβ-induced neurotoxicity [156]. In mouse models of AD and diabetes, GLP-1 analogues attenuate amyloid and tau pathology, reduce inflammation, and improve cognition [54, 157–160]. More recently, they have been shown to reverse cognitive impairment induced by Aβ oligomers in mice, and to provide partial protection against synaptic loss and tau pathology in non-human primates [161]. These encouraging findings together with their safety profiles have prompted current early phase human trials of GLP-1 analogues, although for the moment GLP-1 agonists require subcutaneous administration. However, recent studies have found that long-term treatment with the GLP-1 analogue, liraglutide, provided no benefits in two AD mouse models of cerebral amyloidosis [162]. These seemingly contrasting results highlight the need for a greater understanding of how GLP-1 analogues can offer potential benefits for slowing down progression of AD.

Targeting the same GLP-1/GLP-1R pathway, inhibitors of the enzyme that degrades GLP-1 – dipeptidyl peptidase-4 (DPP-4) – have been found to produce similar results to GLP-1 analogues in laboratory and pre-clinical studies, by stabilising endogenous levels of GLP-1 [163–166]. Saxagliptin and vildagliptin are two DPP-4 inhibitors that have been approved for the treatment of diabetes, and are often used in combination, when other agents such as metformin fail to reduce glucose levels. Some studies have evaluated the benefits of approved DPP-4 inhibitors in AD and vascular dementia models. For example, both saxagliptin and vildagliptin have been shown to reduce amyloid burden, tau phosphorylation, and inflammation, as well as improve cognition, in rats in which brain insulin signalling had been impaired through intracerebral administration of STZ [167, 168]. Later studies in a human neuronal cell line found that another DPP-4 inhibitor, linagliptin, can restore the impaired insulin signalling caused by Aβ in the neuronal cells, thus preventing the downstream activation of GSK3β and tau phosphorylation [169]. In a rat model of vascular endothelial dysfunction and vascular dementia, which involves inducing diabetes (and ultimately the vascular dysfunction) via pancreatectomy, it has been found that the DPP-4 inhibitor vildagliptin can significantly attenuate the pancreatectomy-induced impairments in learning and memory, endothelial function, and BBB permeability [170]. Most recently, linagliptin was administered to 3xTg-AD mice for eight weeks, and the inhibitor was found to mitigate cognitive deficits that normally occur in these mice, as well as improve brain incretin levels, and attenuate Aβ accumulation, tau phosphorylation, and neuroinflammation [171]. These promising findings suggest DPP-4 inhibitors are candidate treatments for AD that should be investigated in clinical trials.

There is evidence that GLP-1 agonists and DPP-4 inhibitors provide beneficial effects on long-term potentiation (LTP) and cognition as well. In one study, intracerebroventricular injection of liraglutide improved LTP; other studies found that the subcutaneous injection of exendin-4 and liraglutide in obese mice improved disturbances in LTP; and the peripheral administration of DPP-4 inhibitors (sitagliptin and vildagliptin) in rats fed a high-fat diet led to improvements in cognitive functioning in several studies (for a review see [166]). In studies of stroke in mice and rats, there is also evidence that GLP-1R agonists reduce oxidative stress and inflammation, both of which are linked to T2D as well as AD pathogenesis [172–174].

4.4 Conclusions

Evidence from epidemiological, clinical, and animal studies has established strong links between T2D and neurodegeneration such as that observed in AD. The precise and most important mechanisms that underpin these links remain to be determined, but are likely to involve impaired insulin signalling, inflammatory, and oxidative stress pathways that occur early in the neurodegenerative process.

The link between T2D and AD is not limited to T2D promoting neurodegeneration, as evidence is mounting for the notion that accumulation of AD proteins could also contribute to insulin resistance and T2D, that could further exacerbate neurodegenerative processes [175]. The Aβ peptide and APP have been suggested to regulate systemic metabolism (reviewed in [176, 177]) and plasma levels of the more pathogenic Aβ42 are increased in type 2 diabetics compared to age-matched controls [178]. Tau has roles in insulin transport and its secretion by the pancreatic β-cells [179, 180], and can modulate insulin-dependent translocation of the glucose transporter, GLUT4 [181, 182], critical for glucose uptake by tissues. The deposition of both Aβ and phosphorylated-tau can be found in post-mortem pancreatic tissue from type 2 diabetics [183], in animal models of AD [62] and in a novel mouse model with overlapping T2D and AD [184]. Studies in AD mouse models have also indicated that Aβ impairs insulin signalling in liver and muscle, contributing to insulin resistance in these mice when fed a high-fat diet [184, 185]. Aβ active immunisation in mice was shown to improve insulin sensitivity and glucose tolerance [184], providing further evidence for Aβ modulating peripheral insulin sensitivity and glucose metabolism. Whether the accumulation of phosphorylated-tau results in similar pathological contributions remains to be determined, but very recent findings show that the KO of tau in mice leads to β-cell dysfunction, impaired glucose-stimulated insulin secretion, and glucose intolerance [186]. Loss of tau also resulted in increased epididymal fat mass and leptin levels, and eventually the onset of diabetes. These results are further support for an important role for tau in insulin transport/secretion; a role that warrants further investigation.

Treatment approaches for managing diabetes have shown efficacy in reducing AD-related neurodegeneration in pre-clinical animal studies, and such treatments are now being assessed as potential therapeutics to prevent or slow the progression to AD in human clinical trials. The management of diabetes can often involve a combination of treatments to control hyperglycaemia and hyperinsulinaemia, as well as treatments to improve peripheral insulin sensitivity. It would be of great interest to determine if such an approach, using a combination of diabetic treatment agents, can also demonstrate enhanced efficacy in preventing or slowing neurodegeneration such as that seen in AD.

References

1 Hoyer, S. and Nitsch, R. (1989). Cerebral excess release of neurotransmitter amino acids subsequent to reduced cerebral glucose metabolism in early-onset dementia of Alzheimer type. *J. Neural Transm.* 75: 227–232.
2 Mayer, G., Nitsch, R., and Hoyer, S. (1990). Effects of changes in peripheral and cerebral glucose metabolism on locomotor activity, learning and memory in adult male rats. *Brain Res.* 532: 95–100.

3 Craft, S., Newcomer, J., Kanne, S. et al. (1996). Memory improvement following induced hyperinsulinemia in Alzheimer's disease. *Neurobiol. Aging* 17: 123–130.

4 Talbot, K., Wang, H.Y., Kazi, H. et al. (2012). Demonstrated brain insulin resistance in Alzheimer's disease patients is associated with IGF-1 resistance, IRS-1 dysregulation, and cognitive decline. *J. Clin. Invest.* 122: 1316–1338.

5 Biessels, G.J., Strachan, M.W., Visseren, F.L. et al. (2014). Dementia and cognitive decline in type 2 diabetes and prediabetic stages: towards targeted interventions. *Lancet Diabetes Endocrinol.* 2: 246–255.

6 Kooistra, M., Geerlings, M.I., Mali, W.P. et al., Group S-MS(2013). Diabetes mellitus and progression of vascular brain lesions and brain atrophy in patients with symptomatic atherosclerotic disease. The SMART-MR study. *J. Neurol. Sci.* 332: 69–74.

7 Moran, C., Phan, T.G., Chen, J. et al. (2013). Brain atrophy in type 2 diabetes: regional distribution and influence on cognition. *Diabetes Care* 36: 4036–4042.

8 Weinstein, G., Maillard, P., Himali, J.J. et al. (2015). Glucose indices are associated with cognitive and structural brain measures in young adults. *Neurology* 84: 2329–2337.

9 Launer, L.J., Miller, M.E., Williamson, J.D. et al., ACCORD MIND investigators (2011). Effects of intensive glucose lowering on brain structure and function in people with type 2 diabetes (ACCORD MIND): a randomised open-label substudy. *Lancet Neurol.* 10: 969–977.

10 Craft, S., Peskind, E., Schwartz, M.W. et al. (1998). Cerebrospinal fluid and plasma insulin levels in Alzheimer's disease: relationship to severity of dementia and apolipoprotein E genotype. *Neurology* 50: 164–168.

11 Duarte, A.I., Moreira, P.I., and Oliveira, C.R. (2012). Insulin in central nervous system: more than just a peripheral hormone. *J. Aging Res.* 2012: 384017.

12 Reger, M.A., Watson, G.S., Green, P.S. et al. (2008). Intranasal insulin administration dose-dependently modulates verbal memory and plasma amyloid-beta in memory-impaired older adults. *J. Alzheimers Dis.* 13: 323–331.

13 Baker, L.D., Cross, D.J., Minoshima, S. et al. (2011). Insulin resistance and Alzheimer-like reductions in regional cerebral glucose metabolism for cognitively normal adults with prediabetes or early type 2 diabetes. *Arch. Neurol.* 68: 51–57.

14 Craft, S. (2007). Insulin resistance and Alzheimer's disease pathogenesis: potential mechanisms and implications for treatment. *Curr. Alzheimer Res.* 4: 147–152.

15 Neumann, K.F., Rojo, L., Navarrete, L.P. et al. (2008). Insulin resistance and Alzheimer's disease: molecular links & clinical implications. *Curr. Alzheimer Res.* 5: 438–447.

16 van Elderen, S.G., de Roos, A., de Craen, A.J. et al. (2010). Progression of brain atrophy and cognitive decline in diabetes mellitus: a 3-year follow-up. *Neurology* 75: 997–1002.

17 Saczynski, J.S., Siggurdsson, S., Jonsson, P.V. et al. (2009). Glycemic status and brain injury in older individuals: the age gene/environment susceptibility-Reykjavik study. *Diabetes Care* 32: 1608–1613.

18 Morris, J.K., Vidoni, E.D., Perea, R.D. et al. (2014). Insulin resistance and gray matter volume in neurodegenerative disease. *Neuroscience* 270: 139–147.

19 Reijmer, Y.D., Brundel, M., de Bresser, J. et al., Utrecht Vascular Cognitive Impairment Study Group(2013). Microstructural white matter abnormalities and cognitive functioning in type 2 diabetes: a diffusion tensor imaging study. *Diabetes Care* 36: 137–144.
20 Roberts, R.O., Knopman, D.S., Geda, Y.E. et al. (2014). Association of diabetes with amnestic and nonamnestic mild cognitive impairment. *Alzheimers Dement.* 10: 18–26.
21 Thambisetty, M., Jeffrey Metter, E., Yang, A. et al. (2013). Glucose intolerance, insulin resistance, and pathological features of Alzheimer disease in the Baltimore Longitudinal Study of Aging. *JAMA Neurol.* 70: 1167–1172.
22 Moran, C., Beare, R., Phan, T.G. et al., Alzheimer's Disease Neuroimaging Initiative (ADNI)(2015). Type 2 diabetes mellitus and biomarkers of neurodegeneration. *Neurology* 85: 1123–1130.
23 Wu, L., Rowley, J., Mohades, S. et al., Alzheimer's Disease Neuroimaging Initiative (ADNI)(2012). Dissociation between brain amyloid deposition and metabolism in early mild cognitive impairment. *PLoS One* 7: e47905.
24 Willette, A.A., Modanlo, N., and Kapogiannis, D., for the Alzheimer's Disease Neuroimaging Initiative(2015). Insulin resistance predicts medial temporal hypermetabolism in MCI conversion to Alzheimer's disease. *Diabetes* 64: 1933–1940.
25 Hoscheidt, S.M., Starks, E.J., Oh, J.M. et al. (2016). Insulin resistance is associated with increased levels of cerebrospinal fluid biomarkers of Alzheimer's disease and reduced memory function in at-risk healthy middle-aged adults. *J. Alzheimers Dis.* 52: 1373–1383.
26 Laws, S.M., Gaskin, S., Woodfield, A. et al. (2017). Insulin resistance is associated with reductions in specific cognitive domains and increases in CSF tau in cognitively normal adults. *Sci. Rep.* 7(1): 9766.
27 Huxley, R., Barzi, F., and Woodward, M. (2006). Excess risk of fatal coronary heart disease associated with diabetes in men and women: meta-analysis of 37 prospective cohort studies. *BMJ* 332: 73–78.
28 Chatterjee, S., Peters, S.A., Woodward, M. et al. (2016). Type 2 diabetes as a risk factor for dementia in women compared with men: a pooled analysis of 2.3 million people comprising more than 100,000 cases of dementia. *Diabetes Care* 39: 300–307.
29 Peters, S.A., Huxley, R.R., and Woodward, M. (2014). Diabetes as a risk factor for stroke in women compared with men: a systematic review and meta-analysis of 64 cohorts, including 775,385 individuals and 12,539 strokes. *Lancet* 383: 1973–1980.
30 Gray, S.M., Meijer, R.I., and Barrett, E.J. (2014). Insulin regulates brain function, but how does it get there? *Diabetes* 63: 3992–3997.
31 Banks, W.A., Jaspan, J.B., and Kastin, A.J. (1997). Selective, physiological transport of insulin across the blood-brain barrier: novel demonstration by species-specific radioimmunoassays. *Peptides* 18: 1257–1262.
32 Banks, W.A., Jaspan, J.B., Huang, W., and Kastin, A.J. (1997). Transport of insulin across the blood-brain barrier: saturability at euglycemic doses of insulin. *Peptides* 18: 1423–1429.

33 Moreira, P.I., Duarte, A.I., Santos, M.S. et al. (2009). An integrative view of the role of oxidative stress, mitochondria and insulin in Alzheimer's disease. *J. Alzheimers Dis.* 16: 741–761.

34 Kuwabara, T., Kagalwala, M.N., Onuma, Y. et al. (2011). Insulin biosynthesis in neuronal progenitors derived from adult hippocampus and the olfactory bulb. *EMBO Mol. Med.* 3: 742–754.

35 Hoyer, S., Henneberg, N., Knapp, S. et al. (1996). Brain glucose metabolism is controlled by amplification and desensitization of the neuronal insulin receptor. *Ann. N.Y. Acad. Sci.* 777: 374–379.

36 Konner, A.C., Janoschek, R., Plum, L. et al. (2007). Insulin action in AgRP-expressing neurons is required for suppression of hepatic glucose production. *Cell Metab.* 5: 438–449.

37 Belgardt, B.F., Husch, A., Rother, E. et al. (2008). PDK1 deficiency in POMC-expressing cells reveals FOXO1-dependent and -independent pathways in control of energy homeostasis and stress response. *Cell Metab.* 7: 291–301.

38 Zhao, W., Wu, X., Xie, H. et al. (2010). Permissive role of insulin in the expression of long-term potentiation in the hippocampus of immature rats. *Neurosignals* 18: 236–245.

39 van der Heide, L.P., Ramakers, G.M., and Smidt, M.P. (2006). Insulin signaling in the central nervous system: learning to survive. *Prog. Neurobiol.* 79: 205–221.

40 Chiu, S.L., Chen, C.M., and Cline, H.T. (2008). Insulin receptor signaling regulates synapse number, dendritic plasticity, and circuit function in vivo. *Neuron* 58: 708–719.

41 Stockhorst, U., de Fries, D., Steingrueber, H.J., and Scherbaum, W.A. (2004). Insulin and the CNS: effects on food intake, memory, and endocrine parameters and the role of intranasal insulin administration in humans. *Physiol. Behav.* 83: 47–54.

42 Hoyer, S. (2004). Glucose metabolism and insulin receptor signal transduction in Alzheimer disease. *Eur. J. Pharmacol.* 490: 115–125.

43 Cohen, A.C., Tong, M., Wands, J.R., and de la Monte, S.M. (2007). Insulin and insulin-like growth factor resistance with neurodegeneration in an adult chronic ethanol exposure model. *Alcohol.: Clin. Exp. Res.* 31: 1558–1573.

44 Apostolatos, A., Song, S., Acosta, S. et al. (2012). Insulin promotes neuronal survival via the alternatively spliced protein kinase CdeltaII isoform. *J. Biol. Chem.* 287: 9299–9310.

45 Frolich, L., Blum-Degen, D., Bernstein, H.G. et al. (1998). Brain insulin and insulin receptors in aging and sporadic Alzheimer's disease. *J. Neural Transm.* 105: 423–438.

46 Steen, E., Terry, B.M., Rivera, E.J. et al. (2005). Impaired insulin and insulin-like growth factor expression and signaling mechanisms in Alzheimer's disease – is this type 3 diabetes? *J. Alzheimers Dis.* 7: 63–80.

47 Moloney, A.M., Griffin, R.J., Timmons, S. et al. (2010). Defects in IGF-1 receptor, insulin receptor and IRS-1/2 in Alzheimer's disease indicate possible resistance to IGF-1 and insulin signalling. *Neurobiol. Aging* 31: 224–243.

48 Ma, Q.L., Yang, F., Rosario, E.R. et al. (2009). Beta-amyloid oligomers induce phosphorylation of tau and inactivation of insulin receptor substrate via c-Jun N-terminal kinase signaling: suppression by omega-3 fatty acids and curcumin. *J. Neurosci.* 29: 9078–9089.

49 Kapogiannis, D., Boxer, A., Schwartz, J.B. et al. (2014). Dysfunctionally phosphorylated type 1 insulin receptor substrate in neural-derived blood exosomes of preclinical Alzheimer's disease. *FASEB J.* 29: 589–596.

50 Lee, S.J., Nam, E., Lee, H.J. et al. (2017). Towards an understanding of amyloid-beta oligomers: characterization, toxicity mechanisms, and inhibitors. *Chem. Soc. Rev.* 46: 310–323.

51 Ling, X., Martins, R.N., Racchi, M. et al. (2002). Amyloid beta antagonizes insulin promoted secretion of the amyloid beta protein precursor. *J. Alzheimers Dis.* 4: 369–374.

52 Akhtar, M.W., Sanz-Blasco, S., Dolatabadi, N. et al. (2016). Elevated glucose and oligomeric β-amyloid disrupt synapses via a common pathway of aberrant protein S-nitrosylation. *Nat Comm.* 7: 10242.

53 De Felice, F.G., Vieira, M.N., Bomfim, T.R. et al. (2009). Protection of synapses against Alzheimer's-linked toxins: insulin signaling prevents the pathogenic binding of Abeta oligomers. *Proc. Natl. Acad. Sci. U.S.A.* 106: 1971–1976.

54 Bomfim, T.R., Forny-Germano, L., Sathler, L.B. et al. (2012). An anti-diabetes agent protects the mouse brain from defective insulin signaling caused by Alzheimer's disease-associated Abeta oligomers. *J. Clin. Invest.* 122: 1339–1353.

55 Pessin, J.E. and Saltiel, A.R. (2000). Signaling pathways in insulin action: molecular targets of insulin resistance. *J. Clin. Invest.* 106: 165–169.

56 Schubert, M., Brazil, D.P., Burks, D.J. et al. (2003). Insulin receptor substrate-2 deficiency impairs brain growth and promotes tau phosphorylation. *J. Neurosci.* 23: 7084–7092.

57 Schubert, M., Gautam, D., Surjo, D. et al. (2004). Role for neuronal insulin resistance in neurodegenerative diseases. *Proc. Natl. Acad. Sci. U.S.A.* 101: 3100–3105.

58 Shankar, G.M., Bloodgood, B.L., Townsend, M. et al. (2007). Natural oligomers of the Alzheimer amyloid-beta protein induce reversible synapse loss by modulating an NMDA-type glutamate receptor-dependent signaling pathway. *J. Neurosci.* 27: 2866–2875.

59 Paula-Lima, A.C., Adasme, T., SanMartin, C. et al. (2011). Amyloid beta-peptide oligomers stimulate RyR-mediated Ca2+ release inducing mitochondrial fragmentation in hippocampal neurons and prevent RyR-mediated dendritic spine remodeling produced by BDNF. *Antioxid. Redox Signaling* 14: 1209–1223.

60 Brito-Moreira, J., Paula-Lima, A.C., Bomfim, T.R. et al. (2011). Abeta oligomers induce glutamate release from hippocampal neurons. *Curr. Alzheimer Res.* 8: 552–562.

61 Zempel, H., Thies, E., Mandelkow, E., and Mandelkow, E.M. (2010). Abeta oligomers cause localized Ca(2+) elevation, missorting of endogenous tau into dendrites, tau phosphorylation, and destruction of microtubules and spines. *J. Neurosci.* 30: 11938–11950.

62 Vandal, M., White, P.J., Tremblay, C. et al. (2014). Insulin reverses the high-fat diet-induced increase in brain Abeta and improves memory in an animal model of Alzheimer disease. *Diabetes* 63: 4291–4301.

63 Son, S.M., Song, H., Byun, J. et al. (2012). Accumulation of autophagosomes contributes to enhanced amyloidogenic APP processing under insulin-resistant conditions. *Autophagy* 8: 1842–1844.

64 Zuroff, L., Daley, D., Black, K.L., and Koronyo-Hamaoui, M. (2017). Clearance of cerebral Abeta in Alzheimer's disease: reassessing the role of microglia and monocytes. *Cell. Mol. Life Sci.* 74: 2167–2201.

65 Morelli, L., Llovera, R.E., Mathov, I. et al. (2004). Insulin-degrading enzyme in brain microvessels: proteolysis of amyloid {beta} vasculotropic variants and reduced activity in cerebral amyloid angiopathy. *J. Biol. Chem.* 279: 56004–56013.

66 Gao, W., Eisenhauer, P.B., Conn, K. et al. (2004). Insulin degrading enzyme is expressed in the human cerebrovascular endothelium and in cultured human cerebrovascular endothelial cells. *Neurosci. Lett.* 371: 6–11.

67 Bernstein, H.G., Ansorge, S., Riederer, P. et al. (1999). Insulin-degrading enzyme in the Alzheimer's disease brain: prominent localization in neurons and senile plaques. *Neurosci. Lett.* 263: 161–164.

68 Leissring, M.A., Farris, W., Chang, A.Y. et al. (2003). Enhanced proteolysis of beta-amyloid in APP transgenic mice prevents plaque formation, secondary pathology, and premature death. *Neuron* 40: 1087–1093.

69 Farris, W., Mansourian, S., Chang, Y. et al. (2003). Insulin-degrading enzyme regulates the levels of insulin, amyloid beta-protein, and the beta-amyloid precursor protein intracellular domain in vivo. *Proc. Natl. Acad. Sci. U.S.A.* 100: 4162–4167.

70 Miller, B.C., Eckman, E.A., Sambamurti, K. et al. (2003). Amyloid-beta peptide levels in brain are inversely correlated with insulysin activity levels *in vivo*. *Proc. Natl. Acad. Sci. U.S.A.* 100: 6221–6226.

71 Vekrellis, K., Ye, Z., Qiu, W.Q. et al. (2000). Neurons regulate extracellular levels of amyloid beta-protein via proteolysis by insulin-degrading enzyme. *J. Neurosci.* 20: 1657–1665.

72 Kim, M., Hersh, L.B., Leissring, M.A. et al. (2007). Decreased catalytic activity of the insulin-degrading enzyme in chromosome 10-linked Alzheimer disease families. *J. Biol. Chem.* 282: 7825–7832.

73 Perez, A., Morelli, L., Cresto, J.C., and Castano, E.M. (2000). Degradation of soluble amyloid beta-peptides 1-40, 1-42, and the Dutch variant 1-40Q by insulin degrading enzyme from Alzheimer disease and control brains. *Neurochem. Res.* 25: 247–255.

74 Qin, W. and Jia, J. (2008). Down-regulation of insulin-degrading enzyme by presenilin 1 V97L mutant potentially underlies increased levels of amyloid beta 42. *Eur. J. Neurosci.* 27: 2425–2432.

75 Zhao, Z., Xiang, Z., Haroutunian, V. et al. (2007). Insulin degrading enzyme activity selectively decreases in the hippocampal formation of cases at high risk to develop Alzheimer's disease. *Neurobiol. Aging* 28: 824–830.

76 Ittner, L.M., Ke, Y.D., Delerue, F. et al. (2010). Dendritic function of tau mediates amyloid-beta toxicity in Alzheimer's disease mouse models. *Cell* 142: 387–397.

77 Doble, B.W. and Woodgett, J.R. (2003). GSK-3: tricks of the trade for a multitasking kinase. *J. Cell Sci.* 116: 1175–1186.

78 Bhat, R., Xue, Y., Berg, S. et al. (2003). Structural insights and biological effects of glycogen synthase kinase 3-specific inhibitor AR-A014418. *J. Biol. Chem.* 278: 45937–45945.

79 Macauley, S.L., Stanley, M., Caesar, E.E. et al. (2015). Hyperglycemia modulates extracellular amyloid-beta concentrations and neuronal activity in vivo. *J. Clin. Invest.* 125: 2463–2467.

80 McArdle, M.A., Finucane, O.M., Connaughton, R.M. et al. (2013). Mechanisms of obesity-induced inflammation and insulin resistance: insights into the emerging role of nutritional strategies. *Front. Endocrinol. (Lausanne)* 4: 52.
81 Nakamura, M. and Watanabe, N. (2010). Ubiquitin-like protein MNSFbeta/endophilin II complex regulates Dectin-1-mediated phagocytosis and inflammatory responses in macrophages. *Biochem. Biophys. Res. Commun.* 401: 257–261.
82 Hirosumi, J., Tuncman, G., Chang, L. et al. (2002). A central role for JNK in obesity and insulin resistance. *Nature* 420: 333–336.
83 Gao, Z., Hwang, D., Bataille, F. et al. (2002). Serine phosphorylation of insulin receptor substrate 1 by inhibitor kappa B kinase complex. *J. Biol. Chem.* 277: 48115–48121.
84 Hotamisligil, G.S., Shargill, N.S., and Spiegelman, B.M. (1993). Adipose expression of tumor necrosis factor-alpha: direct role in obesity-linked insulin resistance. *Science* 259: 87–91.
85 Samad, F., Uysal, K.T., Wiesbrock, S.M. et al. (1999). Tumor necrosis factor alpha is a key component in the obesity-linked elevation of plasminogen activator inhibitor 1. *Proc. Natl. Acad. Sci. U.S.A.* 96: 6902–6907.
86 Bhamra, M.S. and Ashton, N.J. (2012). Finding a pathological diagnosis for Alzheimer's disease: are inflammatory molecules the answer? *Electrophoresis* 33: 3598–3607.
87 Craft, S. (2005). Insulin resistance syndrome and Alzheimer's disease: age- and obesity-related effects on memory, amyloid, and inflammation. *Neurobiol. Aging* 26 (Suppl 1): 65–69.
88 Aisen, P.S. (1997). Inflammation and Alzheimer's disease: mechanisms and therapeutic strategies. *Gerontology* 43: 143–149.
89 Fishel, M.A., Watson, G.S., Montine, T.J. et al. (2005). Hyperinsulinemia provokes synchronous increases in central inflammation and beta-amyloid in normal adults. *Arch. Neurol.* 62: 1539–1544.
90 Sokolova, A., Hill, M.D., Rahimi, F. et al. (2009). Monocyte chemoattractant protein-1 plays a dominant role in the chronic inflammation observed in Alzheimer's disease. *Brain Pathol.* 19: 392–398.
91 Bauer, J., Strauss, S., Schreiter-Gasser, U. et al. (1991). Interleukin-6 and alpha-2-macroglobulin indicate an acute-phase state in Alzheimer's disease cortices. *FEBS Lett.* 285: 111–114.
92 Boura-Halfon, S. and Zick, Y. (2009). Phosphorylation of IRS proteins, insulin action, and insulin resistance. *Am. J. Physiol. Endocrinol. Metab.* 296: E581–E591.
93 Erickson, M.A., Hansen, K., and Banks, W.A. (2012). Inflammation-induced dysfunction of the low-density lipoprotein receptor-related protein-1 at the blood-brain barrier: protection by the antioxidant N-acetylcysteine. *Brain Behav. Immun.* 26: 1085–1094.
94 Donahue, J.E., Flaherty, S.L., Johanson, C.E. et al. (2006). RAGE, LRP-1, and amyloid-beta protein in Alzheimer's disease. *Acta Neuropathol.* 112: 405–415.
95 van Straaten, E.C., Harvey, D., Scheltens, P. et al., Alzheimer's Disease Cooperative Study Group(2008). Periventricular white matter hyperintensities increase the likelihood of progression from amnestic mild cognitive impairment to dementia. *J. Neurol.* 255: 1302–1308.

96 Matrone, C., Djelloul, M., Taglialatela, G., and Perrone, L. (2014). Inflammatory risk factors and pathologies promoting Alzheimer's disease progression: is RAGE the key? *Histol. Histopathol.* 30: 125–139.

97 Byun, K., Yoo, Y., Son, M. et al. (2017). Advanced glycation end-products produced systemically and by macrophages: a common contributor to inflammation and degenerative diseases. *Pharmacol. Ther.* 177: 44–55.

98 Reynaert, N.L., Gopal, P., Rutten, E.P. et al. (2016). Advanced glycation end products and their receptor in age-related, non-communicable chronic inflammatory diseases; overview of clinical evidence and potential contributions to disease. *Int. J. Biochem. Cell Biol.* 81: 403–418.

99 Martins, R.N., Harper, C.G., Stokes, G.B., and Masters, C.L. (1986). Increased cerebral glucose-6-phosphate dehydrogenase activity in Alzheimer's disease may reflect oxidative stress. *J. Neurochem.* 46: 1042–1045.

100 Nunomura, A., Perry, G., Aliev, G. et al. (2001). Oxidative damage is the earliest event in Alzheimer disease. *J. Neuropathol. Exp. Neurol.* 60: 759–767.

101 Butterfield, D.A., Poon, H.F., St Clair, D. et al. (2006). Redox proteomics identification of oxidatively modified hippocampal proteins in mild cognitive impairment: insights into the development of Alzheimer's disease. *Neurobiol. Dis.* 22: 223–232.

102 Marcus, D.L., Thomas, C., Rodriguez, C. et al. (1998). Increased peroxidation and reduced antioxidant enzyme activity in Alzheimer's disease. *Exp. Neurol.* 150: 40–44.

103 Massaad, C.A. (2011). Neuronal and vascular oxidative stress in Alzheimer's disease. *Curr. Neuropharmacol.* 9: 662–673.

104 Butterfield, D.A., Di Domenico, F., and Barone, E. (2014). Elevated risk of type 2 diabetes for development of Alzheimer disease: a key role for oxidative stress in brain. *Biochim. Biophys. Acta* 1842: 1693–1706.

105 Aluise, C.D., Robinson, R.A., Cai, J. et al. (2011). Redox proteomics analysis of brains from subjects with amnestic mild cognitive impairment compared to brains from subjects with preclinical Alzheimer's disease: insights into memory loss in MCI. *J. Alzheimers Dis.* 23: 257–269.

106 Sultana, R., Boyd-Kimball, D., Poon, H.F. et al. (2006). Redox proteomics identification of oxidized proteins in Alzheimer's disease hippocampus and cerebellum: an approach to understand pathological and biochemical alterations in AD. *Neurobiol. Aging* 27: 1564–1576.

107 Chen, Z. and Zhong, C. (2013). Decoding Alzheimer's disease from perturbed cerebral glucose metabolism: implications for diagnostic and therapeutic strategies. *Prog. Neurobiol.* 108: 21–43.

108 Manoharan, S., Guillemin, G.J., Abiramasundari, R.S. et al. (2016). The role of reactive oxygen species in the pathogenesis of Alzheimer's disease, Parkinson's disease, and Huntington's disease: a mini review. *Oxid. Med. Cell. Longevity* 2016: 8590578.

109 Calabrese, V., Cornelius, C., Leso, V. et al. (2012). Oxidative stress, glutathione status, sirtuin and cellular stress response in type 2 diabetes. *Biochim. Biophys. Acta* 1822: 729–736.

110 Sies, H. (2014). Role of metabolic H_2O_2 generation: redox signaling and oxidative stress. *J. Biol. Chem.* 289: 8735–8741.

111 Zamora, M. and Villena, J.A. (2014). Targeting mitochondrial biogenesis to treat insulin resistance. *Curr. Pharm. Des.* 20: 5527–5557.

112 Munkacsy, E. and Rea, S.L. (2014). The paradox of mitochondrial dysfunction and extended longevity. *Exp. Gerontol.* 56: 221–233.

113 Reddy, P.H., Tripathi, R., Troung, Q. et al. (2012). Abnormal mitochondrial dynamics and synaptic degeneration as early events in Alzheimer's disease: implications to mitochondria-targeted antioxidant therapeutics. *Biochim. Biophys. Acta* 1822: 639–649.

114 Yao, J., Irwin, R.W., Zhao, L. et al. (2009). Mitochondrial bioenergetic deficit precedes Alzheimer's pathology in female mouse model of Alzheimer's disease. *Proc. Natl. Acad. Sci. U.S.A.* 106: 14670–14675.

115 De Felice, F.G. and Ferreira, S.T. (2014). Inflammation, defective insulin signaling, and mitochondrial dysfunction as common molecular denominators connecting type 2 diabetes to Alzheimer disease. *Diabetes* 63: 2262–2272.

116 Grunblatt, E., Salkovic-Petrisic, M., Osmanovic, J. et al. (2007). Brain insulin system dysfunction in streptozotocin intracerebroventricularly treated rats generates hyperphosphorylated tau protein. *J. Neurochem.* 101: 757–770.

117 Correia, S.C., Santos, R.X., Santos, M.S. et al. (2013). Mitochondrial abnormalities in a streptozotocin-induced rat model of sporadic Alzheimer's disease. *Curr. Alzheimer Res.* 10: 406–419.

118 Anderson, E.J., Lustig, M.E., Boyle, K.E. et al. (2009). Mitochondrial H_2O_2 emission and cellular redox state link excess fat intake to insulin resistance in both rodents and humans. *J. Clin. Invest.* 119: 573–581.

119 James, D., Kang, S., and Park, S. (2014). Injection of beta-amyloid into the hippocampus induces metabolic disturbances and involuntary weight loss which may be early indicators of Alzheimer's disease. *Aging Clin. Exp. Res.* 93–98.

120 Labuzek, K., Suchy, D., Gabryel, B. et al. (2010). Quantification of metformin by the HPLC method in brain regions, cerebrospinal fluid and plasma of rats treated with lipopolysaccharide. *Pharmacol. Rep.* 62: 956–965.

121 Nath, N., Khan, M., Paintlia, M.K. et al. (2009). Metformin attenuated the autoimmune disease of the central nervous system in animal models of multiple sclerosis. *J. Immunol.* 182: 8005–8014.

122 Gupta, A., Bisht, B., and Dey, C.S. (2011). Peripheral insulin-sensitizer drug metformin ameliorates neuronal insulin resistance and Alzheimer's-like changes. *Neuropharmacology* 60: 910–920.

123 Ahmed, S., Mahmood, Z., Javed, A. et al. (2017). Effect of metformin on adult hippocampal neurogenesis: comparison with donepezil and links to cognition. *J. Mol. Neurosci.* 62: 88–98.

124 Imfeld, P., Bodmer, M., Jick, S.S., and Meier, C.R. (2012). Metformin, other antidiabetic drugs, and risk of Alzheimer's disease: a population-based case-control study. *J. Am. Geriatr. Soc.* 60: 916–921.

125 Moore, E.M., Mander, A.G., Ames, D. et al., AIBL Investigators(2013). Increased risk of cognitive impairment in patients with diabetes is associated with metformin. *Diabetes Care* 36: 2981–2987.

126 Thangthaeng, N., Rutledge, M., Wong, J.M. et al. (2017). Metformin impairs spatial memory and visual acuity in old male mice. *Aging Dis.* 8: 17–30.

127 Landreth, G. (2007). Therapeutic use of agonists of the nuclear receptor PPARgamma in Alzheimer's disease. *Curr. Alzheimer Res.* 4: 159–164.

128 Jiang, Q., Heneka, M., and Landreth, G.E. (2008). The role of peroxisome proliferator-activated receptor-gamma (PPARgamma) in Alzheimer's disease: therapeutic implications. *CNS Drugs* 22: 1–14.

129 Watson, G.S., Cholerton, B.A., Reger, M.A. et al. (2005). Preserved cognition in patients with early Alzheimer disease and amnestic mild cognitive impairment during treatment with rosiglitazone: a preliminary study. *Am. J. Geriatr. Psychiatry* 13: 950–958.

130 Harrington, C., Sawchak, S., Chiang, C. et al. (2011). Rosiglitazone does not improve cognition or global function when used as adjunctive therapy to AChE inhibitors in mild-to-moderate Alzheimer's disease: two phase 3 studies. *Curr. Alzheimer Res.* 8: 592–606.

131 Festuccia, W.T., Oztezcan, S., Laplante, M. et al. (2008). Peroxisome proliferator-activated receptor-gamma-mediated positive energy balance in the rat is associated with reduced sympathetic drive to adipose tissues and thyroid status. *Endocrinology* 149: 2121–2130.

132 Chou, P.S., Ho, B.L., and Yang, Y.H. (2017). Effects of pioglitazone on the incidence of dementia in patients with diabetes. *J. Diabetes Complications* 31: 1053–1057.

133 Sato, T., Hanyu, H., Hirao, K. et al. (2011). Efficacy of PPAR-gamma agonist pioglitazone in mild Alzheimer disease. *Neurobiol. Aging* 32: 1626–1633.

134 Geldmacher, D.S., Fritsch, T., McClendon, M.J., and Landreth, G. (2011). A randomized pilot clinical trial of the safety of pioglitazone in treatment of patients with Alzheimer disease. *Arch. Neurol.* 68: 45–50.

135 Kummer, M.P., Schwarzenberger, R., Sayah-Jeanne, S. et al. (2014). Pan-PPAR modulation effectively protects APP/PS1 mice from amyloid deposition and cognitive deficits. *Mol. Neurobiol.* 51: 661–671.

136 Shingo, A.S., Kanabayashi, T., Kito, S., and Murase, T. (2013). Intracerebroventricular administration of an insulin analogue recovers STZ-induced cognitive decline in rats. *Behav. Brain Res.* 241: 105–111.

137 Guo, Z., Chen, Y., Mao, Y.F. et al. (2017). Long-term treatment with intranasal insulin ameliorates cognitive impairment, tau hyperphosphorylation, and microglial activation in a streptozotocin-induced Alzheimer's rat model. *Sci. Rep.* 7: 45971.

138 Kern, W., Peters, A., Fruehwald-Schultes, B. et al. (2001). Improving influence of insulin on cognitive functions in humans. *Neuroendocrinology* 74: 270–280.

139 Craft, S., Asthana, S., Newcomer, J.W. et al. (1999). Enhancement of memory in Alzheimer disease with insulin and somatostatin, but not glucose. *Arch. Gen. Psychiatry* 56: 1135–1140.

140 Benedict, C., Hallschmid, M., Hatke, A. et al. (2004). Intranasal insulin improves memory in humans. *Psychoneuroendocrinology* 29: 1326–1334.

141 Craft, S., Baker, L.D., Montine, T.J. et al. (2012). Intranasal insulin therapy for Alzheimer disease and amnestic mild cognitive impairment: a pilot clinical trial. *Arch. Neurol.* 69: 29–38.

142 Claxton, A., Baker, L.D., Hanson, A. et al. (2015). Long-acting intranasal insulin detemir improves cognition for adults with mild cognitive impairment or early-stage Alzheimer's disease dementia. *J. Alzheimers Dis.* 44: 897–906.

143 Craft, S., Claxton, A., Baker, L.D. et al. (2017). Effects of regular and long-acting insulin on cognition and Alzheimer's disease biomarkers: a pilot clinical trial. *J. Alzheimers Dis.* 57: 1325–1334.

144 Kim, B., Sullivan, K.A., Backus, C., and Feldman, E.L. (2011). Cortical neurons develop insulin resistance and blunted Akt signaling: a potential mechanism contributing to enhanced ischemic injury in diabetes. *Antioxid. Redox Signaling* 14: 1829–1839.

145 Boland, C.L., Degeeter, M., Nuzum, D.S., and Tzefos, M. (2013). Evaluating second-line treatment options for type 2 diabetes: focus on secondary effects of GLP-1 agonists and DPP-4 inhibitors. *Ann. Pharmacother.* 47: 490–505.

146 Salcedo, I., Tweedie, D., Li, Y., and Greig, N.H. (2012). Neuroprotective and neurotrophic actions of glucagon-like peptide-1: an emerging opportunity to treat neurodegenerative and cerebrovascular disorders. *Br. J. Pharmacol.* 166: 1586–1599.

147 Duarte, A.I., Candeias, E., Correia, S.C. et al. (2013). Crosstalk between diabetes and brain: glucagon-like peptide-1 mimetics as a promising therapy against neurodegeneration. *Biochim. Biophys. Acta* 1832: 527–541.

148 Hunter, K. and Holscher, C. (2012). Drugs developed to treat diabetes, liraglutide and lixisenatide, cross the blood brain barrier and enhance neurogenesis. *BMC Neurosci.* 13: 33.

149 Gao, H., Wang, X., Zhang, Z. et al. (2007). GLP-1 amplifies insulin signaling by up-regulation of IRbeta, IRS-1 and Glut4 in 3T3-L1 adipocytes. *Endocrine* 32: 90–95.

150 Li, L., Yang, G., Li, Q. et al. (2008). Exenatide prevents fat-induced insulin resistance and raises adiponectin expression and plasma levels. *Diabetes Obes. Metab.* 10: 921–930.

151 Lund, A., Knop, F.K., and Vilsboll, T. (2014). Glucagon-like peptide-1 receptor agonists for the treatment of type 2 diabetes: differences and similarities. *Eur. J. Intern. Med.* 25: 407–414.

152 Hamilton, A., Patterson, S., Porter, D. et al. (2011). Novel GLP-1 mimetics developed to treat type 2 diabetes promote progenitor cell proliferation in the brain. *J. Neurosci. Res.* 89: 481–489.

153 Sharma, M.K., Jalewa, J., and Holscher, C. (2014). Neuroprotective and anti-apoptotic effects of liraglutide on SH-SY5Y cells exposed to methylglyoxal stress. *J. Neurochem.* 128: 459–471.

154 Parthsarathy, V. and Holscher, C. (2013). Chronic treatment with the GLP1 analogue liraglutide increases cell proliferation and differentiation into neurons in an AD mouse model. *PLoS One* 8: e58784.

155 McClean, P.L. and Holscher, C. (2014). Lixisenatide, a drug developed to treat type 2 diabetes, shows neuroprotective effects in a mouse model of Alzheimer's disease. *Neuropharmacology* 86: 241–258.

156 Qiu, C., Wang, Y.P., Pan, X.D. et al. (2016). Exendin-4 protects Abeta(1-42) oligomer-induced PC12 cell apoptosis. *Am. J. Transl. Res.* 8: 3540–3548.

157 Xu, W., Yang, Y., Yuan, G. et al. (2014). Exendin-4, a glucagon-like peptide-1 receptor agonist, reduces Alzheimer disease-associated tau hyperphosphorylation in the hippocampus of rats with type 2 diabetes. *J. Invest. Med.* 63: 267–272.

158 Chen, S., An, F.M., Yin, L. et al. (2014). Glucagon-like peptide-1 protects hippocampal neurons against advanced glycation end product-induced tau hyperphosphorylation. *Neuroscience* 256: 137–146.

159 McClean, P.L. and Holscher, C. (2014). Liraglutide can reverse memory impairment, synaptic loss and reduce plaque load in aged APP/PS1 mice, a model of Alzheimer's disease. *Neuropharmacology* 76 (Pt A): 57–67.

160 Yang, Y., Zhang, J., Ma, D. et al. (2013). Subcutaneous administration of liraglutide ameliorates Alzheimer-associated tau hyperphosphorylation in rats with type 2 diabetes. *J. Alzheimers Dis.* 37: 637–648.

161 Batista, A.F., Forny-Germano, L., Clarke, J.R. et al. (2018). The diabetes drug liraglutide reverses cognitive impairment in mice and attenuates insulin receptor and synaptic pathology in a non-human primate model of Alzheimer's disease. *J. Pathol.* 245: 85–100.

162 Hansen, H.H., Fabricius, K., Barkholt, P. et al. (2016). Long-term treatment with liraglutide, a glucagon-like peptide-1 (GLP-1) receptor agonist, has no effect on beta-amyloid plaque load in two transgenic APP/PS1 mouse models of Alzheimer's disease. *PLoS One* 11: e0158205.

163 Drucker, D.J. (2003). Enhancing incretin action for the treatment of type 2 diabetes. *Diabetes Care* 26: 2929–2940.

164 Hansen, L., Deacon, C.F., Orskov, C., and Holst, J.J. (1999). Glucagon-like peptide-1-(7-36)amide is transformed to glucagon-like peptide-1-(9-36)amide by dipeptidyl peptidase IV in the capillaries supplying the L cells of the porcine intestine. *Endocrinology* 140: 5356–5363.

165 Brown, D.X. and Evans, M. (2012). Choosing between GLP-1 receptor agonists and DPP-4 inhibitors: a pharmacological perspective. *J. Nutr. Metab.* 2012: 381713.

166 Groeneveld, O.N., Kappelle, L.J., and Biessels, G.J. (2016). Potentials of incretin-based therapies in dementia and stroke in type 2 diabetes mellitus. *J. Diabetes Investig.* 7: 5–16.

167 Kosaraju, J., Gali, C.C., Khatwal, R.B. et al. (2013). Saxagliptin: a dipeptidyl peptidase-4 inhibitor ameliorates streptozotocin induced Alzheimer's disease. *Neuropharmacology* 72: 291–300.

168 Kosaraju, J., Murthy, V., Khatwal, R.B. et al. (2013). Vildagliptin: an anti-diabetes agent ameliorates cognitive deficits and pathology observed in streptozotocin-induced Alzheimer's disease. *J. Pharm. Pharmacol.* 65: 1773–1784.

169 Kornelius, E., Lin, C.L., Chang, H.H. et al. (2015). DPP-4 inhibitor linagliptin attenuates Abeta-induced cytotoxicity through activation of AMPK in neuronal cells. *CNS Neurosci. Ther.* 21: 549–557.

170 Jain, S. and Sharma, B. (2015). Neuroprotective effect of selective DPP-4 inhibitor in experimental vascular dementia. *Physiol. Behav.* 152: 182–193.

171 Kosaraju, J., Holsinger, R.M., Guo, L., and Tam, K.Y. (2016). Linagliptin, a dipeptidyl peptidase-4 inhibitor, mitigates cognitive deficits and pathology in the 3xTg-AD mouse model of Alzheimer's disease. *Mol. Neurobiol.* 54: 6074–6084.

172 Teramoto, S., Miyamoto, N., Yatomi, K. et al. (2011). Exendin-4, a glucagon-like peptide-1 receptor agonist, provides neuroprotection in mice transient focal cerebral ischemia. *J. Cereb. Blood Flow Metab.* 31: 1696–1705.

173 Sato, K., Kameda, M., Yasuhara, T. et al. (2013). Neuroprotective effects of liraglutide for stroke model of rats. *Int. J. Mol. Sci.* 14: 21513–21524.

174 Darsalia, V., Mansouri, S., Ortsater, H. et al. (2012). Glucagon-like peptide-1 receptor activation reduces ischaemic brain damage following stroke in type 2 diabetic rats. *Clin. Sci. (Lond)* 122: 473–483.

175 Bharadwaj, P., Wijesekara, N., Liyanapathirana, M. et al. (2017). The link between type 2 diabetes and neurodegeneration: roles for amyloid-beta, amylin, and tau proteins. *J. Alzheimers Dis.* 59: 421–432.

176 Czeczor, J.K. and McGee, S.L. (2017). Emerging roles for the amyloid precursor protein and derived peptides in the regulation of cellular and systemic metabolism. *J. Neuroendocrinol.* 29: 1–8.

177 Puig, K.L., Brose, S.A., Zhou, X. et al. (2017). Amyloid precursor protein modulates macrophage phenotype and diet-dependent weight gain. *Sci. Rep.* 7: 43725.

178 Peters, K.E., Davis, W.A., Taddei, K. et al. (2017). Plasma amyloid-beta peptides in type 2 diabetes: a matched case-control study. *J. Alzheimers Dis.* 56: 1127–1133.

179 Maj, M., Gartner, W., Ilhan, A. et al. (2010). Expression of TAU in insulin-secreting cells and its interaction with the calcium-binding protein secretagogin. *J. Endocrinol.* 205: 25–36.

180 Maj, M., Hoermann, G., Rasul, S. et al. (2016). The microtubule-associated protein tau and its relevance for pancreatic beta cells. *J. Diabetes Res.* 2016: 1964634.

181 Emoto, M., Langille, S.E., and Czech, M.P. (2001). A role for kinesin in insulin-stimulated GLUT4 glucose transporter translocation in 3T3-L1 adipocytes. *J. Biol. Chem.* 276: 10677–10682.

182 Liu, L.Z., Cheung, S.C., Lan, L.L. et al. (2013). Microtubule network is required for insulin-induced signal transduction and actin remodeling. *Mol. Cell. Endocrinol.* 365: 64–74.

183 Miklossy, J., Qing, H., Radenovic, A. et al. (2010). Beta amyloid and hyperphosphorylated tau deposits in the pancreas in type 2 diabetes. *Neurobiol. Aging* 31: 1503–1515.

184 Wijesekara, N., Ahrens, R., Sabale, M. et al. (2017). Amyloid-beta and islet amyloid pathologies link Alzheimer's disease and type 2 diabetes in a transgenic model. *FASEB J.* 31: 5409–5418.

185 Zhang, Y., Zhou, B., Zhang, F. et al. (2012). Amyloid-beta induces hepatic insulin resistance by activating JAK2/STAT3/SOCS-1 signaling pathway. *Diabetes* 61: 1434–1443.

186 Wijesekara, N., Goncalves, R.A., Ahrens, R. et al. (2018). Tau ablation in mice leads to pancreatic beta cell dysfunction and glucose intolerance. *FASEB J.* 32: 3166–3173.

5

Diet and Nutrition, and their Influence on Alzheimer's Disease and other Neurodegenerative Diseases

Stephanie R. Rainey-Smith[1,2], Rhona Creegan[3], Stephanie J. Fuller[1], Michele L. Callisaya[4,5] and Velandai Srikanth[5,6]

[1] *Centre of Excellence for Alzheimer's disease Research and Care, School of Medical and Health Sciences, Edith Cowan University, Joondalup, Western Australia, Australia*
[2] *Australian Alzheimer's Research Foundation, Ralph and Patricia Sarich Neuroscience, Research Institute, Nedlands, Australia*
[3] *Omega Nutrition Health, Perth, Western Australia, Australia*
[4] *Menzies Institute for Medical Research, University of Tasmania, Hobart, Tasmania, Australia*
[5] *Peninsula Clinical School, Central Clinical School, Monash University, Melbourne, Victoria, Australia*
[6] *Department of Medicine, Peninsula Health, Melbourne, Victoria, Australia*

5.1 Introduction

Digestive deterioration can occur with age. For example, atrophic gastritis is a process of chronic inflammation of the stomach lining leading to loss of cells, which is common in older adults. This condition affects absorption of essential nutrients, for example vitamin B12 and folate [1, 2], deficiencies of which can result in high levels of the non-protein amino acid homocysteine, which has been associated with an increased risk of Alzheimer's disease (AD) [3, 4]. Protein absorption is also affected by atrophic gastritis, leading to an impaired supply of essential amino acids, including tryptophan and tyrosine, which are necessary for neurotransmitter synthesis [5].

Both metabolic rate and physical activity also decline with age; and with weight gain concerns, older adults are more likely to consume inadequate micronutrients through eating less. Moreover, nutrient status may be further compromised by pharmaceutical agents required for the management of a variety of conditions. For example, cerebrovascular and cardiovascular disease (CVD), obesity, hypertension, dyslipidaemia, and type 2 diabetes mellitus (T2D) frequently require management with pharmaceutical agents. Furthermore, these conditions have related metabolic and physiological abnormalities, which are influenced by diet and possible nutrient deficiencies, and are themselves also well-established risk factors for AD (see [6, 7] for reviews). Several other factors, often overlooked, can also influence diet quality in the elderly: if living alone, this reduces the incentive to eat a varied diet; physical restrictions such as rheumatoid arthritis can limit cooking ability; transport to shops and markets may be limited if not driving; and reduced income can also influence food choices.

5.2 Dietary Patterns

It is important to recognise that an individual's diet usually comprises a myriad of foods, ranging from highly nutritious items to foods of almost no nutritional value. Consequently, when examining the relationship between diet and brain health, it is likely to be more useful to examine indices of food and nutrient intake that express several related aspects of diet concurrently, rather than just focus on consumption of single nutrients [8]: 'Dietary patterns' are examples of such indices. Whilst individual study results are not always consistent, the overarching message from research into dietary patterns is that so called 'healthy' dietary patterns are associated with better brain health outcomes, while the contrary is true of 'unhealthy' eating models.

Adherence to a Mediterranean style diet (MeDi), for example, has been shown to confer a degree of protection against cognitive decline and, ultimately, to reduce risk of AD [9–11]. This style of eating comprises a high intake of nutrient dense, high-fibre foods such as legumes, vegetables, fruits, and cereals. This intake of high-fibre, non-refined carbohydrates contributes to a low glycaemic load eating model, which helps to prevent dyslipidaemia and insulin resistance. Low to moderate intakes of meat, dairy, and poultry are indicative of low to moderate intakes of saturated fatty acids and cholesterol, whilst moderately high intakes of fish, seafood, and olive oil result in favourably high intakes of omega-3 fatty acids and mono-unsaturated fats respectively. Cheese and yoghurt are the main dairy products; and although red wine is consumed regularly, this is in moderation and usually with meals [9, 12]. The MeDi is rich in anti-inflammatory and antioxidant constituents which confer general health benefits, in addition to potentially ameliorating inflammatory and oxidative stress processes specifically associated with AD [13–15]. Notably, some of these anti-inflammatory and antioxidant constituents have also been shown to impact upon gene transcription factors which influence lipid metabolism, energy homeostasis and, potentially, longevity [16–20]. Furthermore, a recent study demonstrated that MeDi adherence is beneficial for maintaining brain health in older adults, by slowing the accumulation of AD pathology. Specifically, the rates of accumulation of Aβ in the brain were assessed over three years. Increasing MeDi adherence was associated with decreasing the rate of brain Aβ accumulation, with each one point MeDi score increase associated with an annual decrease in Aβ accumulation rate. Further evaluation revealed fruit intake to be the individual MeDi score component which contributed most strongly to this relationship, with a high intake of fruit associated with less accumulation of Aβ [21].

Another diet that has been associated with longevity and good cognitive health is the traditional diet of Okinawa, Japan. The main constituents of this traditional diet include root vegetables (mostly sweet potatoes), green and yellow vegetables, soybean-based foods, and medicinal plants. Marine foods, lean meats, fruit, spices, tea, and alcohol are also consumed in moderation [22]. This diet has a lot in common with the MeDi, and similarly emphasises fresh (unprocessed), mostly vegetarian foods, with high antioxidant content, as well as regular intakes of seafood.

The Dietary Approaches to Stop Hypertension (DASH) diet emphasises fruits, vegetables, and low-fat dairy foods; it includes whole grains, poultry, fish, and nuts, and contains smaller amounts of red meat, sweets, and sugar-containing beverages compared to a diet typical of the United States [23]. Consequently, intakes of total and saturated fat and cholesterol are lower than intakes from a typical American diet, whilst intakes of potassium, calcium, magnesium, dietary fibre, and protein are higher [23]. DASH diet adherence has been shown to lower blood pressure and protect against other cardiovascular factors that can adversely affect brain health [23, 24]. Furthermore, a randomised trial has demonstrated the protective effects of DASH against cognitive decline [24], and a recent systematic review has consolidated the concept that both the MeDi and DASH diet reduce AD risk and slow rates of cognitive decline [25].

A recently devised dietary pattern termed the MIND diet (Mediterranean-DASH diet intervention for neurodegenerative delay) is tailored specifically to neuroprotection. The MIND diet is styled after the MeDi and DASH diets but with modifications that reflect the most compelling results of the diet-dementia field. For example, like the MeDi and DASH diet, the MIND diet emphasises limited intake of red meat and foods high in saturated fats, and high intake of natural plant-based foods. However, the MIND diet uniquely specifies intake of berries and green leafy vegetables, and does not specify high fruit, dairy, or potato intake, or more than one serving of fish per week [26]. Significantly, recent results have indicated that adherence to the MIND diet is associated with both slower rates of cognitive decline, and with lower rates of incident AD compared to either the MeDi or DASH diet [26, 27].

In contrast to the MeDi, DASH, and MIND diets, adherence to a western-style diet characterised by high fat, high refined carbohydrates and sugar, low fibre, and high salt, is associated with increased cognitive decline and risk of AD [11, 28]. Numerous studies have confirmed a link between high-fat/high-sugar diets and cognitive decline, thereby intimating a role for insulin resistance and diet-induced endocrine abnormalities [29–32]: these links are discussed in detail in other chapters of this book. Furthermore, diets containing high cholesterol and saturated fat, added sugar, and other high glycaemic load foods have been shown to contribute to dyslipidaemia [33, 34]. It was assumed until recently that the adverse effects of such diets on AD risk were due to negative influences on insulin sensitivity, metabolism, and cardiovascular health: while these are major contributing factors, published studies have also shown direct effects of such diets on the brain. Indeed, a high saturated fat/high refined sugar diet fed to animals has been shown to impair spatial memory through a reduction in brain-derived neurotrophic factor (BDNF) levels in the hippocampus [35]. Signalling molecules downstream of BDNF which are important for neurite outgrowth, neurotransmitter release, as well as learning and memory, were also reduced [35].

Some of the key components of the dietary patterns discussed above, and their contribution to AD risk and pathology, will be discussed in the sections that follow.

5.3 Key Macronutrients

5.3.1 Dietary Fatty Acids

Dietary fatty acids provide energy. Additionally, however, the diverse functions of lipids mean that the quantity and type consumed are important for determining disease risk. Certain fats are essential components of our diet, and are thought to influence cognitive health as well as risk of many age-related diseases; for example omega-3- and omega-6-polyunsaturated fatty acids, described below, and in greater detail in other chapters, such as Chapter 7 on fat and lipid metabolism by Hone et al. Moreover, a high intake of saturated fat is correlated with the development of obesity, dyslipidaemia, insulin resistance, diabetes, and vascular disease, which as mentioned previously are all AD risk factors [36–38]. Some saturated fatty acids have other detrimental effects, for example, palmitic acid has been shown to upregulate ceramide production, which is considered a major contributor to insulin resistance and dyslipidaemia [39, 40]. Toxic ceramides have been proposed to link insulin resistance with excess dietary saturated fatty acids and inflammatory cytokines [41], and elevated levels of ceramides have been measured in post-mortem AD brain tissue [42, 43]. Other AD studies have linked certain ceramide species and their metabolism to accelerated brain Aβ deposition through promotion of insoluble fibril formation [44], and to enhanced tau pathology [45–47].

In general, the involvement of saturated fatty acids in AD pathogenesis is unclear, although it is well-known that a diet with a high ratio of saturated fat to polyunsaturated or mono-unsaturated fats results in a poor plasma cholesterol profile, characterised by higher levels of low-density lipoprotein (LDL) cholesterol and lower levels of high-density lipoprotein (HDL) cholesterol [48]. Such a lipid profile increases the risk of CVD, obesity and T2D, and thus increases AD risk. Much research has centred around cholesterol itself and its potential detrimental effects on AD risk, as well as on the health benefits of certain polyunsaturated fatty acids, as described below.

5.3.2 Cholesterol

Many studies and reviews have covered this topic, and it is also discussed in Chapter 7 on fat and lipid metabolism by Hone et al. It was suggested about 25 years ago that high cholesterol levels may be linked to increased risk of AD, and that statins may reduce this risk (statins are drugs that reduce cholesterol levels by inhibiting the enzyme 3-hydroxy-3-methylglutaryl-Coenzyme A (HMG-CoA) reductase, the first enzyme of the cholesterol biosynthesis pathway). The protein apolipoprotein E (apoE) is a constituent of various classes of lipoproteins in the blood, and is a major cholesterol carrier. In the brain, apoE is produced by astrocytes, and transports cholesterol to cells via apoE receptors; members of the LDL receptor family. ApoE is encoded by the *APOE* gene. In humans there are six possible *APOE* genotypes, coded by two of three possible alleles (ε2, ε3, and ε4), located on chromosome 19. Links between AD and lipid metabolism came to the fore when it was found that carrying an *APOE* ε4 allele increased AD risk considerably, with carrying two alleles posing an even greater risk [49]. ApoE ε4 protein (compared to apoE ε3 and apoE ε2) is associated with hyperlipidaemia and hypercholesterolaemia which can lead to atherosclerosis, coronary heart disease, and stroke. ApoE is also involved in Aβ clearance from the brain, and apoE ε4 has been shown to be less efficient at Aβ clearance; carrying at least one *APOE* ε4 allele is associated with greater brain Aβ deposition in AD, and a greater risk of cerebral amyloid angiopathy (for a review see [50]). Reducing cholesterol levels was suggested to be a potential treatment that would decrease AD risk; however, after many epidemiological and longitudinal studies of a variety of statins, times of treatment, and dosages, the overall conclusions have been mixed, with a recent Cochrane Database Systematic Review concluding that statins given in late life to people at risk of vascular disease do not prevent cognitive decline or dementia [51]. Having said this, statins at earlier stages in life given to improve blood HDL/LDL profiles with the aim of reducing CVD (an AD risk factor), may help reduce risk indirectly, though dietary changes to raise HDL and lower LDL levels would be at least as effective. It can be noted here that MeDi, and DASH diet adherence have both been associated with improved blood cholesterol profiles [52, 53].

5.3.3 Polyunsaturated Fatty Acids

Dietary polyunsaturated fatty acids (PUFA) affect a broad spectrum of physiological processes. Some of these PUFA are converted to prostaglandins, leukotrienes, thromboxanes, and other metabolites through the action of cyclooxygenase (COX) and lipoxygenase enzymes. Several products of PUFA conversion act as signalling molecules which play important roles in cellular function and are consequently at least partially influenced by diet [54]. Conversion of omega-6 PUFA gives rise to signalling molecules which are more atherogenic, pro-thrombotic, and inflammatory compared to those generated during omega-3 PUFA conversion [5]. The essential omega-3 PUFA alpha-linolenic acid (ALA), which is necessary for health, yet cannot be synthesised in the human body, is found in seeds, nuts, and many common vegetable oils, and is the precursor for the longer omega-3 PUFA, eicosapentaenoic acid (EPA) and docosahexaenoic acid (DHA), which play critical roles in many metabolic processes [55]. ALA conversion is negatively impacted by hormone imbalances, diet and nutrient deficiencies [56–58]: although, in addition to synthesis from dietary ALA, both EPA and DHA are readily available in fish and fish oil.

Pro-inflammatory eicosanoids and cytokines are upregulated by high intake of omega-6 PUFA, such as arachidonic acid (AA), which is typically found in meat. AA-enriched diets also lead to elevations in levels of vasoconstrictive non-classical eicosanoids such as isoprostanes [59]. By contrast, DHA-enriched diets promote anti-inflammatory, anti-thrombotic, vasodilatory, and neuroprotective effects through production of docosanoid signalling molecules during metabolism [54, 60] (for a more detailed discussion of research into the influences of omega-3 fatty acids on inflammation, see Chapter 8 on inflammation by Sharman et al.). The ratio of dietary AA to DHA has been proposed to influence several diseases, including AD, and may be important in designing nutrition-based strategies for disease prevention [61]. As discussed in greater detail by Hone et al. in Chapter 7, modern western diets have omega-6 : omega-3 fatty acid intake ratios of approximately 10 : 1 or higher, yet nutritional anthropologists suggest our ancestors would have consumed diets with intake ratios of 1 : 1 [62]. This change in ratio, independent of the number of calories derived from lipids, is thought to lead to dysregulation of lipid homeostasis, and is associated with obesity [62].

AA and DHA are delivered to the brain from the periphery, via plasma lipoproteins and lysophospholipids [5]. Either aberrant biochemical pathways and/or low dietary intakes may account for low DHA levels. While DHA can be obtained from the diet, an adequate supply to the brain also relies on peroxisomal production. EPA is elongated and desaturated in the endoplasmic reticulum, yielding tetracosahexaenoic acid (THA). Following transportation to the peroxisome, THA undergoes a final oxidation step whereby two carbon atoms are removed to yield DHA [63]. This final step has been proposed to be a bottleneck in the ALA to DHA conversion process, and is thought to be the reason supplementary dietary intakes may be necessary to meet the DHA requirements of the brain. Significantly, impaired liver DHA biosynthesis, elevated THA, and reduced expression of peroxisomal proteins required for THA to DHA conversion have all been detected in AD patients [64]. The length of THA molecules means that accumulation can adversely affect mitochondrial function [65]; an important point given that mitochondrial dysfunction and oxidative stress are purportedly early and central events in AD pathogenesis. Impaired activity of the enzymes responsible for fatty acid elongation and desaturation have also been proposed to result in reduced production of longer chain PUFA in AD. Consequences of this impaired enzymatic activity would include reduced cell membrane fluidity and an imbalance in PUFA-derived signalling molecules such as eicosanoids and docosanoids. Indeed, the activity of the enzyme delta 6-desaturase, which ensures the flow of fatty acids into the elongation and desaturation pathways, may be influenced by dietary intakes of fatty acids, various nutrients such as vitamin B6 [56] and metabolic hormones [66, 67]. Furthermore, insulin is known to affect activity of both delta 5- and delta 6-desaturases [57], and if the supply of long-chain PUFA to the brain is reduced as a result of abnormalities in insulin function, this may represent an additional mechanism through which metabolic dysfunction, insulin resistance, and T2D contribute to AD.

One way in which EPA and DHA are able to inhibit different aspects of inflammation including leukocyte chemotaxis, adhesion molecule expression and interactions, and the production of inflammatory cytokines, is through the action of specialised pro-resolving mediators (SPM). SPM from omega-6 fatty acids, such as lipoxins, and from omega-3 fatty acids such as resolvins, protectins, and maresins, act in reducing/resolving the inflammatory process in certain diseases, by stimulating the phases of resolution of inflammation. This discovery has resulted in the resolution of inflammation being considered as an active instead of a passive process [68]. These lipid mediators also help tissue regeneration, whereas their deregulation helps to maintain chronic inflammation and has also been linked to CVD [69], a risk factor for AD. Changes in levels of lipoxins and possibly the other anti-inflammatory lipids (resolvins, protectins, and maresins) are thought to be involved in several other inflammatory conditions, such as rheumatoid arthritis, type 1 diabetes mellitus, multiple sclerosis, and lupus [70]. It is believed that production of these lipid mediators is initiated during lipid-mediator class switching, in which the classic initiators of acute inflammation, prostaglandins, and leukotrienes switch to produce the SPM [71]. Dietary studies and dietary supplementation with omega-3 fatty acids indicate that increasing omega-3 fatty acid intake can improve Aβ phagocytosis and reduce inflammation in people with minor cognitive impairment [72], believed to be due to rises in Resolvin D1. Furthermore, a combination of omega-3 fatty acids, resveratrol, and other antioxidants has been shown to improve cognition in mild cognitive impairment (MCI) patients [73], although this study was small, and larger double-blind, placebo-controlled studies are needed to verify these results. Nevertheless, these studies underscore the importance of aiming for a diet with a greater proportion of omega-3 fatty acids, to maintain a healthy ratio of omega-6 : omega-3 fatty acids.

5.3.4 Dietary Carbohydrates

Carbohydrates encompass the simplest sugars or monosaccharides such as glucose, fructose, and galactose, disaccharides such as table sugar (sucrose) and lactose, as well as the more complex carbohydrates such as the polysaccharides in starch and cellulose. The brain is especially dependent on glucose, and uses about 25% of the body's glucose, despite being only about 2% of a person's weight. The quantity and type of dietary carbohydrate consumed can significantly impact upon glucose regulation and lipid profiles, and consequently can also influence the likelihood of developing AD risk factors such as T2D, obesity, hypertension, and CVD. For example, a sustained intake of high glycaemic load foods from refined carbohydrates and simple sugars can result in insulin resistance and metabolic syndrome [34, 74]. If not addressed early, these signs of metabolic imbalance often lead to the other more serious conditions described above. The digestion of carbohydrates and their influence on cognition are discussed in greater detail in Chapter 6 by Fernando et al.

The fructose and glucose found in fruits are not in high quantities, such that ingestion of one or two pieces of fruit in a single sitting is not going to tax a person's insulin regulation system. However, the ingestion of sucrose in drinks, cakes, and processed foods, which is then rapidly converted to fructose and glucose during digestion, can lead to a high blood glucose level shortly after eating. Regular ingestion of high glycaemic load foods in this manner causes stress to the insulin regulatory cycle, leading to insulin resistance, as well as oxidative stress and disrupted myocardial calcium homeostasis [75]. The same problem occurs following ingestion of refined starchy foods, as the removal of the outer fibrous and protein-rich parts of grains allows for unhealthy fast digestion of the sugars.

Dietary fibre comprises indigestible carbohydrates, which are further classified as insoluble, soluble, and resistant starch. Insoluble fibre slows down the digestive process, allowing the digestive system more time to absorb other nutrients (important in the ageing population where compromised nutrient absorption is prevalent, frequently due to certain medical conditions or medications). Insoluble fibre also provides bulk, and some forms feed the probiotic bacteria in the colon [76]. By modulating food ingestion, digestion, absorption, and metabolism, dietary fibre reduces the risk of hyperlipidaemia, hypercholesterolaemia, and hyperglycaemia, which thereby helps reduce risk of T2D, CVD, and colon cancer [77, 78].

Soluble fibre and resistant starch can also feed probiotic bacteria and improve bowel health. Resistant starch is found in many unprocessed cereals and grains, lentils, as well as cooked-then-cooled potato, rice, and pasta. Other sources of dietary fibre include fruits and vegetables, whole-grain cereals, nuts, and seeds; again foods that feature prominently in the MeDi, DASH, MIND, and Okinawa diets. Some dietary fibre is used by probiotic bacteria to produce short-chain fatty acids (SCFA), which can be absorbed into the bloodstream and provide an alternative source of energy to the brain: recent studies suggest SCFA can benefit AD patients and individuals with MCI [79–81].

Fructose is rapidly absorbed and mostly metabolised by the liver, with consumption of large quantities inducing lipogenesis and triglyceride accumulation. Fructokinase is one of the major enzymes involved in fructose metabolism; it phosphorylates fructose to yield fructose-1-phosphate, which is then metabolised to triose phosphates, glyceraldehydes, and dihydroxyacetone phosphate. When ingesting low quantities, the vast majority of fructose is converted to trioses in the liver, which in turn are released into the bloodstream as lactate for oxidation in extra-hepatic tissues, or converted via gluconeogenesis to glucose, which is released or stored as glycogen [82]. However, the mechanism of fructose metabolism bypasses the main rate-controlling step of glycolysis [83]; consequently, when large quantities are ingested, fructose is continually converted to fat. Indeed, triglycerides form following the conversion of fructose to glycerol-3-phosphate, and esterification with free fatty acids. Triglyceride accumulation contributes to reduced insulin sensitivity, hepatic insulin resistance, and impaired glucose tolerance [84]. It has been suggested that fructose consumption causes increased energy intake and reduced energy expenditure due to its failure to stimulate leptin production, and thus does not lead to satiety. fMRI imaging of the brain has also shown that the brain responds differently to fructose or fructose-containing sugars, when compared to glucose or aspartame [85].

The association of neurogenesis with the chronic ingestion of simple sugars has been investigated using animal studies. Studies of rats fed either sucrose or fructose demonstrated reduced numbers of newly mature neurons in the dentate gyrus, the most prolific neurogenesis region of the hippocampus. Increased numbers of apoptotic cells were also observed. Intriguingly, when the feeds contained either glucose or fructose, enhanced proliferation of new neurons was observed, perhaps in an attempt to compensate for the increased apoptosis. The study authors suggested that elevated tumour necrosis factor alpha (TNFα) levels may be reducing survival of the new neurons by promoting apoptosis and impairing blood brain barrier function [86]. It is worthy of note, however, that elevated inflammatory cytokines (e.g. TNFα) and triglycerides (following fructose conversion to fat) can both compromise blood–brain barrier integrity [87].

Studies have shown that the adipose-derived hormone leptin and gut-derived hormone ghrelin stimulate neurogenesis in regions of the hippocampus, hypothalamus, and brain stem that regulate feeding, as does the vagus nerve connecting the brain and gut [88–92]. Furthermore, it has been shown that a compromised blood–brain barrier can prevent delivery of leptin and ghrelin to the hippocampus and reduce neurogenesis [86], and that chronic ingestion of high-sugar and high-calorie foods reduces the sensitivity of vagal afferent neurons to peripheral signals and their constitutive expression of orexigenic receptors and neuropeptides. This disruption of vagal signalling is sufficient to drive hyperphagia and obesity [93]. These effects apparently relate to fructose and sucrose ingestion only, as they are not seen with glucose consumption. The downregulation of hippocampal neurogenesis also appears to be independent of glucose levels, insulin, insulin-like growth factor-1, and cortisol. Significantly, therefore, whilst fructose is thought to be metabolised mainly by the liver and kidneys, it is apparent that this sugar acts centrally, affecting both neuronal function and neurogenesis [94]. These findings provide plausible links between increased fructose consumption in sweetened foods and drinks, and the increased risk of cognitive impairment and AD in people suffering from obesity, metabolic disease, insulin resistance, and T2D (which are, as previously mentioned, risk factors for AD development).

5.4 Key Micronutrients

Deficiencies in specific nutrients in the elderly may exacerbate developing or existing pathology in the brain, particularly in the presence of other risk factors [95]. The formation and maintenance of neurons relies on an adequate supply of the building blocks and cofactors required for normal functioning of structural and biochemical components, as well as signalling and neurotransmitter pathways, all of which must be obtained from the diet [96]. Moreover, neurons are particularly sensitive to oxidation-induced mitochondrial decay, which is a feature of normal brain ageing and is exacerbated in most neurodegenerative diseases. Thus, it is very important to maintain an adequate supply of nutrients that reduce oxidative stress, and protect mitochondrial enzymes and mitochondrial membranes, to support cellular energy generation and prevent neurological decline [97].

Certain vitamins, minerals, and other metabolites are critical cofactors in the synthesis of mitochondrial enzymes and for the maintenance of other biochemical pathways, and therefore diets that supply inadequate amounts of micronutrients can accelerate mitochondrial decay and neurodegeneration [98]. Nutrients supporting mitochondrial function include B vitamins, vitamin C, ubiquinone (CoQ10), iron, copper, zinc, manganese, and magnesium [98]. Deficiencies in several micronutrients have been linked to dementia, including vitamins A, B6, B12, D, E, K, folate, manganese, magnesium, selenium, and zinc. Some of these dietary constituents will be discussed in the sections that follow.

5.4.1 Water Soluble Vitamins

5.4.1.1 B Vitamins

Through their role as coenzymes in mitochondrial adenosine triphosphate (ATP) generation, the B vitamins are intimately involved in lipid, carbohydrate, and protein metabolism. Vitamin B6 (pyridoxine) metabolism depends on both vitamins B2 (riboflavin) and B3 (niacin). Synthesis of niacin from tryptophan requires the activated form of vitamin B6 (pyridoxal-5′-phosphate, PLP) to act as a cofactor for the enzyme kyureninase [5, 99]. Vitamin B5 (pantothenic acid) is the precursor to coenzyme A (CoA), which forms the key intermediate acetyl-CoA, thereby linking lipid, protein, and carbohydrate metabolism, and serving as the gateway to energy generation via ATP in the tricarboxylic acid (TCA)/oxidative phosphorylation cycle [5]. Thus, the critical role of the B vitamins in mitochondrial function and cell biochemistry in general makes it clear that any dietary or lifestyle factor which reduces availability of these micronutrients, including poor absorption and medication use, increases risk of neurological damage.

Vitamin B1 (Thiamin) Among the elderly, subclinical thiamin deficiency is not uncommon [100]. Numerous thiamin-dependent processes have been shown to be significantly reduced in the AD brain [101, 102] and deficiency has been associated with dementia [103]. The thiamin-dependent enzymes transketolase, pyruvate dehydrogenase, and α-ketoglutarate dehydrogenase have crucial roles in glucose metabolism and energy generation, and reductions in enzyme activity can result in nerve cell damage [104]. The pyruvate dehydrogenase and α-ketoglutarate dehydrogenase enzymes in particular, which play a part in the Krebs cycle, are specifically affected in AD, as many studies have shown in both brain tissue and peripheral tissues that activities of these enzymes are lower in AD, yet the other four Krebs cycle enzymes are unchanged [102, 105–108]. A lower level of transketolase also decreases the production of reducing substances such as reduced nicotinamide adenine dinucleotide phosphate (NADPH) via the pentose phosphate pathway, which is required for lipid synthesis and the removal of reactive oxygen species. A reduction in pentoses, required for nucleic acids, coenzymes, and polysaccharides, is also seen, which can further compromise cellular function [104]. Reduced α-ketoglutarate dehydrogenase activity due to thiamin deficiency may contribute to decreased levels of several neurotransmitters such as γ-amino butyric acid (GABA), glutamate, and aspartate [109], and NMDA (n-methyl D-aspartate) receptor-mediated excitotoxicity may be involved in the neuronal damage seen with thiamin deficiency, although this is yet to be established. Moreover, thiamin deficiency-induced low transketolase activity has been linked to impaired hippocampal neurogenesis [110, 111]. In other studies, increased levels of cerebrospinal fluid (CSF) phosphorylated tau (an AD biomarker) have been measured in cases of thiamin deficiency [112], and *in vitro* and *in vivo* studies have shown thiamin deficiency induces oxidative stress, which promotes amyloidogenic processing of amyloid precursor protein (APP) and subsequent Aβ accumulation [113, 114].

Further clarification of the relationship between thiamin deficiency and AD is required, as it is not known to what extent disturbances in thiamin function are a cause of AD pathogenesis or a consequence of AD pathology. Nevertheless, more recent studies have suggested mechanistic roles for thiamin deficiencies in AD pathogenesis. For example, it has been shown that thiamin is important in the defence against accumulation of advanced glycation end-products (AGE). Plasma AGE are increased in thiamin deficiency, in a dose-dependent fashion [108]. This may be due to disruptions in the glycolytic cycle as a result of the enzyme deficiencies mentioned above, causing higher than normal conversion of glyceraldehyde-3-phosphate into methylglyoxal, which is the most potent precursor of AGE [115]. Thiamin has been shown to inhibit lipid peroxidation in liver microsomes, reduce free radical oxidation of oleic acid in an *in vitro* model, and increase glutathione reductase activity in a rat model of cardiac insufficiency (for a review see [108]). Lower levels of thiamin diphosphate (active form of thiamin) are detected in AD, and recent studies indicate this may be the result of higher activity of the thiamin-metabolising enzymes thiamin diphosphatase and thiamin monophosphatase, which have been detected in blood samples of AD patients [116]. Thus a dietary thiamin deficiency may be compounded by changes in thiamin metabolism, which could also impact glucose metabolism; at this stage, however, it is not known how early in AD pathogenesis this change occurs, or whether these changes are, in fact, a result of glucose metabolism dysregulation (which does occur early in AD pathogenesis). Another recent review has also suggested that thiamin deficiency leads to neurodegeneration due to the interplay between deficiency-induced increased oxidative stress, endoplasmic reticulum stress, and autophagy [117].

Vitamin B2 (Riboflavin)   Riboflavin is a precursor of the coenzymes flavin mononucleotide (FMN) and flavin adenine dinucleotide (FAD), which are both crucial redox cofactors in mitochondrial ATP generation and in other biochemical pathways [97]. As already mentioned in this book, there is substantial evidence that oxidative stress is a contributing factor to both the development and progression of AD [118, 119]. Riboflavin is vital in reducing oxidised glutathione, a major intracellular antioxidant, and restoring its antioxidant capacity [120]. In addition, FAD is a coenzyme for methylene tetrahydrofolate reductase which converts homocysteine to methionine, and xanthine oxidase which produces uric acid [97]. Elevated homocysteine and low levels of reduced glutathione are linked to both ageing and cognitive decline [121–123]. In the case of uric acid, studies have suggested that high levels correlate with risk of hypertension, cerebrovascular and renal disease, and that levels rise with ageing. On the other hand, uric acid is an effective antioxidant and some studies have suggested higher serum uric acid levels slow the rate of cognitive decline. Nevertheless, many other studies suggest the opposite, and recent reports indicate sex-specific associations between serum uric acid levels and cognitive changes or other health indices: for example, higher serum uric acid has been linked to a faster rate of Parkinson's disease progression in women, higher serum uric acid is also more strongly associated with CVD in women than men (for a review see [124]).

Vitamin B3 (Niacin) Niacin or nicotinic acid is required for formation of the ubiquitous mitochondrial redox coenzymes nicotinamide adenine dinucleotide (NAD) and NAD phosphate (NADP), and a severe deficiency of niacin or its precursor tryptophan causes pellagra, in which dementia is a prominent feature [5]. Although the exact mechanism linking niacin deficiency and dementia has not been established, niacin has been shown to be important for DNA synthesis and repair, myelination and dendritic growth, cellular calcium signalling, as well as acting as a potent antioxidant in brain mitochondria [125–128]. Niacin has been included in supplement preparations used in trials, where improvements in cognitive test scores have been reported [129]; and a large prospective study using food frequency questionnaires (FFQs) to estimate niacin intake concluded that dietary niacin may protect against AD and age-related cognitive decline [128]. However, further research is required into the potential cognition-improving roles of specific nutrients such as niacin.

Vitamin B6 (Pyridoxine), Vitamin B12 (Cobalamin), and Folate Vitamins B6, B12, and folate as a group have an important role, as they function together to help reduce homocysteine levels in the body, either by converting to cysteine, or recycling back to methionine. High serum homocysteine levels are linked to several conditions, including CVD, stroke, osteoporosis, Parkinson's disease, AD, and dementia [121–123]. The elderly are more likely to suffer from a B12 deficiency (pernicious anaemia), which can be due to lower meat and dairy intake, or to certain medical conditions or medications impairing absorption during digestion [130]. A recent study involving treatment of people with MCI, AD, and other cognitive disorders (who had high homocysteine levels), with cysteine, methylfolate, and methylcobalamin (B12) showed that such treatment could slow cognitive decline, and that this correlated with reductions in homocysteine levels [131]. Whilst validation via randomised, placebo-controlled trials is required, this suggests B12 supplementation is potentially an effective way to help reduce cognitive decline in susceptible people.

Deficiencies in vitamin B6 have been associated with depression, a decline in cognitive function, and may contribute to AD progression [132]. Approximately 10% of the US population are estimated to consume less than half the recommended dietary intake of vitamin B6 [133], and a low or deficient status is generally common in the elderly [132]. PLP is the active form of vitamin B6, and it is involved in amino acid metabolism of neurotransmitters such as GABA, serotonin, dopamine, and noradrenalin [5].

Methylation reactions in the brain are critical, and therefore an adequate supply of methyl groups provided by folate, vitamin B12, and SAMe (S-adenosyl methionine) is vital. The elderly may be compromised by dietary deficiency, poor absorption, and inadequate inter-conversion of folates, as occurs in people with certain polymorphisms in the methylene tetrahydrofolate reductase (*MTHFR*) gene. The importance of vitamin B12 has been described in relation to methylation reactions, with the production and maintenance of myelin implicated: demyelination is thought to be one mechanism via which vitamin B12 deficiency affects central nervous system (CNS) function [120]. Additionally, adenosylcobalamin, a metabolite of vitamin B12 acts as a mitochondrial cofactor for the production of succinyl-CoA: this is important for converting odd-chain fatty acids (not normally present in cell membranes) from propionate to succinate for oxidation in the TCA cycle. This conversion is inhibited with vitamin B12 deficiency, and can result in odd-chain fatty acids being incorporated into myelin, therefore affecting nerve transmission [134].

Folate status also appears to be associated with tissue levels of DHA, which is concentrated in neural tissue and affects receptor function and cell signalling [135]. Animal studies have shown that concentrations of DHA in platelets, erythrocytes, and intestinal phospholipids are increased in rats fed supplemental folate [136]. Further, animal studies have demonstrated that dietary folate deficiency causes depletion of DHA in neural tissue [137].

5.4.2 Fat Soluble Vitamins

5.4.2.1 Vitamin A (Retinol, Retinal, and Retinoic Acid)

Vitamin A can be described as a group of unsaturated lipid-like compounds that includes retinol, retinal, retinoic acid, and several provitamin A carotenoids including beta-(β) carotene. Retinol is found in foods from animal sources, including dairy products, fish, and meat (especially liver), whereas beta-carotene, which we can convert into active vitamin A, is found in large amounts in orange and green vegetables such as carrots, spinach, kale, and sweet potatoes. Vitamin A functions as an antioxidant, and is required for good vision, and maintenance of the immune system. Furthermore, vitamin A in the form of retinoic acid exerts hormone-like activity via binding to nuclear receptors. This process regulates cell differentiation, proliferation, and apoptosis in adults, and influences binding of many other nuclear receptors involved in a diverse number of processes, including lipid metabolism [120, 138]. Studies in rats have shown that vitamin A deficiency decreases the liver content of phospholipids [139]. This process may adversely affect liver function itself in terms of lipid metabolism and bile production, and it may also affect the supply of crucial phospholipids to other organs, including the brain. Vitamin A plays key roles in α-secretase production, acetylcholine transmission, and in the regulation of excessive microglial activation [140], and vitamin A insufficiency has been shown to influence these processes in AD [141, 142]. There are two binding sites for the retinoic acid receptor just upstream from the α-secretase gene ADAM-10 (A Disintegrin And Metalloproteinase Domain-containing Protein 10), and retinoic acid has been shown to upregulate ADAM-10 expression [143], thereby increasing non-amyloidogenic APP processing. In animal studies, vitamin A deficient mice were shown to have impaired ADAM-10 transcription, and the addition of vitamin A upregulated both ADAM-10 and APP levels, resulting in reduced formation of Aβ and increased formation of the neuroprotective secreted beta-amyloid precursor protein ectodomain sAPPα [144]. Additionally, dietary deficiency of vitamin A in adult rats leads to an increase in deposition of Aβ in cerebral blood vessels [145]. Retinoic acid insufficiency has also been connected to reduced production of acetylcholine transferase, which inhibits the neurotransmitter function of acetylcholine, a common feature of AD [142]. Further, as mentioned previously, inflammation is a key feature of AD, and retinoic acid is a powerful modulator of immune function. It reduces Aβ-induced inflammation via suppression of interleukin-6 (IL-6) and inhibition of TNFα, and increases production of anti-inflammatory cytokines such as IL-10: the net effect is to reduce microglial expression of inducible nitric oxide synthase (iNOS) and hence activation. These effects are thought to be mediated by inhibiting the translocation of nuclear factor kappa beta (NF-κB) [142]. Additionally, retinol has a crucial role in mitochondria as it is an essential cofactor for protein kinase C delta (PKC-delta), which acts as a nutritional sensor to regulate energy homeostasis [146]. Vitamin A deficiency may therefore contribute to the hypometabolism seen in the AD brain [147].

Recent cell culture studies have also found that a form of vitamin A (All-trans-retinoic acid) can reduce expression of beta-site APP cleaving enzyme 1 (BACE1) under inflammatory conditions, via modulation of NFκB signalling [148]. This may explain why a recent report has shown that marginal vitamin A deficiency in an AD mouse model promotes BACE1-mediated Aβ production and amyloid deposition; changes which were accompanied by memory deficits in the mice [149]. In fact, transcription of many AD-relevant genes has been shown to be influenced by vitamin A, including the genes for APP, BACE1 (as mentioned above), the presenilins (PS1 and PS2; components of the γ-secretase enzyme involved in Aβ production), ADAM 10 (which cleaves APP within the Aβ region, also discussed above), and insulin-degrading enzyme (which is a major Aβ-degrading enzyme) (for a review see [150]). The vitamin can also influence the intracellular sorting of APP cleaving enzymes, thereby influencing APP processing and, last but not least, AD transgenic mice studies show it may influence tau phosphorylation, thus reducing aggregation of tau (for a review see [150]).

Vitamin A insufficiency can result from poor dietary intakes of vitamin A rich foods, or from chronic malabsorption of lipids, impaired bile production, zinc deficiency, or heavy smoking and alcohol consumption (both of which place a high demand on antioxidants) [151]. Insufficiency can also occur as a result of two single nucleotide polymorphisms (SNPs) in the gene that converts the vitamin A precursor, β-carotene, to retinol (Beta carotene15,15′-monoxygenase). These SNPs are present in 25–40% of the population and result in reduced enzyme activity and conversion to retinol [152]. Individuals carrying these SNPs may benefit from higher intakes of pre-formed retinol rather than relying on carotenoid sources from plant foods.

5.4.2.2 Vitamin D

Vitamin D, a cholesterol metabolite, plays a significant role in calcium homeostasis and bone health, and increases intestinal absorption of calcium, magnesium, and phosphate. This vitamin has been implicated as a factor in AD, as studies have reported lower serum levels in AD patients [153, 154]. In addition, osteoporosis (associated with vitamin D deficiency) and AD often exist as comorbidities [155, 156], with both conditions being provoked by inflammatory processes and insulin resistance. The ligand-mediated vitamin D receptor (VDR) is a nuclear, ligand-dependent transcription factor that complexes with hormonally active vitamin D (1,25(OH)2D3) to regulate the expression of more than 900 genes involved in a wide array of physiological functions, including calcium/phosphate homeostasis, cellular proliferation and differentiation, and immune responses. The receptor is found in most tissues of the body, including the brain [157, 158]. Reduced mRNA for the VDR has been shown in specific hippocampal regions in AD compared to normal controls [159] and a higher frequency of VDR polymorphisms has also been reported to occur in AD [160]. Vitamin D may protect the structure and integrity of neurons through detoxification pathways, and 1,25(OH)2D3 has also been shown to inhibit iNOS, and therefore reduce inflammation and oxidation and prevent excessive microglial activation. In addition, vitamin D upregulates γ-glutamyl transpeptidase and increases glutathione synthesis (a critical intracellular antioxidant; [161]), and upregulates the synthesis of neurotrophins such as the docosanoid neuroprotectin D1 (NPD1), and glial-derived neurotrophic factor (both necessary for neuronal survival; [157]).

In AD there is loss of hippocampal cells which has been attributed (at least partly) to elevated voltage-gated calcium channels, reduced calcium buffering capacity, and glucocorticoid neurotoxicity. Vitamin D is a major regulator of calcium homeostasis and can protect against excitotoxicity [157], yet a recent review of osteoporosis and dementia, looking at the current published evidence, did not find this aspect of vitamin D function to be related to disease aetiology [162]. However, vitamin D deficiencies have also been linked to reduced physical mobility and function (possibly linked to osteoporosis), which would lead to lower physical strength and reduced cardiovascular health (a condition which has been linked to higher risk of AD). There are also studies that have suggested lower vitamin D levels are associated with depressive symptoms and mood in older adults, although some studies show no association [163].

Interestingly, insulin sensitivity and signalling have been linked to vitamin D [164], and a recent transcriptome analysis of vitamin D-treated AD transgenic mice indicated that vitamin D influences insulin signalling as well as oestrogen signalling [165]. Furthermore, a study of over 2000 men showed a correlation between vitamin D levels and bioavailable testosterone [166]. Testosterone levels drop with ageing, and low levels of testosterone in elderly men have been linked to MCI and AD [167, 168].

Some interventional studies have failed to show improvements in cognitive outcomes following vitamin D supplementation, yet longitudinal studies have often (but not always) shown that low vitamin D levels are associated with greater cognitive decline and that supplementation sometimes improves aspects of cognition [169]. These recent associations of vitamin D with a myriad of signalling and metabolic functions suggest further studies are needed to understand the effects of vitamin D, and to determine (i) whether supplementation is of therapeutic value, and (ii) the best age for such intervention.

5.4.2.3 Vitamin E

There are eight naturally occurring forms of vitamin E, with α-tocopherol being the most biologically active. Dietary sources include vegetable oils (such as sunflower, corn, and soybean oils), nuts (such as almonds, peanuts, and hazelnuts), seeds, green leafy vegetables (such as spinach and broccoli), and fortified (where vitamin E has been added) breakfast cereals, fruit juices, and margarine. Vitamin E is a major component of the body's antioxidant defence system, protecting against lipid peroxidation in cell membranes, reducing the production of prostaglandins, and inhibiting platelet aggregation [170].

Vitamin E levels have been shown to be lower in AD [171], and decreased serum levels have been associated with poor memory in the elderly [172]. In addition to accumulating in circulating lipoproteins, vitamin E is also transported in plasma by phospholipid transfer protein (PLTP). Studies have shown lower CSF PLTP activity levels in AD compared to normal healthy controls, and this may result in reduced vitamin E transport to the brain and increased oxidative stress [173, 174]. In neuronal cultures, vitamin E inhibits Aβ-induced lipid peroxidation and cell death [175, 176].

Apart from its role as an antioxidant, there is increasing evidence that vitamin E may regulate gene activity, as gene array studies have connected vitamin E deficiency with altered gene expression in the hippocampus of rats [177]. This study showed the downregulation of 948 genes including those affecting growth hormone, thyroid hormones, insulin-like growth factor, neuronal growth factor, melatonin, dopaminergic neurotransmission, and clearance of advanced glycation end-products [177]. Also, genes coding for proteins related to Aβ clearance were strongly downregulated in the presence of vitamin E deficiency [177]. Vitamin E also influences cholesterol levels by affecting the SREBP/SCAP system (sterol regulatory element binding protein/SREBP cleavage-activating protein), one of the main systems controlling cellular cholesterol levels. Since APP cleavage occurs in cholesterol-dependent lipid rafts, it is likely that vitamin E can influence Aβ production, with higher cholesterol content in membranes being associated with enhanced Aβ production as well as greater cell membrane internalisation of APP, leading to Aβ overproduction in acidic intracellular compartments. Furthermore, a promotion of Aβ aggregation and Aβ-induced toxicity by cholesterol has been reported (for a review see [150]).

In addition to protecting against lipid peroxidation, influencing cholesterol levels, and modifying gene expression, recent studies have shown that vitamin E can block intracellular accumulation of ceramides [178], this is of note considering ceramide levels are known to be linked to memory impairment, hippocampal volume loss, and increased risk of AD, though possibly only in men [179]. Ceramides also protect BACE1 from breakdown, a process which is thought to occur indirectly via ceramide-mediated promotion of post-translational modification of the enzyme [180].

Trials using supplemental vitamin E, however, have produced conflicting results [14, 181], perhaps due to the varying forms of vitamin E used; naturally occurring vitamin E is a mixture of α- and γ-tocopherols, whilst the commonly used commercial form (d-α-tocopherol) contains just one isomer with activity. Additionally, a single isolated nutrient is less likely to produce a positive outcome due to the synergistic nature of nutrients and the fact that dietary sources contain so many other compounds: this, however, is likely to remain a limitation with respect to many such studies and should not be considered as unique to vitamin E trials. A recent Cochrane Database Systematic Review found no conclusive evidence that vitamin E supplementation improves cognitive function in people with MCI or dementia, or that it prevents progression from MCI to AD, yet the review concluded by saying that the trials were small, dosage needs to be considered, and further research is required [179].

5.4.3 Dietary Minerals

Minerals required in the diet include calcium, iron, phosphorous, magnesium, sodium, potassium, chloride, and sulphur. Some minerals are required in small amounts, such as manganese, zinc, selenium, copper, iodine, and cobalt. All can be obtained from a varied diet that includes a mix of fruits, vegetables, nuts, and protein sources. Some of the minerals known to be relevant to AD are discussed below.

5.4.3.1 Selenium

Selenium functions as an antioxidant and as an important regulator of brain function. In particular, it forms part of several selenoproteins that are important in fighting oxidative stress in the brain. Selenoproteins include the antioxidant enzymes glutathione peroxidases and thioredoxin reductases, as well as selenoprotein P, an extracellular ubiquitously expressed glycoprotein. Many studies have shown that selenium is important in the reduction of oxidative stress and other detrimental agents in AD and Parkinson's disease, as well as in epilepsy, and this mineral has also been shown to be important in mitochondrial function and calcium homeostasis (for reviews see [182, 183]). With respect to brain health and AD pathogenesis, selenium compounds have been shown to inhibit tau hyperphosphorylation, a critical step in the formation of neurofibrillary tangles, whereas selenoprotein P appears to protect APP against excessive copper and iron deposition. Selenoproteins also have anti-inflammatory properties, and protect microtubules in the neuronal cytoskeleton. Decreases in plasma selenium levels and levels of thioredoxin enzymes have been linked to cognitive decline in AD, irrespective of nutritional status, and selenium levels are also lower in AD brain tissue, although not all studies have found such changes [182, 184], and further research is necessary to determine the potential value of selenium supplement therapy. Nevertheless, several recent animal studies have shown promising results using selenium supplements: for example, AD-triple transgenic mice undergoing selenium supplementation demonstrated enhanced autophagy, reduced oxidative stress, lower $A\beta$ and tau pathology, and improved cognitive outcomes [185, 186].

5.4.3.2 Manganese

In the nervous system, manganese is required as a cofactor for certain enzymes, such as astrocytic glutamine synthetase, pyruvate carboxylase, and mitochondrial superoxide dismutase. However, an excess of manganese is toxic, leading to symptoms similar to Parkinson's disease [187]. Studies have implicated abnormal manganese metabolism in AD, such that manganese-superoxide dismutase enzyme levels are reduced in AD, and a dysfunction in this enzyme aids amyloid plaque formation. Manganese homeostasis is also tightly regulated by transporters, thought to be highly relevant in some neurological conditions like Parkinson's disease [188]. A recent meta-analysis reported that significant decreases in serum manganese levels are seen in both MCI and AD compared to age-matched control subjects, though no differences were found between MCI and AD; implying manganese changes may occur early in the disease process, and that a deficiency may be a risk factor for AD [189].

5.4.3.3 Zinc, Iron, Copper, and Calcium

The metals zinc, iron, copper, and calcium are important for neuronal function. Disruptions in levels and the metabolism of one of these elements are frequently accompanied by disruptions in all three others, as seen in several neuropathological conditions including AD, Parkinson's disease, Huntington's disease, and amyotrophic lateral sclerosis. Recently developed imaging techniques have helped to focus on where changes in metal metabolism occur, allowing researchers to decipher pathological pathways and provide potential avenues for therapy [190–194]. In AD, copper, zinc, and iron ions are found in amyloid plaques, and co-localise with $A\beta$ [195, 196]. These ions, particularly zinc and copper, are also known to facilitate $A\beta$ aggregation, and AD-model transgenic mice studies have shown that chelators which remove these ions can reduce $A\beta$ deposition [197].

Zinc Zinc is essential for brain function, as it is important in axonal and synaptic transmission (zinc is found in synaptic vesicles), nucleic acid metabolism, and as a cofactor for several enzymes including copper/zinc superoxide dismutase. Early studies showed zinc (and copper) could accelerate Aβ aggregation, zinc is also known to enhance APP expression, increase Aβ production and plaque deposition, and it has been suggested that chelating agents such as clioquinol may be useful as therapy against the development of AD pathology [198, 199].

However, more recently, a general disruption in zinc homeostasis in the brain, particularly at synapses in glutamatergic nerve terminals, has been identified as being central in the glutamatergic excitotoxic cascade that occurs in AD [200]. Under certain conditions, including hypoxia, hypoglycaemia, and inflammation, zinc is released with glutamate in abnormally high levels into the synaptic cleft, to concentrations of around 0.3 mM, which exceed the binding capacity of carrier proteins. The excess zinc is absorbed by post-synaptic neurons, disrupting zinc homeostasis and disrupting signalling mechanisms. Zinc transporter function is also disturbed, and the aberrant distribution of zinc includes an excess going to mitochondrial compartments, which is thought to contribute to the acetyl-CoA changes that have been noted early in AD, and which in turn are thought to be central to mitochondrial dysfunction, pathological changes to energy (ATP) regulation, and disturbances in acetylcholine synthesis [200–202]. These changes to zinc metabolism do not occur in isolation, they often interact with alterations in copper, calcium, and iron metabolism, and are often linked to oxidative stress, mitochondrial dysfunction, inflammation, and disruptions to brain signalling.

Iron Iron is required in the CNS for oxygen transport, oxidative phosphorylation, myelin production, and for neurotransmitter synthesis. Abnormal iron metabolism has been detected in several neurodegenerative conditions and is characterised by greater hydroxyl radical production, which causes damage to proteins, lipids, and DNA. This process may be exacerbated by age-related changes in iron metabolism, such as the accumulation of iron in ferritin, the major intracellular iron storage protein. Elevated levels of ferritin have been detected in AD, in the vicinity of plaques and neurofibrillary tangles, and this excess ferritin has also been linked to hippocampal tissue damage [194, 203]. High levels of iron have been detected in the substantia nigra in Parkinson's disease patients, and in the hippocampus and cerebral cortex in AD. Furthermore, recent brain imaging studies have shown higher cortical iron levels are associated with higher Aβ deposition levels in MCI, with the iron deposits co-localising with the Aβ plaques [204]. It has been hypothesised that iron fortification in foods may be causing early build-up of iron and excessive iron storage, which may lead to higher risk of Parkinson's disease, and possibly also AD [205], however further research is necessary to confirm this link.

Copper Copper is involved in iron absorption and the production of red blood cells, and it is also a requirement for our immune and nervous systems. Either an excess or a deficiency of copper can affect brain function. Notably, some important enzymes involved in reducing oxidative stress (e.g. superoxide dismutase-1) have copper as a cofactor, thus it is unsurprising that certain brain cells (the astrocytes) are important regulators of copper homeostasis [206].

Disruptions to copper metabolism and distribution throughout the brain occur in AD, and copper has been shown to aid Aβ aggregation [207]. Several studies have investigated copper levels in AD brains, with one study published in the 1990s describing a significant increase [196], whereas others showed no change, or a decrease [208]. With technologies improving over the years, the consensus now seems to be that, unlike iron and zinc, copper levels are substantially decreased in all AD-affected brain regions compared to controls, as shown by recent mass spectrometry studies for example [209]. This finding suggests that chelation therapy to remove excess iron, zinc, and copper from the brain may only add to the metal imbalance that seems to occur early in the AD pathogenic process [208].

Shellfish, whole grains, beans, nuts, seeds, potatoes, and liver are good sources of copper, with sufficient levels usually ingested as part of a healthy diet. However, malnutrition, malabsorption, or excessive zinc intake can lead to a deficiency of copper. Even a marginal copper imbalance has been linked to impaired immune function, bone de-mineralisation, and an increased risk of cardiovascular and neurodegenerative diseases.

Calcium Calcium is required for bone formation, as well as muscle and digestive system function. Calcium is also required in all cells for signal transduction pathways, and in neurons for neurotransmitter release. Disruptions to calcium metabolism are involved in osteoporosis, calcium oxalate (kidney stone) formation, artery plaque formation, certain cancers, and hyperparathyroidism; there are also disruptions to calcium metabolism and function in AD. Studies of presenilin mutation carriers who develop familial AD have shown that these people have synaptic calcium-signalling abnormalities, and disrupted intracellular calcium stores, thought to be due to presenilin functions that are independent of their role as part of the γ-secretase complex [210]. The presenilins and Aβ both seem to affect calcium homeostasis at very early stages of AD pathogenesis, impacting synaptic transmission and function prior to amyloid plaque deposition. Altered calcium signalling also regulates genes such as calcineurin, calmodulin kinase II, and mitogen-activated protein (MAP) kinase, and induces protein modifications and neurite degeneration [211].

Western diets are thought to be deficient in calcium intake, and it has been shown that disruptions to the function of the VDR (mentioned above under vitamin D) and the calcium-sensing receptor, when vitamin D/calcium are insufficient, lead to disruptions in cell metabolism, which increase the risk of osteoporosis, some cancers, metabolic syndrome, T2D, hypertension, and CVD, many of which are risk factors for AD [212, 213]. For example, calcium deficiency has been linked to a high-fat diet-induced non-alcoholic steatohepatitis (NASH), as calcium supplements could reduce NASH in mice fed a high-fat western-style diet. This protective effect was due to calcium-induced changes to the gut microbiota as well as changes in the hepatic bile acid pool [214]. Thus, ensuring an adequate intake of calcium together with vitamin D may be important in preventing many illnesses as well as neurodegeneration.

5.5 Conclusion

The numerous integrated processes leading to the development and proliferation of AD are complex and involve genetics, epigenetics, metabolic dysfunction, hormonal circuits, chronic inflammation and oxidative stress injury. Nutrition, by its influence on all of these contributing factors, is likely to profoundly impact upon AD pathogenesis and risk. Therefore, understanding the effect of macro- and micro-nutrients on neuronal biochemistry and AD pathology will provide opportunities for dietary manipulation to promote neuronal resistance to insults and reduce brain injury. This chapter has highlighted some of the key nutrients involved both directly in neuronal biochemistry and indirectly by influencing peripheral metabolism, which in turn can promote AD pathology. Deficiencies or excesses of nutrients are unlikely to cause AD on their own, but when combined with genetic factors and metabolic disease may accelerate existing pathology. AD pathology develops over many years before clinical symptoms appear, providing the opportunity to develop interventions, including nutritional approaches, which could slow or stop disease progression well before any clinical manifestations are apparent. Such interventions could include the use of dietary phytochemicals and omega-3 fatty acids to activate cell-survival signalling mechanisms and help ameliorate poor metabolic health. Diets composed of energy-dense, nutrient-poor foods and containing high levels of saturated fats and simple sugars, as well as low fibre, will continue to drive metabolic disease and associated morbidities, including AD.

Micronutrient insufficiencies are often present with metabolic disease due to inadequate intakes and increased requirement as part of altered metabolism and medication use. In an ageing individual, intakes and assimilation of nutrients can be compromised, and may partly explain the conflicting results of clinical studies using nutrient interventions. However, nutrient interventions are most likely going to be insufficient in a large proportion of people with unhealthy western-style diets, as the toxic, inflammatory, and calorie-intense nature of many foods regularly eaten cannot be counter-balanced by a few nutrient-dense pills; the overall diet needs to be addressed. In addition, many clinical nutrient intervention studies are inconsistently designed in terms of disease stage and extent of neuronal injury, and further trials need to administer intervention before significant neurodegeneration is present. The profound impact of nutrition on the processes contributing to AD pathology cannot be denied but the lack of consistency in study data highlights the complexity of interpreting results from nutritional intervention trials. Future trials should account for bioavailability of supplements used, the existing diet of the cohort, and the synergistic nature of nutrients in general: nutrients do not exist in isolation in food. Strategies need to be employed to reduce the predicted explosion in the number of AD cases, and as nutrition is emerging as an important part of the complex AD puzzle, one strategy might be assignment of a specialist nutritionist as part of ongoing healthcare of an ageing individual, particularly in those at increased risk of developing this devastating disease.

References

1 van Asselt, D.Z., de Groot, L.C., van Staveren, W.A. et al. (1998). Role of cobalamin intake and atrophic gastritis in mild cobalamin deficiency in older Dutch subjects. *Am. J. Clin. Nutr.* 68: 328–334.
2 Krasinski, S.D., Russell, R.M., Samloff, I.M. et al. (1986). Fundic atrophic gastritis in an elderly population. Effect on hemoglobin and several serum nutritional indicators. *J. Am. Geriatr. Soc.* 34: 800–806.
3 Obeid, R. and Herrmann, W. (2006). Mechanisms of homocysteine neurotoxicity in neurodegenerative diseases with special reference to dementia. *FEBS Lett.* 580: 2994–3005.

4 Tucker, K.L., Qiao, N., Scott, T. et al. (2005). High homocysteine and low B vitamins predict cognitive decline in aging men: the Veterans Affairs Normative Aging Study. *Am. J. Clin. Nutr.* 82: 627–635.
5 Gropper, S.S.J. and Groff, J. (2012). *Advanced Nutrition and Human Metabolism*, 6e. Boston: Thomson Wadsworth.
6 Polidori, M.C., Pientka, L., and Mecocci, P. (2012). A review of the major vascular risk factors related to Alzheimer's disease. *J. Alzheimers Dis.* 32: 521–530.
7 Patterson, C., Feightner, J., Garcia, A., and MacKnight, C. (2007). General risk factors for dementia: a systematic evidence review. *Alzheimers Dement.* 3: 341–347.
8 Kant, A.K. (1996). Indexes of overall diet quality: a review. *J. Am. Diet. Assoc.* 96: 785–791.
9 Scarmeas, N., Stern, Y., Tang, M.X. et al. (2006). Mediterranean diet and risk for Alzheimer's disease. *Ann. Neurol.* 59: 912–921.
10 Gu, Y., Nieves, J.W., Stern, Y. et al. (2010). Food combination and Alzheimer disease risk: a protective diet. *Arch. Neurol.* 67: 699–706.
11 Gardener, S.L., Rainey-Smith, S.R., Barnes, M.B. et al. (2015). Dietary patterns and cognitive decline in an Australian study of ageing. *Mol. Psychiatry* 20: 860–866.
12 Solfrizzi, V., Panza, F., and Capurso, A. (2003). The role of diet in cognitive decline. *J. Neural Transm.* 110: 95–110.
13 Morris, M.C., Evans, D.A., Bienias, J.L. et al. (2002). Dietary intake of antioxidant nutrients and the risk of incident Alzheimer disease in a biracial community study. *JAMA* 287: 3230–3237.
14 Luchsinger, J.A. and Mayeux, R. (2004). Dietary factors and Alzheimer's disease. *Lancet Neurol.* 3: 579–587.
15 Gardener, S.L., Rainey-Smith, S.R., and Martins, R.N. (2015). Diet and inflammation in Alzheimer's disease and related chronic diseases: a review. *J. Alzheimers Dis.* 50: 301–334.
16 Son, T.G., Camandola, S., and Mattson, M.P. (2008). Hormetic dietary phytochemicals. *Neuromolecular Med.* 10: 236–246.
17 Gomez-Pinilla, F. (2008). Brain foods: the effects of nutrients on brain function. *Nat. Rev. Neurosci.* 9: 568–578.
18 Gomez-Pinilla, F. (2008). The influences of diet and exercise on mental health through hormesis. *Ageing Res. Rev.* 7: 49–62.
19 Mattson, M.P. (2008). Hormesis and disease resistance: activation of cellular stress response pathways. *Hum. Exp. Toxicol.* 27: 155–162.
20 Mattson, M.P. (2008). Dietary factors, hormesis and health. *Ageing Res. Rev.* 7: 43–48.
21 Rainey-Smith, S.R., Gu, Y., Gardener, S.L. et al. (2018). Mediterranean diet adherence and rate of cerebral Aβ-amyloid accumulation: data from the Australian imaging, biomarkers and lifestyle study of ageing. *Transl Psychiatry.* 2018 Oct 30; 8(1): 238.
22 Willcox, D.C., Scapagnini, G., and Willcox, B.J. (2014). Healthy aging diets other than the Mediterranean: a focus on the Okinawan diet. *Mech. Ageing Dev.* 136–137: 148–162.
23 Sacks, F.M., Appel, L.J., Moore, T.J. et al. (1999). A dietary approach to prevent hypertension: a review of the Dietary Approaches to Stop Hypertension (DASH) Study. *Clin. Cardiol.* 22: III6–III10.

24 Smith, P.J., Blumenthal, J.A., Babyak, M.A. et al. (2010). Effects of the dietary approaches to stop hypertension diet, exercise, and caloric restriction on neurocognition in overweight adults with high blood pressure. *Hypertension* 55: 1331–1338.

25 Solfrizzi, V., Custodero, C., Lozupone, M. et al. (2017). Relationships of dietary patterns, foods, and micro- and macronutrients with Alzheimer's disease and late-life cognitive disorders: a systematic review. *J. Alzheimers Dis.* 59: 815–849.

26 Morris, M.C., Tangney, C.C., Wang, Y. et al. (2015). MIND diet slows cognitive decline with aging. *Alzheimers Dement.* 11: 1015–1022.

27 Morris, M.C., Tangney, C.C., Wang, Y. et al. (2015). MIND diet associated with reduced incidence of Alzheimer's disease. *Alzheimers Dement.* 11: 1007–1014.

28 Kanoski, S.E. and Davidson, T.L. (2011). Western diet consumption and cognitive impairment: links to hippocampal dysfunction and obesity. *Physiol. Behav.* 103: 59–68.

29 Brayne, C., Gao, L., and Matthews, F., MRC Cognitive Function and Ageing Study(2005). Challenges in the epidemiological investigation of the relationships between physical activity, obesity, diabetes, dementia and depression. *Neurobiol. Aging* 26 (Suppl 1): 6–10.

30 Convit, A. (2005). Links between cognitive impairment in insulin resistance: an explanatory model. *Neurobiol. Aging* 26 (Suppl 1): 31–35.

31 Craft, S. (2005). Insulin resistance syndrome and Alzheimer's disease: age- and obesity-related effects on memory, amyloid, and inflammation. *Neurobiol. Aging* 26 (Suppl 1): 65–69.

32 Greenwood, C.E. and Winocur, G. (2005). High-fat diets, insulin resistance and declining cognitive function. *Neurobiol. Aging* 26 (Suppl 1): 42–45.

33 Brand-Miller, J., Hayne, S., Petocz, P., and Colagiuri, S. (2003). Low-glycemic index diets in the management of diabetes: a meta-analysis of randomized controlled trials. *Diabetes Care* 26: 2261–2267.

34 Brand-Miller, J.C. (2003). Glycemic load and chronic disease. *Nutr. Rev.* 61: S49–S55.

35 Molteni, R., Barnard, R.J., Ying, Z. et al. (2002). A high-fat, refined sugar diet reduces hippocampal brain-derived neurotrophic factor, neuronal plasticity, and learning. *Neuroscience* 112: 803–814.

36 Dietschy, J.M. (1998). Dietary fatty acids and the regulation of plasma low density lipoprotein cholesterol concentrations. *J. Nutr.* 128: 444S–448S.

37 Woollett, L.A., Spady, D.K., and Dietschy, J.M. (1992). Regulatory effects of the saturated fatty acids 6:0 through 18:0 on hepatic low density lipoprotein receptor activity in the hamster. *J. Clin. Invest.* 89: 1133–1141.

38 Woollett, L.A., Spady, D.K., and Dietschy, J.M. (1992). Saturated and unsaturated fatty acids independently regulate low density lipoprotein receptor activity and production rate. *J. Lipid Res.* 33: 77–88.

39 Gill, J.M. and Sattar, N. (2009). Ceramides: a new player in the inflammation-insulin resistance paradigm? *Diabetologia* 52: 2475–2477.

40 Chavez, J.A. and Summers, S.A. (2012). A ceramide-centric view of insulin resistance. *Cell Metab.* 15: 585–594.

41 Summers, S.A. (2006). Ceramides in insulin resistance and lipotoxicity. *Prog. Lipid Res.* 45: 42–72.

42 Han, X. (2005). Lipid alterations in the earliest clinically recognizable stage of Alzheimer's disease: implication of the role of lipids in the pathogenesis of Alzheimer's disease. *Curr. Alzheimer Res.* 2: 65–77.

43 Han, X., M Holtzman, D., DW, M.K. Jr. et al. (2002). Substantial sulfatide deficiency and ceramide elevation in very early Alzheimer's disease: potential role in disease pathogenesis. *J. Neurochem.* 82: 809–818.

44 Matsuzaki, K. (2010). Ganglioside cluster-mediated aggregation and cytotoxicity of amyloid beta-peptide: molecular mechanism and inhibition. *Yakugaku Zasshi* 130: 511–515.

45 He, X., Huang, Y., Li, B. et al. (2010). Deregulation of sphingolipid metabolism in Alzheimer's disease. *Neurobiol. Aging* 31: 398–408.

46 Grimm, M.O., Haupenthal, V.J., Rothhaar, T.L. et al. (2013). Effect of different phospholipids on alpha-secretase activity in the non-amyloidogenic pathway of Alzheimer's disease. *Int. J. Mol. Sci.* 14: 5879–5898.

47 Ahima, R.S. and Antwi, D.A. (2008). Brain regulation of appetite and satiety. *Endocrinol. Metab. Clin. North Am.* 37: 811–823.

48 Mensink, R.P. and Katan, M.B. (1992). Effect of dietary fatty acids on serum lipids and lipoproteins. A meta-analysis of 27 trials. *Arterioscler. Thromb.* 12: 911–919.

49 Corder, E.H., Saunders, A.M., Strittmatter, W.J. et al. (1993). Gene dose of apolipoprotein E type 4 allele and the risk of Alzheimer's disease in late onset families. *Science* 261: 921–923.

50 Liu, C.C., Liu, C.C., Kanekiyo, T. et al. (2013). Apolipoprotein E and Alzheimer disease: risk, mechanisms and therapy. *Nat. Rev. Neurol.* 9: 106–118.

51 McGuinness, B., Craig, D., Bullock, R., and Passmore, P. (2016). Statins for the prevention of dementia. *Cochrane Database Syst. Rev.* (1): CD003160. https://doi.org/10.1002/14651858.CD003160.pub3.

52 Domenech, M., Roman, P., Lapetra, J. et al. (2014). Mediterranean diet reduces 24-hour ambulatory blood pressure, blood glucose, and lipids: one-year randomized, clinical trial. *Hypertension* 64: 69–76.

53 Asemi, Z., Tabassi, Z., Samimi, M. et al. (2013). Favourable effects of the dietary approaches to stop hypertension diet on glucose tolerance and lipid profiles in gestational diabetes: a randomised clinical trial. *Br. J. Nutr.* 109: 2024–2030.

54 Horrocks, L.A. and Farooqui, A.A. (2004). Docosahexaenoic acid in the diet: its importance in maintenance and restoration of neural membrane function. *Prostaglandins Leukot. Essent. Fatty Acids* 70: 361–372.

55 Sastry, P.S. (1985). Lipids of nervous tissue: composition and metabolism. *Prog. Lipid Res.* 24: 69–176.

56 Bordoni, A., Hrelia, S., Lorenzini, A. et al. (1998). Dual influence of aging and vitamin B6 deficiency on delta-6-desaturation of essential fatty acids in rat liver microsomes. *Prostaglandins Leukot. Essent. Fatty Acids* 58: 417–420.

57 Das, U.N. (2010). A defect in Delta6 and Delta5 desaturases may be a factor in the initiation and progression of insulin resistance, the metabolic syndrome and ischemic heart disease in South Asians. *Lipids Health Dis.* 9: 130.

58 Horrobin, D.F. (1981). Loss of delta-6-desaturase activity as a key factor in aging. *Med. Hypotheses* 7: 1211–1220.

59 Montuschi, P., Barnes, P., and Roberts, L.J. 2nd (2007). Insights into oxidative stress: the isoprostanes. *Curr. Med. Chem.* 14: 703–717.

60 Oster, T. and Pillot, T. (2010). Docosahexaenoic acid and synaptic protection in Alzheimer's disease mice. *Biochim. Biophys. Acta* 1801: 791–798.
61 Simopoulos, A.P. (2008). The importance of the omega-6/omega-3 fatty acid ratio in cardiovascular disease and other chronic diseases. *Exp. Biol. Med. (Maywood)* 233: 674–688.
62 Simopoulos, A.P. (2016). An increase in the omega-6/omega-3 fatty acid ratio increases the risk for obesity. *Nutrients* 8: 128.
63 Infante, J.P. and Huszagh, V.A. (1997). On the molecular etiology of decreased arachidonic (20:4n-6), docosapentaenoic (22:5n-6) and docosahexaenoic (22:6n-3) acids in Zellweger syndrome and other peroxisomal disorders. *Mol. Cell. Biochem.* 168: 101–115.
64 Astarita, G., Jung, K.M., Berchtold, N.C. et al. (2010). Deficient liver biosynthesis of docosahexaenoic acid correlates with cognitive impairment in Alzheimer's disease. *PLoS One* 5: e12538.
65 Kou, J., Kovacs, G.G., Hoftberger, R. et al. (2011). Peroxisomal alterations in Alzheimer's disease. *Acta Neuropathol.* 122: 271–283.
66 Cunnane, S.C. (1988). Evidence that adverse effects of zinc deficiency on essential fatty acid composition in rats are independent of food intake. *Br. J. Nutr.* 59: 273–278.
67 Cunnane, S.C. (1988). Role of zinc in lipid and fatty acid metabolism and in membranes. *Prog. Food Nutr. Sci.* 12: 151–188.
68 Molfino, A., Amabile, M.I., Monti, M., and Muscaritoli, M. (2017). Omega-3 polyunsaturated fatty acids in critical illness: anti-inflammatory, proresolving, or both? *Oxid. Med. Cell. Longevity* 2017: 5987082.
69 Capo, X., Martorell, M., Busquets-Cortes, C. et al. (2018). Resolvins as proresolving inflammatory mediators in cardiovascular disease. *Eur. J. Med. Chem.* 153: 123–130.
70 Das, U.N. (2011). Lipoxins as biomarkers of lupus and other inflammatory conditions. *Lipids Health Dis.* 10: 76.
71 Serhan, C.N., Chiang, N., Dalli, J., and Levy, B.D. (2014). Lipid mediators in the resolution of inflammation. *Cold Spring Harbor Perspect. Biol.* 7: a016311.
72 Fiala, M., Terrando, N., and Dalli, J. (2015). Specialized pro-resolving mediators from omega-3 fatty acids improve amyloid-beta phagocytosis and regulate inflammation in patients with minor cognitive impairment. *J. Alzheimers Dis.* 48: 293–301.
73 Famenini, S., Rigali, E.A., Olivera-Perez, H.M. et al. (2017). Increased intermediate M1-M2 macrophage polarization and improved cognition in mild cognitive impairment patients on omega-3 supplementation. *FASEB J.* 31: 148–160.
74 Barclay, A.W., Brand-Miller, J.C., and Mitchell, P. (2003). Glycemic index, glycemic load and diabetes in a sample of older Australians. *Asia Pac. J. Clin. Nutr.* 12 Suppl: S11.
75 Maarman, G.J., Mendham, A.E., Lamont, K., and George, C. (2017). Review of a causal role of fructose-containing sugars in myocardial susceptibility to ischemia/reperfusion injury. *Nutr. Res.* 42: 11–19.
76 Duranti, S., Ferrario, C., van Sinderen, D. et al. (2017). Obesity and microbiota: an example of an intricate relationship. *Genes Nutr.* 12: 18.
77 Kaczmarczyk, M.M., Miller, M.J., and Freund, G.G. (2012). The health benefits of dietary fiber: beyond the usual suspects of type 2 diabetes mellitus, cardiovascular disease and colon cancer. *Metabolism* 61: 1058–1066.

78 McMacken, M. and Shah, S. (2017). A plant-based diet for the prevention and treatment of type 2 diabetes. *J. Geriatr. Cardiol.* 14: 342–354.

79 Lei, E., Vacy, K., and Boon, W.C. (2016). Fatty acids and their therapeutic potential in neurological disorders. *Neurochem. Int.* 95: 75–84.

80 Cunnane, S.C., Courchesne-Loyer, A., Vandenberghe, C. et al. (2016). Can ketones help rescue brain fuel supply in later life? Implications for cognitive health during aging and the treatment of Alzheimer's disease. *Front. Mol. Neurosci.* 9: 53.

81 Zilberter, M., Ivanov, A., Ziyatdinova, S. et al. (2013). Dietary energy substrates reverse early neuronal hyperactivity in a mouse model of Alzheimer's disease. *J. Neurochem.* 125: 157–171.

82 Laughlin, M.R. (2014). Normal roles for dietary fructose in carbohydrate metabolism. *Nutrients* 6: 3117–3129.

83 Havel, P.J. (2005). Dietary fructose: implications for dysregulation of energy homeostasis and lipid/carbohydrate metabolism. *Nutr. Rev.* 63: 133–157.

84 Basciano, H., Federico, L., and Adeli, K. (2005). Fructose, insulin resistance, and metabolic dyslipidemia. *Nutr. Metab. (Lond)* 2: 5.

85 Stanhope, K.L. (2016). Sugar consumption, metabolic disease and obesity: the state of the controversy. *Crit. Rev. Clin. Lab. Sci.* 53: 52–67.

86 van der Borght, K., Kohnke, R., Goransson, N. et al. (2011). Reduced neurogenesis in the rat hippocampus following high fructose consumption. *Regul. Pept.* 167: 26–30.

87 Banks, W.A. (2008). The blood-brain barrier as a cause of obesity. *Curr. Pharm. Des.* 14: 1606–1614.

88 Kokoeva, M.V., Yin, H., and Flier, J.S. (2005). Neurogenesis in the hypothalamus of adult mice: potential role in energy balance. *Science* 310: 679–683.

89 McNay, D.E., Briancon, N., Kokoeva, M.V. et al. (2012). Remodeling of the arcuate nucleus energy-balance circuit is inhibited in obese mice. *J. Clin. Invest.* 122: 142–152.

90 Migaud, M., Batailler, M., Segura, S. et al. (2010). Emerging new sites for adult neurogenesis in the mammalian brain: a comparative study between the hypothalamus and the classical neurogenic zones. *Eur. J. Neurosci.* 32: 2042–2052.

91 Pierce, A.A. and Xu, A.W. (2010). De novo neurogenesis in adult hypothalamus as a compensatory mechanism to regulate energy balance. *J. Neurosci.* 30: 723–730.

92 Kim, C., Kim, S., and Park, S. (2017). Neurogenic effects of ghrelin on the hippocampus. *Int. J. Mol. Sci.* 18 (588): 1–7.

93 de Lartigue, G. (2016). Role of the vagus nerve in the development and treatment of diet-induced obesity. *J. Physiol.* 594: 5791–5815.

94 Funari, V.A., Crandall, J.E., and Tolan, D.R. (2007). Fructose metabolism in the cerebellum. *Cerebellum* 6: 130–140.

95 Dauncey, M.J. (2009). New insights into nutrition and cognitive neuroscience. *Proc. Nutr. Soc.* 68: 408–415.

96 Kamphuis, P.J. and Scheltens, P. (2010). Can nutrients prevent or delay onset of Alzheimer's disease? *J. Alzheimers Dis.* 20: 765–775.

97 Liu, J. and Ames, B.N. (2005). Reducing mitochondrial decay with mitochondrial nutrients to delay and treat cognitive dysfunction, Alzheimer's disease, and Parkinson's disease. *Nutr. Neurosci.* 8: 67–89.

98 Pieczenik, S.R. and Neustadt, J. (2007). Mitochondrial dysfunction and molecular pathways of disease. *Exp. Mol. Pathol.* 83: 84–92.
99 Smith, C., Marks, A.D., and Lieberman, M. (2005). *Basic Medical Biochemistry*. Lippincott Williams & Wilkins.
100 O'Keeffe, S.T. (2000). Thiamine deficiency in elderly people. *Age Ageing* 29: 99–101.
101 Gibson, G.E. and Blass, J.P. (2007). Thiamine-dependent processes and treatment strategies in neurodegeneration. *Antioxid. Redox Signaling* 9: 1605–1619.
102 Gibson, G.E., Sheu, K.F., Blass, J.P. et al. (1988). Reduced activities of thiamine-dependent enzymes in the brains and peripheral tissues of patients with Alzheimer's disease. *Arch. Neurol.* 45: 836–840.
103 Wyatt, D.T., Nelson, D., and Hillman, R.E. (1991). Age-dependent changes in thiamin concentrations in whole blood and cerebrospinal fluid in infants and children. *Am. J. Clin. Nutr.* 53: 530–536.
104 Singleton, C.K. and Martin, P.R. (2001). Molecular mechanisms of thiamine utilization. *Curr. Mol. Med.* 1: 197–207.
105 Heroux, M., Raghavendra Rao, V.L., Lavoie, J. et al. (1996). Alterations of thiamine phosphorylation and of thiamine-dependent enzymes in Alzheimer's disease. *Metab. Brain Dis.* 11: 81–88.
106 Mastrogiacoma, F., Bettendorff, L., Grisar, T., and Kish, S.J. (1996). Brain thiamine, its phosphate esters, and its metabolizing enzymes in Alzheimer's disease. *Ann. Neurol.* 39: 585–591.
107 Mastrogiacoma, F., Lindsay, J.G., Bettendorff, L. et al. (1996). Brain protein and alpha-ketoglutarate dehydrogenase complex activity in Alzheimer's disease. *Ann. Neurol.* 39: 592–598.
108 Chen, Z. and Zhong, C. (2013). Decoding Alzheimer's disease from perturbed cerebral glucose metabolism: implications for diagnostic and therapeutic strategies. *Prog. Neurobiol.* 108: 21–43.
109 Langlais, P.J. and Zhang, S.X. (1993). Extracellular glutamate is increased in thalamus during thiamine deficiency-induced lesions and is blocked by MK-801. *J. Neurochem.* 61: 2175–2182.
110 Zhao, N., Zhong, C., Wang, Y. et al. (2008). Impaired hippocampal neurogenesis is involved in cognitive dysfunction induced by thiamine deficiency at early pre-pathological lesion stage. *Neurobiol. Dis.* 29: 176–185.
111 Zhao, Y., Pan, X., Zhao, J. et al. (2009). Decreased transketolase activity contributes to impaired hippocampal neurogenesis induced by thiamine deficiency. *J. Neurochem.* 111: 537–546.
112 Matsushita, S., Miyakawa, T., Maesato, H. et al. (2008). Elevated cerebrospinal fluid tau protein levels in Wernicke's encephalopathy. *Alcohol. Clin. Exp. Res.* 32: 1091–1095.
113 Zhang, Q., Yang, G., Li, W. et al. (2011). Thiamine deficiency increases beta-secretase activity and accumulation of beta-amyloid peptides. *Neurobiol. Aging* 32: 42–53.
114 Karuppagounder, S.S., Xu, H., Shi, Q. et al. (2009). Thiamine deficiency induces oxidative stress and exacerbates the plaque pathology in Alzheimer's mouse model. *Neurobiol. Aging* 30: 1587–1600.
115 Angeloni, C., Zambonin, L., and Hrelia, S. (2014). Role of methylglyoxal in Alzheimer's disease. *Biomed. Res. Int.* 2014: 238485.

116 Pan, X., Sang, S., Fei, G. et al. (2017). Enhanced activities of blood thiamine diphosphatase and monophosphatase in Alzheimer's disease. *PLoS One* 12: e0167273.

117 Liu, D., Ke, Z., and Luo, J. (2017). Thiamine deficiency and neurodegeneration: the interplay among oxidative stress, endoplasmic reticulum stress, and autophagy. *Mol. Neurobiol.* 54: 5440–5448.

118 Markesbery, W.R. (1997). Oxidative stress hypothesis in Alzheimer's disease. *Free Radical Biol. Med.* 23: 134–147.

119 Perry, G., Cash, A.D., and Smith, M.A. (2002). Alzheimer disease and oxidative stress. *J. Biomed. Biotechnol.* 2: 120–123.

120 University LPIaOS, Micronutrient Information Centre lpi.oregonstate.edu.

121 Seshadri, S., Beiser, A., Selhub, J. et al. (2002). Plasma homocysteine as a risk factor for dementia and Alzheimer's disease. *N. Engl. J. Med.* 346: 476–483.

122 Joseph, J.A., Denisova, N., Fisher, D. et al. (1998). Membrane and receptor modifications of oxidative stress vulnerability in aging. Nutritional considerations. *Ann. N.Y. Acad. Sci.* 854: 268–276.

123 Ames, B.N., Cathcart, R., Schwiers, E., and Hochstein, P. (1981). Uric acid provides an antioxidant defense in humans against oxidant- and radical-caused aging and cancer: a hypothesis. *Proc. Natl. Acad. Sci. U.S.A.* 78: 6858–6862.

124 Beydoun, M.A., Canas, J.A., Dore, G.A. et al. (2016). Serum uric acid and its association with longitudinal cognitive change among urban adults. *J. Alzheimers Dis.* 52: 1415–1430.

125 Hageman, G.J. and Stierum, R.H. (2001). Niacin, poly(ADP-ribose) polymerase-1 and genomic stability. *Mutat. Res.* 475: 45–56.

126 Nakashima, Y. and Suzue, R. (1984). Influence of nicotinic acid on cerebroside synthesis in the brain of developing rats. *J. Nutr. Sci. Vitaminol. (Tokyo)* 30: 525–534.

127 Melo, S.S., Meirelles, M.S., Jordao, A.A. Jr., and Vannucchi, H. (2000). Lipid peroxidation in nicotinamide-deficient and nicotinamide-supplemented rats. *Int. J. Vitam. Nutr. Res.* 70: 321–323.

128 Morris, M.C., Evans, D.A., Bienias, J.L. et al. (2004). Dietary niacin and the risk of incident Alzheimer's disease and of cognitive decline. *J. Neurol. Neurosurg. Psychiatry* 75: 1093–1099.

129 Battaglia, A., Bruni, G., Ardia, A., and Sacchetti, G. (1989). Nicergoline in mild to moderate dementia. A multicenter, double-blind, placebo-controlled study. *J. Am. Geriatr. Soc.* 37: 295–302.

130 Porter, K., Hoey, L., Hughes, C.F. et al. (2016). Causes, consequences and public health implications of low B-vitamin status in ageing. *Nutrients* 8 (725): 1–29.

131 Hara, J., Shankle, W.R., Barrentine, L.W., and Curole, M.V. (2016). Novel therapy of hyperhomocysteinemia in mild cognitive impairment, Alzheimer's disease, and other dementing disorders. *J. Nutr. Health Aging* 20: 825–834.

132 Malouf, R. and Grimley Evans, J. (2003). The effect of vitamin B6 on cognition. *Cochrane Database Syst. Rev.* (4): CD004393. https://doi.org/10.1002/14651858.CD004393.

133 Wakimoto, P. and Block, G. (2001). Dietary intake, dietary patterns, and changes with age: an epidemiological perspective. *J. Gerontol. A Biol. Sci. Med. Sci.* 56 Spec No 2: 65–80.

134 Coker, M., de Klerk, J.B., Poll-The, B.T. et al. (1996). Plasma total odd-chain fatty acids in the monitoring of disorders of propionate, methylmalonate and biotin metabolism. *J. Inherit. Metab. Dis.* 19: 743–751.

135 Umhau, J.C., Dauphinais, K.M., Patel, S.H. et al. (2006). The relationship between folate and docosahexaenoic acid in men. *Eur. J. Clin. Nutr.* 60: 352–357.

136 Pita, M.L. and Delgado, M.J. (2000). Folate administration increases n-3 polyunsaturated fatty acids in rat plasma and tissue lipids. *Thromb. Haemost.* 84: 420–423.

137 Hirono, H. and Wada, Y. (1978). Effects of dietary folate deficiency on developmental increase of myelin lipids in rat brain. *J. Nutr.* 108: 766–772.

138 Balmer, J.E. and Blomhoff, R. (2002). Gene expression regulation by retinoic acid. *J. Lipid Res.* 43: 1773–1808.

139 Khanna, A. and Reddy, T.S. (1983). Effect of undernutrition and vitamin A deficiency on the phospholipid composition of rat tissues at 21 days of age. – I. Liver, spleen and kidney. *Int. J. Vitam. Nutr. Res.* 53: 3–8.

140 Koryakina, A., Aeberhard, J., Kiefer, S. et al. (2009). Regulation of secretases by all-trans-retinoic acid. *FEBS J.* 276: 2645–2655.

141 Goodman, A.B. and Pardee, A.B. (2003). Evidence for defective retinoid transport and function in late onset Alzheimer's disease. *Proc. Natl. Acad. Sci. U.S.A.* 100: 2901–2905.

142 Shudo, K., Fukasawa, H., Nakagomi, M., and Yamagata, N. (2009). Towards retinoid therapy for Alzheimer's disease. *Curr. Alzheimer Res.* 6: 302–311.

143 Tippmann, F., Hundt, J., Schneider, A. et al. (2009). Up-regulation of the alpha-secretase ADAM10 by retinoic acid receptors and acitretin. *FASEB J.* 23: 1643–1654.

144 Corcoran, J.P., So, P.L., and Maden, M. (2004). Disruption of the retinoid signalling pathway causes a deposition of amyloid beta in the adult rat brain. *Eur. J. Neurosci.* 20: 896–902.

145 Husson, M., Enderlin, V., Delacourte, A. et al. (2006). Retinoic acid normalizes nuclear receptor mediated hypo-expression of proteins involved in beta-amyloid deposits in the cerebral cortex of vitamin A deprived rats. *Neurobiol. Dis.* 23: 1–10.

146 Acin-Perez, R., Hoyos, B., Zhao, F. et al. (2010). Control of oxidative phosphorylation by vitamin A illuminates a fundamental role in mitochondrial energy homoeostasis. *FASEB J.* 24: 627–636.

147 Craft, S. (2009). The role of metabolic disorders in Alzheimer disease and vascular dementia: two roads converged. *Arch. Neurol.* 66: 300–305.

148 Wang, R., Chen, S., Liu, Y. et al. (2015). All-trans-retinoic acid reduces BACE1 expression under inflammatory conditions via modulation of nuclear factor kappaB (NFkappaB) signaling. *J. Biol. Chem.* 290: 22532–22542.

149 Zeng, J., Chen, L., Wang, Z. et al. (2017). Marginal vitamin A deficiency facilitates Alzheimer's pathogenesis. *Acta Neuropathol.* 133: 967–982.

150 Grimm, M.O., Mett, J., and Hartmann, T. (2016). The impact of vitamin E and other fat-soluble vitamins on Alzheimer's disease. *Int. J. Mol. Sci.* 17 (1785): 1–18.

151 Russell, R.M. (2000). The vitamin A spectrum: from deficiency to toxicity. *Am. J. Clin. Nutr.* 71: 878–884.

152 Leung, W.C., Hessel, S., Meplan, C. et al. (2009). Two common single nucleotide polymorphisms in the gene encoding beta-carotene 15,15′-monoxygenase alter beta-carotene metabolism in female volunteers. *FASEB J.* 23: 1041–1053.

153 Sato, Y., Asoh, T., and Oizumi, K. (1998). High prevalence of vitamin D deficiency and reduced bone mass in elderly women with Alzheimer's disease. *Bone* 23: 555–557.

154 Scott, T.M., Peter, I., Tucker, K.L. et al. (2006). The Nutrition, Aging, and Memory in Elders (NAME) study: design and methods for a study of micronutrients and cognitive function in a homebound elderly population. *Int. J. Geriatr. Psychiatry* 21: 519–528.

155 Luckhaus, C., Mahabadi, B., Grass-Kapanke, B. et al. (2009). Blood biomarkers of osteoporosis in mild cognitive impairment and Alzheimer's disease. *J. Neural Transm.* 116: 905–911.

156 Tysiewicz-Dudek, M., Pietraszkiewicz, F., and Drozdzowska, B. (2008). Alzheimer's disease and osteoporosis: common risk factors or one condition predisposing to the other? *Ortop. Traumatol. Rehabil.* 10: 315–323.

157 Buell, J.S. and Dawson-Hughes, B. (2008). Vitamin D and neurocognitive dysfunction: preventing "D"ecline? *Mol. Aspects Med.* 29: 415–422.

158 Wang, Y., Zhu, J., and DeLuca, H.F. (2012). Where is the vitamin D receptor? *Arch. Biochem. Biophys.* 523: 123–133.

159 Sutherland, M.K., Somerville, M.J., Yoong, L.K. et al. (1992). Reduction of vitamin D hormone receptor mRNA levels in Alzheimer as compared to Huntington hippocampus: correlation with calbindin-28k mRNA levels. *Brain Res. Mol. Brain Res.* 13: 239–250.

160 Gezen-Ak, D., Dursun, E., Ertan, T. et al. (2007). Association between vitamin D receptor gene polymorphism and Alzheimer's disease. *Tohoku J. Exp. Med.* 212: 275–282.

161 Baas, D., Prufer, K., Ittel, M.E. et al. (2000). Rat oligodendrocytes express the vitamin D(3) receptor and respond to 1,25-dihydroxyvitamin D(3). *Glia* 31: 59–68.

162 Downey, C.L., Young, A., Burton, E.F. et al. (2017). Dementia and osteoporosis in a geriatric population: is there a common link? *World J. Orthop.* 8: 412–423.

163 Houston, D.K. (2015). Vitamin D and age-related health outcomes: movement, mood, and memory. *Curr. Nutr. Rep.* 4: 185–200.

164 Alvarez, J.A. and Ashraf, A. (2010). Role of vitamin D in insulin secretion and insulin sensitivity for glucose homeostasis. *Int. J. Endocrinol.* 2010: 351385.

165 Landel, V., Millet, P., Baranger, K. et al. (2016). Vitamin D interacts with Esr1 and Igf1 to regulate molecular pathways relevant to Alzheimer's disease. *Mol. Neurodegener.* 11: 22.

166 Wehr, E., Pilz, S., Boehm, B.O. et al. (2010). Association of vitamin D status with serum androgen levels in men. *Clin. Endocrinol. (Oxf)* 73: 243–248.

167 Chu, L.W., Tam, S., Lee, P.W. et al. (2008). Bioavailable testosterone is associated with a reduced risk of amnestic mild cognitive impairment in older men. *Clin. Endocrinol. (Oxf)* 68: 589–598.

168 Hogervorst, E., Bandelow, S., Combrinck, M., and Smith, A.D. (2004). Low free testosterone is an independent risk factor for Alzheimer's disease. *Exp. Gerontol.* 39: 1633–1639.

169 Landel, V., Annweiler, C., Millet, P. et al. (2016). Vitamin D, cognition and Alzheimer's disease: the therapeutic benefit is in the D-tails. *J. Alzheimers Dis.* 53: 419–444.

170 Rizvi, S., Raza, S.T., Ahmed, F. et al. (2014). The role of vitamin E in human health and some diseases. *Sultan Qaboos Univ. Med. J.* 14: e157–e165.

171 Jimenez-Jimenez, F.J., de Bustos, F., Molina, J.A. et al. (1997). Cerebrospinal fluid levels of alpha-tocopherol (vitamin E) in Alzheimer's disease. *J. Neural Transm.* 104: 703–710.

172 Perkins, A.J., Hendrie, H.C., Callahan, C.M. et al. (1999). Association of antioxidants with memory in a multiethnic elderly sample using the Third National Health and Nutrition Examination Survey. *Am. J. Epidemiol.* 150: 37–44.

173 Vuletic, S., Peskind, E.R., Marcovina, S.M. et al. (2005). Reduced CSF PLTP activity in Alzheimer's disease and other neurologic diseases; PLTP induces ApoE secretion in primary human astrocytes in vitro. *J. Neurosci. Res.* 80: 406–413.

174 Desrumaux, C., Risold, P.Y., Schroeder, H. et al. (2005). Phospholipid transfer protein (PLTP) deficiency reduces brain vitamin E content and increases anxiety in mice. *FASEB J.* 19: 296–297.

175 Yatin, S.M., Varadarajan, S., and Butterfield, D.A. (2000). Vitamin E prevents Alzheimer's amyloid beta-peptide (1-42)-induced neuronal protein oxidation and reactive oxygen species production. *J. Alzheimers Dis.* 2: 123–131.

176 Butterfield, D.A., Koppal, T., Subramaniam, R., and Yatin, S. (1999). Vitamin E as an antioxidant/free radical scavenger against amyloid beta-peptide-induced oxidative stress in neocortical synaptosomal membranes and hippocampal neurons in culture: insights into Alzheimer's disease. *Rev. Neurosci.* 10: 141–149.

177 Rota, C., Rimbach, G., Minihane, A.M. et al. (2005). Dietary vitamin E modulates differential gene expression in the rat hippocampus: potential implications for its neuroprotective properties. *Nutr. Neurosci.* 8: 21–29.

178 Cutler, R.G., Kelly, J., Storie, K. et al. (2004). Involvement of oxidative stress-induced abnormalities in ceramide and cholesterol metabolism in brain aging and Alzheimer's disease. *Proc. Natl. Acad. Sci. U.S.A.* 101: 2070–2075.

179 Mielke, M.M., Haughey, N.J., Han, D. et al. (2017). The association between plasma ceramides and sphingomyelins and risk of Alzheimer's disease differs by sex and APOE in the Baltimore Longitudinal Study of Aging. *J. Alzheimers Dis.* 60: 819–828.

180 Ko, M.H. and Puglielli, L. (2009). Two endoplasmic reticulum (ER)/ER Golgi intermediate compartment-based lysine acetyltransferases post-translationally regulate BACE1 levels. *J. Biol. Chem.* 284: 2482–2492.

181 Kidd, P.M. (2008). Alzheimer's disease, amnestic mild cognitive impairment, and age-associated memory impairment: current understanding and progress toward integrative prevention. *Altern. Med. Rev.* 13: 85–115.

182 Dominiak, A., Wilkaniec, A., Wroczynski, P., and Adamczyk, A. (2016). Selenium in the therapy of neurological diseases: where is it going? *Curr. Neuropharmacol.* 14: 282–299.

183 Steinbrenner, H. and Sies, H. (2013). Selenium homeostasis and antioxidant selenoproteins in brain: implications for disorders in the central nervous system. *Arch. Biochem. Biophys.* 536: 152–157.

184 Lovell, M.A., Xie, C., Gabbita, S.P., and Markesbery, W.R. (2000). Decreased thioredoxin and increased thioredoxin reductase levels in Alzheimer's disease brain. *Free Radical Biol. Med.* 28: 418–427.

185 Xie, Y., Tan, Y., Zheng, Y. et al. (2017). Ebselen ameliorates beta-amyloid pathology, tau pathology, and cognitive impairment in triple-transgenic Alzheimer's disease mice. *J. Biol. Inorg. Chem.* 22: 851–865.

186 Zhang, Z.H., Wu, Q.Y., Zheng, R. et al. (2017). Selenomethionine mitigates cognitive decline by targeting both tau hyperphosphorylation and autophagic clearance in an Alzheimer's disease mouse model. *J. Neurosci.* 37: 2449–2462.

187 Perl, D.P. and Olanow, C.W. (2007). The neuropathology of manganese-induced parkinsonism. *J. Neuropathol. Exp. Neurol.* 66: 675–682.

188 Chen, P., Chakraborty, S., Mukhopadhyay, S. et al. (2015). Manganese homeostasis in the nervous system. *J. Neurochem.* 134: 601–610.

189 Du, K., Liu, M., Pan, Y. et al. (2017). Association of serum manganese levels with Alzheimer's disease and mild cognitive impairment: a systematic review and meta-analysis. *Nutrients* 9: 231.

190 Barnham, K.J. and Bush, A.I. (2014). Biological metals and metal-targeting compounds in major neurodegenerative diseases. *Chem. Soc. Rev.* 43: 6727–6749.

191 Pfaender, S. and Grabrucker, A.M. (2014). Characterization of biometal profiles in neurological disorders. *Metallomics* 6: 960–977.

192 Cui, Z., Bu, W., Fan, W. et al. (2016). Sensitive imaging and effective capture of Cu(2+): towards highly efficient theranostics of Alzheimer's disease. *Biomaterials* 104: 158–167.

193 Ward, R.J., Zucca, F.A., Duyn, J.H. et al. (2014). The role of iron in brain ageing and neurodegenerative disorders. *Lancet Neurol.* 13: 1045–1060.

194 Cristovao, J.S., Santos, R., and Gomes, C.M. (2016). Metals and neuronal metal binding proteins implicated in Alzheimer's disease. *Oxid. Med. Cell. Longevity* 2016: 9812178.

195 Miller, L.M., Wang, Q., Telivala, T.P. et al. (2006). Synchrotron-based infrared and X-ray imaging shows focalized accumulation of Cu and Zn co-localized with beta-amyloid deposits in Alzheimer's disease. *J. Struct. Biol.* 155: 30–37.

196 Lovell, M.A., Robertson, J.D., Teesdale, W.J. et al. (1998). Copper, iron and zinc in Alzheimer's disease senile plaques. *J. Neurol. Sci.* 158: 47–52.

197 Cherny, R.A., Atwood, C.S., Xilinas, M.E. et al. (2001). Treatment with a copper-zinc chelator markedly and rapidly inhibits beta-amyloid accumulation in Alzheimer's disease transgenic mice. *Neuron* 30: 665–676.

198 Li, L.B. and Wang, Z.Y. (2016). Disruption of brain zinc homeostasis promotes the pathophysiological progress of Alzheimer's disease. *Histol. Histopathol.* 31: 623–627.

199 Bareggi, S.R. and Cornelli, U. (2012). Clioquinol: review of its mechanisms of action and clinical uses in neurodegenerative disorders. *CNS Neurosci. Ther.* 18: 41–46.

200 Szutowicz, A., Bielarczyk, H., Zysk, M. et al. (2017). Early and late pathomechanisms in Alzheimer's disease: from zinc to amyloid-beta neurotoxicity. *Neurochem. Res.* 42: 891–904.

201 Adiele, R.C. and Adiele, C.A. (2016). Mitochondrial regulatory pathways in the pathogenesis of Alzheimer's disease. *J. Alzheimers Dis.* 53: 1257–1270.

202 Szutowicz, A., Bielarczyk, H., Jankowska-Kulawy, A. et al. (2013). Acetyl-CoA the key factor for survival or death of cholinergic neurons in course of neurodegenerative diseases. *Neurochem. Res.* 38: 1523–1542.

203 Quintana, C., Bellefqih, S., Laval, J.Y. et al. (2006). Study of the localization of iron, ferritin, and hemosiderin in Alzheimer's disease hippocampus by analytical microscopy at the subcellular level. *J. Struct. Biol.* 153: 42–54.

204 van Bergen, J.M., Li, X., Hua, J. et al. (2016). Colocalization of cerebral iron with amyloid beta in mild cognitive impairment. *Sci. Rep.* 6: 35514.

205 Hare, D.J., Cardoso, B.R., Raven, E.P. et al. (2017). Excessive early-life dietary exposure: a potential source of elevated brain iron and a risk factor for Parkinson's disease. *NPJ Parkinson's Dis.* 3: 1.

206 Scheiber, I.F., Mercer, J.F., and Dringen, R. (2014). Metabolism and functions of copper in brain. *Prog. Neurobiol.* 116: 33–57.

207 Cuajungco, M.P., Frederickson, C.J., and Bush, A.I. (2005). Amyloid-beta metal interaction and metal chelation. *Subcell Biochem.* 38: 235–254.

208 Drew, S.C. (2017). The case for abandoning therapeutic chelation of copper ions in Alzheimer's disease. *Front. Neurosci.* 11: 317.

209 Xu, J., Church, S.J., Patassini, S. et al. (2017). Evidence for widespread, severe brain copper deficiency in Alzheimer's dementia. *Metallomics* 9: 1106–1119.

210 Woods, N.K. and Padmanabhan, J. (2012). Neuronal calcium signaling and Alzheimer's disease. *Adv. Exp. Med. Biol.* 740: 1193–1217.

211 Popugaeva, E., Pchitskaya, E., and Bezprozvanny, I. (2017). Dysregulation of neuronal calcium homeostasis in Alzheimer's disease – a therapeutic opportunity? *Biochem. Biophys. Res. Commun.* 483: 998–1004.

212 Peterlik, M. and Cross, H.S. (2009). Vitamin D and calcium insufficiency-related chronic diseases: molecular and cellular pathophysiology. *Eur. J. Clin. Nutr.* 63: 1377–1386.

213 Pannu, P.K., Calton, E.K., and Soares, M.J. (2016). Calcium and vitamin D in obesity and related chronic disease. *Adv. Food Nutr. Res.* 77: 57–100.

214 Nadeem Aslam, M., Bassis, C.M., Zhang, L. et al. (2016). Calcium reduces liver injury in mice on a high-fat diet: alterations in microbial and bile acid profiles. *PLoS One* 11: e0166178.

6

Carbohydrate and Protein Metabolism: Influences on Cognition and Alzheimer's Disease

W.M.A.D. Binosha Fernando[1,2], Veer B. Gupta[3], Vijay Jayasena[4], Charles S. Brennan[5,6,7,8] and Ralph N. Martins[1,2,9,10,11]

[1] Centre of Excellence for Alzheimer's Disease Research and Care, School of Medical and Health Sciences, Edith Cowan University, Joondalup, WA, Australia
[2] Australian Alzheimer's Research Foundation, Ralph and Patricia Sarich Neuroscience Research Institute, Nedlands, WA, Australia
[3] School of Medicine, Deakin University, Geelong, VIC, Australia
[4] School of Science and Health, Western Sydney University, Hawkesbury, NSW, Australia
[5] Department of Wine, Food and Molecular Biosciences, Lincoln University, Lincoln, New Zealand
[6] Riddet Institute, Palmerston North, New Zealand
[7] School of Food Science, Tianjin University of Commerce, Tianjin, China
[8] School of Food Science, South China University of Technology, Guangzhou, China
[9] Department of Biomedical Sciences, Macquarie University, Sydney, NSW, Australia
[10] School of Psychiatry and Clinical Neurosciences, University of Western Australia, Perth, WA, Australia
[11] KaRa Institute of Neurological Diseases, Sydney, NSW, Australia

6.1 Carbohydrates

Carbohydrates are a diverse group of compounds, and are also a major source of energy for the human body. They are omnipresent in nature with a range of chemical, physical, and physiological properties. The general molecular formula for larger carbohydrates is $(CH_2O)n$, and carbohydrates can be classified as monosaccharides, disaccharides, oligosaccharides, or polysaccharides (Figure 6.1).

Polysaccharides are used as energy storage (for example the starch in potatoes and glycogen in mammalian liver), or as structural components (for example the cellulose and lignin in plants and chitin in insects). Simple sugars such as fructose, glucose, and sucrose are found in fruits and vegetables mostly, but will be present in all living things as they are basic energy sources.

6.1.1 Carbohydrate Digestion

Following the ingestion of carbohydrates as part of a meal, complex carbohydrates are broken down to some extent in the mouth, with the action of salivary amylase. After swallowing, no further carbohydrate digestion occurs until the carbohydrates reach the small intestine, where pancreatic amylase, as well as small intestine brush border enzymes, continue to break down the carbohydrates. Eventually digestion results in monosaccharides, which are absorbed into the bloodstream. Simple sugars such as sucrose, glucose, and fructose are easily digested and absorbed, or just absorbed

Neurodegeneration and Alzheimer's Disease: The Role of Diabetes, Genetics, Hormones, and Lifestyle,
First Edition. Edited by Ralph N. Martins, Charles S. Brennan, W.M.A.D. Binosha Fernando,
Margaret A. Brennan and Stephanie J. Fuller.
© 2019 John Wiley & Sons Ltd. Published 2019 by John Wiley & Sons Ltd.

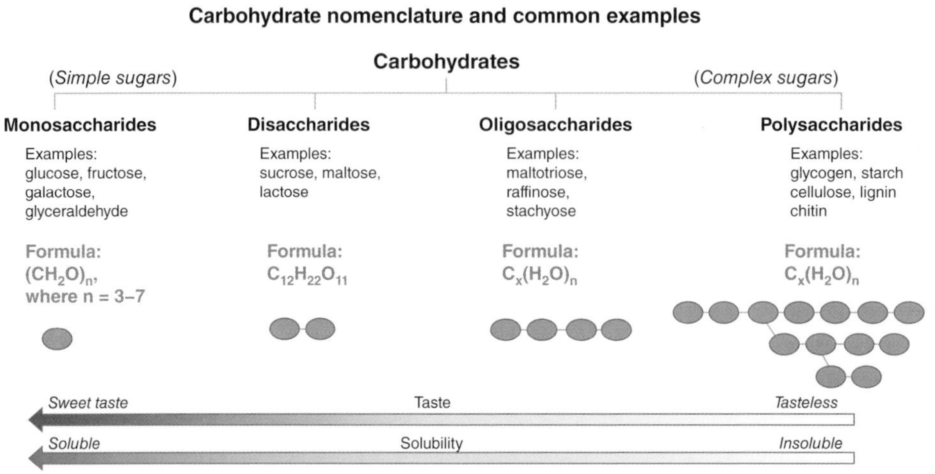

Carbohydrate nomenclature and common examples

Carbohydrates

(Simple sugars) — (Complex sugars)

Monosaccharides	Disaccharides	Oligosaccharides	Polysaccharides
Examples: glucose, fructose, galactose, glyceraldehyde	Examples: sucrose, maltose, lactose	Examples: maltotriose, raffinose, stachyose	Examples: glycogen, starch cellulose, lignin chitin
Formula: $(CH_2O)_n$, where n = 3–7	Formula: $C_{12}H_{22}O_{11}$	Formula: $C_x(H_2O)_n$	Formula: $C_x(H_2O)_n$

Taste: Sweet taste ←→ Tasteless

Solubility: Soluble ←→ Insoluble

Figure 6.1 Classification of carbohydrates.

in the case of monosaccharides, and can raise the blood glucose level rapidly. On the other hand, polysaccharides, which are widely available in fruits, vegetables, and whole grains, require a longer time to digest, typically resulting in a slower rise in blood glucose concentration. However, the speed of glucose absorption is not the only determinant of blood glucose concentration following carbohydrate ingestion, the amount of sugar/carbohydrate is equally important (as well as other foods eaten at the same time), as slower breakdown and absorption of a large quantity of starch can be just as taxing on the glucose regulatory system – these aspects of dietary carbohydrate – speed of absorption and total amount of carbohydrate – lead to the calculations of the glycaemic index and glycaemic load of foods, respectively [1]. Many studies show that higher post-prandial glycaemia is a dominant mechanism for progression of many chronic conditions such as type 2 diabetes, obesity, and cardiovascular disease [2]. As a result, the concepts of low glycaemic index foods, and particularly low glycaemic load foods, are being explained and used in the management of type 2 diabetes as well as cardiovascular diseases.

Not all carbohydrates can be digested by humans however, and the indigestible ones include dietary fibre (soluble and insoluble) as well as resistant starch and some oligosaccharides [3]. These reach our large bowel and are beneficial in that they feed probiotic bacteria: the dietary fibre and resistant starch that enter the colon are fermented by such bacteria, and products include short-chain fatty acids (SCFA) such as acetate, propionate, and butyrate, as well as hydrogen and methane gases and other metabolites. The SCFA can be absorbed by the colonic epithelium, or metabolised by the colonic bacteria [3, 4]. Butyrate is believed to enhance colonic cell health as it provides energy for the epithelial cells, and it also has been shown to inhibit histone deacetylase, thus influencing colonic function, and may reduce inflammation by inhibiting nuclear factor kappa B (NFkB) and upregulating peroxisome proliferator-activated receptor-γ (PPAR-γ) expression [5, 6].

In general, it is now believed that SCFA may suppress inflammation by reducing the migration and growth of immune cells, and reducing levels of cytokines; SCFA can also induce apoptosis in cancer cells. Propionate is absorbed and metabolised aerobically in the liver while acetate passes via the liver into the blood, from where it is used as an energy source. It is interesting to note that propionate may play a direct role in blood glucose control by suppressing the release of plasma triacylglycerols, which contribute to insulin resistance [7]. In addition, other studies have shown that non-starch polysaccharides may reduce the reabsorption of bile acids, inducing synthesis of new bile acids from cholesterol, thus reducing blood cholesterol levels [8]. This is all evidence that increasing or regulating SCFA levels may provide therapeutic strategies to help prevent chronic inflammation [9], reduce cholesterol levels, and reduce risk of type 2 diabetes – all known risk factors for Alzheimer's disease (AD).

6.1.2 Glucose Ingestion and Use

Glucose is the primary fuel for the brain, but unfortunately glucose cannot be stored in the brain [10]. Therefore, the maintenance of glucose at adequate levels is important to support healthy brain function at all times. Glucose is transferred to liver, brain, and other tissues via the blood from the gastrointestinal tract. Unlike the liver though, the brain depends almost entirely on the circulating blood glucose for energy. Excess glucose from the diet, in the presence of high ATP (adenosine triphosphate – unit of energy produced in cells) levels, is converted to glycogen (via glycogenesis) and stored in the muscles and liver. Glycogen can then be converted back to glucose through glycogenolysis and released into the blood as required. When glycogen and glucose levels are too low, or when a person is on a high-fat/low-carbohydrate diet, ketone bodies can be used by the brain. These include acetoacetate (AcAc) and β-hydroxybutyrate, and are obtained from lipid breakdown in the liver. These are discussed in greater detail below.

6.1.3 Glucose and Insulin, Insulin Resistance, and Type 2 Diabetes (Short Summary)

This topic is discussed in greater detail in Chapter 4 of this book, so will only be summarised here.

Blood glucose levels will invariably rise after a meal, which causes insulin to be released from the pancreas, to stimulate muscle, fat, and liver cells, amongst others, to absorb glucose from the bloodstream. This then lowers blood glucose levels back to a normal level. Some of the absorbed glucose will be used for energy in all the body tissues, any excess will be stored as glycogen in muscle and liver cells, or alternatively stored as fat in the long term.

When on a high-sugar/carbohydrate diet, the pancreatic β-cells try to keep up with the increased demand for insulin by producing more, yet high-sugar and high-calorie diet-associated problems like obesity, inflammation, dysregulation of sugar, and lipid metabolism cause negative feedback, reducing the effectiveness of the insulin signal – this is known as insulin resistance. In insulin resistance, muscle, fat, and liver cells do not respond properly to insulin and thus cannot easily absorb glucose from the bloodstream, leading to hyperglycaemia. Eventually, pancreatic β-cells may not be able to produce enough insulin, resulting in type 2 diabetes.

Obesity, especially excess fat around the waist, is a primary cause of insulin resistance. Originally thought just to be an area for fat storage, it is now known that belly fat produces hormones and other substances that can lead to insulin resistance, high blood pressure, disturbed lipid and cholesterol metabolism, and cardiovascular disease. Insulin resistance and hyperglycaemia can also lead to kidney damage, damage to the retina, and neurological damage. When cells lack glucose due to insulin resistance, it can lead to regular breakdown of lipid for energy, which can lead to ketoacidosis – a life-threatening condition.

Insulin and insulin-like growth factor-1 (IGF1) control many biological processes, mostly by acting on two related tyrosine kinase receptors – the insulin receptor (IR) and the insulin-like growth factor-1 receptor (IGF1R). Binding and activating these receptors initiates a cascade of phosphorylation reactions, many of which are points of regulation and negative feedback control points [11]. Normally, insulin and IGF1 effects *in vivo* mostly reflect hormonal concentration and relative expression levels of the receptors in different tissues, rather than the capacity of IR and IGF-1R to convey different signals [12]. However, under certain conditions including hyperglycaemia, inflammation, lipotoxicity, endoplasmic reticulum stress, and mitochondrial dysfunction, Ser/Thr kinases are activated, which then induce inhibitory phosphorylation of IR and insulin receptor substrate (IRS) proteins, leading to insulin resistance [11]. High ceramide levels, often seen in AD, also induces insulin resistance via protein kinase C and c-Jun N-terminal kinase (JNK) activation [13]. Lipotoxicity, hyperglycaemia, and chronic inflammation, all seen in obesity, lead to increased secretion of pro-inflammatory cytokines, such as tumour necrosis factor-α (TNF-α), interleukin-1β (IL-1β), or IL-6, which induce insulin resistance via several mechanisms [13, 14]. Thus it is clear that although glucose is essential for brain function, regularly overtaxing the post-prandial insulin/glucose regulation cycle, as well as a diet too high in calories, can cause disruptions to glucose and lipid metabolism. This eventually leads to a vicious cycle of inflammation, oxidative stress, obesity, and insulin resistance, and increases the risk of many other chronic conditions such as type 2 diabetes and cardiovascular disease, as well as AD.

To produce energy in forms the body can use, most commonly ATP and Nicotinamide adenine dinucleotide phosphate (NADP), glucose is broken down through the glycolysis pathway in the cytoplasm to produce pyruvate in order to generate ATP and NADH; the pyruvate can then be converted to acetyl-CoA and put through the citric acid cycle in the mitochondrial matrix to produce more ATP and NADH. As mentioned above, blood glucose levels need to be maintained within a narrow range for optimal metabolic function, and yet the western diet often causes large surges in glucose, leading to excessive insulin secretion, eventually leading to insulin resistance, and if left untreated, type 2 diabetes.

6.1.4 Relative Intake of Carbohydrate and its Impacts on Neurodegenerative Disease Risk

In 1997, William Grant [15] identified a link between the quantity and type of food consumed in different countries and in different eras, with the prevalence of AD. He noted a positive association between both total calories and total fat, and incidence of AD. However, follow-up studies have only sometimes agreed with this theory, highlighting the difficulties in establishing environmental influences on disease risk.

Studies of the palaeolithic period have suggested dietary intakes consisted of plant:animal ratios of 65:35, yet more recent studies suggest 45–65% of dietary energy came from animal sources, with a fat:protein:carbohydrate intake of around 40:30:30, as a percentage of energy. With respect to food volume, food was largely plant matter, and carbohydrates were released as energy in the form of short-chain fatty acids (from digestion of fibre), thus dietary carbohydrate was also very different from the high glycaemic products found in modern diets [16].

During the Neolithic period, people switched to high-cholesterol (HC) diets. Interestingly, possession of an apolipoprotein E ε4 allele (*APOE ε4*; the major genetic risk factor for AD) is uncommon in populations with a long history of agriculture, which implies that consumption of HC diets may have selected against *APOE ε4* carriers. There are three common allelic variants of *APOE*: ε2, ε3, and ε4. Possession of *APOE ε4* alleles increases the risk of developing AD, in a dose-dependent manner. *APOE ε4* is also a risk factor for cardiovascular disease, thought to be due to the protein apoE ε4's deficiencies in lipid transport and receptor binding, compared to the other apoE proteins.

It is known that HC diets elevate very low density lipoprotein (VLDL) levels [17]. Low-density lipoprotein (LDL) levels are also raised, and Lithell et al. [18] noticed that a HC diet (compared to a high-fat diet) could significantly increase insulin levels and decrease lipase activities. Our bodies preferentially use glucose, thus HC diets constrain the use of fatty acids and increase the retention time of triglyceride-rich lipoproteins. In a similar way, it is thought APOE ε4 protein increases LDL/VLDL retention time by inhibiting lipolysis. For example, studies of subjects consuming high-fat meals have demonstrated elevated TRL (Triglyceride Rich Lipoprotein) in apoE ε3/ε3 and apoE ε3/ε4 individuals, yet in the apoE ε3/ε4 individuals the LDL/VLDL levels remained elevated for a much longer period [19]. It is believed that the suboptimal mechanisms in lipid metabolism that have been demonstrated in *APOE ε4* individuals are similar to what is seen in all people on HC diets, for example concerning inhibition of lipid metabolism, and that this may explain the selection against *APOE ε4* alleles in long-time agricultural societies. In support of this, in countries where diets are low in carbohydrate content, populations have higher *APOE ε4* allele frequencies [20]. Interestingly, possession of the *APOE ε4* allele in such countries is not linked to AD risk, though total calorie intake, obesity, insulin resistance, and cardiovascular disease levels are most likely related to this statistic and just as important in determining AD risk.

A recent study of a cohort of elderly persons showed that a diet with a high percentage of carbohydrate intake was associated with an increased risk of mild cognitive impairment (MCI) [21]. A possible explanation may be disruptions to glucose and insulin metabolism as described above, however overall nutrition may also be involved, as diets high in carbohydrate are often more likely to be lacking in vitamins, antioxidants, and complete protein. Interestingly, the Honolulu Asia [22] ageing study which has 30 years follow-up has detected a positive correlation between carbohydrate intake and the development of Parkinson's disease (PD).

In light of what is known about the digestion and metabolism of carbohydrates, and considering the low quality and increased processing of many western diet carbohydrate sources, it is recommended that carbohydrate intake should include healthier choices such as fresh fruit and vegetables, wholegrain breads, wholegrain cereals and pastas, and should have a significant reduction in the intake of cakes, sweet biscuits, sugary drinks, and confectionery [23, 24]. However, many other aspects of diet, as well as energy metabolism, brain function, neurodegenerative disease pathogenesis, and other chronic health conditions all impact on brain glucose levels and utilisation, some of which are discussed below.

6.1.5 Ketogenic Diets

As many studies have linked AD risk to diet-modifiable conditions, dietary approaches to AD prevention involving low carbohydrate intakes have received great attention. Diets that comprise very low carbohydrate levels result in high levels of ketone bodies such as 3-beta-hydroxybutyrate (3HB), acetoacetate (AcAc), and acetone [25]. This is because glucose reserves become insufficient to supply the brain with glucose, and insufficient to maintain the supply of pyruvate/oxaloacetate to allow normal fat oxidation in the tricarboxylic acid cycle (TCA). Such a diet is referred to as a ketogenic diet [26]. A ketogenic diet has been found to be one of the most effective therapies for drug-resistant epilepsy, and to be of assistance for conditions such as Glucose transporter type 1 (GLUT1) deficiency syndrome, pyruvate dehydrogenase deficiency, myoclonic astatic epilepsy (Doose syndrome), tuberous sclerosis complex, Rett syndrome, and severe myoclonic epilepsy in infancy (Dravet syndrome) [25, 27]. The mechanism responsible for the protective effect of ketogenic diets on neurodegenerative diseases [27] is not completely understood. Nevertheless, it is well documented that a ketogenic diet can stabilise blood glucose, elevate fatty acid levels, and enhance bioenergetics reserves. There are also neuron-specific effects such as modulation of ATP-sensitive potassium channels, enhanced neurotransmission, increased brain derived neurotrophic factor (BDNF) expression due to glycolytic restriction, and reduced neuroinflammation. Ketogenic diets are thought to provide efficient energy sources for neurogeneration involving focal brain hypometabolism, they have been shown to decrease oxidative damage caused by metabolic stress, and to increase mitochondrial biogenesis [28]. In AD, mitochondrial dysfunction is thought to be an early event, and ketones have been shown to reduce amyloid beta (Aβ)-induced toxicity [29], whereas ketogenic diets in animal studies have shown a variety of improvements, including lower Aβ deposition levels, improved cognition, and improved motor function, depending on animal model used [28]. Many studies have shown that ketogenic diets improve glucose homeostasis and reduce insulin resistance [30, 31], however long-term maintenance on a ketogenic diet has also been linked with the development of non-alcoholic fatty liver disease, therefore greater understanding or monitoring of such a diet is needed. It has also been suggested that the accumulation of advanced glycation end-products (AGE) might be reduced by ketogenic diets, though this has yet to be investigated properly.

6.1.6 Glucose and Its Effects on Cognition

Among the carbohydrates, the memory-improving mechanism of glucose has been investigated for more than 20 years. The study of glucose's effects on memory has led to a number of important developments in the understanding of memory, brain physiology, and pathological consequences of impaired glucose tolerance.

The interest in glucose's effect on memory enhancement was partly initiated in 1981 by Lapp, in a study which reported healthy adolescents with higher glucose levels had better recall of word pairs than fasting control adolescents [32]. In 1984, Messier and White revealed that the administration of glucose enhanced memory performance in rats [33]. Foster et al. suggested in 1998 that glucose is more beneficial in older individuals than young adults, and that the improvements seen with glucose are not dependent on baseline glucose levels [34]. Positive effects of glucose on memory have been successfully demonstrated in many animal and human trials [33, 35–38] and glucose-enhanced memory has regularly been demonstrated in healthy elderly subjects as well as in AD patients, schizophrenia patients, and people with memory impairments. Together, glucose appears to improve verbal episodic memory performance, attention, design fluency, verbal fluency, and visual memory.

However, most of the work indicates that glucose-enhanced memory is dependent on the both time of application and the dose (Table 6.1) and that the effect of the dose of glucose on memory enhancement may depend on the age [57, 64], gender [64], body weight [62], and glucose regulatory efficiency [64, 65]. Dose-response studies have observed an inverted-U dose response curve [66], where small (e.g. $10\,mg\,kg^{-1}$) and large (e.g. $500\,mg\,kg^{-1}$) doses have less effect on memory, whereas moderate (e.g. $100\,mg\,kg^{-1}$) doses deliver optimal memory enhancement. In animal studies, optimal doses have ranged from $100\,mg\,kg^{-1}$ to $2\,g\,kg^{-1}$ and in clinical studies, doses of 25–75 g for a 75 kg person have been shown to be effective, which corresponds to doses of $300\,mg\,kg^{-1}$ up to $1\,g\,kg^{-1}$ [67].

In 1993, Manning et al. [68] reported that a 75 g oral glucose dose diminishes discrepancies in episodic memory performance when compared to a saccharin placebo in patients with AD. Craft et al. showed [69, 70] enhanced verbal episodic memory performance in both healthy adults and AD patients after consumption of glucose, irrespective of their glucose regulatory efficiency difference [68], and one characteristic of AD is a relatively weaker glucose regulatory efficiency.

Glucose administration has been shown to decrease cognitive impairment in people with schizophrenia in several studies [71–73]. Most of the studies have observed improved recognition memory and spatial memory following glucose ingestion. For example, recognition memory was enhanced after ingesting a dose of 50 or 75 g glucose in adults with schizophrenia, although it was found that young schizophrenia patients had decreases in attentional performance at the highest (75 g) glucose dose [73]. Fucetola et al. also observed an enhancement of spatial memory upon glucose ingestion [73]. It was suggested that impairment of verbal episodic memory was the main clinical feature of schizophrenia, and in later studies by Stone et al. [72] was noted that glucose could increase verbal episodic memory performance in patients with schizophrenia.

Pettersen and Skelton [74] studied the effect of glucose ingestion on head injuries. In this research, they observed that glucose ingestion resulted in better performance in verbal episodic memory in patients with mild head injuries due to sports. Riby et al. [75] observed similar improvements in verbal memory in older memory-impaired adults as well as healthy elderly controls following 25 g glucose ingestion, though no other significant improvements were seen. Interestingly, they did find that fasting glucose levels, as well as memory performance indices, were significant predictors of cognitive impairment.

Table 6.1 displays the findings of studies which have specifically investigated the effects of glucose on memory enhancement in memory-impaired subjects and in healthy controls. The majority of the studies noted that glucose enhances verbal

Table 6.1 Studies which have investigated effects of glucose on memory enhancement.

Study	Dose	Outcome of the study
Gold [38]	10 or 100 mg kg^{-1}	Enhanced retention performance (Animal)
Messier and Destrade [39]	3 g kg^{-1}	Enhanced retention performance (Animal)
Hall et al. [40]	50 g	Glucose enhanced memory in the elderly (Human)
Messier et al. [41]	3 g kg^{-1}	Enhanced memory of scopolamine-induced amnesia (Animal)
Benton [42]	25 g	Glucose found to be beneficial for small activities (Human)
Azari [43]	30 g	Enhanced memory performance in young, healthy normal adults (Human)
Stone et al. [44]	100 mg kg^{-1}	Glucose influenced a wide range of brain activities (Animal)
Benton and Owens [45]	50 g	Memory enhancement did not occur in those whose blood glucose levels were initially low; rather it occurred irrespective of initial blood glucose level (Human)
Benton et al. [46]	50 – 25 g	Glucose ingestion was associated with better memory and attention (Human)
Rodriguez et al. [47]	320 mg kg^{-1}	Effect of glucose and fructose were similar when injected peripherally (Animal)
Winocur [48]	100 mg kg^{-1}	Improved specific memory function (Animal)
Kopf and Baratti [49]	10–300 mg kg^{-1}	Glucose modulated memory storage (Animal)
Allen et al. [50]	50 g	Enhancement of both memory and fluency performance (Human)
Manning et al. [51]	50 g	Enhanced memory for a declarative/explicit work (Human)
Messier [52]	500 mg kg^{-1}	Improved the memory for the previously observed object (Animal)
Winocur and Gagnon [53]	100 mg kg^{-1}	Cognitive enhancement (Animal)
Manning et al. [54]	50 g	Enhanced both memory storage and retrieval (Human)
Kaplan et al. [55]	50 g	Enhanced cognition (Human)
Greenwood and Winocur [56]	100 mg kg^{-1}	Glucose treatment improved performance (Animal)
Riby [57]	25 g	Memory improvements measured, yet no significant difference between older and younger adults (Meta-analysis)
Salinas and Gold [58]	200 mg kg^{-1}	Post-training glucose injections increased memory formation (Animal)
Riby et al. [59]	25 g	Glucose found to support episodic memory (Human)
Morris [60]	50 g	Low glycaemic index foods may aid in challenging learning situations (Human)
Riby et al. [61]	25–50 g	Found associations between elevated glycaemia and relatively poor cognitive performance (Human)
Sunram et al. [62]	25 g	Study indicated optimal dose might depend on inter-individual differences in glucose regulation and weight (Human)
Scholey et al. [63]	25 g	Glucose found to be cognition enhancer (Human)

episodic memory, mainly in the healthy elderly irrespective of whether glucose is administered as pre-encoding or post-encoding. Post-training administration, which was the main method of glucose administration testing in animal studies, reflects the action of glucose on memory processes that take place after learning a new task. However, in 1997 and 1999 when Flint et al. administered glucose, it was administered either immediately following the training, or delayed, and when administration was delayed there was only a minuscule influence on performance [76, 77]. In clinical studies in 1992, Manning et al. [78], found that ingestion of 50 g glucose either pre- or post-acquisition of a narrative prose passage improved recall 24 hours later. In later studies by the same group, using the same clinical protocol of learning a narrative prose passage, it was found that glucose can enhance both memory storage and retrieval, and that recall was better if glucose was given pre-acquisition [54]. However, it is also important to note that several studies failed to demonstrate any effect of glucose on memory enhancement [67, 79, 80] and positive studies did not indicate the effect of glucose on the pathology of memory impairment. Nevertheless, from Table 6.1, it is clear that many studies have reported improvements in various aspects of memory following glucose ingestion, and this phenomenon has been termed the 'glucose memory facilitation effect'.

6.1.7 Possible Mechanisms Related to Memory Enhancement with Glucose

The glucose requirements of the brain are considerable – although only about 2% of body weight, the brain accounts for around 25% of basal metabolism, and uses approximately 120 g of glucose every day [10]. To supply the brain adequately, blood glucose needs to stay within the normal range of 60–90 mg/100 ml; if below 40 mg ml^{-1}, a person is in a hypoglycaemic condition, and is at risk of confusion, convulsions, coma, or even death. The brain can store glycogen to a very limited extent in astrocytes, but this supply can be exhausted within minutes in time of need, underscoring the need for a constant glucose supply [81]. Although not the same as the acute effects on memory following glucose ingestion mentioned in the studies above, it has been shown in chicken studies that inhibition of glycogenolysis in astrocytes can impair memory consolidation [82].

The studies listed in Table 6.1 show that the best enhancement effects have been observed for verbal declarative memory under a variety of conditions and using various paradigms. This suggests glucose may be providing the most significant effects via the hippocampus, which is particularly important in declarative memory [81]. Glucose is transferred into the brain by crossing the endothelial cells of the blood–brain barrier (BBB), to reach neurons and glial cells. This process requires glucose transporter proteins, and is imperative for normal physiological function and energy metabolism in the brain. The main glucose transport protein in the BBB is GLUT1, whereas GLUT3 is the main facilitative transporter in neurons, and GLUT5 in microglia (GLUT family, gene name SLC2A) [90, 91]. The supply of oxygen is equally important; positron emission tomography (PET) studies have shown that hypoxia can cause reversible deficits in cognitive function, or localised lesions, for example to the medial temporal cortex and its thalamic projection areas. Studies of elderly cognitive decline have suggested this decline can be attributed to impaired oxygen delivery due to reduced blood supply through the cerebral vasculature [92]. Many different mechanisms have been explored to understand the functions related to memory enhancement with glucose once it enters the brain. The most likely explanation is that glucose is required to produce ATP, which is essential for neuronal and glial cellular survival and normal metabolism, as well as for the generation of neurotransmitters. Below are few more specific mechanisms that may explain glucose enhancement of memory.

6.1.7.1 Glucose and the Hippocampus

As mentioned above, many studies suggest that the hippocampus is the region where glucose enhances memory [93]. Research on glucose and memory enhancement has shown that glucose mainly boosts episodic memory, which requires the hippocampus. The 'remember–know' paradigm was used to reveal that glucose ingestion appears to facilitate recognition memory that is accompanied by recollection of contextual details and episodic richness [94], implicating the hippocampus as the brain region that is centrally involved in mediating the glucose memory enhancement effect, rather than medial temporal lobe structures. In studies of schizophrenia, functional magnetic resonance imaging (fMRI) studies [95] have indicated glucose ingestion leads to a higher association with enhanced parahippocampus activation during verbal encoding, relative to placebo. The tasks sometimes used in such studies of glucose administration often specifically require hippocampal function, especially the object-location memory task, however other brain regions can also be required. Riby et al. [75] used event-related potential methodology (ERP) to investigate effects of glucose on cognitive processes, and their results agree with fMRI studies which have shown that, although the hippocampus appears to be the main brain area influenced by the increase in glucose, the medial-temporal lobe and the pre-frontal cortex may also be sensitive to glucose administration. Smith et al. [96] also noticed that glucose could target the brain more globally, when modulating memory. More recent glucose administration studies again support the central role of the hippocampus in object-location memory tasks [97, 98]. Further neuroimaging studies, utilising fMRI and fluorodeoxyglucose-positron emission tomography (FDG-PET) are likely to be useful in determining the specific regions of the brain that are most metabolically active subsequent to glucose ingestion, during cognitive task performance.

6.1.7.2 Glucose Availability in Brain Cells

The studies above of acute memory enhancement following glucose ingestion, as well as the studies below concerning mechanisms whereby glucose may improve brain function, all underscore the importance of maintaining stable glucose levels in the brain, for optimum brain performance and brain cell survival, particularly in the hippocampus. However this is quite a challenge for a person on a diet that regularly causes blood glucose rises that stress and damage the insulin/glucose/IR regulatory system, as in this case, brain glucose levels are disrupted due to chronic inflammation, lipid and glucose dysregulation, and eventually insulin resistance and type 2 diabetes. This results in cellular glucose levels frequently being below levels required for normal cellular function [99]. Neurons are particularly susceptible to such damage, due to their high energy requirements for processes like the generation of action potentials and post-synaptic potentials generated after synaptic events, the maintenance of ion gradients, the production of neurotransmitters, and the transport of proteins and other products down axons and dendrites [100].

In addition to this, entry of neuroactive compounds such as glutamate, aspartate, glycine, and D-serine into the brain is highly restricted by the BBB, therefore these compounds must be synthesised from glucose within the brain. This is because the BBB's glucose transport and other transport properties are very different to the 'barriers' into muscle and liver tissues, that do not have tight junctions between their vascular endothelial cells and have different transporter levels for various compounds, thus enabling these organs to metabolise monocarboxylic acids, fatty acids, amino acids, and ketone bodies, as well as glucose.

6.1.7.3 Glucose and the Central Cholinergic System

The central cholinergic system is one of the neurotransmitter systems in the body, and all regions of the cerebral cortex receive intense cholinergic innervation [101]. Cholinergic receptors (ChR) are usually divided into nicotinic (n-acetylcholine receptors – nAChR) and muscarinic (m-acetylcholine receptors – mAChR) receptors, based on the agonist activities of the natural alkaloids, nicotine, and muscarine [102, 103]. Studies of the cholinergic system in cognitive impairment have suggested that many aspects of cognitive impairments can be explained by a decline in the functional integrity of these cholinergic systems, for example the function of nAChR in particular are believed to be disturbed by pathological Aβ interactions [104]. In AD, one of the few effective drugs that reduce dementia symptoms temporarily acts on the enzyme (cholinesterase) that breaks down acetylcholine (ACh), thus increasing the neurotransmitter's ability to transmit signals at synapses [104]. Acetylcholine is known to play a role in many aspects of learning and memory, and the importance of the cholinergic neurons from the nucleus basalis of Meynert on memory is highlighted by the fact that severe degeneration of these particular neurons takes place in AD [105].

Glucose intake can influence hippocampal acetylcholine levels, as glucose administration can increase the rate of hippocampal acetylcholine (ACh) synthesis [106, 107]. Early *in vivo* microdialysis studies using rats in a maze test identified that glucose could reverse the memory impairment caused by morphine, by increasing the hippocampal acetylcholine output, in a dose-dependent manner [108]. It was also found that the administration of glucose to the hippocampus unilaterally could increase ACh formation in both the ipsilateral and contralateral hippocampus [109]. Kopf et al. [110] also observed memory enhancement in an inhibitory avoidance task, after having a high dose of glucose, as well as increased hippocampal ACh synthesis.

6.1.7.4 ATP-Regulated Potassium (K-ATP) Channels and Brain Control of Glucose Homeostasis

ATP-sensitive potassium (K-ATP) channels are critical for the maintenance of glucose homeostasis. These channels exist in many cells, including cardiac myocytes, pancreatic β-cells, muscle cells; as well as neurons, for example in the cortex, basal ganglia, hippocampus, and hypothalamus of the brain [111]. Glucose metabolism determines the quantity of intracellular ATP, which regulates the opening or closing of neuronal K-ATP channels [112]. Neuronal K-ATP channels in the hypothalamus play an important role in peripheral glucose homeostasis [113]. For example, hypothalamic K-ATP channels have been shown to regulate hepatic glucose output, as the stereotactic infusion of the potassium channel activator diazoxide into the hypothalamus can inhibit hepatic glucose production. Furthermore, mice lacking a regulatory subunit (SUR1) of the K-ATP channel show increased glucose production [114], and insulin has been shown to suppress hepatic glucose output by activating K-ATP channels in agouti-related peptide (AgRP) expressing neurons of the arcuate nucleus of the hypothalamus, indicating that these cells are critical in controlling liver glucose production [115]. More recent studies, however, suggest that neuropeptide Y (NPY) expressing cells are the relevant cells that are critical in mediating effects of insulin signalling. It was suggested that AgRP cells are a subset of NPY producing cells, with NPY neurons regulating appetite and energy balance, and the AgRP cells influencing hepatic glucose production [115]. NPY is known to influence peripheral insulin release indirectly via the parasympathetic pathways, as NPY stimulates insulin release from pancreatic β-cells, and this is followed by negative feedback following insulin action on hypothalamic NPY neurons, to reduce NPY levels. This reciprocal control between the two factors seems to be critical for maintaining a balanced energy homeostasis, and disruptions to this control are believed to occur in insulin resistance [116].

6.1.7.5 Effects of High Fructose Diets

Fructose, commonly known as a fruit sugar, is a monosaccharide with the same molecular formula as glucose ($C_6H_{12}O_6$). It is sweeter than sucrose (although it makes up half of sucrose), it is found naturally in many fruits, honey, and maple syrup, and is often used as a sweetener in soft drinks, baking products, and ice creams. However, the metabolism of fructose is different to that of glucose, and most of it appears to be converted to glucose in the liver, to be used for energy production or possibly to be stored as glycogen; alternatively it may be steered towards triglyceride synthesis [117]. Fructose has a greater likelihood than glucose of undergoing the Maillard reaction, thus forming advanced glycation end products (AGE) which, as we mention in the protein section of this chapter, are associated with oxidative stress, inflammation, diabetic complications, and neurodegeneration.

Studies in animals of short-term [47, 118, 119] and long-term administration [120] of fructose have reported enhancements in cognitive performance, though the level of enhancement varied, depending on the species tested, and sex of the animal. For instance, cognitive testing using an operant barpressing task in fructose-fed (15%, 3 months) mice showed enhanced memory and learning [120], yet no significant weight gain or impaired glucose tolerance. However, this was species-dependent, as studies in hamsters had shown that weight gain and glucose dysregulation can occur on high fructose diets. Bruggeman et al. [121] and Vasudevan et al. [122] demonstrated that fructose-induced cognitive impairments could occur more readily in female than in male rats, suggesting that the metabolism of fructose and the effects of a high fructose diet on cognition may be sex-dependent. In contrast, Ross et al. noticed higher spatial memory impairment in male rats compared to female rats, on a high fructose diet, when compared to placebo [123]. Stranahan et al. [124] identified that rats fed a high fructose diet showed weakened cognitive function, due to the development of insulin resistance. Impaired cognitive function due to a high fructose diet was also reported by Agrawal and Gomez-Pinilla in 2012. Other studies of rats and hamsters have shown that the reduction in cognitive function due to high fructose diets is associated with brain insulin resistance [125, 126]. Therefore it is not surprising that high fructose intake is considered to be a risk factor for AD and dementia [127, 128]. In 2011, Ye et al. [129] found that a higher intake of added sugars (mostly fructose and sucrose) is linked with inferior cognitive function in people: greater intakes of total sugars, added sugars, and sugar-sweetened beverages were all associated with lower mini-mental state examination (MMSE) scores. Apart from fructose and sugar intake, overall diet quality is also important for cognitive function, which is particularly relevant in poor urban settings, where cost and access to good quality food is an issue [130]. Fructose has also been shown to affect neurogenesis, as shown in the work of Borght et al. and Rafati et al. [131, 132]. The work indicated that high fructose and sucrose consumption could significantly reduce hippocampal neurogenesis, while glucose consumption did not have a reducing effect. However, another study of mice compared a diet high in fructose to an isocaloric glucose diet and found that fructose decreased physical activity, increased body fat, yet had no effect on hippocampal neurogenesis or learning [133]. Additional research is needed to understand the underlying mechanisms [134], and studies such as these are further complicated by the finding that levels of spontaneous physical activity as well as basal metabolic rates (in mice) significantly influence fasting blood glucose levels, lipid profiles, fat mass, and other metabolic syndrome indicators, irrespective of whether they were on a high-fat, high-carbohydrate, or control diet [135].

6.1.7.6 Sucrose

Sucrose is the disaccharide we know as table sugar, and consists of fructose attached to glucose. Studies of high-sucrose diets, similar to studies of high-carbohydrate, high-fructose, or high-glucose diets, demonstrate the negative impact of sucrose consumption on metabolic outcomes [136], especially for cognition. For example, rats given a sucrose solution (32%) in addition to chow for eight weeks had a poorer memory in a novel object recognition task compared with rats that only received chow [137]. This result was independent of the effects of the sucrose solution on body weight. A study by Hsu et al. also indicated low hippocampal function [138] in rats fed a high-sucrose diet, compared to a control diet. In another study, young rats fed a supplemental sucrose solution (32%) for six weeks required more time to find a hidden platform in the Morris Water Maze, showing damage to the hippocampus [139, 140]. Furthermore, rats given a high-sucrose diet for six weeks demonstrated relatively poor spatial memory [140], and when the consumption was extended for eight weeks, poor recognition memory performance was observed [137]. Lastly, several animal model experiments have shown that maternal sugar intake during gestation or lactation can have a negative impact on the development of neuronal cells in offspring [141–144].

6.2 Proteins

Dementia involves the gradual deterioration of cognitive and physical functions of an individual [145]. Given the increasing incidence of dementia worldwide, researchers are investigating potential strategies that can initiate changes at both molecular and cellular levels to improve brain function. Recently, a lot of attention has focused on identifying ways to attenuate preclinical stages of AD, such as MCI in the elderly, as this precedes the onset of dementia and AD [146]. Moderating dietary intake, together with ensuring that macronutrient and micronutrient requirements are met, is one such strategy which has shown positive effects on cognitive function in the elderly, both in epidemiological studies and clinical studies [147–150]. Research shows a strong association between weight gain, obesity and associated disorders, and cognitive decline [151]. Experts emphasise the importance of maintaining a healthy weight, yet in western countries especially, increasingly sedentary lifestyles and inappropriate intakes of unhealthy and/or processed foods is increasing the number of people with chronic health problems related to diet [152, 153]. Many dietary strategies have been proposed in order to maintain healthy weight, and high-protein/low-carbohydrate diets are among those approaches [154]. Such diets would reduce blood glucose fluctuations whilst ensuring adequate protein intake, though it must be remembered that many diets known to promote longevity and healthy brain function (such as the Mediterranean and Okinawa diets) have low protein content. Studies of such diets have shown a strong link between diet and cognition [155]. A low-calorie, low-fat diet is believed to be good for delaying the onset of AD [156]. However, it is important to ensure adequate good quality protein is consistently present in the diet to maintain healthy cognitive performance, particularly in the elderly who often have reduced appetites and less efficient digestive systems [157, 158]. For example a study by Jakobsen et al. [159] showed that a high-protein diet led to improved cognitive function along with increased levels of phenylalanine and other branched chain amino acids in the plasma [159].

6.2.1 Protein Metabolism in General

The proteins in the body are molecules which have essential roles to play, maintaining the body's function and physiology [160]. They consist of smaller subunits, the amino acids, that join together in different permutations and combinations [161], with individual protein sequences determined by the genetic code that contains the specific information about the composition of a required protein [162].

The amount of dietary protein required by an individual as part of the diet depends on body weight and stage in growth cycles; thus the nutritional requirements of children and adults are different [163–165]. Furthermore, older adults often require a higher protein intake due to reduced digestive capabilities, or to promote muscle protein synthesis. The requirement for adults is usually 1 g of protein for every kilogram of bodyweight, and a balanced diet generally covers the standard needs of both adults and children [166, 167]. The major sources of protein include foods such as meat, fish, poultry, eggs, and dairy, and plant sources such as nuts, grains, and pulses [168].

The proteins consumed as part of food are broken down by digestive juices in our body into smaller subunits called amino acids [169]. Most commonly, non-specific endo- and exo-proteases carry out most of the protein catabolism, and amino acids are recycled as they are used to produce new proteins [170]. Excess protein can be deaminated, and converted into glucose through gluconeogenesis, or can be modified to become a substrate for the citric acid cycle (also known as the tricarboxylic acid cycle – TCA) and get utilised as another source of energy for the body. When amino acids get deaminated in these conversions, the amine group of the amino acid gets converted to ammonia which is removed by the liver in the formation of urea. The resultant deaminated amino acids get converted into pyruvate, acetylcoenzyme A (acetylCoA), oxaloacetate, fumarate, succinyl CoA, or α-ketoglutarate, all of which can enter the TCA cycle for energy production. These amino acid conversions can happen during periods of need or stress, or when excess protein is eaten. Alanine for example is converted to pyruvate via alanine aminotransferase, and arginine, proline, histidine, and glutamine can all be converted to glutamate, then to α-ketoglutarate [171]. If these deaminated amino acids are not required for energy production, they are converted to fat.

The above paragraph highlights the fact that excess protein can be a source of unwanted calories in a diet. Recent transgenic mice studies have shown that a diet high in calories, whether the source is from protein, fat, or carbohydrate, increases AD pathology and cognitive deficits, when compared to a lower calorie diet [172]. It has also been shown that a low-fat protein diet can lead to lower levels of aggregated phospho-tau in a mouse model of tauopathy, when compared to the same mice on a standard chow diet [173]. A high calorie diet has already been linked with AD in many epidemiological studies, as well as in animal research, thought to be due to the resulting obesity, cardiovascular problems, and glucose/insulin dysregulation [174]. Thus although complete protein (containing all essential amino acids) is required in the diet, a moderate intake is recommended, in a diet that does not lead to an overall gain in weight [175].

6.2.2 Links Between Specific Amino Acids and Brain Function

It is well-known that the brain is separated from other organs via the brain capillary endothelial cells which form the blood brain barrier (BBB). This barrier is very selective about which amino acids enter and leave the brain [176–178]. The amino acids present in proteins are required for healthy brain function, and a lack of these can impair normal brain functioning and lead to cognitive impairment [179]. In addition, various amino acids are precursors for certain neurotransmitters in the brain, and transport mechanisms exist to carry these specific amino acids across the BBB [180, 181]. In particular, the amino acids tyrosine, histidine, tryptophan, and arginine are essential for neurotransmitter synthesis in the brain [182, 183]. The BBB cells are polarised, such that there is a polar distribution of transport proteins that mediate amino acid homeostasis in the brain. There are facilitative transporters and Na(+) dependent transporters to help transport amino acids from one side to the other, depending on needs. This way the BBB helps to regulate amino acid content in the brain, for example it helps maintain neutral amino acid concentration at about 10% of levels found in the circulation [178], and small neutral amino acids such as glycine and alanine are known to get actively pumped across the BBB [184–186]. The brain requirements for all the individual essential amino acids are not known, however the concentration of different amino acids in blood, the health of the BBB, toxic build-up of waste products, and certain medications can all influence the transport of amino acids across the BBB, and can thus influence normal cognitive functioning [183, 187].

The large neutral amino acids tyrosine and tryptophan form the main precursors for various neurotransmitters essential for brain function [188, 189]. Cognitive health is influenced by levels of these two amino acids, as modifications in the brain levels of tyrosine and tryptophan by increased dietary intake has been shown to modify levels of their resultant neurotransmitters [189–193]. These neurotransmitters are involved in a number of neuronal functions including stress responses and working memory, and inadequate levels of these neurotransmitters have been linked to depression, ageing, and impaired cognitive functioning [194].

6.2.2.1 Tryptophan
Tryptophan is involved in several vital processes in the body. It is present in a variety of foods, and it is one of the essential amino acids, yet it is at the lowest concentration in the human body, compared to the other amino acids. The neurotransmitter serotonin is derived from tryptophan, and it is crucial for the functioning of the serotonergic system. A study by Mendelsohn et al. [195] showed the importance of tryptophan in cognitive functioning by acute tryptophan depletion (ATD). ATD specifically resulted in

the impairment of episodic memory, and in fact, the deficiency of tryptophan can cause mood and behaviour changes in individuals, including depression (as mentioned above) and aversion, etc. [196]. Young [196] showed that the changes in cognitive function resulted from changes in the levels of tryptophan in the periphery. Another symptom of tryptophan deficiency is the dysregulation of pain sensitivity, which has been shown in animal models as well as humans [197–199]. In early studies, Hartmann [200] and Spinweber [201] demonstrated that the artificial administration of tryptophan can alleviate the symptoms brought about by tryptophan deprivation, thus the tryptophan increased sleepiness and decreased pain sensitivity. This has been supported by animal studies which showed changes in serotonin levels one hour post injection of this amino acid [202]. A very well-established role of tryptophan is the regulation of mood [188]. A diet deficient in tryptophan can lead to alteration in levels of depression and changes in the state of an individual's mood [203]. However, although low tryptophan levels have been linked to the onset of depression, increasing tryptophan intake has had limited success in treating depression through increasing serotonin production [204].

Aggression or violent behaviour is another symptom of tryptophan deficiency [205]. Cleare and Bond [206] found that lower levels of tryptophan in the diet could lead to a person being aggressive, and in their studies, the administration of dietary tryptophan could reduce such aggressive behaviour. These changes are all thought to be due to serotonin neurotransmitter functions in the central nervous system (CNS) [207, 208]. Tryptophan is also required for the synthesis of tryptamine – a neuromodulator of serotonin, melatonin, the vitamin niacin, and NAD/NADP, and has been trialled for the treatment of many conditions and disorders, including major depression, pain, insomnia, attention deficit/hyperactivity disorder (ADHD), and chronic fatigue, amongst others [209]. In most cases, treatment has produced mixed results, though the therapeutic combination of tryptophan with mono-amine oxidase inhibitors has been quite successful in the treatment of depression [209]. Interestingly, a recent study showed that modulation of the tryptophan/serotonin pathway in HIV+ve patients by probiotic supplementation resulted in decreased tryptophan yet increased serotonin levels, which suggests another aspect of digestion and metabolism that needs further study [210]. It is interesting that tryptophan degradation via the kynurenine pathway, which accounts for about 90% of its catabolism, results in the production of several neuroactive metabolites. These metabolites have recently been linked to neurodevelopment and pathophysiology of psychiatric disorders such as schizophrenia, and they are also thought to play a role in immunity and inflammation. Enzymes in this pathway are being considered as therapeutic targets in various conditions, but this is beyond the scope of this review [211].

6.2.2.2 Tyrosine

Tyrosine is another important neutral amino acid, as it is the precursor of various neurotransmitters known as catecholamines, including dopamine, epinephrine, and norepinephrine [212, 213]. Tyrosine can be synthesised from phenylalanine to some extent, however the brain is not able to meet all its needs from tyrosine derived from phenylalanine [214]. Most protein-rich foods can supply enough tyrosine for the body, yet being another large neutral amino acid like tryptophan, tyrosine competes with tryptophan to cross the BBB using specific transport proteins [215]. An abundant supply of tyrosine is required by the brain as tyrosine is believed to play an important role in regulating certain important physiological functions following exposure to different kinds of stress inducers such as exposure to heat and cold [216]. This is because the brain's response requires the neurotransmitters norepinephrine (noradrenalin), epinephrine (adrenalin) or dopamine, depending on the source of stress [217]. Many studies have been carried out to investigate the ability of tyrosine to reduce the symptoms and negative effects of low dopamine level-related pathologies such as Parkinson's disease, depression, and phenylketonuria. Others have noticed that in otherwise healthy people, stress caused by cognitively demanding tasks can lead to impairments in working memory and attentional tasks, and that tyrosine can reduce the impairments. Learning and memory are also improved upon administration of tyrosine [218, 219]. Furthermore, tyrosine has also been found to have beneficial effects in humans in improving cognition [220, 221]. A number of other clinical and animal studies have linked tyrosine with brain function and cognition, showing a number of beneficial effects related to cognition and proper behavioural function of the individual [219, 222, 223]. In addition, rat studies have shown beneficial effects on brain function when administering tyrosine to reduce the stress response to cold and restraint stress [182]; similarly, humans and rats that were pre-administered tyrosine were less affected following exposure to the stress factors [224, 225].

More recent studies have shown that even without obvious stress, tyrosine administration has sometimes been found to have an acute beneficial effect, assumed to be due to raising dopamine levels, for example in performing multiple tasks simultaneously [226], updating working memory [227], and inhibitory control [227], although all these situations could be considered to be cognitively stressful. A recent study by some of the same researchers has demonstrated dopamine to be directly involved in improving working memory performance, following tyrosine administration [228]. It also appears that optimum dopamine levels, and thus the requirement for tyrosine, is dependent on the individual, thus individual demands need to be assessed, if considering administering tyrosine to improve cognition [229].

6.2.3 Clinical Studies of Protein Supplementation

A number of studies have been conducted to evaluate the association between dietary protein intake and cognitive functioning (Table 6.2). Rue et al. [83, 230] conducted one of the earlier studies, involving a cohort of 304 healthy individuals aged between 66 and 90 years in a 6-year longitudinal study, and found a positive association between protein intake and cognitive functioning test scores. However, another study [84] showed no significant association between dietary protein intake and cognitive decline. The measurement of cognition in this study was done by MMSE scores on 125 community-dwelling healthy elderly people aged over 68 years. The effect of dietary protein intake in the form of meat was evaluated in a population of more than 8000 healthy elderly people aged over 65 years, using the Diagnostic and Statistical Manual of Mental Disorders (DSM_IV) cognitive test [85]. There was no significant association found between meat consumption (2–3 times/week and 4–6 times/week) and a reduced risk of dementia. Another study [86] was conducted to test the improvement in cognition in response to dietary protein intake using MMSE scores. This study was conducted on 187 free-living elderly participants with normal cognition aged more than 65 years; yet again, no significant association between dietary protein intake and improvement in cognition was found. In a woman-only cohort, where all the participants had normal

Table 6.2 Clinical studies which investigated the association between dietary protein intake and cognitive functioning in elderly individuals.

Author	Population studied	Outcome of the study
La Rue et al. [83]	Healthy elderly individuals (aged 66–90 years)	Positive association between dietary protein intake and cognitive functioning
Deschamp et al. [84]	Non-demented elderly individuals (aged >68 years)	No association between dietary protein intake and cognitive functioning
Barberger Gateau et al. [85]	Non-demented elderly individuals (aged >65 years)	No association between meat consumption and reduction of dementia risk
Velho et al. [86]	Healthy elderly participants (aged >65 years)	No association between dietary protein intake and cognitive functioning
Vercambre et al. [87]	Elderly women (63–68 years)	No association between dietary protein intake and cognitive functioning
Roberts et al. [21]	Healthy aged participants (aged between 70 and 89 years)	A significant association between dietary protein intake and reduced risk of dementia
Aparicio Vizuete et al. [88]	Elderly healthy individuals (aged ≥65 years)	A significant association between dietary protein intake and better cognitive functioning
Guligowska et al. [89]	Comparison of depressed and control elderly people (average age 71)	An association of depression with a combination of low dietary protein, fibre, vitamin B6, and other nutrients was found

cognition and were aged between 63 and 68 years, effects of dietary intake of beef, pork, lamb, and poultry intake were evaluated on the Détérioration Cognitive Observée scale (DECO) scale of cognition [87]. A significant association was only found between higher poultry intake and cognition in this study. A significant association between dietary protein intake and reduced risk of MCI/AD was observed in a study on 937 cognitively normal participants aged between 70 and 89 years, evaluated using clinical dementia rating (CDR) and a range of other cognitive tests based on memory, executive function, and language [21]. In contrast, one study showed a significant negative association between higher protein intake in the form of meat and cognitive functioning [88]. These studies clearly highlight that there is currently inconclusive evidence to support an association between higher protein intake and better cognitive functioning. It is more likely that high protein intake is associated with overall good nutritional status, which is indirectly correlated with good cognitive function. A high-protein diet has been shown to improve both physical and cognitive functioning in young healthy men [159]. The increased intake of protein when combined with other strategies such as resistance training (discussed further in chapter 13) has been shown to improve cognitive function via pathways involving increased levels of growth and neurotrophic factors such as IGF-1, BDNF, decreased levels of IL-6, and also via modulation of body inflammation [159, 231]. These studies demonstrate that protein in the diet may influence cognitive health, yet that so many other physiological aspects such as digestion, exercise, overall mental health, medications, and nutritional status will influence any effects. Importantly, dietary studies should evaluate a whole diet, including carbohydrate, fruit, vegetable, processed foods and total calorie intake, not just protein intake, as other dietary components also influence cognition.

6.2.4 Links Between Loss of Protein Function and Neurodegeneration

Neurodegenerative disorders are highly complex diseases involving a combination of changes at the molecular, cellular, and clinical level. In the case of AD, oxidative stress, mitochondrial dysfunction, and chronic inflammation are believed to be early changes, with many enzymes, membrane proteins, lipid transporters, lipids, and cellular mechanisms functioning abnormally. AD is also specifically known to involve changes in the processing of the Aβ peptide and the tau microtubule-associated protein [232]. In addition, as discussed in Chapter 2, AD and many other neurodegenerative disorders are commonly called proteopathies, as most are associated with the loss of function/gain of function of one or more proteins resulting from the misfolding, aggregation, and toxic build-up of the proteins [233]. Aβ peptides are normal proteolytic products to be found in the body, yet in AD, Aβ peptides are found in higher than normal levels, facilitating aggregation in the brain to form toxic oligomers which disrupt synapses and membrane function [234]. The peptides aggregate further to form the major protein component of senile plaques in the AD brain. Aβ is derived from a larger protein called the amyloid-β precursor protein (APP) [234], a transmembrane protein found in most tissues, and required for neuronal growth and survival. APP can be processed by an amyloidogenic pathway (produces Aβ) or a non-amyloidogenic pathway (no Aβ production), and it is believed that in AD more APP is processed through the amyloidogenic pathway to result in higher than normal Aβ peptide levels. Alternatively, or in addition, clearance mechanisms are less efficient, allowing the build-up of toxic Aβ aggregates [235]. Tau is another protein with disturbed metabolism in AD – it is hyperphosphorylated, and is the main component of neurofibrillary tangles (NFT) seen in AD, as well as some other neurodegenerative conditions [236]. Other protein aggregates are seen in other conditions (see chapter 2), for example in the neurodegenerative conditions Lewy body disease, multiple system atrophy disease, and Parkinson's disease, alpha-synuclein aggregates are formed, and deposit in the form of fibrils [237]. Alpha-synuclein is often seen in association with ubiquitin in damaged neurons [238]. In Parkinson's disease, this protein accumulation has been shown to cause the death of dopaminergic neurons, and is considered to be the result of defective protein transport between the endoplasmic reticulum and the Golgi apparatus [239]. In Lewy body disease, the accumulation of the alpha-synuclein is due to impaired axonal transport of the protein [240]. Mutations in a protein called huntingtin are responsible for the pathogenesis of Huntington's disease [241]. The mutant forms of huntingtin have polyglutamine (polyQ) repeats that cause the protein to fold incorrectly, aggregate, and eventually form insoluble deposits, resulting in the inability of transport and clearance mechanisms to remove the aggregates; this eventually prevents normal ubiquitin proteasome function and is toxic to the cells [242]. In another neurodegenerative disorder, namely amyotrophic lateral sclerosis (ALS, also known as Lou Gehrig's disease, or motor neuron disease), about 20% of inherited forms and 5% of sporadic cases are due to mutations in the antioxidant enzyme Cu/Zn superoxide dismutase 1 (SOD1). These mutations lead to the selective degeneration of neurons, most likely due to increased oxidative stress and aggregated mutant SOD1 disrupting mitochondria and proteasomes [243]. Mutations in many other genes such as the TDP-43 (transactive response DNA binding protein-43) and fusedin-sarcoma protein (FUS) (an RNA-binding protein) genes are known to be involved in ALS, where abnormal protein aggregates and deposits have also been found; yet for each ALS mutant protein, the age of onset as well as the symptoms can be different [244]. Prion protein (PrP) is the key protein responsible for prion diseases or transmissible spongiform encephalopathies such as Creutzfeldt-Jakob disease and Kuru. PrP is unique as it is believed to fold in a specific abnormal manner to convert into an infectious 'prion' protein, which triggers further abnormal folding. These folded prion proteins accumulate and aggregate, leading to a deadly neurodegenerative disease [245].

Various intracellular mechanisms involving protein metabolism are understood to be impaired in most of these neurodegenerative diseases [246] or, at the very least, are not efficient in clearing the abnormal toxic aggregates. The toxic proteins or aggregates accumulate in various regions of the cell such as the cytosol, nucleus, endoplasmic reticulum, and even extracellular locations [247]. Therefore, one of the underlying causes of proteinopathies is the inability to remove the toxic protein build-up.

6.2.5 Clearance Mechanisms Associated with Proteinopathies Involved in Neurodegeneration

Cells use various mechanisms to get rid of damaged, abnormally aggregated, oxidised, or unwanted proteins [248]. In the case of AD, the excess Aβ peptides, as well as oligomeric and fibrillar aggregates of Aβ are all unwanted, and there are various mechanism for Aβ clearance. The main mechanisms involve either Aβ removal to the peripheral blood and lymphatic systems or degradation within the CNS tissues. Aβ can reach the peripheral circulation via chaperone-mediated (CM) transport across the BBB, perivascular drainage, or via the glymphatic system. In the brain parenchyma, cells can phagocytose fibrillar forms of Aβ, possibly also the more toxic soluble aggregates [249–251]. Intracellular Aβ peptide degradation, undertaken by cells that either absorb or engulf Aβ forms, involves autophagy, endosomal/lysosomal degradation, and the ubiquitin-proteasome system (UPS). By reducing intracellular build-up, this helps prevent or reduce intracellular protein aggregation, thus reducing the neurotoxicity of cytosolic Aβ. Extracellular Aβ can be degraded by one of several metalloendopeptidases. These degradation systems are discussed in more detail below.

The UPS is one major degradative pathway, required for the degradation of about 80% of intracellular proteins in eucaryotes, and which utilises the protein ubiquitin to remove protein build-up such as unwanted phosphorylated tau, polyQ repeats, or alpha-synuclein aggregates [252]. In neurodegenerative conditions it is believed that, over the years, the enzymes of the proteasome, the E1, E2, and E3 ligases that are responsible for ubiquitination of unwanted proteins, as well as the proteolytic steps in the proteasome, are not able to function properly in the cell, eventually resulting in accumulation of these toxic proteins. Ubiquitin has been found in the intracellular inclusions of amyloid plaques, NFT, Lewy bodies in Parkinson's, and in the intranuclear inclusions in polyQ disorders [253, 254]. Another process for degradation is the autophagy-lysosome system; this is the principal system for degrading proteins with long half-lives, and is the only system that degrades organelles and large protein aggregates or inclusions. Thus this system would be also needed to remove aggregated proteins of the above-mentioned neurodegenerative conditions [255]. It is thought that when the UPS is overloaded, the lysosome-autophagy system removes protein aggregates and dysfunctional proteasomes [256, 257]. Chaperone-mediated (CM) autophagy [59] is another form of autophagy where proteins are targeted to lysosomes for degradation. However, defective proteins can sometimes bind to the CM pathway receptors on the membranes of lysosomes, thus preventing their own degradation and resulting in toxic build-up [258].

The oxidative stress and inflammation of ageing, as well as chronic conditions like type 2 diabetes and obesity, cause microglia to be chronically activated. They are often associated with senile plaques, and although some studies have shown microglia to be detrimental in that they increase the inflammatory response, these cells are also known to phagocytose and degrade Aβ peptides and aggregates [259]. Monocyte-derived macrophages are also involved in Aβ removal; yet, more controversially, there is now evidence that monocyte infiltration from the periphery may occur, most likely due to a leaky BBB [249].

Secreted enzymes also play a major role in degrading Aβ peptides, and the enzymes responsible include insulin-degrading enzyme, neprilysin, angiotensin-converting enzyme, endothelin converting enzymes, and matrix metalloproteinase-9. These are all zinc-dependent proteases, and there is much evidence that all are involved in Aβ clearance. Some are influenced or induced by immune response changes, for example matrix metalloproteinase-9 has been shown to be involved in both TNFα-mediated pro-inflammatory and anti-inflammatory signalling in activated macrophages and microglia [249, 250].

In the late-onset, most common form of AD, Aβ buildup is attributed to defective clearance, rather than to its overproduction. The above Aβ peptide clearance methods have been studied at length in various animal models of AD, and disruptions to most of these clearance avenues have been detected. It is believed that modulating these clearance mechanisms, for example targeting the immune response in the brain, may be an important early strategy for curtailing Aβ accumulation and disease progression [249, 251].

When cellular processes cannot cope with the Aβ-induced toxicity and/or oxidative stress in AD, apoptosis can occur. Programmed cell death (PCD), an intracellular program, is activated in neurodegenerative diseases such as Parkinson's disease, amyotrophic lateral sclerosis, AD, and Huntington's disease. Apoptosis is a form of PCD and involves a series of biochemical processes leading to cell death [260]. Apoptosis can be extrinsic or intrinsic, depending upon the location of proteins involved. In the case of extrinsic apoptotic pathways, cell-surface death receptors such as Fas cause the activation of caspase-8 or -10 [261]. The intrinsic apoptotic pathway results from mitochondrial permeabilisation, the mitochondrial release of cytochrome c, and activation of proteins like caspase-9 to initiate the caspase pathway [262]. Similarly, other forms of PCD can be observed in neurodegenerative disorders, such as cytoplasmic PCD, or a combination of apoptosis and necrosis [263].

6.2.6 Role of Protein Crosslinking and Inflammation in Neurodegeneration and AD

Protein turnover is known to slow down with ageing, resulting in an increased amount of old and damaged protein in the body. One of the major deleterious changes that can occur is the non-enzymatic glucose-protein condensation reaction, which leads to products or 'adducts' called advanced glycation end-products (AGE) (AGE also discussed in Chapters 4 and 8). Lipids and nucleic acids can also be affected. These reactions are mostly irreversible, leading to an accumulation of AGE [264]. An excess level of free radicals and reactive carbonyl compounds in the body increases the formation of AGE [265]. AGE cause widespread intracellular damage and apoptosis, they are known to accelerate physiological ageing processes, and are considered to be pro-inflammatory mediators in the development of various conditions including cardiovascular diseases, stroke, insulin resistance, and AD [266, 267]. The formation of AGE is also accelerated under hyperglycaemic and oxidative stress conditions – both of which are known to increase the risk of AD [268]. The accumulation of AGE is part of the normal ageing process of the body, but is accelerated in AD. AGE can be found in the pathological deposits of AD such as the amyloid plaques and NFT. For example, Aβ is known to co-localise with AGE in the brain temporal gyrus region in aged individuals as well as AD patients [269]. AGE are also known to play a role in the formation of higher molecular weight oligomers of Aβ from monomeric forms [270]. Loske et al. showed that the oligomerisation process of Aβ gets fast-tracked because of crosslinking through AGE, suggesting AGE play a pivotal role in the early process of Aβ deposition and plaque formation in AD [271]. The number of AGE-positive neurons is directly linked with both the age and the progression of the disease. In addition, the paired helical filaments of tau can become glycated, further exacerbating tangle formation in AD [272]. Recently it has been recognised that diet is a major source of AGE that could cause inflammatory reactions and organ damage [268, 273].

The toxic effects of AGE involve the promotion of further oxidative stress and inflammation, by binding to cell surface receptors or cross-linking with other proteins, altering their structure and reducing their normal function. The best-known receptor that AGE bind to is the receptor for advanced glycation end products (RAGE), a protein that belongs to the immunoglobulin family. Binding to RAGE induces oxidative stress and activates inflammatory cascades, starting with the NF-κB pathway and inflammatory mediators like TNF-α, IL-6, and C-reactive protein (CRP) [274], and hence contributing to various age-related chronic inflammatory diseases.

One of the mechanisms through which AGE cause damage is via reactive oxygen species (ROS) [275]. ROS cause oxidation of sugars and proteins, and protein glycation in turn increases the rate of ROS production. There is also evidence of RAGE upregulation by its own ligands, as increased levels of RAGE mRNA have been observed in human osteoblasts after AGE treatment [276]. The defective Aβ clearance in AD further increases the AGE formation due to the increased half-life of these peptides. In addition, AGE make it difficult for microglia to clear plaques, as AGE crosslink to Aβ, which further impairs the degradation of Aβ by lysosomal proteases. RAGE–Aβ interactions at the BBB lead to oxidative stress, inflammatory responses, and reduced cerebral blood flow, and RAGE can also transfer circulating Aβ across the BBB to the brain [277]. AGE and RAGE also form a strong biochemical link between type 2 diabetes and AD through the development of increased oxidative stress, chronic inflammation and neuronal damage. Hyperglycaemia, a major feature of type 2 diabetes, enhances the production of AGE and causes vascular complications, all of which contribute towards AD pathogenesis. Both AGE and RAGE are considered important drug targets in AD and many RAGE antagonists are currently being studied that can attenuate neuroinflammation and hence slow the disease progression [277]. Recent studies have shown that activated macrophages are a major source of AGE, and anti-inflammatory molecules that inhibit AGE have been shown to be good candidates for ameliorating diabetic complications as well as neurodegenerative diseases such as AD and Parkinson's disease [278].

6.3 Conclusion

Identifying associations between macronutrient intake and neurodegenerative diseases will help to explain the important role of diet in neuronal integrity, brain function, and late-life cognitive impairment. The literature reviewed in this chapter indicates there are important metabolic relationships between protein and carbohydrate intake and cognitive performance. However, these relationships are complex, and are influenced by many other factors, including other dietary components, total calorie intake, genetic make-up, physical exercise levels, and other environmental factors. More work is needed, particularly in relation to long-term studies of dietary intake across the lifespan, to further enhance our understanding of these associations. Further study of protein processing and protein aggregate removal from cells would also improve our understanding of the pathological mechanisms associated with neurodegenerative diseases.

References

1 Venn, B.J. and Green, T.J. (2007). Glycemic index and glycemic load: measurement issues and their effect on diet-disease relationships. *Eur. J. Clin. Nutr.* 61 (Suppl 1): S122–S131.
2 Barclay, A.W., Petocz, P., McMillan-Price, J. et al. (2008). Glycemic index, glycemic load, and chronic disease risk – a meta-analysis of observational studies. *Am. J. Clin. Nutr.* 87: 627–637.
3 Bach Knudsen, K.E. (2015). Microbial degradation of whole-grain complex carbohydrates and impact on short-chain fatty acids and health. *Adv. Nutr.* 6: 206–213.
4 Kumar, V., Sinha, A.K., Makkar, H.P. et al. (2012). Dietary roles of non-starch polysaccharides in human nutrition: a review. *Crit. Rev. Food Sci. Nutr.* 52: 899–935.
5 Kinoshita, M., Suzuki, Y., and Saito, Y. (2002). Butyrate reduces colonic paracellular permeability by enhancing PPARγ activation. *Biochem. Biophys. Res. Commun.* 293: 827–831.
6 Hamer, H.M., Jonkers, D., Venema, K. et al. (2008). Review article: the role of butyrate on colonic function. *Aliment. Pharmacol. Ther.* 27: 104–119.
7 Nilsson, A.C., Ostman, E.M., Holst, J.J., and Bjorck, I.M. (2008). Including indigestible carbohydrates in the evening meal of healthy subjects improves glucose tolerance, lowers inflammatory markers, and increases satiety after a subsequent standardized breakfast. *J. Nutr.* 138: 732–739.
8 Theuwissen, E. and Mensink, R.P. (2008). Water-soluble dietary fibers and cardiovascular disease. *Physiol. Behav.* 94: 285–292.

9 Ohira, H., Tsutsui, W., and Fujioka, Y. (2017). Are short chain fatty acids in gut microbiota defensive players for inflammation and atherosclerosis? *J. Atheroscler. Thromb.* 24: 660–672.

10 Sieber, F.E. and Traystman, R.J. (1992). Special issues: glucose and the brain. *Crit. Care Med.* 20: 104–114.

11 Boucher, J., Kleinridders, A., and Kahn, C.R. (2014). Insulin receptor signaling in normal and insulin-resistant states. *Cold Spring Harb. Perspect. Biol.* 6: a009191.

12 Boucher, J., Tseng, Y.H., and Kahn, C.R. (2010). Insulin and insulin-like growth factor-1 receptors act as ligand-specific amplitude modulators of a common pathway regulating gene transcription. *J. Biol. Chem.* 285: 17235–17245.

13 Schenk, S., Saberi, M., and Olefsky, J.M. (2008). Insulin sensitivity: modulation by nutrients and inflammation. *J. Clin. Invest.* 118: 2992–3002.

14 Osborn, O. and Olefsky, J.M. (2012). The cellular and signaling networks linking the immune system and metabolism in disease. *Nat. Med.* 18: 363–374.

15 Grant, W.B. (1997). Dietary links to Alzheimer's disease. *Alzheimers Dis. Rev.* 2: 42–55.

16 Cummings, J.H. (1981). Short chain fatty acids in the human colon. *Gut* 22: 763–779.

17 Parks, E.J. and Hellerstein, M.K. (2000). Carbohydrate-induced hypertriacylglycerolemia: historical perspective and review of biological mechanisms. *Am. J. Clin. Nutr.* 71: 412–433.

18 Lithell, H., Jacobs, I., Vessby, B. et al. (1982). Decrease of lipoprotein lipase activity in skeletal muscle in man during a short-term carbohydrate-rich dietary regime: with special reference to HDL-cholesterol, apolipoprotein and insulin concentrations. *Metabolism* 31: 994–998.

19 Bergeron, N. and Havel, R.J. (1996). Prolonged postprandial responses of lipids and apolipoproteins in triglyceride-rich lipoproteins of individuals expressing an apolipoprotein ∈4 allele. *J. Clin. Invest.* 97: 65–72.

20 Osuntokun, B.O., Sahota, A., Ogunniyi, A.O. et al. (1995). Lack of an association between apolipoprotein E ε4 and Alzheimer's disease in elderly Nigerians. *Ann. Neurol.* 38: 463–465.

21 Roberts, R.O., Roberts, L.A., Geda, Y.E. et al. (2012). Relative intake of macronutrients impacts risk of mild cognitive impairment or dementia. *J. Alzheimers Dis.* 32: 329–339.

22 Ross, G.W., Abbott, R.D., Petrovitch, H. et al. (2012). Pre-motor features of Parkinson's disease: the Honolulu-Asia aging study experience. *Parkinsonism Relat. Disord.* 18 (Supplement 1): S199–S202.

23 Institute of Medicine (2002). *Dietary Reference Intakes for Energy, Carbohydrate, Fiber, Fat, Fatty Acids, Cholesterol, Protein and Amino Acids (Macronutrients)*. Washington, DC: The National Academies Press https://doi.org/10.17226/10490.

24 Jankovic, N., Geelen, A., Streppel, M.T. et al. (2014). Adherence to a healthy diet according to the World Health Organization guidelines and all-cause mortality in elderly adults from Europe and the United States. *Am. J. Epidemiol.* 180: 978–988.

25 Freeman, J.M. and Kossoff, E.H. (2010). Ketosis and the ketogenic diet, 2010: advances in treating epilepsy and other disorders. *Adv. Pediatr.* 57: 315–329.

26 Hampel, H., Burger, K., Teipel, S.J. et al. (2008). Core candidate neurochemical and imaging biomarkers of Alzheimer's disease. *Alzheimers Dement.* 4: 38–48.

27 Imamura, K., Takeshima, T., Kashiwaya, Y. et al. (2006). D-beta-hydroxybutyrate protects dopaminergic SH-SY5Y cells in a rotenone model of Parkinson's disease. *J. Neurosci. Res.* 84: 1376–1384.

28 Paoli, A., Bianco, A., Damiani, E., and Bosco, G. (2014). Ketogenic diet in neuromuscular and neurodegenerative diseases. *BioMed Res. Int.* 2014: 10.

29 Kashiwaya, Y., Bergman, C., Lee, J.H. et al. (2013). A ketone ester diet exhibits anxiolytic and cognition-sparing properties, and lessens amyloid and tau pathologies in a mouse model of Alzheimer's disease. *Neurobiol. Aging* 34: 1530–1539.

30 Dashti, H.M., Mathew, T.C., Khadada, M. et al. (2007). Beneficial effects of ketogenic diet in obese diabetic subjects. *Mol. Cell. Biochem.* 302: 249–256.

31 Schugar, R.C. and Crawford, P.A. (2012). Low-carbohydrate ketogenic diets, glucose homeostasis, and nonalcoholic fatty liver disease. *Curr. Opin. Clin. Nutr. Metab. Care* 15: 374–380.

32 Lapp, J.E. (1981). Effects of glycemic alterations and noun imagery on the learning of paired associates. *J. Learn. Disabil.* 14: 35–38.

33 Messier, C. and White, N.M. (1984). Contingent and non-contingent actions of sucrose and saccharin reinforcers: effects on taste preference and memory. *Physiol. Behav.* 32: 195–203.

34 Foster, J.K., Lidder, P.G., and Sunram, S.I. (1998). Glucose and memory: fractionation of enhancement effects? *Psychopharmacology (Berl)* 137: 259–270.

35 Flint, R.W. (2004). Emotional arousal, blood glucose levels, and memory modulation: three laboratory exercises in cognitive neuroscience. *J. Undergrad. Neurosci. Educ.* 3: A16–A23.

36 Mohanty, A. and Flint, R.W. Jr. (2001). Differential effects of glucose on modulation of emotional and nonemotional spatial memory tasks. *Cogn. Affect. Behav. Neurosci.* 1: 90–95.

37 Sunram-Lea, S.I., Foster, J.K., Durlach, P., and Perez, C. (2001). Glucose facilitation of cognitive performance in healthy young adults: examination of the influence of fast-duration, time of day and pre-consumption plasma glucose levels. *Psychopharmacology (Berl)* 157: 46–54.

38 Gold, P.E. (1986). Glucose modulation of memory storage processing. *Behav. Neural Biol.* 45: 342–349.

39 Messier, C. and Destrade, C. (1988). Improvement of memory for an operant response by post-training glucose in mice. *Behav. Brain Res.* 31: 185–191.

40 Hall, J.L., Gonder-Frederick, L.A., Chewning, W.W. et al. (1989). Glucose enhancement of performance of memory tests in young and aged humans. *Neuropsychologia* 27: 1129–1138.

41 Messier, C., Durkin, T., Mrabet, O., and Destrade, C. (1990). Memory-improving action of glucose: indirect evidence for a facilitation of hippocampal acetylcholine synthesis. *Behav. Brain Res.* 39: 135–143.

42 Benton, D. (1990). The impact of increasing blood glucose on psychological functioning. *Biol. Psychol.* 30: 13–19.

43 Azari, N.P. (1991). Effects of glucose on memory processes in young adults. *Psychopharmacology (Berl)* 105: 521–524.

44 Stone, W., Rudd, R., and Gold, P. (1992). Glucose attenuation of scopolamine- and age-induced deficits in spontaneous alternation behavior and regional brain [3H]2-deoxyglucose uptake in mice. *Psychobiology* 20: 270–279.

45 Benton, D. and Owens, D.S. (1993). Blood glucose and human memory. *Psychopharmacology (Berl)* 113: 83–88.
46 Benton, D., Owens, D.S., and Parker, P.Y. (1994). Blood glucose influences memory and attention in young adults. *Neuropsychologia* 32: 595–607.
47 Rodriguez, W.A., Horne, C.A., Mondragon, A.N., and Phelps, D.D. (1994). Comparable dose-response functions for the effects of glucose and fructose on memory. *Behav. Neural Biol.* 61: 162–169.
48 Winocur, G. (1995). Glucose-enhanced performance by aged rats on a test of conditional discrimination learning. *Psychobiology* 23: 270–276.
49 Kopf, S.R. and Baratti, C.M. (1996). Effects of posttraining administration of glucose on retention of a habituation response in mice: participation of a central cholinergic mechanism. *Neurobiol. Learn. Mem.* 65: 253–260.
50 Allen, J.B., Gross, A.M., Aloia, M.S., and Billingsley, C. (1996). The effects of glucose on nonmemory cognitive functioning in the elderly. *Neuropsychologia* 34: 459–465.
51 Manning, C.A., Parsons, M.W., Cotter, E.M., and Gold, P.E. (1997). Glucose effects on declarative and nondeclarative memory in healthy elderly and young adults. *Psychobiology* 25: 103–108.
52 Messier, C. (1997). Object recognition in mice: improvement of memory by glucose. *Neurobiol. Learn. Mem.* 67: 172–175.
53 Winocur, G. and Gagnon, S. (1998). Glucose treatment attenuates spatial learning and memory deficits of aged rats on tests of hippocampal function. *Neurobiol. Aging* 19: 233–241.
54 Manning, C.A., Stone, W.S., Korol, D.L., and Gold, P.E. (1998). Glucose enhancement of 24-h memory retrieval in healthy elderly humans. *Behav. Brain Res.* 93: 71–76.
55 Kaplan, R.J., Greenwood, C.E., Winocur, G., and Wolever, T.M. (2000). Cognitive performance is associated with glucose regulation in healthy elderly persons and can be enhanced with glucose and dietary carbohydrates. *Am. J. Clin. Nutr.* 72: 825–836.
56 Greenwood, C.E. and Winocur, G. (2001). Glucose treatment reduces memory deficits in young adult rats fed high-fat diets. *Neurobiol. Learn. Mem.* 75: 179–189.
57 Riby, L.M. (2004). The impact of age and task domain on cognitive performance: a meta-analytic review of the glucose facilitation effect. *Brain Impairment* 5: 145–165.
58 Salinas, J.A. and Gold, P.E. (2005). Glucose regulation of memory for reward reduction in young and aged rats. *Neurobiol. Aging* 26: 45–52.
59 Riby, L.M., McMurtrie, H., Smallwood, J. et al. (2006). The facilitative effects of glucose ingestion on memory retrieval in younger and older adults: is task difficulty or task domain critical? *Br. J. Nutr.* 95: 414–420.
60 Morris, N. (2008). Elevating blood glucose level increases the retention of information from a public safety video. *Biol. Psychol.* 78: 188–190.
61 Riby, L.M., McLaughlin, J., Riby, D.M., and Graham, C. (2008). Lifestyle, glucose regulation and the cognitive effects of glucose load in middle-aged adults. *Br. J. Nutr.* 100: 1128–1134.

62 Sunram-Lea, S.I., Owen, L., Finnegan, Y., and Hu, H. (2011). Dose-response investigation into glucose facilitation of memory performance and mood in healthy young adults. *J. Psychopharmacol.* 25: 1076–1087.

63 Scholey, A.B., Sunram-Lea, S.I., Greer, J. et al. (2009). Glucose administration prior to a divided attention task improves tracking performance but not word recognition: evidence against differential memory enhancement? *Psychopharmacology (Berl)* 202: 549–558.

64 Craft, S., Murphy, C., and Wemstrom, J. (1994). Glucose effects on complex memory and nonmemory tasks: the influence of age, sex, and glucoregulatory response. *Psychobiology* 22: 95–105.

65 Smith, M.A. and Foster, J.K. (2008). Glucoregulatory and order effects on verbal episodic memory in healthy adolescents after oral glucose administration. *Biol. Psychol.* 79: 209–215.

66 Parsons, M.W. and Gold, P.E. (1992). Glucose enhancement of memory in elderly humans: an inverted-U dose-response curve. *Neurobiol. Aging* 13: 401–404.

67 Messier, C. (1998). The absence of effect of glucose on memory is associated with low susceptibility to the amnestic effects of scopolamine in a strain of mice. *Behav. Brain Res.* 96: 47–57.

68 Manning, C.A., Ragozzino, M.E., and Gold, P.E. (1993). Glucose enhancement of memory in patients with probable senile dementia of the Alzheimer's type. *Neurobiol. Aging* 14: 523–528.

69 Craft, S., Zallen, G., and Baker, L.D. (1992). Glucose and memory in mild senile dementia of the Alzheimer type. *J. Clin. Exp. Neuropsychol.* 14: 253–267.

70 Craft, S., Dagogo-Jack, S.E., Wiethop, B.V. et al. (1993). Effects of hyperglycemia on memory and hormone levels in dementia of the Alzheimer type: a longitudinal study. *Behav. Neurosci.* 107: 926–940.

71 Stone, W.S. and Seidman, L.J. (2008). Toward a model of memory enhancement in schizophrenia: glucose administration and hippocampal function. *Schizophr. Bull.* 34: 93–108.

72 Stone, W.S., Seidman, L.J., Wojcik, J.D., and Green, A.I. (2003). Glucose effects on cognition in schizophrenia. *Schizophr. Res.* 62: 93–103.

73 Fucetola, R., Newcomer, J.W., Craft, S., and Melson, A.K. (1999). Age- and dose-dependent glucose-induced increases in memory and attention in schizophrenia. *Psychiatry Res.* 88: 1–13.

74 Pettersen, J. and Skelton, R. (2000). Glucose enhances long-term declarative memory in mildly head-injured varsity rugby players. *Psychobiology* 28: 81–89.

75 Riby, L.M., Marriott, A., Bullock, R. et al. (2009). The effects of glucose ingestion and glucose regulation on memory performance in older adults with mild cognitive impairment. *Eur. J. Clin. Nutr.* 63: 566–571.

76 Flint, R.W. Jr. and Riccio, D.C. (1999). Post-training glucose administration attenuates forgetting of passive-avoidance conditioning in 18-day-old rats. *Neurobiol. Learn. Mem.* 72: 62–67.

77 Flint, R.W. Jr. and Riccio, D.C. (1997). Pretest administration of glucose attenuates infantile amnesia for passive avoidance conditioning in rats. *Dev. Psychobiol.* 31: 207–216.

78 Manning, C.A., Parsons, M.W., and Gold, P.E. (1992). Anterograde and retrograde enhancement of 24-h memory by glucose in elderly humans. *Behav. Neural Biol.* 58: 125–130.

79 Means, L.W. and Edmonds, S.M. (1998). Glucose minimally attenuates scopolamine- but not morphine-induced deficits on a water maze alternation task. *J. Neural Transm.* 105: 1171–1185.

80 Means, L.W., Holsten, R.D., Long, M., and High, K.M. (1996). Scopolamine- and morphine-induced deficits in water maze alternation: failure to attenuate with glucose. *Neurobiol. Learn. Mem.* 66: 167–175.

81 Owen, L. and Sunram-Lea, S.I. (2011). Metabolic agents that enhance ATP can improve cognitive functioning: a review of the evidence for glucose, oxygen, pyruvate, creatine, and L-carnitine. *Nutrients* 3: 735–755.

82 Gibbs, M.E., Anderson, D.G., and Hertz, L. (2006). Inhibition of glycogenolysis in astrocytes interrupts memory consolidation in young chickens. *Glia* 54: 214–222.

83 La Rue, A., Koehler, K.M., Wayne, S.J. et al. (1997). Nutritional status and cognitive functioning in a normally aging sample: a 6-y reassessment. *Am. J. Clin. Nutr.* 65: 20–29.

84 Deschamps, V., Astier, X., Ferry, M. et al. (2002). Nutritional status of healthy elderly persons living in Dordogne, France, and relation with mortality and cognitive or functional decline. *Eur. J. Clin. Nutr.* 56: 305–312.

85 Barberger-Gateau, P., Raffaitin, C., Letenneur, L. et al. (2007). Dietary patterns and risk of dementia: the Three-City cohort study. *Neurology* 69: 1921–1930.

86 Velho, S., Marques-Vidal, P., Baptista, F., and Camilo, M.E. (2008). Dietary intake adequacy and cognitive function in free-living active elderly: a cross-sectional and short-term prospective study. *Clin. Nutr.* 27: 77–86.

87 Vercambre, M.N., Boutron-Ruault, M.C., Ritchie, K. et al. (2009). Long-term association of food and nutrient intakes with cognitive and functional decline: a 13-year follow-up study of elderly French women. *Br. J. Nutr.* 102: 419–427.

88 Aparicio Vizuete, A., Robles, F., Rodriguez-Rodriguez, E. et al. (2010). Association between food and nutrient intakes and cognitive capacity in a group of institutionalized elderly people. *Eur. J. Nutr.* 49: 293–300.

89 Guligowska, A., Piglowska, M., Fife, E. et al. (2016). Inappropriate nutrients intake is associated with lower functional status and inferior quality of life in older adults with depression. *Clin. Interv. Aging* 11: 1505–1517.

90 Mueckler, M. (1994). Facilitative glucose transporters. *Eur. J. Biochem.* 219: 713–725.

91 Joost, H.G. and Thorens, B. (2001). The extended GLUT-family of sugar/polyol transport facilitators: nomenclature, sequence characteristics, and potential function of its novel members (review). *Mol. Membr. Biol.* 18: 247–256.

92 Eustache, F., Rioux, P., Desgranges, B. et al. (1995). Healthy aging, memory subsystems and regional cerebral oxygen consumption. *Neuropsychologia* 33: 867–887.

93 Shastri, L. (2002). Episodic memory and cortico–hippocampal interactions. *Trends Cogn. Sci.* 6: 162–168.

94 Sunram-Lea, S.I., Dewhurst, S.A., and Foster, J.K. (2008). The effect of glucose administration on the recollection and familiarity components of recognition memory. *Biol. Psychol.* 77: 69–75.

95 Stone, W.S., Thermenos, H.W., Tarbox, S.I. et al. (2005). Medial temporal and prefrontal lobe activation during verbal encoding following glucose ingestion in schizophrenia: a pilot fMRI study. *Neurobiol. Learn. Mem.* 83: 54–64.

96 Smith, M.A., Riby, L.M., Sunram-Lea, S.I. et al. (2009). Glucose modulates event-related potential components of recollection and familiarity in healthy adolescents. *Psychopharmacology (Berl)* 205: 11–20.

97 Stollery, B. and Christian, L. (2016). Glucose improves object-location binding in visual-spatial working memory. *Psychopharmacology (Berl)* 233: 529–547.

98 Stollery, B. and Christian, L. (2015). Glucose, relational memory, and the hippocampus. *Psychopharmacology (Berl)* 232: 2113–2125.

99 Sunram-Lea, S.I. and Owen, L. (2017). The impact of diet-based glycaemic response and glucose regulation on cognition: evidence across the lifespan. *Proc. Nutr. Soc.* 76: 466–477.

100 Mergenthaler, P., Lindauer, U., Dienel, G.A., and Meisel, A. (2013). Sugar for the brain: the role of glucose in physiological and pathological brain function. *Trends Neurosci.* 36: 587–597.

101 Bartus, R.T., Dean, R.L. 3rd, Beer, B., and Lippa, A.S. (1982). The cholinergic hypothesis of geriatric memory dysfunction. *Science* 217: 408–414.

102 Graham, A.J., Ray, M.A., Perry, E.K. et al. (2003). Differential nicotinic acetylcholine receptor subunit expression in the human hippocampus. *J. Chem. Neuroanat.* 25: 97–113.

103 Perry, E., Walker, M., Grace, J., and Perry, R. (1999). Acetylcholine in mind: a neurotransmitter correlate of consciousness? *Trends Neurosci.* 22: 273–280.

104 Lombardo, S. and Maskos, U. (2015). Role of the nicotinic acetylcholine receptor in Alzheimer's disease pathology and treatment. *Neuropharmacology* 96: 255–262.

105 Ferreira-Vieira, T.H., Guimaraes, I.M., Silva, F.R., and Ribeiro, F.M. (2016). Alzheimer's disease: targeting the cholinergic system. *Curr. Neuropharmacol.* 14: 101–115.

106 Ragozzino, M.E., Unick, K.E., and Gold, P.E. (1996). Hippocampal acetylcholine release during memory testing in rats: augmentation by glucose. *Proc. Natl. Acad. Sci. U.S.A.* 93: 4693–4698.

107 Dienel, G.A. (2012). Fueling and imaging brain activation. *ASN Neuro* 4 (5): e00093. https://doi.org/10.1042/AN20120021.

108 Ragozzino, M.E. and Gold, P.E. (1994). Task-dependent effects of intra-amygdala morphine injections: attenuation by intra-amygdala glucose injections. *J. Neurosci.* 14: 7478–7485.

109 Ragozzino, M.E., Pal, S.N., Unick, K. et al. (1998). Modulation of hippocampal acetylcholine release and spontaneous alternation scores by intrahippocampal glucose injections. *J. Neurosci.* 18: 1595–1601.

110 Kopf, S.R., Buchholzer, M.L., Hilgert, M. et al. (2001). Glucose plus choline improve passive avoidance behaviour and increase hippocampal acetylcholine release in mice. *Neuroscience* 103: 365–371.

111 Wang, S., Hu, L.F., Yang, Y. et al. (2005). Studies of ATP-sensitive potassium channels on 6-hydroxydopamine and haloperidol rat models of Parkinson's disease: implications for treating Parkinson's disease? *Neuropharmacology* 48: 984–992.

112 Amoroso, S., Schmid-Antomarchi, H., Fosset, M., and Lazdunski, M. (1990). Glucose, sulfonylureas, and neurotransmitter release: role of ATP-sensitive K+ channels. *Science* 247: 852–854.

113 Miki, T. and Seino, S. (2005). Roles of KATP channels as metabolic sensors in acute metabolic changes. *J. Mol. Cell. Cardiol.* 38: 917–925.

114 Pocai, A., Lam, T.K., Gutierrez-Juarez, R. et al. (2005). Hypothalamic K(ATP) channels control hepatic glucose production. *Nature* 434: 1026–1031.

115 Konner, A.C., Janoschek, R., Plum, L. et al. (2007). Insulin action in AgRP-expressing neurons is required for suppression of hepatic glucose production. *Cell Metab.* 5: 438–449.

116 Turner, N., Cooney, G.J., Kraegen, E.W., and Bruce, C.R. (2014). Fatty acid metabolism, energy expenditure and insulin resistance in muscle. *J. Endocrinol.* 220: T61–T79.

117 Sun, S.Z. and Empie, M.W. (2012). Fructose metabolism in humans – what isotopic tracer studies tell us. *Nutr. Metab.* 9: 89–89.

118 Messier, C. and White, N.M. (1987). Memory improvement by glucose, fructose, and two glucose analogs: a possible effect on peripheral glucose transport. *Behav. Neural Biol.* 48: 104–127.

119 Rodriguez, W.A., Horne, C.A., and Padilla, J.L. (1999). Effects of glucose and fructose on recently reactivated and recently acquired memories. *Prog. Neuropsychopharmacol. Biol. Psychiatry* 23: 1285–1317.

120 Messier, C., Whately, K., Liang, J. et al. (2007). The effects of a high-fat, high-fructose, and combination diet on learning, weight, and glucose regulation in C57BL/6 mice. *Behav. Brain Res.* 178: 139–145.

121 Bruggeman, E.C., Li, C., Ross, A.P. et al. (2011). A high fructose diet does not affect amphetamine self-administration or spatial water maze learning and memory in female rats. *Pharmacol. Biochem. Behav.* 99: 356–364.

122 Vasudevan, H., Xiang, H., and McNeill, J.H. (2005). Differential regulation of insulin resistance and hypertension by sex hormones in fructose-fed male rats. *Am. J. Physiol. Heart Circ. Physiol.* 289: H1335–H1342.

123 Ross, A.P., Bartness, T.J., Mielke, J.G., and Parent, M.B. (2009). A high fructose diet impairs spatial memory in male rats. *Neurobiol. Learn. Mem.* 92: 410–416.

124 Stranahan, A.M., Norman, E.D., Lee, K. et al. (2008). Diet-induced insulin resistance impairs hippocampal synaptic plasticity and cognition in middle-aged rats. *Hippocampus* 18: 1085–1088.

125 Mielke, J.G., Taghibiglou, C., Liu, L. et al. (2005). A biochemical and functional characterization of diet-induced brain insulin resistance. *J. Neurochem.* 93: 1568–1578.

126 Agrawal, R. and Gomez-Pinilla, F. (2012). 'Metabolic syndrome' in the brain: deficiency in omega-3 fatty acid exacerbates dysfunctions in insulin receptor signalling and cognition. *J. Physiol.* 590: 2485–2499.

127 Siervo, M., Wells, J.C., Brayne, C., and Stephan, B.C. (2011). Reemphasizing the role of fructose intake as a risk factor for dementia. *J. Gerontol. A Biol. Sci. Med. Sci.* 66: 534–536.

128 Stephan, B.C., Wells, J.C., Brayne, C. et al. (2010). Increased fructose intake as a risk factor for dementia. *J. Gerontol. A Biol. Sci. Med. Sci.* 65: 809–814.

129 Ye, X., Gao, X., Scott, T., and Tucker, K.L. (2011). Habitual sugar intake and cognitive function among middle-aged and older Puerto Ricans without diabetes. *Br. J. Nutr.* 106: 1423–1432.

130 Wright, R.S., Gerassimakis, C., Bygrave, D., and Waldstein, S.R. (2017). Dietary factors and cognitive function in poor urban settings. *Curr. Nutr. Rep.* 6: 32–40.

131 van der Borght, K., Kohnke, R., Goransson, N. et al. (2011). Reduced neurogenesis in the rat hippocampus following high fructose consumption. *Regul. Pept.* 167: 26–30.

132 Rafati, A., Anvari, E., and Noorafshan, A. (2013). High fructose solution induces neuronal loss in the nucleus of the solitary tract of rats. *Folia Neuropathol.* 51: 214–221.

133 Rendeiro, C., Masnik, A.M., Mun, J.G. et al. (2015). Fructose decreases physical activity and increases body fat without affecting hippocampal neurogenesis and learning relative to an isocaloric glucose diet. *Sci. Rep.* 5: 9589.

134 Lowette, K., Roosen, L., Tack, J., and Vanden Berghe, P. (2015). Effects of high-fructose diets on central appetite signaling and cognitive function. *Front. Nutr.* 2: 5.

135 Sadowska, J., Gebczynski, A.K., and Konarzewski, M. (2017). Metabolic risk factors in mice divergently selected for BMR fed high fat and high carb diets. *PLoS One* 12: e0172892.

136 Goran, M.I., Dumke, K., Bouret, S.G. et al. (2013). The obesogenic effect of high fructose exposure during early development. *Nat. Rev. Endocrinol.* 9: 494–500.

137 Jurdak, N. and Kanarek, R.B. (2009). Sucrose-induced obesity impairs novel object recognition learning in young rats. *Physiol. Behav.* 96: 1–5.

138 Hsu, T.M., Konanur, V.R., Taing, L. et al. (2015). Effects of sucrose and high fructose corn syrup consumption on spatial memory function and hippocampal neuroinflammation in adolescent rats. *Hippocampus* 25: 227–239.

139 D'Hooge, R. and De Deyn, P.P. (2001). Applications of the Morris water maze in the study of learning and memory. *Brain Res. Brain Res. Rev.* 36: 60–90.

140 Jurdak, N., Lichtenstein, A.H., and Kanarek, R.B. (2008). Diet-induced obesity and spatial cognition in young male rats. *Nutr. Neurosci.* 11: 48–54.

141 Jen, K.L., Rochon, C., Zhong, S.B., and Whitcomb, L. (1991). Fructose and sucrose feeding during pregnancy and lactation in rats changes maternal and pup fuel metabolism. *J. Nutr.* 121: 1999–2005.

142 Rawana, S., Clark, K., Zhong, S. et al. (1993). Low dose fructose ingestion during gestation and lactation affects carbohydrate metabolism in rat dams and their offspring. *J. Nutr.* 123: 2158–2165.

143 Vickers, M.H., Clayton, Z.E., Yap, C., and Sloboda, D.M. (2011). Maternal fructose intake during pregnancy and lactation alters placental growth and leads to sex-specific changes in fetal and neonatal endocrine function. *Endocrinology* 152: 1378–1387.

144 Sun, B., Purcell, R.H., Terrillion, C.E. et al. (2012). Maternal high-fat diet during gestation or suckling differentially affects offspring leptin sensitivity and obesity. *Diabetes* 61: 2833–2841.

145 Gulpers, B., Ramakers, I., Hamel, R. et al. (2016). Anxiety as a predictor for cognitive decline and dementia: a systematic review and meta-analysis. *Am. J. Geriatr. Psychiatry* 24: 823–842.

146 Panza, F., D'Introno, A., Colacicco, A.M. et al. (2005). Current epidemiology of mild cognitive impairment and other predementia syndromes. *Am. J. Geriatr. Psychiatry* 13: 633–644.

147 Gillette-Guyonnet, S., Secher, M., and Vellas, B. (2013). Nutrition and neurodegeneration: epidemiological evidence and challenges for future research. *Br. J. Clin. Pharmacol.* 75: 738–755.

148 Ortega, R.M., Requejo, A.M., Andres, P. et al. (1997). Dietary intake and cognitive function in a group of elderly people. *Am. J. Clin. Nutr.* 66: 803–809.

149 Solfrizzi, V., Panza, F., Frisardi, V. et al. (2011). Diet and Alzheimer's disease risk factors or prevention: the current evidence. *Expert Rev. Neurother.* 11: 677–708.

150 Otaegui-Arrazola, A., Amiano, P., Elbusto, A. et al. (2014). Diet, cognition, and Alzheimer's disease: food for thought. *Eur. J. Nutr.* 53: 1–23.

151 Hargrave, S.L., Jones, S., and Davidson, T.L. (2016). The outward spiral: a vicious cycle model of obesity and cognitive dysfunction. *Curr. Opin. Behav. Sci.* 9: 40–46.

152 Aalbers, T., Qin, L., Baars, M.A. et al. (2016). Changing behavioral lifestyle risk factors related to cognitive decline in later life using a self-motivated eHealth intervention in Dutch adults. *J. Med. Internet Res.* 18: e171.

153 Xu, S. and Xue, Y. (2016). Protein intake and obesity in young adolescents. *Exp. Ther. Med.* 11: 1545–1549.

154 Wahl, D., Cogger, V.C., Solon-Biet, S.M. et al. (2016). Nutritional strategies to optimise cognitive function in the aging brain. *Ageing Res. Rev.* 31: 80–92.

155 Safouris, A., Tsivgoulis, G., Sergentanis, T.N., and Psaltopoulou, T. (2015). Mediterranean diet and risk of dementia. *Curr. Alzheimer Res.* 12: 736–744.

156 Pedrini, S., Thomas, C., Brautigam, H. et al. (2009). Dietary composition modulates brain mass and solubilizable Abeta levels in a mouse model of aggressive Alzheimer's amyloid pathology. *Mol. Neurodegener.* 4: 40.

157 Tieland, M., van de Rest, O., Dirks, M.L. et al. (2012). Protein supplementation improves physical performance in frail elderly people: a randomized, double-blind, placebo-controlled trial. *J. Am. Med. Dir. Assoc.* 13: 720–726.

158 Soultoukis, G.A. and Partridge, L. (2016). Dietary protein, metabolism, and aging. *Annu. Rev. Biochem.* 85: 5–34.

159 Jakobsen, L.H., Kondrup, J., Zellner, M. et al. (2011). Effect of a high protein meat diet on muscle and cognitive functions: a randomised controlled dietary intervention trial in healthy men. *Clin. Nutr.* 30: 303–311.

160 Alberts, B.J.A., Bray, D., Watson, J. et al. (2002). *Molecular Biology of the Cell*. New York: Garland Science.

161 Brehm, B.J. and D'Alessio, D.A. (2008). Benefits of high-protein weight loss diets: enough evidence for practice? *Curr. Opin. Endocrinol. Diabetes Obes.* 15: 416–421.

162 Bilsborough, S. and Mann, N. (2006). A review of issues of dietary protein intake in humans. *Int. J. Sport Nutr. Exerc. Metab.* 16: 129–152.

163 Siegel, G.J. and Agranoff, B.W. (1999). *Basic Biochemistry: Molecular, Cellular and Medical Aspects*. Philadelphia: Lippincott-Raven.

164 Rocks, T., Pelly, F., Slater, G., and Martin, L.A. (2016). The relationship between dietary intake and energy availability, eating attitudes and cognitive restraint in students enrolled in undergraduate nutrition degrees. *Appetite* 107: 406–414.

165 Baum, J.I., Kim, I.Y., and Wolfe, R.R. (2016). Protein consumption and the elderly: what is the optimal level of intake? *Nutrients* 8: 359.

166 Courtney-Martin, G., Ball, R.O., Pencharz, P.B., and Elango, R. (2016). Protein requirements during aging. *Nutrients* 8: 492.
167 Phillips, S.M., Chevalier, S., and Leidy, H.J. (2016). Protein 'requirements' beyond the RDA: implications for optimizing health. *Appl. Physiol. Nutr. Metab.* 41: 565–572.
168 Volterman, K.A. and Atkinson, S.A. (2016). Protein needs of physically active children. *Pediatr. Exerc. Sci.* 28: 187–193.
169 Goisser, S., Guyonnet, S., and Volkert, D. (2016). The role of nutrition in frailty: an overview. *J. Frailty Aging* 5: 74–77.
170 Wolfe, R.R., Rutherfurd, S.M., Kim, I.Y., and Moughan, P.J. (2016). Protein quality as determined by the digestible indispensable amino acid score: evaluation of factors underlying the calculation. *Nutr. Rev.* 74: 584–599.
171 Barichella, M., Cereda, E., Cassani, E. et al. (2016). Dietary habits and neurological features of Parkinson's disease patients: implications for practice. *Clin. Nutr.* 36: 1054–1061.
172 Kadish, I., Kumar, A., Beitnere, U. et al. (2016). Dietary composition affects the development of cognitive deficits in WT and Tg AD model mice. *Exp. Gerontol.* 86: 39–49.
173 Buccarello, L., Grignaschi, G., Di Giancamillo, A. et al. (2017). Neuroprotective effects of low fat-protein diet in the P301L mouse model of tauopathy. *Neuroscience* 354: 208–220.
174 Kang, S., Lee, Y.H., and Lee, J.E. (2017). Metabolism-centric overview of the pathogenesis of Alzheimer's disease. *Yonsei. Med. J.* 58: 479–488.
175 Hu, N., Yu, J.T., Tan, L. et al. (2013). Nutrition and the risk of Alzheimer's disease. *Biomed. Res. Int.* 2013: 524820.
176 Betz, A.L., Keep, R.F., Beer, M.E., and Ren, X.D. (1994). Blood-brain barrier permeability and brain concentration of sodium, potassium, and chloride during focal ischemia. *J. Cereb. Blood Flow Metab.* 14: 29–37.
177 Pardridge, W.M. and Oldendorf, W.H. (1977). Transport of metabolic substrates through the blood–brain barrier. *J. Neurochem.* 28: 5–12.
178 Hawkins, R.A., O'Kane, R.L., Simpson, I.A., and Vina, J.R. (2006). Structure of the blood–brain barrier and its role in the transport of amino acids. *J. Nutr.* 136: 218s–226s.
179 Fernstrom, J.D. (2013). Large neutral amino acids: dietary effects on brain neurochemistry and function. *Amino Acids* 45: 419–430.
180 Mans, A.M., Biebuyck, J.F., and Hawkins, R.A. (1983). Ammonia selectively stimulates neutral amino acid transport across blood-brain barrier. *Am. J. Physiol.* 245: C74–C77.
181 James, J.H. and Fischer, J.E. (1981). Transport of neutral amino acids at the blood–brain barrier. *Pharmacology* 22: 1–7.
182 Choi, S., Disilvio, B., Fernstrom, M.H., and Fernstrom, J.D. (2009). Meal ingestion, amino acids and brain neurotransmitters: effects of dietary protein source on serotonin and catecholamine synthesis rates. *Physiol. Behav.* 98: 156–162.
183 Fernstrom, J.D. (2005). Branched-chain amino acids and brain function. *J. Nutr.* 135: 1539S–1546S.
184 Pardridge, W.M. (1977). Kinetics of competitive inhibition of neutral amino acid transport across the blood–brain barrier. *J. Neurochem.* 28: 103–108.

185 Lefauconnier, J.M. (1989). Transport processes through the blood–brain barrier. *Reprod. Nutr. Dev.* 29: 689–702.

186 Smith, Q.R. (2000). Transport of glutamate and other amino acids at the blood–brain barrier. *J. Nutr.* 130: 1016S–1022S.

187 Campos-Bedolla, P., Walter, F.R., Veszelka, S., and Deli, M.A. (2014). Role of the blood–brain barrier in the nutrition of the central nervous system. *Arch. Med. Res.* 45: 610–638.

188 Jenkins, T.A., Nguyen, J.C., Polglaze, K.E., and Bertrand, P.P. (2016). Influence of tryptophan and serotonin on mood and cognition with a possible role of the gut–brain axis. *Nutrients* 8 (1): 56. https://doi.org/10.3390/nu8010056.

189 Hommes, F.A. and Lee, J.S. (1990). The control of 5-hydroxytryptamine and dopamine synthesis in the brain: a theoretical approach. *J. Inherit. Metab. Dis.* 13: 37–57.

190 O'Mahony, S.M., Clarke, G., Borre, Y.E. et al. (2015). Serotonin, tryptophan metabolism and the brain–gut–microbiome axis. *Behav. Brain Res.* 277: 32–48.

191 Ashcroft, G.W., Eccleston, D., and Crawford, T.B. (1965). 5-hydroxyindole metabolism in rat brain: a study of intermediate metabolism using the technique of tryptophan loading. I. Methods. *J. Neurochem.* 12: 483–492.

192 Fernstrom, M.H. and Fernstrom, J.D. (1987). Protein consumption increases tyrosine concentration and in vivo tyrosine hydroxylation rate in the light-adapted rat retina. *Brain Res.* 401: 392–396.

193 Fernstrom, M.H. and Fernstrom, J.D. (1995). Brain tryptophan concentrations and serotonin synthesis remain responsive to food consumption after the ingestion of sequential meals. *Am. J. Clin. Nutr.* 61: 312–319.

194 Tam, S.Y. and Roth, R.H. (1997). Mesoprefrontal dopaminergic neurons: can tyrosine availability influence their functions? *Biochem. Pharmacol.* 53: 441–453.

195 Mendelsohn, D., Riedel, W.J., and Sambeth, A. (2009). Effects of acute tryptophan depletion on memory, attention and executive functions: a systematic review. *Neurosci. Biobehav. Rev.* 33: 926–952.

196 Young, V.R. (1990). Amino acids and proteins in relation to the nutrition of elderly people. *Age Ageing* 19: S10–S24.

197 Lieberman, H.R., Corkin, S., Spring, B.J. et al. (1985). The effects of dietary neurotransmitter precursors on human behavior. *Am. J. Clin. Nutr.* 42: 366–370.

198 Sharp, T., Bramwell, S.R., and Grahame-Smith, D.G. (1992). Effect of acute administration of L-tryptophan on the release of 5-HT in rat hippocampus in relation to serotoninergic neuronal activity: an in vivo microdialysis study. *Life Sci.* 50: 1215–1223.

199 Luciana, M., Burgund, E.D., Berman, M., and Hanson, K.L. (2001). Effects of tryptophan loading on verbal, spatial and affective working memory functions in healthy adults. *J. Psychopharmacol.* 15: 219–230.

200 Hartmann, E.L. (1986). Effect of L-tryptophan and other amino acids on sleep. *Nutr. Rev.* 44 (Suppl): 70–73.

201 Spinweber, C.L. (1981). Daytime effects of L-tryptophan [proceedings]. *Psychopharmacol. Bull.* 17: 81–82.

202 Sharp, T., McQuade, R., Bramwell, S., and Hjorth, S. (1993). Effect of acute and repeated administration of 5-HT1A receptor agonists on 5-HT release in rat brain in vivo. *Naunyn Schmiedebergs Arch. Pharmacol.* 348: 339–346.

203 Strasser, B., Gostner, J.M., and Fuchs, D. (2016). Mood, food, and cognition: role of tryptophan and serotonin. *Curr. Opin. Clin. Nutr. Metab. Care* 19: 55–61.
204 Parker, G. and Brotchie, H. (2011). Mood effects of the amino acids tryptophan and tyrosine: 'Food for Thought' III. *Acta Psychiatr. Scand.* 124: 417–426.
205 Gibson, E.L., Vargas, K., Hogan, E. et al. (2014). Effects of acute treatment with a tryptophan-rich protein hydrolysate on plasma amino acids, mood and emotional functioning in older women. *Psychopharmacology (Berl)* 231: 4595–4610.
206 Cleare, A.J. and Bond, A.J. (1995). The effect of tryptophan depletion and enhancement on subjective and behavioural aggression in normal male subjects. *Psychopharmacology (Berl)* 118: 72–81.
207 Markus, C.R., Olivier, B., Panhuysen, G.E. et al. (2000). The bovine protein alpha-lactalbumin increases the plasma ratio of tryptophan to the other large neutral amino acids, and in vulnerable subjects raises brain serotonin activity, reduces cortisol concentration, and improves mood under stress. *Am. J. Clin. Nutr.* 71: 1536–1544.
208 Markus, C.R. (2008). Dietary amino acids and brain serotonin function: implications for stress-related affective changes. *Neuromolecular Med.* 10: 247–258.
209 Richard, D.M., Dawes, M.A., Mathias, C.W. et al. (2009). L-tryptophan: basic metabolic functions, behavioral research and therapeutic indications. *Int. J. Tryptophan Res.* 2: 45–60.
210 Scheri, G.C., Fard, S.N., Schietroma, I. et al. (2017). Modulation of tryptophan/serotonin pathway by probiotic supplementation in human immunodeficiency virus-positive patients: preliminary results of a new study approach. *Int. J. Tryptophan Res.* 10, 1178646917710668.
211 Notarangelo, F.M. and Pocivavsek, A. (2017). Elevated kynurenine pathway metabolism during neurodevelopment: implications for brain and behavior. *Neuropharmacology* 112: 275–285.
212 Jongkees, B.J., Hommel, B., Kuhn, S., and Colzato, L.S. (2015). Effect of tyrosine supplementation on clinical and healthy populations under stress or cognitive demands – a review. *J. Psychiatr. Res.* 70: 50–57.
213 Fernstrom, J.D. and Fernstrom, M.H. (2007). Tyrosine, phenylalanine, and catecholamine synthesis and function in the brain. *J. Nutr.* 137: 1539S–1547S; discussion 1548S.
214 Hase, A., Jung, S.E., and aan het Rot, M. (2015). Behavioral and cognitive effects of tyrosine intake in healthy human adults. *Pharmacol. Biochem. Behav.* 133: 1–6.
215 Fernstrom, J.D. (1977). Effects on the diet on brain neurotransmitters. *Metabolism* 26: 207–223.
216 Wurtman, R.J., Hefti, F., and Melamed, E. (1980). Precursor control of neurotransmitter synthesis. *Pharmacol. Rev.* 32: 315–335.
217 Wurtman, R.J. (1983). Food consumption, neurotransmitter synthesis, and human behaviour. *Experientia Suppl.* 44: 356–369.
218 Reinstein, D.K., Lehnert, H., Scott, N.A., and Wurtman, R.J. (1984). Tyrosine prevents behavioral and neurochemical correlates of an acute stress in rats. *Life Sci.* 34: 2225–2231.
219 Morilak, D.A., Barrera, G., Echevarria, D.J. et al. (2005). Role of brain norepinephrine in the behavioral response to stress. *Prog. Neuropsychopharmacol. Biol. Psychiatry* 29: 1214–1224.

220 Rauch, T.M. and Lieberman, H.R. (1990). Tyrosine pretreatment reverses hypothermia-induced behavioral depression. *Brain Res. Bull.* 24: 147–150.

221 Shukitt-Hale, B., Stillman, M.J., and Lieberman, H.R. (1996). Tyrosine administration prevents hypoxia-induced decrements in learning and memory. *Physiol. Behav.* 59: 867–871.

222 Shurtleff, D., Thomas, J.R., Ahlers, S.T., and Schrot, J. (1993). Tyrosine ameliorates a cold-induced delayed matching-to-sample performance decrement in rats. *Psychopharmacology (Berl)* 112: 228–232.

223 Shurtleff, D., Thomas, J.R., Schrot, J. et al. (1994). Tyrosine reverses a cold-induced working memory deficit in humans. *Pharmacol. Biochem. Behav.* 47: 935–941.

224 Fernstrom, J.D., Wurtman, R.J., Hammarstrom-Wiklund, B. et al. (1979). Diurnal variations in plasma concentrations of tryptophan, tryosine, and other neutral amino acids: effect of dietary protein intake. *Am. J. Clin. Nutr.* 32: 1912–1922.

225 Lehnert, H., Reinstein, D.K., Strowbridge, B.W., and Wurtman, R.J. (1984). Neurochemical and behavioral consequences of acute, uncontrollable stress: effects of dietary tyrosine. *Brain Res.* 303: 215–223.

226 Thomas, J.R., Lockwood, P.A., Singh, A., and Deuster, P.A. (1999). Tyrosine improves working memory in a multitasking environment. *Pharmacol. Biochem. Behav.* 64: 495–500.

227 Colzato, L.S., Jongkees, B.J., Sellaro, R., and Hommel, B. (2013). Working memory reloaded: tyrosine repletes updating in the N-back task. *Front. Behav. Neurosci.* 7: 200.

228 Jongkees, B.J., Sellaro, R., Beste, C. et al. (2017). l-Tyrosine administration modulates the effect of transcranial direct current stimulation on working memory in healthy humans. *Cortex* 90: 103–114.

229 Jongkees, B.J., Hommel, B., and Colzato, L.S. (2014). People are different: tyrosine's modulating effect on cognitive control in healthy humans may depend on individual differences related to dopamine function. *Front. Psychol.* 5: 1101.

230 Lanaro, A.E., Irizarry, S., Haddock, L., and Paniagua, M.E. (1964). Clinical evaluation of thyroid function tests with I-131. *Bol. Asoc. Med. P. R.* 56: 499–507.

231 Daly, R.M., Gianoudis, J., Prosser, M. et al. (2015). The effects of a protein enriched diet with lean red meat combined with a multi-modal exercise program on muscle and cognitive health and function in older adults: study protocol for a randomised controlled trial. *Trials* 16: 339.

232 Kepp, K.P. (2016). Alzheimer's disease due to loss of function: a new synthesis of the available data. *Prog. Neurobiol.* 143: 36–60.

233 Storey, E. and Cappai, R. (1999). The amyloid precursor protein of Alzheimer's disease and the Abeta peptide. *Neuropathol. Appl. Neurobiol.* 25: 81–97.

234 Haass, C. (1996). The molecular significance of amyloid beta-peptide for Alzheimer's disease. *Eur. Arch. Psychiatry Clin. Neurosci.* 246: 118–123.

235 Octave, J.N. (1995). The amyloid peptide and its precursor in Alzheimer's disease. *Rev. Neurosci.* 6: 287–316.

236 Frankfort, S.V., Tulner, L.R., van Campen, J.P. et al. (2008). Amyloid beta protein and tau in cerebrospinal fluid and plasma as biomarkers for dementia: a review of recent literature. *Curr. Clin. Pharmacol.* 3: 123–131.

237 Valera, E., Monzio Compagnoni, G., and Masliah, E. (2016). Review: novel treatment strategies targeting alpha-synuclein in multiple system atrophy as a model of synucleinopathy. *Neuropathol. Appl. Neurobiol.* 42: 95–106.

238 Brudek, T., Winge, K., Rasmussen, N.B. et al. (2016). Altered alpha-synuclein, parkin, and synphilin isoform levels in multiple system atrophy brains. *J. Neurochem.* 136: 172–185.

239 Szargel, R., Rott, R., and Engelender, S. (2008). Synphilin-1 isoforms in Parkinson's disease: regulation by phosphorylation and ubiquitylation. *Cell. Mol. Life Sci.* 65: 80–88.

240 Eyal, A. and Engelender, S. (2006). Synphilin isoforms and the search for a cellular model of lewy body formation in Parkinson's disease. *Cell Cycle* 5: 2082–2086.

241 Landles, C. and Bates, G.P. (2004). Huntingtin and the molecular pathogenesis of Huntington's disease: fourth in molecular medicine review series. *EMBO Rep.* 5: 958–963.

242 Truant, R., Atwal, R.S., and Burtnik, A. (2007). Nucleocytoplasmic trafficking and transcription effects of huntingtin in Huntington's disease. *Prog. Neurobiol.* 83: 211–227.

243 Ogawa, M. and Furukawa, Y. (2014). A seeded propagation of Cu, Zn-superoxide dismutase aggregates in amyotrophic lateral sclerosis. *Front. Cell. Neurosci.* 8: 83.

244 Tapia, R. (2014). Cellular and molecular mechanisms of motor neuron death in amyotrophic lateral sclerosis: a perspective. *Front. Cell. Neurosci.* 8: 241.

245 Erana, H., Venegas, V., Moreno, J., and Castilla, J. (2016). Prion-like disorders and transmissible spongiform encephalopathies: an overview of the mechanistic features that are shared by the various disease-related misfolded proteins. *Biochem. Biophys. Res. Commun.* 483: 1125–1136.

246 Verma, A. (2016). Prions, prion-like prionoids, and neurodegenerative disorders. *Ann. Indian Acad. Neurol.* 19: 169–174.

247 Cushman, M., Johnson, B.S., King, O.D. et al. (2010). Prion-like disorders: blurring the divide between transmissibility and infectivity. *J. Cell Sci.* 123: 1191–1201.

248 Rubinsztein, D.C. (2006). The roles of intracellular protein-degradation pathways in neurodegeneration. *Nature* 443: 780–786.

249 Zuroff, L., Daley, D., Black, K.L., and Koronyo-Hamaoui, M. (2017). Clearance of cerebral Abeta in Alzheimer's disease: reassessing the role of microglia and monocytes. *Cell. Mol. Life Sci.* 74: 2167–2201.

250 Ries, M. and Sastre, M. (2016). Mechanisms of Abeta clearance and degradation by glial cells. *Front. Aging Neurosci.* 8: 160.

251 Tarasoff-Conway, J.M., Carare, R.O., Osorio, R.S. et al. (2015). Clearance systems in the brain-implications for Alzheimer disease. *Nat. Rev. Neurol.* 11: 457–470.

252 Hol, E.M., Fischer, D.F., Ovaa, H., and Scheper, W. (2006). Ubiquitin proteasome system as a pharmacological target in neurodegeneration. *Expert Rev. Neurother.* 6: 1337–1347.

253 Todi, S.V. and Paulson, H.L. (2011). Balancing act: deubiquitinating enzymes in the nervous system. *Trends Neurosci.* 34: 370–382.

254 Zheng, Q., Huang, T., Zhang, L. et al. (2016). Dysregulation of ubiquitin-proteasome system in neurodegenerative diseases. *Front. Aging Neurosci.* 8: 303.

255 Dohm, C.P., Kermer, P., and Bahr, M. (2008). Aggregopathy in neurodegenerative diseases: mechanisms and therapeutic implication. *Neurodegener. Dis.* 5: 321–338.

256 Vila, M. and Przedborski, S. (2003). Targeting programmed cell death in neurodegenerative diseases. *Nat. Rev. Neurosci.* 4: 365–375.

257 Offen, D., Elkon, H., and Melamed, E. (2000). Apoptosis as a general cell death pathway in neurodegenerative diseases. *J. Neural Transm. Suppl.* 58: 153–166.

258 Gao, X. and Hu, H. (2008). Quality control of the proteins associated with neurodegenerative diseases. *Acta Biochim. Biophys. Sin. (Shanghai)* 40: 612–618.

259 Mosher, K.I. and Wyss-Coray, T. (2014). Microglial dysfunction in brain aging and Alzheimer's disease. *Biochem. Pharmacol.* 88: 594–604.

260 Bredesen, D.E., Rao, R.V., and Mehlen, P. (2006). Cell death in the nervous system. *Nature* 443: 796–802.

261 Troy, C.M., Akpan, N., and Jean, Y.Y. (2011). Regulation of caspases in the nervous system implications for functions in health and disease. *Prog. Mol. Biol. Transl. Sci.* 99: 265–305.

262 Ribe, E.M., Serrano-Saiz, E., Akpan, N., and Troy, C.M. (2008). Mechanisms of neuronal death in disease: defining the models and the players. *Biochem. J.* 415: 165–182.

263 Graeber, M.B. and Moran, L.B. (2002). Mechanisms of cell death in neurodegenerative diseases: fashion, fiction, and facts. *Brain Pathol.* 12: 385–390.

264 Vistoli, G., De Maddis, D., Cipak, A. et al. (2013). Advanced glycoxidation and lipoxidation end products (AGEs and ALEs): an overview of their mechanisms of formation. *Free Radic. Res.* 47 (Suppl 1): 3–27.

265 Srikanth, V., Maczurek, A., Phan, T. et al. (2011). Advanced glycation endproducts and their receptor RAGE in Alzheimer's disease. *Neurobiol. Aging* 32: 763–777.

266 Chen, X., Walker, D.G., Schmidt, A.M. et al. (2007). RAGE: a potential target for Abeta-mediated cellular perturbation in Alzheimer's disease. *Curr. Mol. Med.* 7: 735–742.

267 Clynes, R., Moser, B., Yan, S.F. et al. (2007). Receptor for AGE (RAGE): weaving tangled webs within the inflammatory response. *Curr. Mol. Med.* 7: 743–751.

268 Yamagishi, S. and Matsui, T. (2016). Pathologic role of dietary advanced glycation end products in cardiometabolic disorders, and therapeutic intervention. *Nutrition* 32: 157–165.

269 Deane, R., Du Yan, S., Submamaryan, R.K. et al. (2003). RAGE mediates amyloid-beta peptide transport across the blood-brain barrier and accumulation in brain. *Nat. Med.* 9: 907–913.

270 Do, T.M., Dodacki, A., Alata, W. et al. (2016). Age-dependent regulation of the blood–brain barrier influx/efflux equilibrium of amyloid-beta peptide in a mouse model of Alzheimer's disease (3xTg-AD). *J. Alzheimers Dis.* 49: 287–300.

271 Loske, C., Gerdemann, A., Schepl, W. et al. (2000). Transition metal-mediated glycoxidation accelerates cross-linking of beta-amyloid peptide. *Eur. J. Biochem.* 267: 4171–4178.

272 Luth, H.J., Ogunlade, V., Kuhla, B. et al. (2005). Age- and stage-dependent accumulation of advanced glycation end products in intracellular deposits in normal and Alzheimer's disease brains. *Cereb. Cortex* 15: 211–220.

273 Abate, G., Marziano, M., Rungratanawanich, W. et al. (2017). Nutrition and AGE-ing: focusing on Alzheimer's disease. *Oxid. Med. Cell. Longev.* 2017: 7039816.

274 Shi, Z.M., Han, Y.W., Han, X.H. et al. (2016). Upstream regulators and downstream effectors of NF-kappaB in Alzheimer's disease. *J. Neurol. Sci.* 366: 127–134.
275 Ortwerth, B.J., James, H., Simpson, G., and Linetsky, M. (1998). The generation of superoxide anions in glycation reactions with sugars, osones, and 3-deoxyosones. *Biochem. Biophys. Res. Commun.* 245: 161–165.
276 Schubert, M., Gautam, D., Surjo, D. et al. (2004). Role for neuronal insulin resistance in neurodegenerative diseases. *Proc. Natl. Acad. Sci. U.S.A.* 101: 3100–3105.
277 Deane, R.J. (2012). Is RAGE still a therapeutic target for Alzheimer's disease? *Future Med. Chem.* 4: 915–925.
278 Byun, K., Yoo, Y., Son, M. et al. (2017). Advanced glycation end-products produced systemically and by macrophages: a common contributor to inflammation and degenerative diseases. *Pharmacol. Ther.* 177: 44–55.

7

Fat and Lipid Metabolism and the Involvement of Apolipoprotein E in Alzheimer's Disease

Eugene Hone[1,2], Florence Lim[1,2] and Ian J. Martins[1,2]

[1] Centre of Excellence for Alzheimer's Disease Research and Care, School of Medical and Health Sciences, Edith Cowan University, Joondalup, WA, Australia
[2] Cooperative Research Centre for Mental Health, Carlton, VIC, Australia

7.1 Introduction

Dysregulated lipid and cholesterol homeostasis in the body, and particularly in the brain, has been demonstrated in neurodegenerative diseases such as Alzheimer's disease (AD), as well as Parkinson's disease (PD) and Huntington's disease (HD). These changes in lipid metabolism may be a consequence of the disease process, or part of the pathogenic mechanism, or both. More importantly perhaps, with respect to AD, is the mounting evidence that dyslipidaemia helps to drive production or reduce clearance of Aβ, the amyloidogenic peptide believed to be central in AD pathogenesis. Furthermore, other dyslipidaemia-related conditions have also been linked to AD pathogenesis, including obesity, hypertension, inflammation, insulin resistance, and type 2 diabetes. Apart from advancing age, the carriage of one or two copies of the *APOE ε4* alleles is one of the biggest risk factors for developing late-onset (sporadic) AD. The product of this gene is apoE, a protein involved in the transport of lipids. Possession of *APOE ε4* alleles also predisposes individuals to a higher risk of cardiovascular disease. Here we discuss lipid and cholesterol metabolism, and we give an overview of the various lipid and cholesterol metabolic pathways and changes that have been linked to AD, particularly the influence of the different forms of apoE on lipid, cholesterol, and Aβ metabolism.

7.2 Alzheimer's Disease

AD is the most common type of dementia, characterised by the progressive loss of memory and other cognitive functions of the brain. An affected individual gradually becomes totally dependent upon others, culminating in their death approximately 3–10 years after diagnosis. The neurodegenerative changes that are characteristic of an AD brain include widespread synaptic and neuronal loss, the accumulation of extracellular Aβ fibrils and plaques, intracellular neurofibrillary tangles (NFT) composed of hyper-phosphorylated tau filaments, microglial infiltration, and brain atrophy,

---

Neurodegeneration and Alzheimer's Disease: The Role of Diabetes, Genetics, Hormones, and Lifestyle,
First Edition. Edited by Ralph N. Martins, Charles S. Brennan, W.M.A.D. Binosha Fernando,
Margaret A. Brennan and Stephanie J. Fuller.
© 2019 John Wiley & Sons Ltd. Published 2019 by John Wiley & Sons Ltd.

particularly in the regions important for memory, such as the hippocampus, amygdala, and frontal cortex [1]. Genetic mutations in genes whose proteins are involved in the processing of the amyloid precursor protein (APP) to Aβ peptides, such as presenilin-1 (PS1) and presenilin-2 (PS2), as well as AD-related APP mutations, are predisposing risk factors for AD. However, these mutations are involved only in early-onset familial Alzheimer's disease (EOAD) which occurs before age 65, but sometimes as young as 30. These cases are relatively rare and account for less than 5% of all AD cases.

The main risk factor linked to the much more common late-onset form of Alzheimer's disease (LOAD) is *APOE ε4* allele status [2–7]. Other significant risk factors include dyslipidemia, hypertension, obesity, chronic inflammation, insulin resistance, and type 2 diabetes. All of these are also risk factors for cardiovascular disease. When these conditions occur together, this is termed 'metabolic syndrome' [8, 9]. It is believed that metabolic changes caused by these conditions lead to a greater production or reduced clearance (or both) of Aβ peptides. Many of these risk factors can be prevented by altering diet and physical exercise, which are known to reduce the risk of cardiovascular disease. There is a growing body of evidence that reducing these same risk factors would considerably slow or possibly prevent AD pathogenesis [10, 11].

7.3 Cholesterol and Lipid Metabolism

There is increasing evidence that alterations in the metabolism of lipids, particularly cholesterol, are involved in the pathogenesis of many neurodegenerative disorders including AD. This section describes cholesterol synthesis and metabolism. It is followed by some basic information concerning lipid transport and metabolism, to help explain the normal roles of these lipids in the body and the brain. Some changes in lipid metabolism which have been detected in AD are also mentioned.

7.3.1 Cholesterol Synthesis and Metabolism

Cholesterol plays a fundamental role in the structure and function of cell membranes. It influences the rigidity of lipid bilayers, which then affects transport and processing through the membrane. Cholesterol in the brain accounts for 25% of the total body cholesterol [12–14]. Within the brain, about 70% of its cholesterol is present in the myelin, 20% is present in the glial cells, while the remaining 10% is present in the neurons [15]. The cholesterol requirements in the body are met by dietary intake of animal fats, or by synthesis. Cholesterol synthesis is initiated when acetyl-CoA is converted into 3-hydroxy-3-methylglutaryl-CoA (HMG-CoA). Cholesterol is formed when its precursor lanosterol is channelled into either the Bloch pathway [16] or Kandutsch-Russel pathway [17] to generate desmosterol or lathosterol respectively, these are then converted to cholesterol.

Cholesterol is used extensively in the body, particularly in cell membrane structure. Other important physiological functions include the production of bile by the liver and hormone synthesis. Brain cholesterol metabolism is different and independent from that of peripheral tissues, due to the blood–brain barrier (BBB) preventing rapid transport into and out of the brain. Here in the CNS, cholesterol is primarily supplied by local synthesis. In the adult brain, cholesterol is mostly found in non-esterified form, with the rest being in the form of desmosterol and cholesteryl esters. The majority of cholesterol in the adult brain (about 70–80%) is contained in the myelin sheaths formed by oligodendrocytes to insulate axons. The rest is located in the plasma membranes of astrocytes and neurons, where it maintains cellular morphology, plays important roles in lipid rafts, and helps synaptic transmission [18, 19]. After adolescence, a period when higher cholesterol synthesis rates occur for myelin sheath formation in the growing brain, cholesterol turnover is very slow, with the half-life being somewhere between six months and five years. This contrasts greatly with the turnover that occurs in the general circulation, which is in the order of days [18, 19].

Cells can process excess cholesterol either by intracellular storage following esterification, or it can be excreted via ATP-binding cassette transporters such as ABCA1, ABCG1, and ABCG4 [20–23], which are expressed on many cells including neurons and glia in the brain. Subsequent cholesterol removal from the CNS into the periphery is another complex process. Because the CNS is protected from peripheral substances by the BBB, cholesterol must be in a form which can traverse this tightly regulated checkpoint. In this case it is converted into an oxysterol known as 24S-hydroxycholesterol by the enzyme 24S-hydroxylase [24, 25].

7.3.2 Oxysterols

The conversion of cholesterol to oxysterols is a major pathway for excretion of cholesterol from the brain, as oxysterols can pass through the BBB [12, 26] and into the circulation. Oxysterols can be divided into two categories, sterol-ring oxidised cholesterol metabolites and side-chain oxidised cholesterol metabolites [27]. The side-chain oxidised cholesterol metabolites are commonly produced in the body and synthesised either enzymatically, or non-enzymatically by reactive oxygen species. Oxysterols such as 24S-hydroxycholesterol (24-OH-Chol) are produced mainly by the brain-specific enzyme 24S-hydroxylase (encoded by CYP46A1, a member of the cytochrome P450 family). Interestingly, expression of this enzyme is mostly restricted to the pyramidal cells of the cortex and Purkinje cells of the cerebellum, whilst almost none is produced in glial cells [19]. In addition to being permitted passage out of the brain and into the circulation, 24-OH-Chol also activates nuclear transcription factors such as liver X receptors, which increase the expression of cholesterol transport proteins including ABCA1 and apoE in astrocytes. Both of these mechanisms increase cholesterol efflux out of the brain [19, 28–30]. Another oxysterol found in the brain is 27-hydroxycholesterol (27-OH-Chol), produced by sterol 27-hydroxylase in the periphery, mainly by the liver. This can then be transformed into 7α-hydroxy-3-oxo-4-cholestenoic acid (7-OH-4-Chol) by the enzyme 25-hydroxycholesterol 7-alpha-hydroxylase. This metabolite is usually further degraded by the liver. The peripherally produced 27-OH-Chol can cross the BBB directly via diffusion and enter the brain, whereas 24-OH-Chol diffuses from the brain, across the BBB, into the circulation [31].

7.3.2.1 Oxysterols in AD

Multiple studies have shown that oxysterol levels are altered in AD [32–35]. A longitudinal study even found that raised plasma 24-OH-Chol increases the likelihood of developing cognitive impairment within eight years [36]. An extensive review of similar studies [37] has shown that plasma levels of 24-OH-Chol may be used to differentiate AD patients from other neurodegenerative diseases. The review also suggested that plasma levels correlate with the stage of disease, with elevated levels being seen in early neurodegenerative stages when myelin loss is likely to occur. At the later disease stages, low levels of 24-OH-Chol were generally found. They surmised that this is possibly due to neuronal loss which results in less 24-OH-Chol production.

Influx of the oxysterol 27-OH-Chol into the brain has been implicated in AD [38, 39] and PD [40]. Levels of 27-OH-Chol are significantly increased in post-mortem AD brains, where a greater influx of 27-OH-Chol than efflux of 24-OH-Chol was found [39]. This is due to a greater or an altered permeability of the BBB, with this impairment thought to be caused by hypercholesterolaemia, inflammatory responses, and oxidative stress [12]. Interestingly, in HD individuals, Leoni and colleagues have noted lower plasma levels of cholesterol precursors (lanosterol and lathosterols) and its metabolites (24-OH-Chol and 27-OH-Chol) [41], an indication that whole-body cholesterol homeostasis is impaired.

Non-enzymatic oxidation of the sterol rings mainly occurs at position 7 [27] and examples of these oxysterols include 7β-hydroxycholesterol and 7-ketocholesterol. Other oxysterols include 4β-hydroxycholesterol (4β-OH), 5α,6α-epoxycholesterol (α-epoxy), and 5β,6β-epoxycholesterol (β-epoxy), and all of these oxysterols have been detected in AD brains [42]. In relation to AD, oxysterol formation can be catalysed by Aβ [43], with 7β-hydroxycholesterol production increased by interaction with APP and Aβ [43]. Importantly, several oxysterols including 24-OH-Chol and 27-OH-Chol have been reported to modulate protein aggregation and to accelerate Aβ misfolding [27, 44], thus being involved in the amyloid cascade. Increases in brain levels of the oxysterols have also been linked with neuroinflammation markers [31], and higher brain levels of 27-OH-Chol in particular, are thought to help drive AD pathogenesis [45].

In the periphery, secreted cholesterol attaches to lipid-free apoA-1 or apoE for the generation of high density lipoprotein (HDL)-like particles, whereas in the brain this is mostly through apoE [46, 47]. These lipoprotein particles can be removed from the brain via the low-density lipoprotein receptor-related protein-1 (LRP-1) (discussed in greater detail below), and also scavenger receptor class B1 (SRB1), as these receptors are expressed on the brain capillary endothelial cells. The cholesterol may also be transported from glial cells to neurons, as neurons have a greater need for cholesterol in membrane growth and repair [19].

7.3.3 Pathways of Dietary (Exogenous) Lipid Homeostasis

Lipoproteins are particles which carry cholesterol and lipid around the body via the bloodstream. They consist of an outer shell of polar phospholipid surrounding a core of comparatively non-polar cholesteryl esters and triacylglycerols. They are primarily classified by their density, which somewhat reflects their contents (Table 7.1).

Typically, dietary lipids and cholesterol are transported on the least dense of the lipoproteins, known as chylomicrons, which are formed predominantly in the small intestine (Figure 7.1). Each chylomicron is assembled around a molecule of apolipoprotein B48 (apoB48) [48] whilst it is still being translated within the lumen of the endoplasmic reticulum (ER). Chylomicron assembly is mediated by microsomal triacylglycerol transfer protein (MTP). MTP directly interacts with apoB48 [49] and

Table 7.1 Composition of the major lipoprotein classes.

	Chylomicron	Remnant	VLDL	LDL	IDL	HDL
Density (g/ml)	<0.94	<1.006	0.94–1.006	1.006–1.063	1.006–1.019	1.063–1.210
Diameter (nm)	600–200	30–50	60	25	30	7–12
Total lipid (%w/w)	98–99	96–99	90–92	75–80	74–77	40–48
Triacylglycerol	81–89	79	50–58	7–11	27–25	6–7
Cholesteryl ester	2–4	12–13	15–23	47–51	28–31	24–45
Cholesterol	1–3	3–4	4–9	10–12	6–7	6–8
Phospholipid	7–9	2–4	19–21	28–30	13–14	42–51

A summary of the major lipoprotein classes in the body. Their lipid compositions are expressed as a percentage of total weight. Chylomicrons and remnants are derived from dietary lipid, whilst VLDL, LDL, IDL, and HDL are mostly from endogenous sources as part of normal lipid homeostasis.
Source: Adapted from Redgrave, Skipski et al., and Sutherland et al. [14, 53, 54].

is thought to transfer lipid from the endoplasmic reticular membrane to nascent apoB48 [50, 51], where there is further binding of lipid. By the time the particle leaves the intestine for the lymphatic circulation, the nascent chylomicron is typically a complex of >200 000 molecules of triacylglycerol, ~35 000 of phospholipid, ~11 000 of cholesterol ester, ~8000 of free cholesterol, ~60 copies of apolipoprotein A-I, ~15 copies of apolipoprotein A-IV, and ~16 copies of apolipoprotein A-II [52].

Nascent chylomicrons acquire apoC-II from circulating plasma high density lipoprotein (HDL), completing their conversion into mature chylomicron particles [55, 56]. Chylomicrons also acquire apoE which is necessary for the clearance of most lipoproteins from the circulation by the liver. Multiple copies of each apolipoprotein are usually acquired, and this typically amounts to approximately 25 copies of apoE and 180 copies of apoC [57]. Mature chylomicrons then enter the bloodstream and undergo hydrolysis by the enzyme lipoprotein lipase (LPL), to release triglyceride and fatty acids for use as a source of energy by cells [55]. LPL is anchored to the capillary endothelial cell membranes by highly charged heparin sulphate proteoglycan (HSPG) chains [58] where the reaction is controlled by apoC-II and apoC-III [59, 60]. The chylomicron eventually becomes depleted of triglyceride from repeated interactions with LPL (Figure 7.1). The triglyceride-depleted chylomicron then transfers apoC and apoA-I back to the HDL, though the mechanism of this apolipoprotein transfer is not fully understood [52]. This process transforms the particle into a chylomicron remnant which is usually rapidly processed in the liver by receptor-mediated endocytosis [61].

7.3.4 Pathways of Endogenous Lipid Homeostasis

Triacylglycerols and cholesterol (which is synthesised endogenously or needs to be mobilised from the liver) are packaged into very low density lipoprotein (VLDL) particles (Figure 7.1). These are assembled in the ER, and thought to mature in the Golgi complex of the hepatocytes prior to secretion [62]. Up to 30% of their lipids can be of dietary origin [63–66] and they are formed around a molecule of apolipoprotein B100 (apoB100) The initial synthesis of apoB100 begins in the rough ER [67]. At the junction between smooth and rough ER, the growing VLDL acquire the apoB100

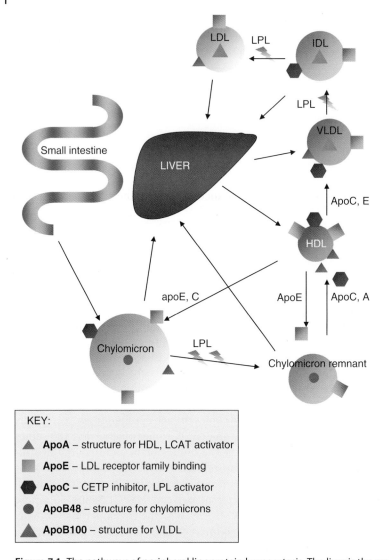

Figure 7.1 The pathways of peripheral lipoprotein homeostasis. The liver is the main site of clearance for the majority of lipoprotein traffic, however triglycerides and fatty acids are released from the lipoproteins by interaction with cell surface-bound LPL (lipoprotein lipase) as they circulate throughout the body. The exact mechanism controlling the transfer of apolipoproteins is yet to be fully understood. (*See color plate section for the color representation of this figure.*)

[68], then are moved to a pre-Golgi compartment that is similar to smooth ER, and finally to the Golgi for secretion [69]. The VLDL may acquire apoE, apoCI, apoCII, and apoCIII, from either the hepatocytes or from circulating HDL once they enter the bloodstream [70], presumably via similar pathways by which chylomicrons acquire their apolipoproteins [55, 56, 71].

Similar to chylomicrons, VLDL particles are hydrolysed by LPL which releases free fatty acids for cellular metabolism [55]. However due to their initial compositions, the triglyceride-depleted particles still contain significant amounts of cholesterol and so fall into a higher-density range (1.006–1.02 g ml^{-1}) and are therefore classed as intermediate density lipoprotein (IDL) [72]. These are usually removed from the circulation by the liver, but if they are not cleared, further interactions of the IDL with LPL take place to almost completely deplete the lipoproteins of triglyceride. The resultant particle is enriched in cholesterol (Figure 7.1) and is classified as LDL (low-density lipoprotein) [73], which circulates in the blood until finally being removed and processed by the liver.

7.3.5 Peripheral Clearance of Lipoproteins and Reverse Cholesterol Transport

The liver is responsible for the peripheral clearance of most of the chylomicron remnants and indeed the majority of all lipoproteins from the peripheral circulation [74, 75]. HDL particles in particular are the main lipoproteins involved in removing cholesterol. These act as cholesterol scavengers, facilitating transport to the liver for conversion to bile acids and secretion (or recycling). Cholesterol can be removed from cells by efflux, through the ABCA1 transporter proteins that facilitate its release to apoA-I (and apoE) containing HDL, which are the extracellular acceptors. The cholesterol-laden HDL then circulate to the liver for processing. This role of HDL is known as reverse cholesterol transport [76]. The apoE contained on some lipoproteins, including VLDL, remnant lipoproteins, and a subset of HDL, interacts with receptors such as the LDL receptor and LRP-1, as well as with HSPG, promoting the endocytic clearance of the lipoproteins in the liver [77, 78].

ApoE binds to LDL receptors which have clustered in pits (Figure 7.2) on the cell surface [79]. These clathrin-coated pits pinch off from the cell membrane to form coated vesicles which envelop their extracellular contents inside the cell [80–82], the clathrin-coated pits also serve as gathering places for receptors destined for endocytosis [79, 83]. Apart from its role in lipid homeostasis, this pathway is also a commonly used internalisation process for several extracellular molecules utilising their respective receptors, such as insulin [84], epidermal growth factor [85], and several others [86].

Current observations indicate that whilst HDL is an acceptor of cellular cholesterol and lipid [87–90], its presence can actually stimulate the release of previously internalised apoE and cholesterol [91–94]. These molecules appear to be sourced specifically from the early endosomes, as indicated by the co-localisation of apoE and cholesterol with early endosome antigen 1 containing vesicles [94], rather than from the plasma membrane pools [89], indicating that this transfer out of the cell is specifically targeted and likely to be a receptor-mediated process. There is compelling evidence the ATP-binding cassette transporter (ABCA1) is involved, which relies on extracellular lipid-free, apoA-I [95]. In the lipid-free state, apoA-I can acquire cholesterol and phospholipid from cells, resulting in the formation of nascent HDL-like particles [96, 97]. Only a small fraction of apoA-I is found in lipid-free form, implying that the lipid-binding process is very rapid [98]. Upon acquiring lecithin : cholesterol acyltransferase (LCAT) and apoE, these particles are released into the bloodstream (Figure 7.2) where they collect cholesterol from cells around the body through esterification into cholesteryl ester, which is then packaged into the core of the particle. These cholesteryl ester-rich HDL are then rapidly removed from circulation by the liver through receptor-mediated endocytosis.

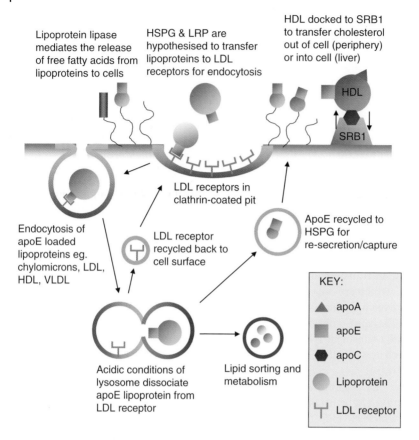

Figure 7.2 Conceptual diagram of lipoprotein clearance by cells. The LDL receptor is usually recycled back to the surface, whilst apoE is either metabolised or recycled via HSPG for a lipoprotein secretion/capture role. Note that since apoE ε4 binds with high affinity to the LDL receptor, this may not permit dissociation from the receptor which traps the complex within the cell leading to raised cellular cholesterol. (*See color plate section for the color representation of this figure.*)

Alternatively, the scavenger receptor class B type1 (SRB1) binds HDL (Figure 7.2) with high affinity [99] and early studies suggested it promoted cellular efflux of cholesterol to HDL [100]. However, more recent evidence indicates that the major function of SRB1 is likely to be a receptor whose purpose is to enable cholesteryl ester-laden HDL to offload their cargo to hepatocytes for processing [101]. This multifunctional receptor is also important in the uptake of lipid-soluble vitamins, and is involved in pathogen recognition. Expression of SRB1 can be modulated by lipopolysaccharides and oxidative stress [102].

An important feature of the LDL receptors is the ability to be recycled [103] which allows for a constant and rapid clearance of lipoprotein from the extracellular space (Figure 7.2). This is made possible by the dissociation of the receptors from their ligands by acidic conditions in the endosomes [104]. After dissociation, the receptors are sent back to the surface where the whole cycle repeats [103]. With the receptor dissociated and recycled, the lipoprotein-apoE complex is then routed to the lysosomal compartments where hydrolysis occurs [105]. Not all of the apoE is immediately degraded in the lysosomal compartment (Figure 7.2). ApoE is somewhat resistant to digestion and accumulates in various intracellular compartments [106, 107], whilst the lipoprotein itself is delivered to the lysosomal compartments [108]. The portion of apoE which does escape degradation has been found to be re-secreted [91, 92, 109, 110] and recent findings suggest that this occurs in all cells in the body [111].

7.3.5.1 Lipoproteins in the CNS

The lipid environment of the CNS is different to the periphery, for example the cholesterol turnover is so much slower (as mentioned earlier), and there is limited circulating triglyceride. In human cerebrospinal fluid (CSF), most of the apolipoprotein content, apoE, apoA-I, and A-II, is present on astrocyte-secreted lipoproteins [112, 113]. The largest particles carry almost exclusively apoE, in contrast to the smaller particles which carry mostly apoA-I and apoA-II [114]. CSF lipoproteins are similar to plasma HDL in composition and relative density, and like nascent HDL in the periphery, nascent astrocyte-derived HDL is largely devoid of core cholesteryl esters and carry apoE and clusterin (apolipoprotein J) [115]. Despite many differences, the metabolism of lipoproteins in the brain has many similarities to that in the periphery. This, as well as other aspects of apoE metabolism, are discussed further in the next section.

7.4 Apolipoprotein E Alleles and Isoforms

As mentioned previously, the apoE protein plays a central role in lipid transport while possession of the *APOE ε4* allele influences AD risk. Additionally, many aspects of Aβ metabolism appear to be influenced by apoE. Therefore, we will now discuss apoE and the variety of ways in which it has been implicated in AD pathogenesis.

The human *APOE* gene is located on chromosome 19, and its three most common alleles are designated ε2, ε3, and ε4. Of these, ε3 is the most common allele in humans (78%) followed by ε4 (14%), then ε2 (8%) [5]. Whilst these figures are derived from a sample of the Australian population, most studies around the world agree that the order of *APOE* allele frequency is ε3 > ε4 > ε2 [5, 116–119].

Differences in apoE protein isoforms, which are the result of the amino acid substitutions at residues 112 and 158, lead to differences in their function or metabolism, including lipoprotein clearance. In the periphery, the amino acid changes cause the apoE molecule to have different affinities for the LDL receptor, where the apoE ε2 isoform exhibits markedly decreased binding compared with apoE ε3, which in turn is less than apoE ε4 [120–122]. This reduced binding results in delayed receptor-mediated clearance of plasma lipoprotein that in rare circumstances can sometimes be exacerbated by dietary or genetic influences, or a combination of both, and can eventually lead to the development of type III hyperlipidemia [120, 123].

However it is usually apoE ε4 which is associated with increased levels of circulating LDL cholesterol, higher triglyceride levels, and a greater risk of coronary artery disease [124–126]. This is despite apoE ε4 having higher affinity for the LDL receptors than apoE ε3 and ε2, and increased levels of lipoprotein internalisation [127–129]. The increased affinity of apoE ε4 for the LDL receptor in the periphery may be a limiting factor for cellular processing of lipoproteins, for it has been observed that apoE ε4 is poorly recycled by cells, yet is readily internalised which results in raised intracellular cholesterol levels [129]. This observation led to the proposal that this increased rate of internalisation may saturate the lipoprotein-processing machinery, leading to the accumulation of intracellular cholesterol. It has been suggested that the binding to this receptor may be too effective, such that apoE ε4 is trapped in the cell (Figure 7.2), leading to poor mobilisation of cholesterol and apoE ε4 [130]. However, this does not seem to be the case in the brain. In *APOE* knock-in animals, it was found that brain levels of apoE ε4 were lower relative to apoE ε3 and apoE ε2 [131], and this was shown to be due to the preferential degradation of apoE ε4 by astrocytes. Such differences in the apoE isoforms are discussed further below.

7.4.1 ApoE in the Brain

The presence of both apoE-containing lipoproteins in the CSF [112, 132] and members of the LDL receptor family on several types of cells in the CNS [113, 133] indicates that apoE performs a similar function in the brain to that in the periphery, the mediation of uptake and redistribution of cholesterol [74, 113, 134]. Indeed it has been demonstrated that lipoprotein homeostasis via apoE and its receptors is essential for healthy neurite outgrowth, plasticity [133, 135–139] and repair [140, 141]. The absence of apoE or LDL receptors has been shown in transgenic mice to severely impact synaptic density and cause severe deficits in working and associative memory [142, 143].

Whilst apoE is clearly a molecule of great importance in the CNS, it is not imported from the periphery [144], where the liver produces it in the largest amounts. Rather it is synthesised locally by astrocytes in significant quantities [132, 145]. Here in the CNS, as in the periphery, apoE binds to the LDL receptor family as a ligand, including LDL receptor and LDL receptor-like proteins (LRP-1, LRP-2/megalin, and others). LRP-1 is primarily expressed in neurons, whereas glial cells mostly express the LDL-receptor. These receptors (particularly LRP-1) are not only used for lipoprotein metabolism, they also bind some proteins involved in brain development (e.g. Sonic Hedgehog, Wnt, and reelin), as well as proteases, protease inhibitors, vitamin transporters, and pro-inflammatory molecules [146]. Following receptor-mediated endocytosis, vesicles deliver lipid particles to late endosomes or lysosomes. Immediately after endocytosis, apoE is detached from the lipid components and is not sent to lysosomes but recycled back to the plasma membrane [91, 147].

While it is known that the strongest genetic modifier for AD risk currently identified is the *APOE* ε4 allele, the mechanism is not well understood. A study that examined the physical distribution of the resultant apoE ε4 protein shows that it gravitates towards the larger, less dense particles of CNS lipoprotein whereas apoE ε2 and apoE ε3 tend to associate with smaller, denser lipoprotein fractions [148]. Like their peripheral counterparts, the CNS apoE proteins have differential effects, where apoE ε2 and apoE ε3 appear to be more effective than apoE ε4 [149–152]. The following sections will detail how the function of apoE, as a lipid transport molecule and its involvement in Aβ clearance and/or aggregation, may explain the genetic association between the *APOE* gene and AD.

7.4.2 Apolipoprotein E and Alzheimer's Disease

Several epidemiological studies have consistently demonstrated that individuals carrying the *APOE* ε4 allele have increased risk for developing AD [2–7, 153], making *APOE* genotype a de facto standard for inclusion in the prediction for developing sporadic AD.

However, while there is an over-representation of *APOE ε4* amongst AD-affected individuals, carriage of the *APOE ε4* allele does not always lead to development of AD, and despite many studies on the subject, the conveyance of risk by the *APOE ε4* allele is still not well understood.

Early studies showed that plasma levels of apoE may be an important factor in AD, as higher levels were observed in the plasma of AD individuals relative to non-AD individuals [154]. Other early studies suggested that polymorphisms in the *APOE* promoter region may influence the probability of developing AD [155–158]. This region, which belongs to the TATA box family, regulates the production of apoE protein where a genotype of -491TT produces much less apoE than -491AT and -491AA. The initial studies demonstrated that the *APOE* -491AT and AA genotypes lead to increased risk for AD independent of *APOE* allele [155, 157]. It was soon realised that the risk for AD may be compounded when *APOE ε4* alleles and the -491AA genotype are combined [158]. These results suggested that the increased production of the apoE protein may boost disease progression, but did not account for any mechanism(s) of action in AD by the apoE ε4 protein itself.

However, more recent studies now suggest that low plasma apoE levels increase the risk of AD [159]. Furthermore, other studies have suggested that CNS and peripheral apoE levels are not correlated, and that the CNS apoE levels correlate better with CSF Aβ levels, which may be more relevant to AD risk [160]. Overall, apoE levels in CSF from AD individuals have been found to be lower [161], and post-mortem studies [162] have found reduced apoE levels in AD-affected brain regions, with the lowest levels being found in *APOE ε4* carriers. It is likely that peripheral and CSF apoE levels change over the course of AD neurodegeneration, and that the levels that may increase risk of AD pathogenesis may not be related to levels once neurodegeneration is established, and it is hoped that further studies will determine the influence of apoE levels on AD risk.

Studies of brain apoE levels have led to contradictory results. An early study in the APPV717F transgenic mouse model demonstrated that expression of mouse *APOE* resulted in deposition of Aβ [163]. However, lower levels of apoE were detected in AD brain when compared to age-matched controls, particularly in *APOE ε4* carriers. Therefore it was suggested that reduced apoE levels in the CNS helped facilitate the increased deposition of Aβ. However, a later study in mice that lacked APOE expression resulted in more diffuse plaque formation with little neuritic degeneration [164], suggesting that the apoE protein was contributing to neuritic plaque formation, whilst expression of human *APOE ε3* or *ε4* resulted in fibrillar Aβ deposition with severe neuritic degeneration. This latter result demonstrated that apoE was in fact required for Aβ toxicity and deposition. It should however be noted that a lack of the apoE protein would have other severe consequences relating to lipid metabolism in the brain, and therefore interpretation of the results in these animals is difficult.

7.4.2.1 ApoE Binding to Aβ

Early histological studies indicated that apoE was associated with Aβ plaques [165], but it was at least another two years before the epidemiological linkage of *APOE* genotype with AD was confirmed [2–7, 153]. Attention soon turned towards the involvement of the apoE protein with Aβ at the molecular level. It was then shown that apoE could bind Aβ, whether in purified form [166], or native form [167–170]. The work investigating binding of Aβ by purified apoE indicated that apoE ε4 bound more rapidly to Aβ compared with apoE ε3 [7] which led to speculation that apoE ε4 facilitates Aβ deposition via its rapid binding to Aβ. The authors noted that residues 12–28 of Aβ peptide and 244–272 of purified apoE were important for complex formation [166]. However, these particular amino acids of apoE are encompassed within the previously characterised C-terminal region that anchors the apoE molecule to the lipoprotein [171–173]. This region is generally inaccessible for most proteins unless they possess lipophilic domains. It was later determined using apoE in a native and theoretically more physiological form that in fact, apoE ε4 had weaker binding affinity to Aβ than the other apoE isoforms [167–170]. There is also evidence of the importance of the apoE ε3 Cys-112 residue (present also in apoE ε2, but not apoE ε4) for binding Aβ [174]. More recent studies using Pittsburgh Compound B positron emission tomography (PiB-PET) have provided further evidence of the association of apoE with Aβ in plaques and shown that Aβ deposition follows a strong *APOE* allele-dependent pattern (ε4 > ε3 > ε2) [175, 176].

In vitro studies led to the hypothesis that apoE might be able to neutralise Aβ toxicity by direct interaction between the two proteins, thus delaying fibril formation [177] and preventing toxic interaction with neurons [178]. It was also thought that this might slow the formation of Aβ oligomers which have been demonstrated to be a more toxic species than monomeric Aβ [179, 180]. More recently though, it has been shown that apoE, especially apoE ε4, increases the oligomerisation of Aβ. Specifically, the levels of Aβ oligomers in the brains of AD patients homozygous for *APOE ε4* were found to be 2.7 times higher than in the brains of AD patients homozygous for *APOE ε3*, when matched for total plaque burden [181]. This might explain the faster cognitive decline of *APOE ε4* allele-carrying AD patients than those with *APOE ε3* alleles. However, the higher levels of these oligomers in *APOE ε4* patients may also be a consequence of reduced Aβ clearance by the CNS as discussed below.

7.4.2.2 ApoE in the Cellular Clearance of Aβ

Another early hypothesis concerning Aβ metabolism was that its cellular uptake and clearance in the brain would provide some neuroprotective effects [182]. Early studies indicated that intracellular uptake of Aβ occurs in an apoE isoform-specific manner, where apoE ε4 was less effective than apoE ε3 and apoE ε2 [183]. Other studies suggested the heparan-sulphate proteoglycans (HSPG)/ LRP-1 system was involved [184] due to the fact that apoE [185–187] and Aβ [188–191] both possess heparin binding domains. However, there was some disagreement regarding the mechanisms of action. One study indicated that Aβ competes with apoE for receptor binding sites and no difference in Aβ uptake was observed with respect to apoE isoform [184], whereas another study showed that Aβ uptake is dependent on apoE isoform [183]. More recently it has been confirmed that LRP-1 mediates Aβ1-42 uptake and lysosomal trafficking [192], and also that HSPG serves as a major Aβ binding receptor on the cell surface [193], where LRP-1 then mediates its endocytosis, following the formation of LRP-1-HSPG complexes. While apoE and Aβ can interact with each other, they also share common receptors including LRP-1, LDL receptor, and HSPG on the cell surface. ApoE likely competes with Aβ for receptor binding, but can also facilitate cellular Aβ uptake by forming complexes with Aβ depending on parameters such as concentrations, apoE isoforms involved, lipidation status, Aβ aggregation status, and receptor distribution patterns [194, 195]. Interestingly, α-2 macroglobulin which is one of the many LRP-1 ligands, also associates with Aβ and may influence its uptake. Other LRP-1 ligands can bind Aβ, and many of these, like α-2 macroglobulin, also bind HSPG. Further studies of these interactions may provide insight into how all these ligands and receptors influence Aβ metabolism [194].

One intriguing aspect of receptor-mediated uptake, aside from being processed locally by cells, is the prospect of facilitating clearance by translocation of Aβ from the brain through the BBB [196–198]. The apoE isoforms also show differential effects on this efflux of brain Aβ into the periphery. Here, it has been shown in mice that apoE ε4–Aβ complexes seem to be diverted to clear via the slower VLDL receptor (VLDLR) pathway. However, when Aβ is complexed with apoE ε3 and apoE ε2, there is evidence of Aβ transit through an additional LRP-1 pathway [199]. This is thought to be because apoE ε4–Aβ complexes have greater affinity for the VLDL receptor whereas the other isoforms favour LRP-1 [199–201], demonstrating that apoE ε4 may increase the risk for AD due to reduced Aβ clearance efficiency. Furthermore, it has already been shown in mice that Aβ is cleared rapidly from the periphery, with the bulk of it being processed by the liver [202, 203] and that the apoE isoforms also exhibit differential effects in this process too [204].

Whatever the role of apoE, there is much evidence that LRP-1 is involved in Aβ clearance. Neurons typically express LRP-1, but when this receptor is deleted from neurons in adult mice, the half-life of Aβ in the interstitial fluid increases, causing greater levels of amyloid pathology [205]. Uptake of Aβ by cells is usually followed by lysosomal degradation, and when this pathway is disturbed, or if the lysosomal enzymes cathepsin B and D are reduced, this results in Aβ accumulation in the lysosomes of AD-model transgenic mice [206, 207]. Interestingly it has also been shown that internalised Aβ can be transported to neighbouring neurons following secretion in exosomes [208], and this may also occur via LRP-1, but is yet to be confirmed [195].

7.4.2.3 ApoE and Antioxidant Properties

Some studies have suggested that apoE has antioxidant properties [209–211] where its proposed mechanism of action is through the binding of copper species, and also by direct absorption of any generated free radicals [209]. There is evidence which indicates that the receptor domain of apoE, particularly regions rich in lysine and arginine residues, is an effective Cu(II) binding site which prevents subsequent Cu(II) mediated redox reactions [212]. This work suggests that apoE could sequester Cu(II) and possibly other metal ions [209] to prevent their interaction with Aβ, reducing the probability of free radical production, which is another possible mechanism to prevent neurotoxicity. More recent studies support this as it has been shown that the co-localisation of Aβ and a high concentration of copper in lipid rafts encourages the formation of neurotoxic Aβ-copper complexes [213]. These complexes can oxidise cholesterol to generate hydrogen peroxide, oxysterols, and other lipid peroxidation products, which have been shown to accumulate in the brains of AD patients and transgenic mouse models. Tau is also sensitive to interactions with copper and cholesterol, as this can trigger a cascade of hyperphosphorylation and aggregation preceding the generation of NFT [214].

7.4.2.4 ApoE and Tissue Transglutaminase

Another pathological change that most likely influences the function of apoE in AD is the post-translational cross-linking of the protein by the enzyme tissue transglutaminase (TTG). Levels of TTG are increased in the AD brain, where its cross-linking has been associated with amyloid deposits and lesion-associated astrocytes in AD [215]. TTG can cause cross-linking, protein complex formation, and reduce protein bioactivity, and it has been shown that apoE and Aβ are both substrates for TTG [216]. Cerebral amyloid angiopathy (CAA) is a pathological hallmark of AD characterised by Aβ deposition and smooth muscle cell death in the walls of the cerebral vasculature. Studies have shown that apoE cross-linking by TTG is significantly greater in these cells of the AD brain compared to those in the healthy brain [216]. TTG enzyme activity has also been shown to be increased in the brains of both MCI and AD individuals, when compared to cognitively normal subjects [217]. Furthermore, transgenic mouse AD models show age-associated increases in TTG levels, with the majority of the enzyme being found in the hippocampus [217], suggesting that this enzyme is not as well regulated in the ageing brain. TTG activity has been shown to increase in inflammatory conditions such as multiple sclerosis and coeliac disease, and is inducible via certain pro-inflammatory pathways such as that of the transcription factor, nuclear factor kappa beta (NFkB). Interestingly, NFkB signalling in turn, appears to be modulated by TTG [218, 219]. AD is characterised by neuroinflammation, apoE dysfunction, as well as reduced Aβ clearance and TTG appears to be involved in all three of these pathogenic mechanisms.

7.4.2.5 Apolipoprotein J (Clusterin, CLU)
Another apolipoprotein that has gained the attention of AD research is apoJ, otherwise known as clusterin (CLU). Attention was focused on this glycoprotein when it was found to have altered expression in the hippocampal tissue of AD brains [220]. ApoJ (or CLU) is found in most physiological fluids [221] and has a diverse range of functions [222–226]. Its role in lipid metabolism is yet to be fully understood, however the evidence currently indicates that it has roles in the transport of lipid and cholesterol from the periphery, back to the liver. ApoJ is known to be carried on HDL particles in the peripheral circulation [227], where it readily associates with apoA-I-carrying lipoproteins [228]. In the brain, it is carried on HDL-like particles secreted from astrocytes [115].

ApoJ has specific affinity for an HDL subclass that contains cholesteryl ester-transfer protein (CETP). This subclass is thought to account for only about 2% of all HDL in the circulation [227]. CETP is an important molecule which collects triglycerides from VLDL or LDL and exchanges them for cholesteryl esters from HDL [229, 230]. Studies of CETP suggest that it can promote atherosclerosis due to this transfer of cholesterol back to these apoB lipoproteins [231–234]. However, the exact role of apoJ and its affinity for these CETP-carrying HDL is not well understood.

It has been suggested that apoJ may have anti-atherogenic properties since paraoxonase, an enzyme that hydrolyses lipid peroxide, is almost exclusively carried by apoJ-associated HDL and it can protect LDL from oxidation [235]. A number of studies have associated the paraoxonase-1 gene (*PON1*) with atherosclerotic disease and stroke but the *PON2* member of the family is expressed in brain, particularly in astrocytes [236]. While it is not known if paraoxonase-2 is carried on apoJ–associated lipoproteins in the CNS, its presence here suggests that it may form one of many layers of defence against oxidative damage [237] in addition to the protein chaperone mechanisms of apoJ itself [238].

ApoJ has been demonstrated to promote cholesterol efflux from macrophage foam cells [239] *in vitro*. Whether this is its major role in other cells, such as the neurons or glia of the CNS, is not known. It shares some receptors with apoE [240] but again, its role in AD is currently unclear. Intriguingly, apoJ has a high affinity for Aβ, and it has been suggested that it may play a role in AD by interacting with apoE (or alone), by affecting Aβ clearance and/or aggregation [241]. ApoJ appears to bind specifically to Aβ1-40, and differences in its levels seem to affect the aggregation of Aβ [242, 243]. A recent study has shown that the lack of apoJ in a transgenic AD mouse model shifts the deposition of amyloid from the brain parenchyma to the cerebrovasculature, due to disruption of apoJ chaperone activity [244]. Thus, current evidence indicates that apoJ plays a role in Aβ clearance, and that alterations in the concentration or effectiveness of such amyloid-chaperone proteins (like apoE) are highly important in AD pathogenesis.

7.5 LRP-1 in the Brain and Its Role in Aβ Clearance

As mentioned earlier, the predominant lipoprotein receptor in the brain is LRP-1 [245, 246]. This receptor accepts over 30 different ligands [247] including apoE and Aβ. Interest in this receptor grew when a genetic link with LOAD was found, where LRP-1 genotype differences were associated with differences in senile plaque deposition levels [248]. It is now believed that LRP-1 is the predominant Aβ clearance protein in the vascular-mediated clearance of Aβ from the brain [249]. Factors that influence this clearance include its expression levels, post-translational modifications, and a process known as LRP-1 shedding.

Interestingly, this shedding process can be carried out by proteases involved in APP cleavage, proteases including β-secretase 1 (BACE-1) and the ADAM-10, ADAM-12 and ADAM-17 enzymes (a disintegrin and metalloprotease). Shedding of LRP-1 produces a soluble form, sLRP-1. This can also sequester free Aβ from the blood as well as in CSF. It is thought that high levels of blood sLRP-1 act as a sink or gradient to draw out Aβ from the brain. Removal of Aβ-associated sLRP-1 from the circulation then occurs via the liver, kidney, and spleen [249–251]. Expression levels of LRP-1 have been shown to be reduced in AD brains, as well as in MCI [249, 252], relative to controls. While LRP-1 levels decrease with normal ageing, plasma levels of Aβ-sLRP-1 were shown to be reduced. However, levels of free Aβ1-40 and Aβ1-42 in plasma were found to be raised in MCI and AD individuals [253], suggesting that sLRP-1 might play a significant role in sequestering Aβ proteins from the circulation. Experiments in mice indicate that only the binding domains, particularly cluster IV of sLRP-1, were sufficient to bind plasma Aβ [250].

The expression of LRP-1 is also known to be negatively regulated by the transcription factor, sterol regulatory element binding protein 2 (SREBP2) [254, 255], which primarily functions to regulate the synthesis and cellular uptake of cholesterol and fatty acids. Furthermore, LRP-1 expression is under the influence of the glucose transporter GLUT1, where lower GLUT1 levels result in lower LRP-1 levels [256]. Reduced levels of glucose transporters and particularly glucose usage have been well-reported in AD and MCI [257–259], suggesting that lower brain glucose utilisation could also reduce Aβ clearance by LRP-1.

7.5.1 LDL, HDL, and AD

Recent population-based prospective cohort studies have found that higher LDL cholesterol levels are associated with a higher risk of AD [260], whilst other studies have shown that higher levels of HDL cholesterol are associated with lower AD risk [261]. Higher LDL cholesterol and total cholesterol levels have also been found to be associated with a faster cognitive decline in patients who develop AD [262]. Interestingly, a history of type 2 diabetes was found to strengthen this association, yet levels of HDL cholesterol were not found to influence the rate of cognitive decline in this study. It is well accepted that high LDL and low HDL levels are associated with cardiovascular disease and are risk factors for AD. Furthermore, it has been found that high LDL cholesterol levels are associated with risk of dementia with stroke (vascular dementia) [263].

The criteria concerning AD diagnosis now acknowledges the many years of disease pathogenesis before symptoms appear [264]. Therefore, some recent studies have examined the possible associations earlier in the disease progression. A review of such studies concluded that high mid-life total cholesterol increases the risk of late-onset AD, and may correlate with the onset of AD pathology. The review also indicated that high mid-life total cholesterol levels are associated with an increased risk of MCI and cognitive decline [265]. However, there was insufficient data to examine any other associations, indicating there are still gaps in the literature concerning the influence of serum cholesterol levels on brain health and disease pathogenesis. Another earlier review found consistent associations between high mid-life total cholesterol and an increased risk of AD, as well as an increased risk of other forms of dementia [266]. This association was not found with high late-life total cholesterol, supporting the concept that abnormal lipid and cholesterol metabolism that is linked to cardiovascular disease, obesity, and hypertension is most likely involved in the early stages of disease pathogenesis. However, not all studies agree on the influence of HDL cholesterol and risk of dementia. For example another review of longitudinal prospective studies found no significant association overall with HDL cholesterol levels [267]. Interestingly, this review indicated that in some cases, when a particular study sample was restricted to individuals without cardio- or cerebrovascular ailments and/or treatment, participants with the lowest quartile of HDL cholesterol levels had an increased risk for dementia [268]. This study also found that low HDL cholesterol and high triglyceride levels were associated with higher incidence of dementia (but not AD) in men. In comparison, women exhibited an association between low triglyceride levels and a lower incidence of AD dementia. Such studies indicate that more information is needed to clearly understand the links between lipid metabolism, hormonal differences, vascular disease, and the development of dementia.

Population studies concerning circulating cholesterol levels are complicated by the fact that many people with high total cholesterol or LDL cholesterol are treated with statins. These are medications that inhibit HMG-CoA-reductase, thus reducing the production of cholesterol. Some (but not all) long-term observational studies of statin use have found that an unintended effect includes a reduction in the risk of dementia and cognitive decline, though probably only if taken around mid-life [269].

7.5.2 Statins, Cholesterol, and AD

Brain and plasma levels of cholesterol and its metabolites will be influenced by statin use, and the extent to which levels are affected depends upon the BBB permeability of the statin prescribed [37]. Statins are known to reduce cholesterol levels and many studies have tried to determine whether statin use decreases the risk of AD. This topic is not covered here as there are many reviews of such studies. However, we will mention that there is a growing consensus that administering statins to the elderly with vascular disease will not protect them from cognitive decline or dementia. This is because of studies such as

McGuinness et al., which showed little benefit from statin use by those with dementia [270]. However, statin intake before disease onset might have a preventative effect. In some subgroups of people, such as those with *APOE ε4* alleles, recent studies suggest certain statins such as simvastatin may slow cognitive decline [271, 272]. Cochrane reviews of studies involving statins suggest that these medications do not prevent cognitive decline or dementia, yet authors commented that participants in the reviewed studies were of moderate to high vascular risk. Furthermore, there were also limitations concerning the cognitive assessments used [270]. More recent studies suggest that a multifaceted intervention comprising regular exercise and healthy diet (which would lower cholesterol levels naturally in most people), along with the reduction of vascular risk factors, psychosocial stress, and major depressive episodes may help prevent cognitive decline [11, 273].

7.6 The Role of Lipid Rafts in Neurodegenerative Diseases

Lipid rafts are buoyant membrane glycolipoprotein microdomains rich in cholesterol and sphingolipids [274–277]. Lipid rafts provide the structural framework for signalling molecules and other proteins on the cell surface and are involved in protein trafficking, signal transduction, immunoglobulin function, neurotransmission, and many ligand-receptor interactions. Lipid rafts have also been linked to various conditions and diseases including cardiovascular disease and certain cancers. They are also important for the entry, replication, assembly, and budding of various types of viruses [278]. Some well-characterised proteins that concentrate on lipid rafts include GPI-anchored proteins, Src family kinases, components of the heterotrimeric G-proteins, and many of the proteins linked to AD, especially those linked with the metabolism of APP [279]. Some of the latter include the γ-secretase complex (processes over 20 proteins, including γ-site cleavage of APP), BACE-1 (β-site APP cleaving enzyme, the enzyme responsible for β-site APP cleavage), ADAM10 (A Disintegrin And Metalloprotease-10, enzyme which cleaves APP at the α-site, also cleaves TNF-α and E-cadherin), and neprilysin, an Aβ-degrading enzyme [279].

Studies have demonstrated that by increasing the dietary cholesterol content, Aβ production can be elevated [280–282]. In animal studies where rabbits were placed on a high-cholesterol diet, a greater level of brain Aβ accumulation was found [282]. In our own mouse studies, we have shown that a high-fat, high-cholesterol (HFHC) diet results in a significant increase in brain cholesterol esters, with a more profound effect in older *APOE ε4*-knock-in mice compared to *APOE ε3* mice [283]. Conversely, the reduction of cell membrane cholesterol has been shown to reduce γ-secretase activity [284] and also to increase the non-amyloidogenic α-secretase cleavage of APP [285, 286]. More recent studies have shown that the membrane lipid content near lipid rafts, from early stage AD brain frontal and entorhinal cortex tissue, has greater microviscosity which correlated with BACE-1/APP interaction levels [287, 288]. This was found not to be due to increased cholesterol or sphingomyelin levels, but due to a lower content of unsaturated fats [287]. This adds to the evidence that dyslipidaemia is central in AD neurodegeneration and that a diet high in polyunsaturated fatty acids may provide benefit in slowing or preventing AD pathogenesis. Transgenic AD mouse models and mathematical modelling studies support this theory, with evidence suggesting that increasing the cholesterol and long-chain polyunsaturated fatty acid (mainly DHA) content of membranes may delay the onset and/or progression of AD [289].

7.7 Changes to Glycerophospholipids in Alzheimer's Disease

Glycerophospholipids include derivatives of glycerol with phosphate groups attached as an ester at one carbon, and one or two lipid moieties attached at the other two carbons, as O-acyl, O-alkyl, or O-alk-1'- enyl residues. The glycerophosphate end of the molecule is polar, whilst the lipid chains are non-polar, thus glycerophospholipids are amphipathic. This property explains their presence and abundance in membrane lipid bilayers. The extracellular surface of the lipid bilayer comprises mainly phosphatidylcholine (PC) and sphingomyelin, while the cytosolic surface of the lipid bilayer comprises phosphatidylethanolamine (PE), phosphatidylinositol, and phosphatidylserine. Almost 30% of the glycerophospholipids in the adult human brain and up to 70% of myelin sheath ethanolamine glycerophospholipids are plasmalogens [290]. These are a subset of glycerophospholipids where the first carbon of the glycerol molecule has the lipid chain attached via an ether linkage rather than an ester bond, whereas the second carbon atom has a fatty acid linked by an ester (as in PC and PE). In AD, major changes in glycerophospholipids have been reported [291–294]. One type of plasmalogen is phosphatidylethanolamine plasmalogen (PEp) and its content in white matter has been reported to decrease during very mild dementia. During AD progression, this decline in PEp levels has also been observed in the grey matter [292]. Similarly, a decline in serum PEp levels has been associated with AD severity [291, 295]. Furthermore, levels of PCp (phosphatidylcholine plasmalogen) have been reported to be significantly decreased in AD prefrontal cortex compared to controls [293]. However, in a further in-depth study, levels of ePC 34:0p, 34:1 p and 32:1e were found to be upregulated while levels of lyso PC, lyso ether PC and PC 34:0e were decreased in the human prefrontal cortex [294]. Lower lyso PC concentrations have also been observed in the CSF of AD individuals compared to controls [296]. Phosphoinositide (PI) had been linked to various human diseases [297–300] including type 2 diabetes [301] which is a risk factor for sporadic AD. An imbalance in phosphatidylinositol 4,5 biphosphate metabolism has also been observed in the presence of Presenilin 1 and Presenilin 2 familial early-onset AD mutations [302]. These changes were shown in fibroblast cells from familial early-onset AD individuals, indicating these changes might also be detectable in peripheral cells, including those from the circulation. These changes in lipid molecules detected in the circulation during the early stages of AD may be useful as disease biomarkers.

Plasmalogens play an important role against oxidation, and have also been shown to reduce γ-secretase activity and therefore influence Aβ production. The vinyl ether bond present in plasmalogens is the proposed reason behind why plasmalogens are less susceptible to polyunsaturated fatty acids oxidation [303]. This process seems to be disrupted in AD, with lower levels of plasmalogens being observed in brain and serum [291, 292, 295]. However, the roles of plasmalogens are still not fully elucidated.

7.7.1 Omega-3 and Omega-6 Fatty Acids

Plasmalogens also contain a fatty alcohol with the vinyl-ether bond located at the sn-1 position, and fatty acids, such as docosahexaenoic acid (DHA, omega-3 fatty acid, 22:6n-3) or arachidonic acid (ARA, omega-6 fatty acid, 20:4n-6), located at the sn-2 position of the glycerol backbone [304]. At the sn-3 position, the carbon links to an ethanolamine (ethanolamine plasmalogen) or a choline (choline plasmalogen) by means of a phosphate ester bond [305].

DHA, ARA, and EPA (eicosapentaenoic acid, omega-3 fatty acid, 20:5n-3) and their transformation into bioactive lipid mediators have been studied considerably in the past couple of decades. The precursors to these fatty acids, ALA (alpha-linolenic acid, 18:3n-3) and LA (linoleic acid, 18:2n-6), are essential dietary fatty acids since the human body cannot produce them [306]. The supply of these fatty acids in the diet has come under scrutiny, as the evolution of modern diets including the increased intake of processed foods has resulted in a large increase in the intake of omega-6 fatty acids, while that of omega-3 fatty acids has decreased. As a result, the ratio of omega-6/omega-3 fatty acids has substantially risen from 1 : 1 in our ancestral diets, to around 8–20 : 1 in today's western diets [307]. This change coincides with a significant increase in the prevalence of obesity [308], as well as a range of inflammatory conditions. This change in ratio has also been linked to systemic inflammation and disruptions to the brain–gut–adipose tissue axis. In particular, omega-6 fatty acids are considered to be pro-inflammatory [307], whereas there is a lot of evidence that omega-3 fatty acids are anti-inflammatory [309]. This is partly because the eicosanoid products derived from omega-6 fatty acids (such as prostaglandin E2 and leukotriene B4 produced from ARA) are more potent mediators of thrombosis and inflammation than similar products derived from omega-3 fatty acids (prostaglandin E3 and leukotriene B5 made from EPA) [307, 310]. This is a major reason high omega-6/omega-3 ratio has been linked to the promotion of many chronic conditions including obesity, atherosclerosis, type 2 diabetes, and cardiovascular disease [307, 311, 312], as well as a raft of autoimmune disorders including lupus, psoriasis, and rheumatoid arthritis.

Other mechanisms underlying the anti-inflammatory effects of EPA and DHA include the alteration of cell-membrane fatty-acid composition. Changes here in the cell membrane have wide-ranging consequences. Examples include altered lipid-raft function, pro-inflammatory nuclear-transcription-factor kappa B (NF-κB), transcription-factor NR1C3 (or peroxisome-proliferator-activated receptor-γ, PPARγ [313]), and G-protein-coupled receptor GPR120, a protein involved in appetite control and insulin sensitisation [314, 315]. One important issue concerning the omega-6/omega-3 ratio is that there is competition between these two fatty-acid types for two desaturation enzymes. These enzymes are required for rate-limiting steps in the conversion of LA to ARA and for ALA to be converted to EPA (and then DHA) [307]. Both fatty acid desaturase 1 (FADS1) and fatty acid desaturase 2 (FADS2) have greater affinity for ALA than LA [316]. However, western diets have caused such an increase in LA intake that it overwhelms these enzymes involved in the desaturation and elongation of ALA [307, 317]. In addition, further interference with this process occurs with dietary intake of excess trans-fatty acids, which are commonly found in processed foods and overheated cooking oils. The changes to the omega-6/omega-3 fatty-acid ratio in western diets is partly due to modern agricultural practices, which have influenced both plant and animal produce, including fish [318, 319]. During the Palaeolithic period, the diets of humans included equal amounts of both omega-6 and omega-3 fatty acids, sourced from plants (LA + ALA) and the fat of land animals and fish (ARA + EPA + DHA) [319–321]. There is considerable evidence from animal studies that a diet with a high omega-6/omega-3 fatty-acid ratio results in several changes to lipid metabolism which increase the risk of atherosclerosis, inflammation and fat deposition, leading to type 2 diabetes and resistance to the signalling of leptin, often referred to as the satiety hormone [307].

7.7.1.1 Omega-3 Fatty Acids, Modern Diets, and Health Implications

Omega-3 fatty acid supplementation is being recommended to try to counteract this imbalance in dietary omega-3/omega-6 fatty-acid intake and studies suggest that such supplements do provide some benefits. However, without concomitant reduction of dietary omega-6, the effects are limited [322]. The traditional Mediterranean diet, widely acknowledged to be healthy, has a high content of seafood and little animal fat, low sugar, and an emphasis on fresh seasonal produce that are typically high in vitamins and antioxidants. It is likely that moving towards such a diet could significantly reduce some of the chronic conditions linked to the high omega-6/omega-3 fatty acid ratios and low-nutrient foods that are common in western diets [307, 323, 324]. There is evidence indicating that the neuroprotective effects provided by DHA are not limited to reducing or slowing AD pathogenesis. DHA intake and its derivative lipid mediators have also been reported to benefit patients with other neurological problems including major depressive and bipolar disorders, Parkinson's disease, and amyotrophic lateral sclerosis [325–328].

7.8 Sphingolipids

Sphingolipids are found in neuronal membranes and play an important role in signal transmission. There are three main types of sphingolipids: ceramides (Cer), sphingomyelins (SM), and glycosphingolipids. Sphingolipid synthesis begins with condensation of palmitoyl-coenzyme A and L-serine to form 3-dehydrosphinganine. This is subsequently metabolised by several enzymes to produce Cer [329, 330], which are in turn processed by SM synthase to produce SM [329].

7.8.1 Ceramides

Changes in Cer levels have been found in AD. Levels of Cer 24:0 and galactosylceramides have been found to increase significantly in the middle frontal gyrus in AD individuals compared to controls [331]. In very early AD cases (Clinical Dementia Rating 0.5), Cer content in the white matter has been found to be elevated, but declines as the dementia progresses beyond the mild cognitive impairment stage [332]. Higher Cer levels have been shown in CSF of moderate AD cases when compared to either mildly or severely affected AD cases [333]. This alteration in sphingomyelin metabolism, often linked to chronic inflammation, ER stress, and oxidative stress, is believed to lead to neuronal degeneration [334]. In particular, Cer promotes the production of Aβ and leads to further oxidative stress. This oxidation of lipids to produce Cer is particularly important in AD [335]. Furthermore, decreases in certain plasma sphingomyelin species as well as increases in plasma Cer (N16:0 and N21:0) levels are considered good potential biomarkers of AD [336]. Cer are also important secondary lipid messengers associated with apoptosis. In fact, Cer can regulate neurotransmitter release and synaptic vesicle fusion, implying that higher levels may lead to synaptic dysfunction [337]. It must be noted that not all ceramides are equal, as some with very long-chain fatty acids are abundant in myelin and considered to be beneficial with respect to AD, whereas other ceramide species trigger inflammatory and apoptotic processes [338]. Other links between sphingolipids and AD include the fact that autophagocytic clearance of Aβ involves sphingomyelinase activities [339].

7.8.2 Sulfatides

Sulfatides (SL), also known as 3-O-sulfogalactosylceramides, are mostly synthesised in oligodendrocytes by two transferases (ceramide galactosyltransferase and cerebroside sulfotransferase) from ceramides and are degraded by a sulfatase (arylsulfatase A). Sulfatides are multifunctional molecules with roles in the nervous system (signal transduction, cell growth, and neuronal plasticity), insulin secretion, the immune system, and haemostasis/thrombosis [340]. Sulfatides have been found by early lipidomics studies of AD to be depleted (up to 90%) in grey matter and approximately 50% in white matter in all cerebral regions examined [332]. Interestingly, in a more recent study by the same authors, it was revealed that brain samples from subjects with Parkinson's disease and dementia with Lewy bodies had either no changes or raised sulfatide levels compared to control samples, suggesting that sulfatide reduction is a specific event in AD [341]. Other recent studies by the same group have shown that reduced SL levels can be detected in pre-clinical stages of AD [342]. Increases in Cer content have been observed in very mild AD subjects and this was found to be related to SL depletion [343]. ApoE has been associated with the transport of SL via lipoprotein metabolism pathways, and thus apoE is believed to help mediate SL homeostasis in the CNS. Furthermore, cell culture studies have shown that sulfatides facilitate apoE-mediated Aβ clearance (particularly Aβ 1–42) in cells [344]. A transgenic mouse study demonstrated that the age-dependent decline in cortical SL concentrations was found to be totally abolished in *APOE*-knockout animals [345], suggesting a role for apoE in the regulation of cerebral SL levels. This study also showed that apoE isoform influenced the level of sulfatide reduction, with apoE ε4 exhibiting a greater depletion. In contrast, in our own studies investigating the effects of a high-fat, high-cholesterol diet on lipid profiles in young and aged *APOE* ε3 and ε4 knock-in mice, we found that SL levels were increased in the aged animals, regardless of their *APOE* genotype or diet [283].

7.8.3 Gangliosides

The glucosylceramide-synthase (GCS) enzyme adds glucose to ceramide, thus generating a precursor for the gangliosides. Gangliosides are a class of glycosphingolipids that contain sialic acid and are expressed in the outer layer of the plasma membrane of all vertebrate cells. Aβ oligomerisation has been found to accelerate in the presence of lipid vesicles containing GM1 gangliosides. These molecules are concentrated in microdomains or lipid rafts. In AD brains, a complex of GM1 and Aβ, termed 'GAβ', has been found to accumulate [346, 347], suggesting that GM1 may influence the pathogenesis of AD.

It has been shown that lipid rafts act as surface catalysts to accelerate the aggregation of Aβ [347] and it has been proposed that these GAβ complexes act as seeds for further β sheet-like aggregation of Aβ [348]. Condensed membrane nano- or microdomains formed by sphingolipids and cholesterol are privileged sites for the binding and oligomerisation of amyloidogenic proteins and it has been suggested that by controlling the balance between unstructured Aβ monomers and α or β conformers, sphingolipids can either inhibit or stimulate the oligomerisation of amyloidogenic proteins [349].

APP processing has been reported to regulate the GCS enzyme [350], as well as another enzyme in the ganglioside pathway – GD3-synthase [351]. In particular, GM3, the substrate for GD3-synthase decreases Aβ generation, whereas the product GD3 enhances Aβ generation [351]. In fact, when AD-transgenic mice are bred with GD3 synthase-deficient mice (which have lower GD3 levels), their progeny show a reduced plaque burden and better cognitive abilities [352]. High levels of GD3 have also previously been linked to mitochondrial damage and apoptosis, in both neurodegenerative disorders and certain cancers [353].

7.9 Conclusions

Lipidomics and genomics studies have made it very clear that lipids and their metabolism are central in AD pathogenesis. This review has described many of the lipid-related changes that occur in AD, demonstrating the wide range of such changes and, in some cases, listing potential therapeutic treatments. Reducing the risk of AD will involve dietary changes and healthy lifestyles that can reduce the risk of dyslipidaemia, insulin resistance, type 2 diabetes, cardiovascular disease, and chronic inflammation, which are all known risk factors for AD. Despite the many studies on the influence of the *APOE ε4* allele on Aβ aggregation, binding, and clearance, the overall pathological effect of this allele is still not known. Further studies will consolidate these findings and hopefully clarify which changes in lipid metabolism are most relevant in AD pathogenesis. It is hoped this will pave the way towards effective treatments, whilst highlighting the importance of preventing dyslipidaemia.

References

1 Serrano-Pozo, A., Frosch, M.P., Masliah, E., and Hyman, B.T. (2011). Neuropathological alterations in Alzheimer disease. *Cold Spring Harb. Perspect. Med.* 1: a006189.
2 Corder, E.H., Saunders, A.M., Strittmatter, W.J. et al. (1993). Gene dose of apolipoprotein E type 4 allele and the risk of Alzheimer's disease in late onset families. *Science* 261: 921–923.
3 Houlden, H., Crook, R., Hardy, J. et al. (1994). Confirmation that familial clustering and age of onset in late onset Alzheimer's disease are determined at the apolipoprotein E locus. *Neurosci. Lett.* 174: 222–224.

4 Hyman, B.T., Gomez-Isla, T., Briggs, M. et al. (1996). Apolipoprotein E and cognitive change in an elderly population. *Ann. Neurol.* 40: 55–66.
5 Martins, R.N., Clarnette, R., Fisher, C. et al. (1995). ApoE genotypes in Australia: roles in early and late onset Alzheimer's disease and Down's syndrome. *Neuroreport* 6: 1513–1516.
6 Saunders, A.M., Strittmatter, W.J., Schmechel, D. et al. (1993). Association of apolipoprotein E allele epsilon 4 with late-onset familial and sporadic Alzheimer's disease. *Neurology* 43: 1467–1472.
7 Strittmatter, W.J., Saunders, A.M., Schmechel, D. et al. (1993). Apolipoprotein E: high-avidity binding to beta-amyloid and increased frequency of type 4 allele in late-onset familial Alzheimer disease. *Proc. Natl. Acad. Sci. U.S.A.* 90: 1977–1981.
8 Razay, G., Vreugdenhil, A., and Wilcock, G. (2007). The metabolic syndrome and Alzheimer disease. *Arch. Neurol.* 64: 93–96.
9 Sorrentino, M.J. (2005). Implications of the metabolic syndrome: the new epidemic. *Am. J. Cardiol.* 96: 3E–7E.
10 Dye, L., Boyle, N.B., Champ, C., and Lawton, C. (2017). The relationship between obesity and cognitive health and decline. *Proc. Nutr. Soc.* 76: 443–454.
11 Solfrizzi, V., Panza, F., Frisardi, V. et al. (2011). Diet and Alzheimer's disease risk factors or prevention: the current evidence. *Expert Rev. Neurother.* 11: 677–708.
12 Bjorkhem, I. (2006). Crossing the barrier: oxysterols as cholesterol transporters and metabolic modulators in the brain. *J. Intern. Med.* 260: 493–508.
13 Thelen, K.M., Falkai, P., Bayer, T.A., and Lutjohann, D. (2006). Cholesterol synthesis rate in human hippocampus declines with aging. *Neurosci. Lett.* 403: 15–19.
14 Sutherland, W.H., Restieaux, N.J., Nye, E.R. et al. (1998). IDL composition and angiographically determined progression of atherosclerotic lesions during simvastatin therapy. *Arterioscler. Thromb. Vasc. Biol.* 18: 577–583.
15 Leoni, V., Solomon, A., and Kivipelto, M. (2010). Links between ApoE, brain cholesterol metabolism, tau and amyloid beta-peptide in patients with cognitive impairment. *Biochem. Soc. Trans.* 38: 1021–1025.
16 Bloch, K. (1965). The biological synthesis of cholesterol. *Science* 150: 19–28.
17 Kandutsch, A.A. and Russell, A.E. (1960). Preputial gland tumor sterols: 3. A metabolic pathway from lanosterol to cholesterol. *J. Biol. Chem.* 235: 2256–2261.
18 Dietschy, J.M. and Turley, S.D. (2004). Thematic review series: brain lipids. Cholesterol metabolism in the central nervous system during early development and in the mature animal. *J. Lipid Res.* 45: 1375–1397.
19 Zhang, J. and Liu, Q. (2015). Cholesterol metabolism and homeostasis in the brain. *Protein Cell* 6: 254–264.
20 Kobayashi, A., Takanezawa, Y., Hirata, T. et al. (2006). Efflux of sphingomyelin, cholesterol, and phosphatidylcholine by ABCG1. *J. Lipid Res.* 47: 1791–1802.
21 Terasaka, N., Wang, N., Yvan-Charvet, L., and Tall, A.R. (2007). High-density lipoprotein protects macrophages from oxidized low-density lipoprotein-induced apoptosis by promoting efflux of 7-ketocholesterol via ABCG1. *Proc. Natl. Acad. Sci. U.S.A.* 104: 15093–15098.
22 Wang, N., Lan, D., Chen, W. et al. (2004). ATP-binding cassette transporters G1 and G4 mediate cellular cholesterol efflux to high-density lipoproteins. *Proc. Natl. Acad. Sci. U.S.A.* 101: 9774–9779.

23 Wang, N., Yvan-Charvet, L., Lutjohann, D. et al. (2008). ATP-binding cassette transporters G1 and G4 mediate cholesterol and desmosterol efflux to HDL and regulate sterol accumulation in the brain. *FASEB J.* 22: 1073–1082.

24 Saint-Pol, J., Vandenhaute, E., Boucau, M.C. et al. (2012). Brain pericytes ABCA1 expression mediates cholesterol efflux but not cellular amyloid-beta peptide accumulation. *J. Alzheimers Dis.* 30: 489–503.

25 Wang, Y., Muneton, S., Sjovall, J. et al. (2008). The effect of 24S-hydroxycholesterol on cholesterol homeostasis in neurons: quantitative changes to the cortical neuron proteome. *J. Proteome Res.* 7: 1606–1614.

26 Vaya, J. and Schipper, H.M. (2007). Oxysterols, cholesterol homeostasis, and Alzheimer disease. *J. Neurochem.* 102: 1727–1737.

27 Brown, J. 3rd, Theisler, C., Silberman, S. et al. (2004). Differential expression of cholesterol hydroxylases in Alzheimer's disease. *J. Biol. Chem.* 279: 34674–34681.

28 Matsuda, A., Nagao, K., Matsuo, M. et al. (2013). 24(S)-hydroxycholesterol is actively eliminated from neuronal cells by ABCA1. *J. Neurochem.* 126: 93–101.

29 Liang, Y., Lin, S., Beyer, T.P. et al. (2004). A liver X receptor and retinoid X receptor heterodimer mediates apolipoprotein E expression, secretion and cholesterol homeostasis in astrocytes. *J. Neurochem.* 88: 623–634.

30 Pfrieger, F.W. and Ungerer, N. (2011). Cholesterol metabolism in neurons and astrocytes. *Prog. Lipid Res.* 50: 357–371.

31 Testa, G., Staurenghi, E., Zerbinati, C. et al. (2016). Changes in brain oxysterols at different stages of Alzheimer's disease: their involvement in neuroinflammation. *Redox Biol.* 10: 24–33.

32 Lutjohann, D., Papassotiropoulos, A., Bjorkhem, I. et al. (2000). Plasma 24S-hydroxycholesterol (cerebrosterol) is increased in Alzheimer and vascular demented patients. *J. Lipid Res.* 41: 195–198.

33 Papassotiropoulos, A., Lutjohann, D., Bagli, M. et al. (2002). 24S-hydroxycholesterol in cerebrospinal fluid is elevated in early stages of dementia. *J. Psychiatr. Res.* 36: 27–32.

34 Schonknecht, P., Lutjohann, D., Pantel, J. et al. (2002). Cerebrospinal fluid 24S-hydroxycholesterol is increased in patients with Alzheimer's disease compared to healthy controls. *Neurosci. Lett.* 324: 83–85.

35 Shafaati, M., Solomon, A., Kivipelto, M. et al. (2007). Levels of ApoE in cerebrospinal fluid are correlated with tau and 24S-hydroxycholesterol in patients with cognitive disorders. *Neurosci. Lett.* 425: 78–82.

36 Hughes, T.M., Kuller, L.H., Lopez, O.L. et al. (2012). Markers of cholesterol metabolism in the brain show stronger associations with cerebrovascular disease than Alzheimer's disease. *J. Alzheimers Dis.* 30: 53–61.

37 Hughes, T.M., Rosano, C., Evans, R.W., and Kuller, L.H. (2013). Brain cholesterol metabolism, oxysterols, and dementia. *J. Alzheimers Dis.* 33: 891–911.

38 Shafaati, M., Marutle, A., Pettersson, H. et al. (2011). Marked accumulation of 27-hydroxycholesterol in the brains of Alzheimer's patients with the Swedish APP 670/671 mutation. *J. Lipid Res.* 52: 1004–1010.

39 Heverin, M., Bogdanovic, N., Lutjohann, D. et al. (2004). Changes in the levels of cerebral and extracerebral sterols in the brain of patients with Alzheimer's disease. *J. Lipid Res.* 45: 186–193.

40 Marwarha, G., Rhen, T., Schommer, T., and Ghribi, O. (2011). The oxysterol 27-hydroxycholesterol regulates alpha-synuclein and tyrosine hydroxylase expression levels in human neuroblastoma cells through modulation of liver X receptors and estrogen receptors – relevance to Parkinson's disease. *J. Neurochem.* 119: 1119–1136.

41 Leoni, V., Mariotti, C., Nanetti, L. et al. (2011). Whole body cholesterol metabolism is impaired in Huntington's disease. *Neurosci. Lett.* 494: 245–249.

42 Hascalovici, J.R., Vaya, J., Khatib, S. et al. (2009). Brain sterol dysregulation in sporadic AD and MCI: relationship to heme oxygenase-1. *J. Neurochem.* 110: 1241–1253.

43 Nelson, T.J. and Alkon, D.L. (2005). Oxidation of cholesterol by amyloid precursor protein and beta-amyloid peptide. *J. Biol. Chem.* 280: 7377–7387.

44 Famer, D., Meaney, S., Mousavi, M. et al. (2007). Regulation of alpha- and beta-secretase activity by oxysterols: cerebrosterol stimulates processing of APP via the alpha-secretase pathway. *Biochem. Biophys. Res. Commun.* 359: 46–50.

45 Gamba, P., Testa, G., Gargiulo, S. et al. (2015). Oxidized cholesterol as the driving force behind the development of Alzheimer's disease. *Front. Aging Neurosci.* 7: 119.

46 Yu, C., Youmans, K.L., and LaDu, M.J. (2010). Proposed mechanism for lipoprotein remodelling in the brain. *Biochim. Biophys. Acta* 1801: 819–823.

47 Koldamova, R., Fitz, N.F., and Lefterov, I. (2014). ATP-binding cassette transporter A1: from metabolism to neurodegeneration. *Neurobiol. Dis.* 72 (Pt A): 13–21.

48 Phillips, M.L., Pullinger, C., Kroes, I. et al. (1997). A single copy of apolipoprotein B-48 is present on the human chylomicron remnant. *J. Lipid Res.* 38: 1170–1177.

49 Wu, X., Zhou, M., Huang, L.-S. et al. (1996). Demonstration of a physical interaction between microsomal triglyceride transfer protein and Apolipoprotein B during the assembly of ApoB-containing lipoproteins. *J. Biol. Chem.* 271: 10277–10281.

50 Wetterau, J.R., Aggerbeck, L.P., Bouma, M.E. et al. (1992). Absence of microsomal triglyceride transfer protein in individuals with abetalipoproteinemia. *Science* 258: 999–1001.

51 Narcisi, T.M., Shoulders, C.C., Chester, S.A. et al. (1995). Mutations of the microsomal triglyceride-transfer-protein gene in abetalipoproteinemia. *Am. J. Hum. Genet.* 57: 1298–1310.

52 Havel, R.J. and Kane, J.P. (2001). Introduction: structure and metabolism of plasma lipoproteins. In: *The Metabolic and Molecular Bases of Inherited Disease* (ed. C.R. Scriver and W.S. Sly), 2705–2716. New York: McGraw-Hill Professional.

53 Redgrave, T.G. (1970). Formation of cholesteryl ester-rich particulate lipid during metabolism of chylomicrons. *J. Clin. Invest.* 49: 465–471.

54 Skipski, V.P., Barclay, M., Barclay, R.K. et al. (1967). Lipid composition of human serum lipoproteins. *Biochem. J* 104: 340–352.

55 Havel, R.J., Kane, J.P., and Kashyap, M.L. (1973). Interchange of apolipoproteins between chylomicrons and high density lipoproteins during alimentary lipemia in man. *J. Clin. Invest.* 52: 32–38.

56 Bisgaier, C.L. and Glickman, R.M. (1983). Intestinal synthesis, secretion, and transport of lipoproteins. *Annu. Rev. Physiol.* 45: 625–636.

57 Bhattacharya, S. and Redgrave, T.G. (1981). The content of apolipoprotein B in chylomicron particles. *J. Lipid Res.* 22: 820–828.

58 Braun, J.E. and Severson, D.L. (1992). Regulation of the synthesis, processing and translocation of lipoprotein lipase. *Biochem. J* 287 (Pt 2): 337–347.

59 Jackson, R.L., Tajima, S., Yamamura, T. et al. (1986). Comparison of apolipoprotein C-II-deficient triacylglycerol-rich lipoproteins and trioleoylglycerol/phosphatidylcholine-stabilized particles as substrates for lipoprotein lipase. *Biochim. Biophys. Acta Lipids Lipid Metab.* 875: 211–219.

60 Brown, W.V. and Baginsky, M.L. (1972). Inhibition of lipoprotein lipase by an apoprotein of human very low density lipoprotein. *Biochem. Biophys. Res. Commun.* 46: 375–382.

61 Brown, M.S., Kovanen, P.T., and Goldstein, J.L. (1981). Regulation of plasma cholesterol by lipoprotein receptors. *Science* 212: 628–635.

62 Olofsson, S.O., Bjursell, G., Bostrom, K. et al. (1987). Apolipoprotein B: structure, biosynthesis and role in the lipoprotein assembly process. *Atherosclerosis* 68: 1–17.

63 Fungwe, T.V., Cagen, L., Wilcox, H.G., and Heimberg, M. (1992). Regulation of hepatic secretion of very low density lipoprotein by dietary cholesterol. *J. Lipid Res.* 33: 179–191.

64 Khan, B., Wilcox, H.G., and Heimberg, M. (1989). Cholesterol is required for secretion of very-low-density lipoprotein by rat liver. *Biochem. J.* 258: 807–816.

65 Khan, B.V., Fungwe, T.V., Wilcox, H.G., and Heimberg, M. (1990). Cholesterol is required for the secretion of the very-low-density lipoprotein: in vivo studies. *Biochim. Biophys. Acta* 1044: 297–304.

66 Ross, A.C. and Zilversmit, D.B. (1977). Chylomicron remnant cholesteryl esters as the major constituent of very low density lipoproteins in plasma of cholesterol-fed rabbits. *J. Lipid Res.* 18: 169–181.

67 Palade, G. (1975). Intracellular aspects of the process of protein synthesis. *Science* 189: 347–358.

68 Alexander, C.A., Hamilton, R.L., and Havel, R.J. (1976). Subcellular localization of B apoprotein of plasma lipoproteins in rat liver. *J. Cell Biol.* 69: 241–263.

69 Boren, J., Wettesten, M., Sjoberg, A. et al. (1990). The assembly and secretion of apoB 100 containing lipoproteins in Hep G2 cells: evidence for different sites for protein synthesis and lipoprotein assembly. *J. Biol. Chem.* 265: 10556–10564.

70 Rustaeus, S., Lindberg, K., Stillemark, P. et al. (1999). Assembly of very low density lipoprotein: a two-step process of apolipoprotein B core lipidation. *J. Nutr.* 129: 463s–466s.

71 Golan, D.E., Tashjian, A.H.J., Armstrong, E.J., and Armstrong, A.W. (2004). Pharmacology of cholesterol and lipid metabolism. In: *Principles of Pharmacology: The Pathophysiologic Basis of Drug Therapy*, 417–438. Baltimore and Philadelphia: Lippincott Williams and Wilkins.

72 Eisenberg, S. and Levy, R.I. (1975). Lipoprotein Metabolism. In: *Advances in Lipid Research* (ed. R. Paoletti and D. Kritchevsky), 1. New York: Academic Press.

73 Packard, C.J., Demant, T., Stewart, J.P. et al. (2000). Apolipoprotein B metabolism and the distribution of VLDL and LDL subfractions. *J. Lipid Res.* 41: 305–318.

74 Mahley, R.W. (1988). Apolipoprotein E: cholesterol transport protein with expanding role in cell biology. *Science* 240: 622–630.

75 Mahley, R.W., Hui, D.Y., Innerarity, T.L., and Beisiegel, U. (1989). Chylomicron remnant metabolism. Role of hepatic lipoprotein receptors in mediating uptake. *Arteriosclerosis* 9: I14–I18.

76 Schmitz, G. and Grandl, M. (2009). The molecular mechanisms of HDL and associated vesicular trafficking mechanisms to mediate cellular lipid homeostasis. *Arterioscler. Thromb. Vasc. Biol.* 29: 1718–1722.

77 Getz, G.S. and Reardon, C.A. (2009). Apoprotein E as a lipid transport and signaling protein in the blood, liver, and artery wall. *J. Lipid Res.* 50 (Suppl): S156–S161.

78 Mahley, R.W. and Ji, Z.S. (1999). Remnant lipoprotein metabolism: key pathways involving cell-surface heparan sulfate proteoglycans and apolipoprotein E. *J. Lipid Res.* 40: 1–16.

79 Anderson, R.G., Goldstein, J.L., and Brown, M.S. (1976). Localization of low density lipoprotein receptors on plasma membrane of normal human fibroblasts and their absence in cells from a familial hypercholesterolemia homozygote. *Proc. Natl. Acad. Sci. U.S.A.* 73: 2434–2438.

80 Roth, T.F. and Porter, K.R. (1964). Yolk protein uptake in the oocyte of the mosquito Aedes Aegypti. L. *J. Cell Biol.* 20: 313–332.

81 Pearse, B.M. (1975). Coated vesicles from pig brain: purification and biochemical characterization. *J. Mol. Biol.* 97: 93–98.

82 Pearse, B.M. (1976). Clathrin: a unique protein associated with intracellular transfer of membrane by coated vesicles. *Proc. Natl. Acad. Sci. U.S.A.* 73: 1255–1259.

83 Anderson, R.G., Goldstein, J.L., and Brown, M.S. (1977). A mutation that impairs the ability of lipoprotein receptors to localise in coated pits on the cell surface of human fibroblasts. *Nature* 270: 695–699.

84 Terris, S. and Steiner, D.F. (1975). Binding and degradation of 125I-insulin by rat hepatocytes. *J. Biol. Chem.* 250: 8389–8398.

85 Carpenter, G. and Cohen, S. (1976). 125I-labeled human epidermal growth factor: binding, internalization, and degradation in human fibroblasts. *J. Cell Biol.* 71: 159–171.

86 Pastan, I.H. and Willingham, M.C. (1981). Journey to the center of the cell: role of the receptosome. *Science* 214: 504–509.

87 Aviram, M., Bierman, E.L., and Oram, J.F. (1989). High-density lipoprotein stimulates sterol translocation between intracellular and plasma-membrane pools in human monocyte-derived macrophages. *J. Lipid Res.* 30: 65–76.

88 Mendez, A.J., Oram, J.F., and Bierman, E.L. (1991). Protein-kinase-C as a mediator of high-density-lipoprotein receptor-dependent efflux of intracellular cholesterol. *J. Biol. Chem.* 266: 10104–10111.

89 Oram, J.F., Mendez, A.J., Slotte, J.P., and Johnson, T.F. (1991). High density lipoprotein apolipoproteins mediate removal of sterol from intracellular pools but not from plasma membranes of cholesterol-loaded fibroblasts. *Arterioscler. Thromb.* 11: 403–414.

90 von Eckardstein, A., Huang, Y., Wu, S. et al. (1995). Reverse cholesterol transport in plasma of patients with different forms of familial HDL deficiency. *Arterioscler. Thromb. Vasc. Biol.* 15: 691–703.

91 Rensen, P.C., Jong, M.C., van Vark, L.C. et al. (2000). Apolipoprotein E is resistant to intracellular degradation in vitro and in vivo: evidence for retroendocytosis. *J. Biol. Chem.* 275: 8564–8571.

92 Heeren, J., Weber, W., and Beisiegel, U. (1999). Intracellular processing of endocytosed triglyceride-rich lipoproteins comprises both recycling and degradation. *J. Cell Sci.* 112: 349–359.

93 Heeren, J., Grewal, T., Jackle, S., and Beisiegel, U. (2001). Recycling of apolipoprotein E and lipoprotein lipase through endosomal compartments in vivo. *J. Biol. Chem.* 276: 42333–42338.

94 Heeren, J., Grewal, T., Laatsch, A. et al. (2003). Recycling of apoprotein E is associated with cholesterol efflux and high density lipoprotein internalization. *J. Biol. Chem.* 278: 14370–14378.

95 Gursky, O. and Atkinson, D. (1996). Thermal unfolding of human high-density apolipoprotein A-1: implications for a lipid-free molten globular state. *Proc. Natl. Acad. Sci. U.S.A.* 93: 2991–2995.

96 Hara, H. and Yokoyama, S. (1991). Interaction of free apolipoproteins with macrophages: formation of high density lipoprotein-like lipoproteins and reduction of cellular cholesterol. *J. Biol. Chem.* 266: 3080–3086.

97 Takahashi, Y. and Smith, J.D. (1999). Cholesterol efflux to apolipoprotein AI involves endocytosis and resecretion in a calcium-dependent pathway. *Proc. Natl. Acad. Sci. U.S.A.* 96: 11358–11363.

98 Brouillette, C.G., Anantharamaiah, G.M., Engler, J.A., and Borhani, D.W. (2001). Structural models of human apolipoprotein A-I: a critical analysis and review. *Biochim. Biophys. Acta* 1531: 4–46.

99 Acton, S., Rigotti, A., Landschulz, K.T. et al. (1996). Identification of scavenger receptor SR-BI as a high density lipoprotein receptor. *Science* 271: 518–520.

100 Ji, Y., Jian, B., Wang, N. et al. (1997). Scavenger receptor BI promotes high density lipoprotein-mediated cellular cholesterol efflux. *J. Biol. Chem.* 272: 20982–20985.

101 Ajees, A.A., Anantharamaiah, G.M., Mishra, V.K. et al. (2006). Crystal structure of human apolipoprotein A-I: insights into its protective effect against cardiovascular diseases. *Proc. Natl. Acad. Sci. U.S.A.* 103: 2126–2131.

102 Valacchi, G., Sticozzi, C., Lim, Y., and Pecorelli, A. (2011). Scavenger receptor class B type I: a multifunctional receptor. *Ann. N.Y. Acad. Sci.* 1229: E1–E7.

103 Goldstein, J.L., Basu, S.K., Brunschede, G.Y., and Brown, M.S. (1976). Release of low density lipoprotein from its cell surface receptor by sulfated glycosaminoglycans. *Cell* 7: 85–95.

104 Marsh, M., Bolzau, E., and Helenius, A. (1983). Penetration of Semliki Forest virus from acidic prelysosomal vacuoles. *Cell* 32: 931–940.

105 Brown, M.S. and Goldstein, J.L. (1979). Receptor-mediated endocytosis: insights from the lipoprotein receptor system. *Proc. Natl. Acad. Sci. U.S.A.* 76: 3330–3337.

106 Tabas, I., Myers, J.N., Innerarity, T.L. et al. (1991). The influence of particle size and multiple apoprotein E-receptor interactions on the endocytic targeting of beta-VLDL in mouse peritoneal macrophages. *J. Cell Biol.* 115: 1547–1560.

107 Tabas, I., Lim, S., Xu, X.X., and Maxfield, F.R. (1990). Endocytosed beta-VLDL and LDL are delivered to different intracellular vesicles in mouse peritoneal macrophages. *J. Cell Biol.* 111: 929–940.

108 Myers, J.N. (1993). Beta-very low density lipoprotein is sequestered in surface-connected tubules in mouse peritoneal macrophages. *J. Cell Biol.* 123: 1389–1402.

109 Fazio, S., Linton, M.F., Hasty, A.H., and Swift, L.L. (1999). Recycling of apolipoprotein E in mouse liver. *J. Biol. Chem.* 274: 8247–8253.

110 Swift, L.L., Farkas, M.H., Major, A.S. et al. (2001). A recycling pathway for resecretion of internalized apolipoprotein E in liver cells. *J. Biol. Chem.* 276: 22965–22970.

111 Farkas, M.H., Swift, L.L., Hasty, A.H. et al. (2003). The recycling of apolipoprotein E in primary cultures of mouse hepatocytes evidence for a physiologic connection to high density lipoprotein metabolism. *J. Biol. Chem.* 278: 9412–9417.

112 Roheim, P.S., Carey, M., Forte, T., and Vega, G.L. (1979). Apolipoproteins in human cerebrospinal fluid. *Proc. Natl. Acad. Sci. U.S.A.* 76: 4646–4649.

113 Pitas, R.E., Boyles, J.K., Lee, S.H. et al. (1987). Lipoproteins and their receptors in the central-nervous-system – characterization of the lipoproteins in cerebrospinal-fluid and identification of Apolipoprotein-B,E(Ldl) receptors in the brain. *J. Biol. Chem.* 262: 14352–14360.

114 Guyton, J.R., Miller, S.E., Martin, M.E. et al. (1998). Novel large apolipoprotein E-containing lipoproteins of density 1.006-1.060 g/ml in human cerebrospinal fluid. *J. Neurochem.* 70: 1235–1240.

115 LaDu, M.J., Gilligan, S.M., Lukens, J.R. et al. (1998). Nascent astrocyte particles differ from lipoproteins in CSF. *J. Neurochem.* 70: 2070–2081.

116 Kamboh, M.I., Sepehrnia, B., and Ferrell, R.E. (1989). Genetic studies of human apolipoproteins: VI. Common polymorphism of apolipoprotein E in blacks. *Dis. Markers* 7: 49–55.

117 Kamboh, M.I., Weiss, K.M., and Ferrell, R.E. (1991). Genetic studies of human apolipoproteins: XVI. APOE polymorphism and cholesterol levels in the Mayans of the Yucatan Peninsula, Mexico. *Clin. Genet.* 39: 26–32.

118 Tsukamoto, K., Watanabe, T., Matsushima, T. et al. (1993). Determination by PCR-RFLP of apo E genotype in a Japanese population. *J. Lab. Clin. Med.* 121: 598–602.

119 Gerdes, L.U., Klausen, I.C., Sihm, I., and Faergeman, O. (1992). Apolipoprotein E polymorphism in a Danish population compared to findings in 45 other study populations around the world. *Genet. Epidemiol.* 9: 155–167.

120 Schneider, W.J., Kovanen, P.T., Brown, M.S. et al. (1981). Familial dysbetalipoproteinemia: abnormal binding of mutant apoprotein E to low density lipoprotein receptors of human fibroblasts and membranes from liver and adrenal of rats, rabbits, and cows. *J. Clin. Invest.* 68: 1075–1085.

121 Rall, S.C. Jr., Weisgraber, K.H., Innerarity, T.L., and Mahley, R.W. (1982). Structural basis for receptor binding heterogeneity of apolipoprotein E from type III hyperlipoproteinemic subjects. *Proc. Natl. Acad. Sci. U.S.A.* 79: 4696–4700.

122 Gregg, R.E., Zech, L.A., Schaefer, E.J., and Brewer, H.B. Jr. (1981). Type III hyperlipoproteinemia: defective metabolism of an abnormal apolipoprotein E. *Science* 211: 584–586.

123 Brown, M.S. and Goldstein, J.L. (1983). Lipoprotein receptors in the liver: control signals for plasma cholesterol traffic. *J. Clin. Invest.* 72: 743–747.

124 Bennet, A.M., Di Angelantonio, E., Ye, Z. et al. (2007). Association of apolipoprotein E genotypes with lipid levels and coronary risk. *JAMA* 298: 1300–1311.

125 Eto, M., Watanabe, K., and Ishii, K. (1986). Reciprocal effects of apolipoprotein E alleles (epsilon 2 and epsilon 4) on plasma lipid levels in normolipidemic subjects. *Clin. Genet.* 29: 477–484.

126 Bredie, S.J., Vogelaar, J.M., Demacker, P.N., and Stalenhoef, A.F. (1996). Apolipoprotein E polymorphism influences lipid phenotypic expression, but not the low density lipoprotein subfraction distribution in familial combined hyperlipidemia. *Atherosclerosis* 126: 313–324.

127 Bohnet, K., Pillot, T., Visvikis, S. et al. (1996). Apolipoprotein (apo) E genotype and apoE concentration determine binding of normal very low density lipoproteins to HepG2 cell surface receptors. *J. Lipid Res.* 37: 1316–1324.

128 Mamotte, C.D., Sturm, M., Foo, J.I. et al. (1999). Comparison of the LDL-receptor binding of VLDL and LDL from apoE4 and apoE3 homozygotes. *Am. J. Physiol.* 276: E553–E557.

129 Heeren, J., Grewal, T., Laatsch, A. et al. (2004). Impaired recycling of apolipoprotein E4 is associated with intracellular cholesterol accumulation. *J. Biol. Chem.* 279: 55483–55492.

130 Malloy, S.I., Altenburg, M.K., Knouff, C. et al. (2004). Harmful effects of increased LDLR expression in mice with human APOE*4 but not APOE*3. *Arterioscler. Thromb. Vasc. Biol.* 24: 91–97.

131 Riddell, D.R., Zhou, H., Atchison, K. et al. (2008). Impact of apolipoprotein E (ApoE) polymorphism on brain ApoE levels. *J. Neurosci.* 28: 11445–11453.

132 Pitas, R.E., Boyles, J.K., Lee, S.H. et al. (1987). Astrocytes synthesize apolipoprotein E and metabolize apolipoprotein E-containing lipoproteins. *Biochim. Biophys. Acta* 917: 148–161.

133 Holtzman, D.M., Pitas, R.E., Kilbridge, J. et al. (1995). Low density lipoprotein receptor-related protein mediates apolipoprotein E-dependent neurite outgrowth in a central nervous system-derived neuronal cell line. *Proc. Natl. Acad. Sci. U.S.A.* 92: 9480–9484.

134 Weisgraber, K.H. and Mahley, R.W. (1996). Human apolipoprotein E: the Alzheimer's disease connection. *FASEB J.* 10: 1485–1494.

135 Bellosta, S., Nathan, B.P., Orth, M. et al. (1995). Stable expression and secretion of apolipoproteins E3 and E4 in mouse neuroblastoma cells produces differential effects on neurite outgrowth. *J. Biol. Chem.* 270: 27063–27071.

136 DeMattos, R.B., Curtiss, L.K., and Williams, D.L. (1998). A minimally lipidated form of cell-derived apolipoprotein E exhibits isoform-specific stimulation of neurite outgrowth in the absence of exogenous lipids or lipoproteins. *J. Biol. Chem.* 273: 4206–4212.

137 Ignatius, M.J., Shooter, E.M., Pitas, R.E., and Mahley, R.W. (1987). Lipoprotein uptake by neuronal growth cones in vitro. *Science* 236: 959–962.

138 Nathan, B.P., Bellosta, S., Sanan, D.A. et al. (1994). Differential effects of apolipoproteins E3 and E4 on neuronal growth in vitro. *Science* 264: 850–852.

139 Weeber, E.J., Beffert, U., Jones, C. et al. (2002). Reelin and ApoE receptors cooperate to enhance hippocampal synaptic plasticity and learning. *J. Biol. Chem.* 277: 39944–39952.

140 Ignatius, M.J., Gebicke-Harter, P.J., Skene, J.H. et al. (1986). Expression of apolipoprotein E during nerve degeneration and regeneration. *Proc. Natl. Acad. Sci. U.S.A.* 83: 1125–1129.

141 Ignatius, M.J., Gebicke-Haerter, P.J., Pitas, R.E., and Shooter, E.M. (1987). Apolipoprotein E in nerve injury and repair. *Prog. Brain Res.* 71: 177–184.

142 Mulder, M., Jansen, P.J., Janssen, B.J. et al. (2004). Low-density lipoprotein receptor-knockout mice display impaired spatial memory associated with a decreased synaptic density in the hippocampus. *Neurobiol. Dis.* 16: 212–219.

143 Oitzl, M.S., Mulder, M., Lucassen, P.J. et al. (1997). Severe learning deficits in apolipoprotein E-knockout mice in a water maze task. *Brain Res.* 752: 189–196.

144 Linton, M.F., Gish, R., Hubl, S.T. et al. (1991). Phenotypes of apolipoprotein B and apolipoprotein E after liver transplantation. *J. Clin. Invest.* 88: 270–281.

145 Boyles, J.K., Pitas, R.E., Wilson, E. et al. (1985). Apolipoprotein E associated with astrocytic glia of the central nervous system and with nonmyelinating glia of the peripheral nervous system. *J. Clin. Invest.* 76: 1501–1513.

146 Lane-Donovan, C., Philips, G.T., and Herz, J. (2014). More than cholesterol transporters: lipoprotein receptors in CNS function and neurodegeneration. *Neuron* 83: 771–787.

147 Petrov, A.M., Kasimov, M.R., and Zefirov, A.L. (2016). Brain cholesterol metabolism and its defects: linkage to neurodegenerative diseases and synaptic dysfunction. *Acta Nat.* 8: 58–73.

148 Yamauchi, K., Tozuka, M., Hidaka, H. et al. (1999). Characterization of apolipoprotein E-containing lipoproteins in cerebrospinal fluid: effect of phenotype on the distribution of apolipoprotein E. *Clin. Chem.* 45: 1431–1438.

149 Ji, Z.-S., Pitas, R.E., and Mahley, R.W. (1998). Differential cellular accumulation/retention of Apolipoprotein E mediated by cell surface Heparan Sulfate proteoglycans. *J. Biol. Chem.* 273: 13452–13460.

150 Maezawa, I., Zaja-Milatovic, S., Milatovic, D. et al. (2006). Apolipoprotein E isoform-dependent dendritic recovery of hippocampal neurons following activation of innate immunity. *J. Neuroinflamm.* 3: 21.

151 Maezawa, I., Maeda, N., Montine, T.J., and Montine, K.S. (2006). Apolipoprotein E-specific innate immune response in astrocytes from targeted replacement mice. *J. Neuroinflamm.* 3: 10.

152 Maezawa, I., Nivison, M., Montine, K.S. et al. (2006). Neurotoxicity from innate immune response is greatest with targeted replacement of E4 allele of apolipoprotein E gene and is mediated by microglial p38MAPK. *Faseb J.* 20: 797–799.

153 Dai, X.Y., Nanko, S., Hattori, M. et al. (1994). Association of apolipoprotein E4 with sporadic Alzheimer's disease is more pronounced in early onset type. *Neurosci. Lett.* 175: 74–76.

154 Taddei, K., Clarnette, R., Gandy, S.E., and Martins, R.N. (1997). Increased plasma apolipoprotein E (apoE) levels in Alzheimer's disease. *Neurosci. Lett.* 223: 29–32.

155 Bullido, M.J., Artiga, M.J., Recuero, M. et al. (1998). A polymorphism in the regulatory region of APOE associated with risk for Alzheimer's dementia. *Nat. Genet.* 18: 69–71.

156 Lambert, J.C., Pasquier, F., Cottel, D. et al. (1998). A new polymorphism in the APOE promoter associated with risk of developing Alzheimer's disease. *Hum. Mol. Genet.* 7: 533–540.

157 Laws, S.M., Taddei, K., Martins, G. et al. (1999). The —491AA polymorphism in the APOE gene is associated with increased plasma apoE levels in Alzheimer's disease. *NeuroReport* 10: 879–882.

158 Laws, S.M., Clarnette, R.M., Taddei, K. et al. (2002). APOE- E4 and APOE -491A polymorphisms in individuals with subjective memory loss. *Mol. Psychiatry* 7: 768–775.

159 Rasmussen, K.L., Tybjaerg-Hansen, A., Nordestgaard, B.G., and Frikke-Schmidt, R. (2018). Plasma apolipoprotein E levels and risk of dementia: a Mendelian randomization study of 106,562 individuals. *Alzheimers Dement.* 14: 71–80.

160 Baker-Nigh, A.T., Mawuenyega, K.G., Bollinger, J.G. et al. (2016). Human central nervous system (CNS) ApoE isoforms are increased by age, differentially altered by amyloidosis, and relative amounts reversed in the CNS compared with plasma. *J. Biol. Chem.* 291: 27204–27218.

161 Lehtimaki, T., Pirttila, T., Mehta, P.D. et al. (1995). Apolipoprotein E (apoE) polymorphism and its influence on ApoE concentrations in the cerebrospinal fluid in Finnish patients with Alzheimer's disease. *Hum. Genet.* 95: 39–42.

162 Beffert, U., Cohn, J.S., Petit-Turcotte, C. et al. (1999). Apolipoprotein E and beta-amyloid levels in the hippocampus and frontal cortex of Alzheimer's disease subjects are disease-related and apolipoprotein E genotype dependent. *Brain Res.* 843: 87–94.

163 Bales, K.R., Verina, T., Dodel, R.C. et al. (1997). Lack of apolipoprotein E dramatically reduces amyloid beta-peptide deposition. *Nat. Genet.* 17: 263–264.

164 Holtzman, D.M., Bales, K.R., Tenkova, T. et al. (2000). Apolipoprotein E isoform-dependent amyloid deposition and neuritic degeneration in a mouse model of Alzheimer's disease. *Proc. Natl. Acad. Sci. U.S.A.* 97: 2892–2897.

165 Namba, Y., Tomonaga, M., Kawasaki, H. et al. (1991). Apolipoprotein E immunoreactivity in cerebral amyloid deposits and neurofibrillary tangles in Alzheimer's disease and kuru plaque amyloid in Creutzfeldt-Jakob disease. *Brain Res.* 541: 163–166.

166 Strittmatter, W.J., Weisgraber, K.H., Huang, D.Y. et al. (1993). Binding of human apolipoprotein E to synthetic amyloid beta peptide: isoform-specific effects and implications for late-onset Alzheimer disease. *Proc. Natl. Acad. Sci. U.S.A.* 90: 8098–8102.

167 LaDu, M.J., Falduto, M.T., Manelli, A.M. et al. (1994). Isoform-specific binding of apolipoprotein E to beta-amyloid. *J. Biol. Chem.* 269: 23403–23406.

168 LaDu, M.J., Pederson, T.M., Frail, D.E. et al. (1995). Purification of apolipoprotein E attenuates isoform-specific binding to beta-amyloid. *J. Biol. Chem.* 270: 9039–9042.

169 LaDu, M.J., Lukens, J.R., Reardon, C.A., and Getz, G.S. (1997). Association of human, rat, and rabbit apolipoprotein E with beta-amyloid. *J. Neurosci. Res.* 49: 9–18.

170 Yang, D.S., Smith, J.D., Zhou, Z. et al. (1997). Characterization of the binding of amyloid-beta peptide to cell culture-derived native apolipoprotein E2, E3, and E4 isoforms and to isoforms from human plasma. *J. Neurochem.* 68: 721–725.

171 Wetterau, J.R., Aggerbeck, L.P., Rall, S.C. Jr., and Weisgraber, K.H. (1988). Human apolipoprotein E3 in aqueous solution: I. Evidence for two structural domains. *J. Biol. Chem.* 263: 6240–6248.

172 Aggerbeck, L.P., Wetterau, J.R., Weisgraber, K.H. et al. (1988). Human apolipoprotein E3 in aqueous solution: II. Properties of the amino- and carboxyl-terminal domains. *J. Biol. Chem.* 263: 6249–6258.

173 Westerlund, J.A. and Weisgraber, K.H. (1993). Discrete carboxyl-terminal segments of apolipoprotein E mediate lipoprotein association and protein oligomerization. *J. Biol. Chem.* 268: 15745–15750.

174 Bentley, N.M., Ladu, M.J., Rajan, C. et al. (2002). Apolipoprotein E structural requirements for the formation of SDS-stable complexes with beta-amyloid-(1-40): the role of salt bridges. *Biochem. J.* 366: 273–279.

175 Kok, E., Haikonen, S., Luoto, T. et al. (2009). Apolipoprotein E-dependent accumulation of Alzheimer disease-related lesions begins in middle age. *Ann. Neurol.* 65: 650–657.

176 Morris, J.C., Roe, C.M., Xiong, C. et al. (2010). APOE predicts amyloid-beta but not tau Alzheimer pathology in cognitively normal aging. *Ann. Neurol.* 67: 122–131.

177 Naiki, H., Hasegawa, K., Yamaguchi, I. et al. (1998). Apolipoprotein E and antioxidants have different mechanisms of inhibiting Alzheimer's β-amyloid fibril formation in vitro†. *Biochemistry* 37: 17882–17889.

178 Drouet, B., Fifre, A., Pincon-Raymond, M. et al. (2001). ApoE protects cortical neurones against neurotoxicity induced by the non-fibrillar C-terminal domain of the amyloid-beta peptide. *J. Neurochem.* 76: 117–127.

179 Walsh, D.M., Klyubin, I., Fadeeva, J.V. et al. (2002). Naturally secreted oligomers of amyloid beta protein potently inhibit hippocampal long-term potentiation in vivo. *Nature* 416: 535–539.

180 Dahlgren, K.N., Manelli, A.M., Stine, W.B. Jr. et al. (2002). Oligomeric and fibrillar species of amyloid-beta peptides differentially affect neuronal viability. *J. Biol. Chem.* 277: 32046–32053.

181 Hashimoto, T., Serrano-Pozo, A., Hori, Y. et al. (2012). Apolipoprotein E, especially apolipoprotein E4, increases the oligomerization of amyloid beta peptide. *J. Neurosci.* 32: 15181–15192.

182 Jordan, J., Galindo, M.F., Miller, R.J. et al. (1998). Isoform-specific effect of apolipoprotein E on cell survival and beta-amyloid-induced toxicity in rat hippocampal pyramidal neuronal cultures. *J. Neurosci.* 18: 195–204.

183 Yang, D.S., Small, D.H., Seydel, U. et al. (1999). Apolipoprotein E promotes the binding and uptake of beta-amyloid into Chinese hamster ovary cells in an isoform-specific manner. *Neuroscience* 90: 1217–1226.

184 Winkler, K., Scharnagl, H., Tisljar, U. et al. (1999). Competition of Abeta amyloid peptide and apolipoprotein E for receptor-mediated endocytosis. *J. Lipid Res.* 40: 447–455.

185 Rall, S.C. Jr., Weisgraber, K.H., and Mahley, R.W. (1982). Human apolipoprotein E: the complete amino acid sequence. *J. Biol. Chem.* 257: 4171–4178.

186 Weisgraber, K.H., Rall, S.C. Jr., Mahley, R.W. et al. (1986). Human apolipoprotein E. Determination of the heparin binding sites of apolipoprotein E3. *J. Biol. Chem.* 261: 2068–2076.

187 Cardin, A.D., Hirose, N., Blankenship, D.T. et al. (1986). Binding of a high reactive heparin to human apolipoprotein E: identification of two heparin-binding domains. *Biochem. Biophys. Res. Commun.* 134: 783–789.

188 Gupta-Bansal, R., Frederickson, R.C., and Brunden, K.R. (1995). Proteoglycan-mediated inhibition of a beta proteolysis: a potential cause of senile plaque accumulation. *J. Biol. Chem.* 270: 18666–18671.

189 Talafous, J., Marcinowski, K.J., Klopman, G., and Zagorski, M.G. (1994). Solution structure of residues 1-28 of the amyloid beta-peptide. *Biochemistry* 33: 7788–7796.

190 Buee, L., Ding, W., Anderson, J.P. et al. (1993). Binding of vascular heparan sulfate proteoglycan to Alzheimer's amyloid precursor protein is mediated in part by the N-terminal region of A4 peptide. *Brain Res.* 627: 199–204.

191 Buee, L., Ding, W., Delacourte, A., and Fillit, H. (1993). Binding of secreted human neuroblastoma proteoglycans to the Alzheimer's amyloid A4 peptide. *Brain Res.* 601: 154–163.

192 Fuentealba, R.A., Liu, Q., Zhang, J. et al. (2010). Low-density lipoprotein receptor-related protein 1 (LRP1) mediates neuronal Abeta42 uptake and lysosomal trafficking. *PLoS One* 5: e11884.

193 Kanekiyo, T., Zhang, J., Liu, Q. et al. (2011). Heparan sulphate proteoglycan and the low-density lipoprotein receptor-related protein 1 constitute major pathways for neuronal amyloid-beta uptake. *J. Neurosci.* 31: 1644–1651.

194 Kanekiyo, T., Xu, H., and Bu, G. (2014). ApoE and Abeta in Alzheimer's disease: accidental encounters or partners? *Neuron* 81: 740–754.

195 Kanekiyo, T. and Bu, G. (2014). The low-density lipoprotein receptor-related protein 1 and amyloid-beta clearance in Alzheimer's disease. *Front. Aging Neurosci.* 6: 93.

196 Castellano, J.M., Deane, R., Gottesdiener, A.J. et al. (2012). Low-density lipoprotein receptor overexpression enhances the rate of brain-to-blood Abeta clearance in a mouse model of beta-amyloidosis. *Proc. Natl. Acad. Sci. U.S.A.* 109: 15502–15507.

197 Cirrito, J.R., Deane, R., Fagan, A.M. et al. (2005). P-glycoprotein deficiency at the blood–brain barrier increases amyloid-beta deposition in an Alzheimer disease mouse model. *J. Clin. Invest.* 115: 3285–3290.

198 Shibata, M., Yamada, S., Kumar, S.R. et al. (2000). Clearance of Alzheimer's amyloid-ss(1-40) peptide from brain by LDL receptor-related protein-1 at the blood-brain barrier. *J. Clin. Invest.* 106: 1489–1499.

199 Deane, R., Sagare, A., Hamm, K. et al. (2008). apoE isoform-specific disruption of amyloid beta peptide clearance from mouse brain. *J. Clin. Invest.* 118: 4002–4013.

200 Nazer, B., Hong, S., and Selkoe, D.J. (2008). LRP promotes endocytosis and degradation, but not transcytosis, of the amyloid-beta peptide in a blood–brain barrier in vitro model. *Neurobiol. Dis.* 30: 94–102.

201 Salameh, T.S., Rhea, E.M., Banks, W.A., and Hanson, A.J. (2016). Insulin resistance, dyslipidemia, and apolipoprotein E interactions as mechanisms in cognitive impairment and Alzheimer's disease. *Exp. Biol. Med. (Maywood)* 241: 1676–1683.

202 Hone, E., Martins, I.J., Fonte, J., and Martins, R.N. (2003). Apolipoprotein E influences amyloid-beta clearance from the murine periphery. *J. Alzheimers Dis.* 5: 1–8.

203 Ghiso, J., Shayo, M., Calero, M. et al. (2004). Systemic catabolism of Alzheimer's Abeta40 and Abeta42. *J. Biol. Chem.* 279: 45897–45908.

204 Sharman, M.J., Morici, M., Hone, E. et al. (2010). APOE genotype results in differential effects on the peripheral clearance of amyloid-beta42 in APOE knock-in and knock-out mice. *J. Alzheimers Dis.* 21: 403–409.

205 Kanekiyo, T., Cirrito, J.R., Liu, C.C. et al. (2013). Neuronal clearance of amyloid-beta by endocytic receptor LRP1. *J. Neurosci.* 33: 19276–19283.

206 Eimer, W.A. and Vassar, R. (2013). Neuron loss in the 5XFAD mouse model of Alzheimer's disease correlates with intraneuronal Abeta42 accumulation and Caspase-3 activation. *Mol. Neurodegener.* 8: 2.

207 Li, J., Kanekiyo, T., Shinohara, M. et al. (2012). Differential regulation of amyloid-beta endocytic trafficking and lysosomal degradation by apolipoprotein E isoforms. *J. Biol. Chem.* 287: 44593–44601.

208 Song, H.L., Shim, S., Kim, D.H. et al. (2014). Beta-amyloid is transmitted via neuronal connections along axonal membranes. *Ann. Neurol.* 75: 88–97.

209 Miyata, M. and Smith, J.D. (1996). Apolipoprotein E allele-specific antioxidant activity and effects on cytotoxicity by oxidative insults and beta-amyloid peptides. *Nat. Genet.* 14: 55–61.

210 Lauderback, C.M., Kanski, J., Hackett, J.M. et al. (2002). Apolipoprotein E modulates Alzheimer's Abeta(1-42)-induced oxidative damage to synaptosomes in an allele-specific manner. *Brain Res.* 924: 90–97.

211 Mabile, L., Lefebvre, C., Lavigne, J. et al. (2003). Secreted apolipoprotein E reduces macrophage-mediated LDL oxidation in an isoform-dependent way. *J. Cell Biochem.* 90: 766–776.

212 Pham, T., Kodvawala, A., and Hui, D.Y. (2005). The receptor binding domain of apolipoprotein E is responsible for its antioxidant activity. *Biochemistry* 44: 7577–7582.

213 Hung, Y.H., Robb, E.L., Volitakis, I. et al. (2009). Paradoxical condensation of copper with elevated beta-amyloid in lipid rafts under cellular copper deficiency conditions: implications for Alzheimer disease. *J. Biol. Chem.* 284: 21899–21907.

214 Hung, Y.H., Bush, A.I., and La Fontaine, S. (2013). Links between copper and cholesterol in Alzheimer's disease. *Front. Physiol.* 4: 111.

215 Wilhelmus, M.M., de Jager, M., Smit, A.B. et al. (2016). Catalytically active tissue transglutaminase colocalises with Abeta pathology in Alzheimer's disease mouse models. *Sci. Rep.* 6: 20569.

216 de Jager, M., Drukarch, B., Hofstee, M. et al. (2015). Tissue transglutaminase-catalysed cross-linking induces Apolipoprotein E multimers inhibiting Apolipoprotein E's protective effects towards amyloid-beta-induced toxicity. *J. Neurochem.* 134: 1116–1128.

217 Zhang, J., Wang, S., Huang, W. et al. (2016). Tissue Transglutaminase and its product Isopeptide are increased in Alzheimer's disease and APPswe/PS1dE9 double transgenic mice brains. *Mol. Neurobiol.* 53: 5066–5078.

218 Feola, J., Barton, A., Akbar, A. et al. (2017). Transglutaminase 2 modulation of NF-kappaB signaling in astrocytes is independent of its ability to mediate astrocytic viability in ischemic injury. *Brain Res.* 1668: 1–11.

219 Ientile, R., Curro, M., and Caccamo, D. (2015). Transglutaminase 2 and neuroinflammation. *Amino Acids* 47: 19–26.

220 May, P.C., Lampert-Etchells, M., Johnson, S.A. et al. (1990). Dynamics of gene expression for a hippocampal glycoprotein elevated in Alzheimer's disease and in response to experimental lesions in rat. *Neuron* 5: 831–839.

221 Shannan, B., Seifert, M., Leskov, K. et al. (2006). Challenge and promise: roles for clusterin in pathogenesis, progression and therapy of cancer. *Cell Death Differ.* 13: 12–19.

222 Bailey, R.W., Aronow, B., Harmony, J.A., and Griswold, M.D. (2002). Heat shock-initiated apoptosis is accelerated and removal of damaged cells is delayed in the testis of clusterin/ApoJ knock-out mice. *Biol. Reprod.* 66: 1042–1053.

223 Fritz, I.B., Burdzy, K., Setchell, B., and Blaschuk, O. (1983). Ram rete testis fluid contains a protein (clusterin) which influences cell-cell interactions in vitro. *Biol. Reprod.* 28: 1173–1188.

224 Mishima, K., Inoue, H., Nishiyama, T. et al. (2012). Transplantation of side population cells restores the function of damaged exocrine glands through clusterin. *Stem Cells* 30: 1925–1937.

225 Park, S., Mathis, K.W., and Lee, I.K. (2014). The physiological roles of apolipoprotein J/clusterin in metabolic and cardiovascular diseases. *Rev. Endocr. Metab. Disord.* 15: 45–53.

226 Trougakos, I.P., So, A., Jansen, B. et al. (2004). Silencing expression of the clusterin/apolipoprotein j gene in human cancer cells using small interfering RNA induces spontaneous apoptosis, reduced growth ability, and cell sensitization to genotoxic and oxidative stress. *Cancer Res.* 64: 1834–1842.

227 de Silva, H.V., Stuart, W.D., Duvic, C.R. et al. (1990). A 70-kDa apolipoprotein designated ApoJ is a marker for subclasses of human plasma high density lipoproteins. *J. Biol. Chem.* 265: 13240–13247.

228 Stuart, W.D., Krol, B., Jenkins, S.H., and Harmony, J.A. (1992). Structure and stability of apolipoprotein J-containing high-density lipoproteins. *Biochemistry* 31: 8552–8559.

229 Zilversmit, D.B., Hughes, L.B., and Balmer, J. (1975). Stimulation of cholesterol ester exchange by lipoprotein-free rabbit plasma. *Biochim. Biophys. Acta* 409: 393–398.

230 Pattnaik, N.M. and Zilversmit, D.B. (1979). Interaction of cholesteryl ester exchange protein with human plasma lipoproteins and phospholipid vesicles. *J. Biol. Chem.* 254: 2782–2786.

231 Brown, M.L., Inazu, A., Hesler, C.B. et al. (1989). Molecular basis of lipid transfer protein deficiency in a family with increased high-density lipoproteins. *Nature* 342: 448–451.

232 Inazu, A., Brown, M.L., Hesler, C.B. et al. (1990). Increased high-density lipoprotein levels caused by a common cholesteryl-ester transfer protein gene mutation. *N. Engl. J. Med.* 323: 1234–1238.

233 Moriyama, Y., Okamura, T., Inazu, A. et al. (1998). A low prevalence of coronary heart disease among subjects with increased high-density lipoprotein cholesterol levels, including those with plasma cholesteryl ester transfer protein deficiency. *Prev. Med.* 27: 659–667.

234 Zhang, J., Niimi, M., Yang, D. et al. (2017). Deficiency of cholesteryl ester transfer protein protects against atherosclerosis in rabbits. *Arterioscler. Thromb. Vasc. Biol.* 37: 1068–1075.

235 Navab, M., Hama-Levy, S., Van Lenten, B.J. et al. (1997). Mildly oxidized LDL induces an increased apolipoprotein J/paraoxonase ratio. *J. Clin. Invest.* 99: 2005–2019.

236 Costa, L.G., de Laat, R., Dao, K. et al. (2014). Paraoxonase-2 (PON2) in brain and its potential role in neuroprotection. *Neurotoxicology* 43: 3–9.

237 Ng, C.J., Wadleigh, D.J., Gangopadhyay, A. et al. (2001). Paraoxonase-2 is a ubiquitously expressed protein with antioxidant properties and is capable of preventing cell-mediated oxidative modification of low density lipoprotein. *J. Biol. Chem.* 276: 44444–44449.

238 Humphreys, D.T., Carver, J.A., Easterbrook-Smith, S.B., and Wilson, M.R. (1999). Clusterin has chaperone-like activity similar to that of small heat shock proteins. *J. Biol. Chem.* 274: 6875–6881.

239 Gelissen, I.C., Hochgrebe, T., Wilson, M.R. et al. (1998). Apolipoprotein J (clusterin) induces cholesterol export from macrophage-foam cells: a potential anti-atherogenic function? *Biochem. J.* 331 (Pt 1: 231–237.

240 Leeb, C., Eresheim, C., and Nimpf, J. (2014). Clusterin is a ligand for apolipoprotein E receptor 2 (ApoER2) and very low density lipoprotein receptor (VLDLR) and signals via the Reelin-signaling pathway. *J. Biol. Chem.* 289: 4161–4172.

241 DeMattos, R.B., Cirrito, J.R., Parsadanian, M. et al. (2004). ApoE and clusterin cooperatively suppress Abeta levels and deposition: evidence that ApoE regulates extracellular Abeta metabolism in vivo. *Neuron* 41: 193–202.

242 Howlett, D.R., Hortobagyi, T., and Francis, P.T. (2013). Clusterin associates specifically with Abeta40 in Alzheimer's disease brain tissue. *Brain Pathol.* 23: 623–632.

243 Wilson, M.R., Yerbury, J.J., and Poon, S. (2008). Potential roles of abundant extracellular chaperones in the control of amyloid formation and toxicity. *Mol. Biosyst.* 4: 42–52.

244 Wojtas, A.M., Kang, S.S., Olley, B.M. et al. (2017). Loss of clusterin shifts amyloid deposition to the cerebrovasculature via disruption of perivascular drainage pathways. *Proc. Natl. Acad. Sci. U.S.A.* 114: E6962–E6971.

245 Wolf, B.B., Lopes, M.B., VandenBerg, S.R., and Gonias, S.L. (1992). Characterization and immunohistochemical localization of alpha 2-macroglobulin receptor (low-density lipoprotein receptor-related protein) in human brain. *Am. J. Pathol.* 141: 37–42.

246 Bu, G., Maksymovitch, E.A., Nerbonne, J.M., and Schwartz, A.L. (1994). Expression and function of the low density lipoprotein receptor-related protein (LRP) in mammalian central neurons. *J. Biol. Chem.* 269: 18521–18528.

247 Lillis, A.P., Mikhailenko, I., and Strickland, D.K. (2005). Beyond endocytosis: LRP function in cell migration, proliferation and vascular permeability. *J. Thromb. Haemost.* 3: 1884–1893.

248 Kang, D.E., Saitoh, T., Chen, X. et al. (1997). Genetic association of the low-density lipoprotein receptor-related protein gene (LRP), an apolipoprotein E receptor, with late-onset Alzheimer's disease. *Neurology* 49: 56–61.

249 Ramanathan, A., Nelson, A.R., Sagare, A.P., and Zlokovic, B.V. (2015). Impaired vascular-mediated clearance of brain amyloid beta in Alzheimer's disease: the role, regulation and restoration of LRP1. *Front. Aging Neurosci.* 7: 136.

250 Sagare, A., Deane, R., Bell, R.D. et al. (2007). Clearance of amyloid-beta by circulating lipoprotein receptors. *Nat. Med.* 13: 1029–1031.

251 Tamaki, C., Ohtsuki, S., Iwatsubo, T. et al. (2006). Major involvement of low-density lipoprotein receptor-related protein 1 in the clearance of plasma free amyloid beta-peptide by the liver. *Pharm. Res.* 23: 1407–1416.

252 Donahue, J.E., Flaherty, S.L., Johanson, C.E. et al. (2006). RAGE, LRP-1, and amyloid-beta protein in Alzheimer's disease. *Acta Neuropathol.* 112: 405–415.

253 Sagare, A.P., Deane, R., Zetterberg, H. et al. (2011). Impaired lipoprotein receptor-mediated peripheral binding of plasma amyloid-beta is an early biomarker for mild cognitive impairment preceding Alzheimer's disease. *J. Alzheimers Dis.* 24: 25–34.

254 Llorente-Cortes, V., Costales, P., Bernues, J. et al. (2006). Sterol regulatory element-binding protein-2 negatively regulates low density lipoprotein receptor-related protein transcription. *J. Mol. Biol.* 359: 950–960.

255 Llorente-Cortes, V., Royo, T., Otero-Vinas, M. et al. (2007). Sterol regulatory element binding proteins downregulate LDL receptor-related protein (LRP1) expression and LRP1-mediated aggregated LDL uptake by human macrophages. *Cardiovasc. Res.* 74: 526–536.

256 Winkler, E.A., Nishida, Y., Sagare, A.P. et al. (2015). GLUT1 reductions exacerbate Alzheimer's disease vasculo-neuronal dysfunction and degeneration. *Nat. Neurosci.* 18: 521–530.

257 Kalaria, R.N. and Harik, S.I. (1989). Reduced glucose transporter at the blood-brain barrier and in cerebral cortex in Alzheimer disease. *J. Neurochem.* 53: 1083–1088.

258 Kato, T., Inui, Y., Nakamura, A., and Ito, K. (2016). Brain fluorodeoxyglucose (FDG) PET in dementia. *Ageing Res. Rev.* 30: 73–84.

259 Simpson, I.A., Chundu, K.R., Davies-Hill, T. et al. (1994). Decreased concentrations of GLUT1 and GLUT3 glucose transporters in the brains of patients with Alzheimer's disease. *Ann. Neurol.* 35: 546–551.

260 Schilling, S., Tzourio, C., Soumare, A. et al. (2017). Differential associations of plasma lipids with incident dementia and dementia subtypes in the 3C study: a longitudinal, population-based prospective cohort study. *PLoS Med.* 14: e1002265.

261 Reitz, C., Tang, M.X., Schupf, N. et al. (2010). Association of higher levels of high-density lipoprotein cholesterol in elderly individuals and lower risk of late-onset Alzheimer disease. *Arch. Neurol.* 67: 1491–1497.

262 Helzner, E.P., Luchsinger, J.A., Scarmeas, N. et al. (2009). Contribution of vascular risk factors to the progression in Alzheimer disease. *Arch. Neurol.* 66: 343–348.

263 Moroney, J.T., Tang, M.X., Berglund, L. et al. (1999). Low-density lipoprotein cholesterol and the risk of dementia with stroke. *JAMA* 282: 254–260.

264 Sperling, R.A., Aisen, P.S., Beckett, L.A. et al. (2011). Toward defining the preclinical stages of Alzheimer's disease: recommendations from the National Institute on Aging-Alzheimer's Association workgroups on diagnostic guidelines for Alzheimer's disease. *Alzheimers Dement.* 7: 280–292.

265 Anstey, K.J., Ashby-Mitchell, K., and Peters, R. (2017). Updating the evidence on the association between serum cholesterol and risk of late-life dementia: review and meta-analysis. *J. Alzheimers Dis.* 56: 215–228.

266 Anstey, K.J., Lipnicki, D.M., and Low, L.F. (2008). Cholesterol as a risk factor for dementia and cognitive decline: a systematic review of prospective studies with meta-analysis. *Am. J. Geriat. Psychiatry* 16: 343–354.

267 Koch, M. and Jensen, M.K. (2016). HDL-cholesterol and apolipoproteins in relation to dementia. *Curr. Opin. Lipidol.* 27: 76–87.

268 Ancelin, M.L., Ripoche, E., Dupuy, A.M. et al. (2013). Sex differences in the associations between lipid levels and incident dementia. *J. Alzheimers Dis.* 34: 519–528.

269 Macedo, A.F., Taylor, F.C., Casas, J.P. et al. (2014). Unintended effects of statins from observational studies in the general population: systematic review and meta-analysis. *BMC Med.* 12: 51.

270 McGuinness, B., Craig, D., Bullock, R., and Passmore, P. (2016). Statins for the prevention of dementia. *Cochrane Database Syst. Rev.* CD003160. https://doi.org/10.1002/14651858.CD003160.pub3.

271 Geifman, N., Brinton, R.D., Kennedy, R.E. et al. (2017). Evidence for benefit of statins to modify cognitive decline and risk in Alzheimer's disease. *Alzheimers Res. Ther.* 9: 10.

272 Shinohara, M., Sato, N., Shimamura, M. et al. (2014). Possible modification of Alzheimer's disease by statins in midlife: interactions with genetic and non-genetic risk factors. *Front. Aging Neurosci.* 6: 71.

273 Rakesh, G., Szabo, S.T., Alexopoulos, G.S., and Zannas, A.S. (2017). Strategies for dementia prevention: latest evidence and implications. *Ther. Adv. Chronic Dis.* 8: 121–136.

274 Simons, K. and Ehehalt, R. (2002). Cholesterol, lipid rafts, and disease. *J. Clin. Invest.* 110: 597–603.

275 Schneider, A., Schulz-Schaeffer, W., Hartmann, T. et al. (2006). Cholesterol depletion reduces aggregation of amyloid-beta peptide in hippocampal neurons. *Neurobiol. Dis.* 23: 573–577.

276 Allen, J.A., Halverson-Tamboli, R.A., and Rasenick, M.M. (2007). Lipid raft microdomains and neurotransmitter signalling. *Nat. Rev. Neurosci.* 8: 128–140.

277 Reed, T., Perluigi, M., Sultana, R. et al. (2008). Redox proteomic identification of 4-hydroxy-2-nonenal-modified brain proteins in amnestic mild cognitive impairment: insight into the role of lipid peroxidation in the progression and pathogenesis of Alzheimer's disease. *Neurobiol. Dis.* 30: 107–120.

278 Suzuki, T. and Suzuki, Y. (2006). Virus infection and lipid rafts. *Biol. Pharm. Bull.* 29: 1538–1541.

279 Hicks, D.A., Nalivaeva, N.N., and Turner, A.J. (2012). Lipid rafts and Alzheimer's disease: protein-lipid interactions and perturbation of signaling. *Front. Physiol.* 3: 189.

280 Shie, F.S., Jin, L.W., Cook, D.G. et al. (2002). Diet-induced hypercholesterolemia enhances brain a beta accumulation in transgenic mice. *Neuroreport* 13: 455–459.

281 Refolo, L.M., Malester, B., LaFrancois, J. et al. (2000). Hypercholesterolemia accelerates the Alzheimer's amyloid pathology in a transgenic mouse model. *Neurobiol. Dis.* 7: 321–331.

282 Sparks, D.L., Scheff, S.W., Hunsaker, J.C. et al. (1994). Induction of Alzheimer-like beta-amyloid immunoreactivity in the brains of rabbits with dietary cholesterol. *Exp. Neurol.* 126: 88–94.

283 Lim, W.L., Lam, S.M., Shui, G. et al. (2013). Effects of a high-fat, high-cholesterol diet on brain lipid profiles in apolipoprotein E epsilon3 and epsilon4 knock-in mice. *Neurobiol. Aging* 34: 2217–2224.

284 Wahrle, S., Das, P., Nyborg, A.C. et al. (2002). Cholesterol-dependent gamma-secretase activity in buoyant cholesterol-rich membrane microdomains. *Neurobiol. Dis.* 9: 11–23.

285 Simons, M., Keller, P., De Strooper, B. et al. (1998). Cholesterol depletion inhibits the generation of beta-amyloid in hippocampal neurons. *Proc. Natl. Acad. Sci. U.S.A.* 95: 6460–6464.

286 Kojro, E., Gimpl, G., Lammich, S. et al. (2001). Low cholesterol stimulates the non-amyloidogenic pathway by its effect on the alpha -secretase ADAM 10. *Proc. Natl. Acad. Sci. U.S.A.* 98: 5815–5820.

287 Diaz, M., Fabelo, N., Martin, V. et al. (2015). Biophysical alterations in lipid rafts from human cerebral cortex associate with increased BACE1/AbetaPP interaction in early stages of Alzheimer's disease. *J. Alzheimers Dis.* 43: 1185–1198.

288 Fabelo, N., Martin, V., Marin, R. et al. (2014). Altered lipid composition in cortical lipid rafts occurs at early stages of sporadic Alzheimer's disease and facilitates APP/BACE1 interactions. *Neurobiol. Aging* 35: 1801–1812.

289 Santos, G., Diaz, M., and Torres, N.V. (2016). Lipid raft size and lipid mobility in non-raft domains increase during aging and are exacerbated in APP/PS1 mice model of Alzheimer's disease: predictions from an agent-based mathematical model. *Front. Physiol.* 7: 90.

290 Farooqui, A.A. and Horrocks, L.A. (2001). Plasmalogens: workhorse lipids of membranes in normal and injured neurons and glia. *Neuroscientist* 7: 232–245.

291 Goodenowe, D.B., Cook, L.L., Liu, J. et al. (2007). Peripheral ethanolamine plasmalogen deficiency: a logical causative factor in Alzheimer's disease and dementia. *J. Lipid Res.* 48: 2485–2498.

292 Han, X., Holtzman, D.M., and McKeel, D.W. Jr. (2001). Plasmalogen deficiency in early Alzheimer's disease subjects and in animal models: molecular characterization using electrospray ionization mass spectrometry. *J. Neurochem.* 77: 1168–1180.

293 Igarashi, M., Ma, K., Gao, F. et al. (2011). Disturbed choline plasmalogen and phospholipid fatty acid concentrations in Alzheimer's disease prefrontal cortex. *J. Alzheimers Dis.* 24: 507–517.

294 Chan, R.B., Oliveira, T.G., Cortes, E.P. et al. (2012). Comparative lipidomic analysis of mouse and human brain with Alzheimer disease. *J. Biol. Chem.* 287: 2678–2688.

295 Wood, P.L., Mankidy, R., Ritchie, S. et al. (2010). Circulating plasmalogen levels and Alzheimer disease assessment scale-cognitive scores in Alzheimer patients. *J. Psychiatry Neurosci.* 35: 59–62.

296 Mulder, C., Wahlund, L.O., Teerlink, T. et al. (2003). Decreased lysophosphatidylcholine/phosphatidylcholine ratio in cerebrospinal fluid in Alzheimer's disease. *J. Neural. Transm. (Vienna)* 110: 949–955.

297 Li, J., Yen, C., Liaw, D. et al. (1997). PTEN, a putative protein tyrosine phosphatase gene mutated in human brain, breast, and prostate cancer. *Science* 275: 1943–1947.

298 Lee, J.W., Soung, Y.H., Kim, S.Y. et al. (2005). PIK3CA gene is frequently mutated in breast carcinomas and hepatocellular carcinomas. *Oncogene* 24: 1477–1480.

299 Suchy, S.F. and Nussbaum, R.L. (2002). The deficiency of PIP2 5-phosphatase in Lowe syndrome affects actin polymerization. *Am. J. Hum. Genet.* 71: 1420–1427.

300 Zhang, X., Jefferson, A.B., Auethavekiat, V., and Majerus, P.W. (1995). The protein deficient in Lowe syndrome is a phosphatidylinositol-4,5-bisphosphate 5-phosphatase. *Proc. Natl. Acad. Sci. U.S.A.* 92: 4853–4856.

301 Marion, E., Kaisaki, P.J., Pouillon, V. et al. (2002). The gene INPPL1, encoding the lipid phosphatase SHIP2, is a candidate for type 2 diabetes in rat and man. *Diabetes* 51: 2012–2017.

302 Landman, N., Jeong, S.Y., Shin, S.Y. et al. (2006). Presenilin mutations linked to familial Alzheimer's disease cause an imbalance in phosphatidylinositol 4,5-bisphosphate metabolism. *Proc. Natl. Acad. Sci. U.S.A.* 103: 19524–19529.

303 Nagan, N. and Zoeller, R.A. (2001). Plasmalogens: biosynthesis and functions. *Prog. Lipid Res.* 40: 199–229.

304 Messias, M.C.F., Mecatti, G.C., Priolli, D.G., and de Oliveira Carvalho, P. (2018). Plasmalogen lipids: functional mechanism and their involvement in gastrointestinal cancer. *Lipids Health Dis.* 17: 41.

305 Maeba, R., Nishimukai, M., Sakasegawa, S. et al. (2015). Plasma/serum Plasmalogens: methods of analysis and clinical significance. *Adv. Clin. Chem.* 70: 31–94.

306 Anderson, B.M. and Ma, D.W. (2009). Are all n-3 polyunsaturated fatty acids created equal? *Lipids Health Dis.* 8: 33.

307 Simopoulos, A.P. (2016). An increase in the Omega-6/Omega-3 fatty acid ratio increases the risk for obesity. *Nutrients* 8: 128.

308 Massiera, F., Barbry, P., Guesnet, P. et al. (2010). A western-like fat diet is sufficient to induce a gradual enhancement in fat mass over generations. *J. Lipid Res.* 51: 2352–2361.

309 Chen, X., Chen, C., Fan, S. et al. (2018). Omega-3 polyunsaturated fatty acid attenuates the inflammatory response by modulating microglia polarization through SIRT1-mediated deacetylation of the HMGB1/NF-kappaB pathway following experimental traumatic brain injury. *J. Neuroinflamm.* 15: 116.

310 Kang, J.X. (2003). The importance of omega-6/omega-3 fatty acid ratio in cell function: the gene transfer of omega-3 fatty acid desaturase. *World Rev. Nutr. Diet.* 92: 23–36.

311 Kromhout, D. and de Goede, J. (2014). Update on cardiometabolic health effects of omega-3 fatty acids. *Curr. Opin. Lipidol.* 25: 85–90.

312 Simopoulos, A.P. (2008). The importance of the omega-6/omega-3 fatty acid ratio in cardiovascular disease and other chronic diseases. *Exp. Biol. Med. (Maywood)* 233: 674–688.

313 Kim, J.H., Song, J., and Park, K.W. (2015). The multifaceted factor peroxisome proliferator-activated receptor gamma (PPARgamma) in metabolism, immunity, and cancer. *Arch. Pharmacal Res.* 38: 302–312.

314 Im, D.S. (2017). FFA4 (GPR120) as a fatty acid sensor involved in appetite control, insulin sensitivity and inflammation regulation. *Mol. Aspects Med.*

315 Zarate, R., El Jaber-Vazdekis, N., Tejera, N. et al. (2017). Significance of long chain polyunsaturated fatty acids in human health. *Clin. Transl. Med.* 6: 25.

316 de Gomez Dumm, I.N. and Brenner, R.R. (1975). Oxidative desaturation of alpha-linoleic, linoleic, and stearic acids by human liver microsomes. *Lipids* 10: 315–317.

317 Hagve, T.A. and Christophersen, B.O. (1984). Effect of dietary fats on arachidonic acid and eicosapentaenoic acid biosynthesis and conversion to C22 fatty acids in isolated rat liver cells. *Biochim. Biophys. Acta* 796: 205–217.

318 Simopoulos, A.P. (2011). Evolutionary aspects of diet: the omega-6/omega-3 ratio and the brain. *Mol. Neurobiol.* 44: 203–215.

319 van Vliet, T. and Katan, M.B. (1990). Lower ratio of n-3 to n-6 fatty acids in cultured than in wild fish. *Am. J. Clin. Nutr.* 51: 1–2.

320 Guil-Guerrero, J.L., Tikhonov, A., Rodriguez-Garcia, I. et al. (2014). The fat from frozen mammals reveals sources of essential fatty acids suitable for Palaeolithic and Neolithic humans. *PLoS One* 9: e84480.

321 Kuipers, R.S., Luxwolda, M.F., Dijck-Brouwer, D.A. et al. (2010). Estimated macronutrient and fatty acid intakes from an east African Paleolithic diet. *Br. J. Nutr.* 104: 1666–1687.

322 Enos, R.T., Velazquez, K.T., McClellan, J.L. et al. (2014). Reducing the dietary omega-6:omega-3 utilizing alpha-linolenic acid; not a sufficient therapy for attenuating high-fat-diet-induced obesity development nor related detrimental metabolic and adipose tissue inflammatory outcomes. *PLoS One* 9: e94897.

323 Di Daniele, N., Noce, A., Vidiri, M.F. et al. (2017). Impact of Mediterranean diet on metabolic syndrome, cancer and longevity. *Oncotarget* 8: 8947–8979.

324 Serra-Majem, L., Roman, B., and Estruch, R. (2006). Scientific evidence of interventions using the Mediterranean diet: a systematic review. *Nutr. Rev.* 64: S27–S47.

325 Dyall, S.C. (2015). Long-chain omega-3 fatty acids and the brain: a review of the independent and shared effects of EPA, DPA and DHA. *Front. Aging Neurosci.* 7: 52.

326 Fitzgerald, K.C., O'Reilly, E.J., Falcone, G.J. et al. (2014). Dietary omega-3 polyunsaturated fatty acid intake and risk for amyotrophic lateral sclerosis. *JAMA Neurol.* 71: 1102–1110.

327 McNamara, R.K. (2016). Role of omega-3 fatty acids in the etiology, treatment, and prevention of depression: current status and future directions. *J. Nutr. Intermed. Metab.* 5: 96–106.

328 Saunders, E.F., Ramsden, C.E., Sherazy, M.S. et al. (2016). Omega-3 and omega-6 polyunsaturated fatty acids in bipolar disorder: a review of biomarker and treatment studies. *J. Clin. Psychiatry* 77: e1301–e1308.

329 Futerman, A.H. and Riezman, H. (2005). The ins and outs of sphingolipid synthesis. *Trends Cell Biol.* 15: 312–318.

330 Zinser, E.G., Hartmann, T., and Grimm, M.O. (2007). Amyloid beta-protein and lipid metabolism. *Biochim. Biophys. Acta* 1768: 1991–2001.

331 Cutler, R.G., Kelly, J., Storie, K. et al. (2004). Involvement of oxidative stress-induced abnormalities in ceramide and cholesterol metabolism in brain aging and Alzheimer's disease. *Proc. Natl. Acad. Sci. U.S.A.* 101: 2070–2075.

332 Han, X., D, M.H., McKeel, D.W. Jr. et al. (2002). Substantial sulfatide deficiency and ceramide elevation in very early Alzheimer's disease: potential role in disease pathogenesis. *J. Neurochem.* 82: 809–818.

333 Satoi, H., Tomimoto, H., Ohtani, R. et al. (2005). Astroglial expression of ceramide in Alzheimer's disease brains: a role during neuronal apoptosis. *Neuroscience* 130: 657–666.

334 Haughey, N.J., Bandaru, V.V., Bae, M., and Mattson, M.P. (2010). Roles for dysfunctional sphingolipid metabolism in Alzheimer's disease neuropathogenesis. *Biochim. Biophys. Acta* 1801: 878–886.

335 Alessenko, A.V., Bugrova, A.E., and Dudnik, L.B. (2004). Connection of lipid peroxide oxidation with the sphingomyelin pathway in the development of Alzheimer's disease. *Biochem. Soc. Trans.* 32: 144–146.

336 Han, X., Rozen, S., Boyle, S.H. et al. (2011). Metabolomics in early Alzheimer's disease: identification of altered plasma sphingolipidome using shotgun lipidomics. *PLoS One* 6: e21643.

337 Fonteh, A.N., Ormseth, C., Chiang, J. et al. (2015). Sphingolipid metabolism correlates with cerebrospinal fluid beta amyloid levels in Alzheimer's disease. *PLoS One* 10: e0125597.

338 Puglielli, L., Ellis, B.C., Saunders, A.J., and Kovacs, D.M. (2003). Ceramide stabilizes beta-site amyloid precursor protein-cleaving enzyme 1 and promotes amyloid beta-peptide biogenesis. *J. Biol. Chem.* 278: 19777–19783.

339 Young, M.M., Kester, M., and Wang, H.G. (2013). Sphingolipids: regulators of crosstalk between apoptosis and autophagy. *J. Lipid Res.* 54: 5–19.

340 Takahashi, T. and Suzuki, T. (2012). Role of sulfatide in normal and pathological cells and tissues. *J. Lipid Res.* 53: 1437–1450.

341 Cheng, H., Xu, J., McKeel, D.W. Jr., and Han, X. (2003). Specificity and potential mechanism of sulfatide deficiency in Alzheimer's disease: an electrospray ionization mass spectrometric study. *Cell Mol. Biol. (Noisy-le-grand)* 49: 809–818.

342 Cheng, H., Wang, M., Li, J.L. et al. (2013). Specific changes of sulfatide levels in individuals with pre-clinical Alzheimer's disease: an early event in disease pathogenesis. *J. Neurochem.* 127: 733–738.

343 Han, X. (2007). Potential mechanisms contributing to sulfatide depletion at the earliest clinically recognizable stage of Alzheimer's disease: a tale of shotgun lipidomics. *J. Neurochem.* 103 (Suppl 1): 171–179.

344 Zeng, Y. and Han, X. (2008). Sulfatides facilitate apolipoprotein E-mediated amyloid-beta peptide clearance through an endocytotic pathway. *J. Neurochem.* 106: 1275–1286.

345 Cheng, H., Zhou, Y., Holtzman, D.M., and Han, X. (2010). Apolipoprotein E mediates sulfatide depletion in animal models of Alzheimer's disease. *Neurobiol. Aging* 31: 1188–1196.

346 Hoshino, T., Mahmood, M.I., Mori, K., and Matsuzaki, K. (2013). Binding and aggregation mechanism of amyloid beta-peptides onto the GM1 ganglioside-containing lipid membrane. *J. Phys. Chem. B* 117: 8085–8094.

347 Kakio, A., Nishimoto, S., Kozutsumi, Y., and Matsuzaki, K. (2003). Formation of a membrane-active form of amyloid beta-protein in raft-like model membranes. *Biochem. Biophys. Res. Commun.* 303: 514–518.

348 Ariga, T., McDonald, M.P., and Yu, R.K. (2008). Role of ganglioside metabolism in the pathogenesis of Alzheimer's disease – a review. *J. Lipid Res.* 49: 1157–1175.

349 Fantini, J. and Yahi, N. (2010). Molecular insights into amyloid regulation by membrane cholesterol and sphingolipids: common mechanisms in neurodegenerative diseases. *Expert Rev. Mol. Med.* 12: e27.

350 Grimm, M.O., Zinser, E.G., Grosgen, S. et al. (2012). Amyloid precursor protein (APP) mediated regulation of ganglioside homeostasis linking Alzheimer's disease pathology with ganglioside metabolism. *PLoS One* 7: e34095.

351 Grimm, M.O., Hundsdorfer, B., Grosgen, S. et al. (2014). PS dependent APP cleavage regulates glucosylceramide synthase and is affected in Alzheimer's disease. *Cell Physiol. Biochem.* 34: 92–110.

352 Bernardo, A., Harrison, F.E., McCord, M. et al. (2009). Elimination of GD3 synthase improves memory and reduces amyloid-beta plaque load in transgenic mice. *Neurobiol. Aging* 30: 1777–1791.

353 Malisan, F. and Testi, R. (2002). GD3 ganglioside and apoptosis. *Biochim. Biophys. Acta* 1585: 179–187.

8

Inflammation in Alzheimer's Disease, and Prevention with Antioxidants and Phenolic Compounds – What Are the Most Promising Candidates?

Matthew J. Sharman[1], Giuseppe Verdile[2,3,4], Shanmugam Kirubakaran[5] and Gerald Münch[5]

[1] School of Health Sciences, University of Tasmania, Locked Bag 1322, Launceston, TAS, Australia
[2] School of Pharmacy and Biomedical Sciences, Faculty of Health Sciences, Curtin Health Innovation Research Institute, Curtin University, Bentley, WA, Australia
[3] Centre of Excellence for Alzheimer's Disease Research and Care, School of Medical and Health Sciences, Edith Cowan University, Joondalup, Australia
[4] Australian Alzheimer's Research Foundation, Ralph and Patricia Sarich Neuroscience Research Institute, Nedlands, Australia
[5] Department of Pharmacology and Molecular Medicine Research Group, School of Medicine, Western Sydney University, NSW, Australia

8.1 Introduction

Alzheimer's disease (AD) is the most common age-related neurodegenerative disorder, which currently affects about 30 million people worldwide. The brain pathology in AD that ultimately leads to cognitive decline and profound dementia is characterised by extensive synaptic and neuronal loss, the formation of intracellular neurofibrillary tangles (NFT) and the extracellular deposition of Aβ fibrils and plaques in susceptible regions of the brain. This is accompanied by a chronic inflammatory response including microglial infiltration, as well as extensive oxidative damage. Mitochondrial damage, oxidative stress, and inflammation may be initiating factors of AD, and/or possibly the overproduction or reduced clearance of toxic Aβ peptides and aggregates. Importantly, a destructive cycle begins with this pathology, as oxidative stress and inflammation promote Aβ production and hyperphosphorylation of tau, and in turn, these pathologies also increase oxidative stress and inflammation. As a result of the involvement of the two proteins Aβ and microtubule-associated protein tau (MAP-tau) in AD pathology, therapeutic mechanisms to reduce the development of these two main disease pathologies have been studied at length over the past three decades [1, 2]. Unfortunately, such studies have not led to an FDA (US Food and Drug Administration)-approved treatment yet. In this book chapter, we will focus on neuroinflammation as the major therapeutic target.

8.2 Inflammation and the Immune Response in AD

8.2.1 The Role of Microglia and Astrocytes in Chronic Inflammation in AD

The two major types of brain cells that participate in the immune/inflammatory response are astrocytes and microglia. Microglia and astrocytes are often found

Neurodegeneration and Alzheimer's Disease: The Role of Diabetes, Genetics, Hormones, and Lifestyle,
First Edition. Edited by Ralph N. Martins, Charles S. Brennan, W.M.A.D. Binosha Fernando, Margaret A. Brennan and Stephanie J. Fuller.
© 2019 John Wiley & Sons Ltd. Published 2019 by John Wiley & Sons Ltd.

associated with Alzheimer's amyloid plaques. These cells function together in response to brain injury. This occurs through gliosis, one inflammatory response present in AD, where fibrous astrocytes become more numerous, and become activated and involved in prostaglandin/arachidonic acid-mediated inflammation. Microglial proliferation and activation are then thought to be further promoted, or microglial cytotoxic activity is modulated, by the growth factors produced by astrocyte reactions. Glial cells generate many molecules associated with inflammatory and immune functions. Inflammatory cytokines and other microglia-derived factors account for the neurotoxicity in gliosis, while reactive astrocyte products overall tend to be neuroprotective [3].

The inflammatory response at the site of injury, however, also represents a source of numerous growth factors and cytokines, with trophic, mitogenic, chemotactic, and angiogenic activities (Table 8.1), in addition to reactive oxygen species and reactive nitrogen species (ROS/RNS) [3].

It is well understood that the overproduction of microglial pro-inflammatory mediators is neurotoxic, which is why it is believed by many that systemic inflammation

Table 8.1 Secretory products of microglia and astrocytes that may have damaging or protective functions in AD.

Factor	Microglia	Astrocytes
Cytokines	IL-1α & β, IL-3, IL-5, IL-6, IL-8, IL-12, IL-18, INF-α, INF-γ; TNF-α	IL-1α & β, IL-3, IL-5, IL-6, IL-8, IL-12, IL-18, INF-γ, CSF-1, GSF, CSF, TNF-α
Coagulation factors	Plasminogen and urokinase type plasminogen activator	Tissue plasminogen and urokinase type plasminogen activator
Complement proteins	C1, C3, C4	C3, C4, C6, C7, C8, C9, Factor B, Factor I, membrane cofactor protein, CD46, clusterin, vitronectin
Eicosanoides	Prostaglandin D2, leucotriene C4	
Growth factors	NGF, TGF-α &-β, Basic FGF	NGF, TGF-α &-β, Basic FGF, CNTF, IGF-1, GDNF
Reactive N_2 intermediates	Nitric oxide	Nitric oxide
Reactive O_2 intermediates	Superoxide ions	
Proteases and protease inhibitors	Metalloproteinase inhibitors TIMP-1 and TIMP-2	Protease nexin 1, α-1-antichymotrypsin, α-2-macroglobulin, cathepsin G
Transport proteins		Apolipoprotein D, apolipoprotein B
Matrix proteins		Laminin, fibronectin, tenascin, heparan-, chondroitin-, and dermatin-sulfate proteoglycans
Adhesion factors		VCAM-1, NCAM, NCAM-1 and ICAM-2

Abbreviations: IL, interleukin; INF-α, interferon-α; TNF-α, tumour necrosis factor-α; NGF, nerve growth factor; TGF-α &-β, transforming growth factor α & β; Basic FGF, basic fibroblast growth factor; CNTF, ciliary neurotrophic factor; CSF-1, colony stimulating factor-1; TIMP, tissue inhibitor of metalloproteinase; VCAM-1, vascular cell adhesion molecule-1; NCAM, neural cell adhesion molecule; ICAM-2, intercellular adhesion molecule-2; IGF-1, insulin-like growth factor-1; GDNF, glial derived neurotrophic factor
Source: Adapted from [3–5].

(that also escalates with ageing) exacerbates or possibly triggers neurological diseases such as AD, Parkinson's disease, and motor neuron disease. As mentioned above, Aβ is able to activate microglia, initiating or aggravating an inflammatory response; and inflammation in turn can increase Aβ production.

Recent studies have suggested there are two types of activated microglia, namely the M1 and M2 phenotype microglia, with the M1 microglia inducing a pro-inflammatory response, and the M2 cells having a neuroprotective role – reducing inflammation, phagocytosing Aβ, and reducing Aβ-mediated toxicity [6–9]. The polarisation and balance of microglia in the CNS is important, as it has been shown to influence learning and memory [10]. Clearly microglia are not always harmful – there is evidence they may reduce AD pathogenic mechanisms by contributing to the clearance of Aβ, since they phagocytose Aβ and release enzymes responsible for Aβ degradation. Microglia also secrete growth factors and anti-inflammatory cytokines, which are neuroprotective. These will most likely be the M2 microglial cells. The normal microglial phagocytosis of damaged cells is also important for maintaining a healthy brain environment, as damaged cells can become potent inflammatory stimuli, resulting in further tissue damage. On the other hand, microglia become less efficient at these processes as people age; they can also become overactive in response to stimulation, for example by higher levels of Aβ, or due to chronic age-related conditions such as type 2 diabetes, cardiovascular disease, and obesity. Furthermore, phagocytosis by microglia can also activate a respiratory 'burst', which produces toxic ROS [11]. A respiratory burst (sometimes called oxidative burst) is the rapid release of ROS (superoxide radicals and hydrogen peroxide) from cells.

Mouse models of AD have recently provided further evidence of the overstimulation and ageing aspects of microglia. For example, studies of AD-model brain slice cultures have demonstrated that the addition of young microglia or their conditioned medium could induce microglial proliferation and reduce amyloid plaque size [12]. Other studies have shown that microglia isolated from aged mouse brains have a gene expression pattern aimed at pro-inflammatory processes, phagocytosis, and lipid homeostasis. Furthermore, studies of middle-aged people's brains have shown that signs of inflammation are already present, by the age-dependent increases in CD68 (associated with phagocytosis) and HLA-DR (associated with antigen presentation) seen in microglia of white matter [13], and increased microglial activity is also detectable in early-onset AD brain tissue, as well as in late-onset AD cases [13].

Tau hyperphosphorylation and NFT formation, which occur in several neurodegenerative conditions, have traditionally been considered to be a cause of neuroinflammation, yet as we have mentioned above, more recent studies indicate chronic inflammation is likely to be an initiating factor in these pathologies. For example, gene variants that have been linked to AD involve many genes that impact microglial function and complement signalling (reviewed in [14, 15]). Furthermore, studies of traumatic brain injury, a well-known precursor to NFT formation in later life, have shown that the neuroinflammation that occurs after injury can persist for years post-injury, and that any future injuries tend to provoke over-reactive glial responses in later years, most likely increasing tau pathology (for reviews see [16, 17]).

Although astrocytes are important in maintaining neuronal health by reacting as part of the normal immune responses of the brain, astrogliosis can also contribute to neuronal inflammation. As can be seen in Table 8.1, many signals and cytokines secreted by microglia are also secreted by astrocytes. However, some microglial products such as IL-1β, TNF-α, IL-6, and C1q have been shown to co-activate astrocytes which can lead to neuronal dysfunction and death. Recently it was shown that microglia can activate a subtype of astrocytes, these 'A1' astrocytes lose their ability to promote neuronal survival, growth, synaptogenesis, and phagocytosis, and are also highly toxic to neurons, though the exact mechanism of toxicity is still unknown [18]. These astrocytes have been detected in several neurodegenerative conditions including AD, Huntington's disease, Parkinson's disease, multiple sclerosis, and amyotrophic lateral sclerosis, underscoring the central role of chronic microglial and astrocyte activation in neurodegenerative conditions. The A1 astrocytes were shown to be induced specifically by microglial secretion of interleukin 1-α (IL-1α), tumour necrosis factor-α (TNF-α), and C1q (first subcomponent of C1 complex in complement activation) [18].

Interestingly, the common occurrence of an over-reactive microglial response has also been shown in retinal neurodegeneration, which occurs in glaucoma. Furthermore, AD, Parkinson's disease, and glaucoma all have Aβ, α-synuclein, and phospho-tau deposits in the eye, and primary open-angle glaucoma has recently been found to be a risk factor for AD [19–21]. These findings should be explored further, as the eye is obviously easily accessible and is being investigated for the purposes of diagnosis of neurodegenerative conditions.

Other recent studies have shown that microglia may be influenced by adiponectin in AD. Adiponectin is an adipokine derived from adipose tissue, that can regulate inflammation and control macrophages during conditions of oxidative stress. Although in much lower concentrations in the brain, adiponectin receptors are expressed in many regions such as the hypothalamus, hippocampus, and cortex, and adiponectin in the brain is involved in lipid and glucose metabolism, the regulation of food intake, as well as neurogenesis (for a review see [22]). An adiponectin deficiency is strongly related to type 2 diabetes (a risk factor for AD), yet studies of adiponectin levels in AD have found both increased and decreased levels [23–25], compared to controls.

Studies of aged adiponectin-knockout mice suggest that adiponectin deficiency leads to cognitive impairments and AD-related pathologies through AMP-activated protein kinase (AMPK) inactivation and cerebral insulin resistance [26], and other studies have shown that adiponectin regulates the polarisation of microglia towards the M2 anti-inflammatory subtype via peroxisome proliferator-activated receptor-α (PPAR-α) signalling, when microglia are exposed to toxic oligomers of Aβ [27]. Adiponectin signalling using AMPK and PPAR-α occurs via the AdipoR2 and AdipoR1 receptors, with AMPK being the main downstream effector. It has been shown that obesity, insulin resistance, and type 2 diabetes are associated with reduced levels of adiponectin, indicating another link between these chronic conditions, increased inflammation, and AD, and a recent review suggests adiponectin replacement therapy may benefit these conditions [28], and therefore possibly also reduce AD risk.

8.3 Oxidative Stress

Oxidative stress results from the imbalance between the production of ROS and a biological system's ability to neutralise these ROS, detoxify the reactive intermediates, or easily repair the resulting damage. Oxidative stress can cause cell death, whereas

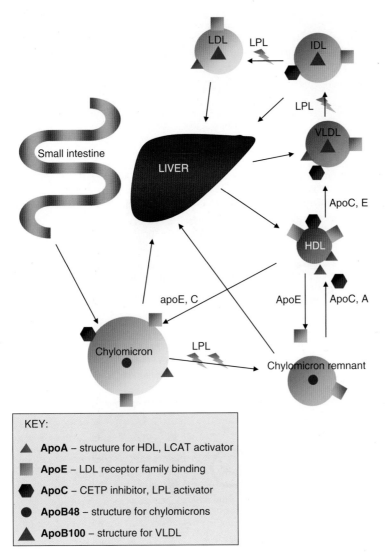

Figure 7.1 The pathways of peripheral lipoprotein homeostasis. The liver is the main site of clearance for the majority of lipoprotein traffic, however triglycerides and fatty acids are released from the lipoproteins by interaction with cell surface-bound LPL (lipoprotein lipase) as they circulate throughout the body. The exact mechanism controlling the transfer of apolipoproteins is yet to be fully understood.

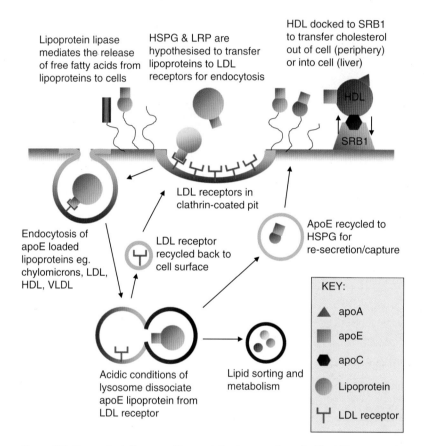

Figure 7.2 Conceptual diagram of lipoprotein clearance by cells. The LDL receptor is usually recycled back to the surface, whilst apoE is either metabolised or recycled via HSPG for a lipoprotein secretion/capture role. Note that since apoE ε4 binds with high affinity to the LDL receptor, this may not permit dissociation from the receptor which traps the complex within the cell leading to raised cellular cholesterol.

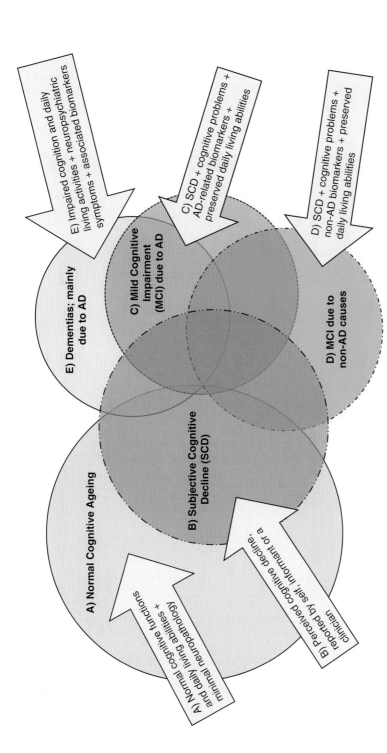

Figure 9.1 The interrelationship between normal cognitive ageing, subjective cognitive decline, and neuropathological conditions. The figure shows five potential scenarios of cognitive ageing. Some individuals live long without significant pathological cognitive impairment or concerns affecting their independent lifestyle and daily living activities (A). A group of older adults may report noticeable decline in cognition (SCD), (B) [48]. In fact up to 27% of older adults aged 60 years old and over may report serious concerns about their cognitive changes [11]. Individuals reporting SCD are twice as likely to develop dementia as compared to those without such complaints [48]. A group of individuals with SCD will develop cognitive decline that can be detected by objective measures (MCI; C and D). The prevalence of MCI [49] amongst older adults is about 16% and it is considered as a prodromal condition with increased risk of developing dementia [34]. Dementia due to AD (E) is very common [50] and can be seen in up to 50% of older adults, depending on age, genetic risk factors, sex, ethno-racial group, and education level. Each arrow corresponds to a brief description of the core criteria for diagnosing each stage of the cognitive decline progression. The dashed barriers emphasize the permeability between conditions while the solid line indicates the irreversibility of the AD neuropathological changes based on our current knowledge. Source: This figure is adapted and modified from: [51].

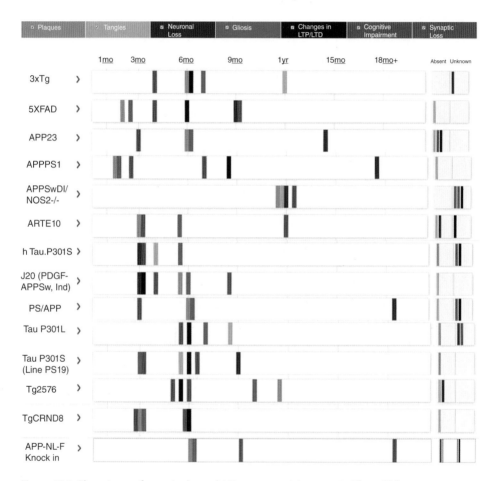

Figure 10.1 Phenotypes of commonly used AD mouse models generated from Alzforum.

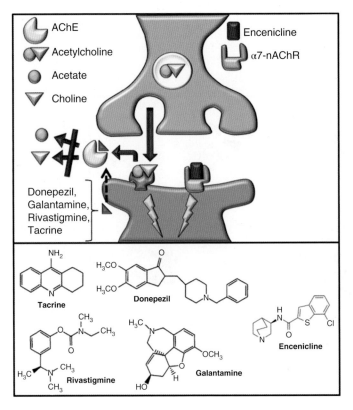

Figure 14.1 Diagram of synapse and site of action of commonly used AD drugs, and structure of commonly used AD drugs.

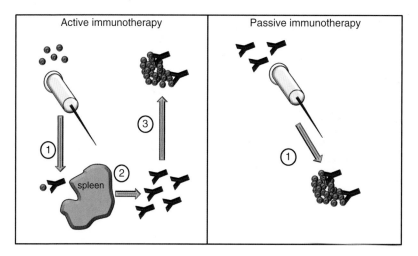

Figure 14.2 Active and passive immunotherapy.

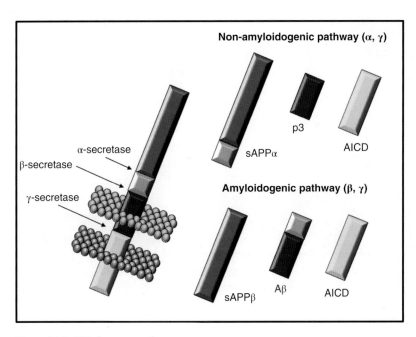

Figure 14.3 APP cleavage pathways.

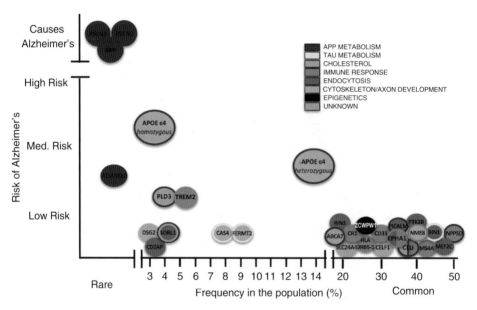

Figure 15.2 Rare and common genetic variants which contribute to Alzheimer's disease risk. Distributed by frequency in population and AD risk-effect size. Genes are colour-coded by probable pathway through which they are involved in AD pathogenesis. Source: Modified from Karch and Goate, 2015 [7].

moderate oxidation can trigger cell apoptosis and more intense stress may cause necrosis [29]. The peroxidation of polyunsaturated fatty acids, or lipid peroxidation, is especially important, because it is a self-propagating reaction that will continue until it is terminated by defences or until the substrate is exhausted. Free radical attack on polyunsaturated fatty acids leads to structural damage to cell membranes. It also generates several aldehyde byproducts, including malondialdehyde and C_3-C_{10} straight-chain aldehydes, as well as α,β-unsaturated aldehydes such as 4-hydroxynonenal (HNE) and acrolein. Of these, the α,β-unsaturated aldehydes in particular may be primary effectors of tissue damage. They show high reactivity with nucleophiles, including sulfhydryl groups of cysteine, histidine, and lysine, and they also impair key neuronal processes [30]. Lipid peroxidation also produces oxidised and endocyclised products of arachidonic acid (F_2-isoprostanes or F_2-IsoPs) or docosahexaenoic acid (F_4-neuroprostanes or F_4-NeuroPs) that are quantitative *in vivo* biomarkers of free-radical damage [30].

Free radicals, particularly the hydroxyl radicals, also attack nucleic acids. This leads to strand breaks, cross-linking, and base modifications and these may contribute to alterations in protein production and ultimately instigate neuron dysfunction and death. Mitochondrial DNA (mtDNA) is more susceptible to free-radical-mediated damage than nuclear DNA (nDNA), as a result of its proximity to the site of ROS production. It also lacks protective histones and significant noncoding sequences, and has limited repair capacity. As Dizdaroglu et al. argue in their review, DNA attack by ROS can lead to the generation of more than 20 oxidised base adducts, with 8-hydroxydeoxyguanine (8-OHdG) the most prominent because of the relatively low oxidation potential of guanine [31]. In addition to direct oxidation by ROS, DNA can also be modified by α,β-unsaturated aldehyde byproducts of lipid peroxidation through an initial addition of the exocyclic amino group [32].

These adducts are potentially biologically relevant, because they may promote DNA–DNA and DNA–protein cross-linking that can limit transcription. Similar to the products of lipid peroxidation, protein oxidation is not simply a reflection of damaged tissue, but an effector of cellular dysfunction [33].

Mitochondria are particularly vulnerable to oxidative stress, as energy production, the production of antioxidant enzymes, and the maintenance of membrane potential are all decreased. This can cause a further increase in ROS, leading to cell death by caspase activation and apoptosis [34, 35]. Calcium metabolism and metal (in particular iron, zinc, and copper) homeostasis are also disturbed by oxidative stress. These changes together with the reduction in antioxidant defence, the dysfunction in energy metabolism and mitochondrial function, disruptions in cellular trafficking, and stress on the proteasomal degradation system all lead to disruption in synaptic activity, neuronal damage, and eventually cell death [36].

8.3.1 Advanced Glycation End Products

The advanced glycation end-products (AGE) are a heterogenous group of compounds that occur due to the non-enzymatic glycation of free amino groups on protein, lipids, or nucleic acids, by reducing sugars and reactive aldehydes [37]. They are more often formed under hyperglycaemic and/or oxidative stress conditions, and some AGE are also derived from the diet, particularly from foods fried or roasted at very high temperature, meat and processed meat products, and full-fat cheese. AGE have toxic effects related to their ability to promote oxidative stress and inflammation, following binding to cell-surface receptors or cross-linking with other proteins, altering their structure and function [37]. A major AGE receptor is RAGE, which is found throughout the body including the brain, and levels of RAGE are increased in AD [38]. AGE binding to RAGE induces the activation of various intracellular cascades, which involve the NF-κB pathway and inflammatory mediators like TNF-α, IL-6, and C-reactive protein, all of which are linked to increased inflammation and oxidative stress. RAGE has also been implicated in cardiovascular diseases and type 2 diabetes, both known risk factors for AD [39], and recent studies have found many links between AGE, RAGE, microglial activation, and disrupted Aβ metabolism, including the excessive transfer of Aβ from the blood to the brain via RAGE on the blood–brain barrier [40].

8.3.2 Involvement of the Complement System in AD

The complement system involves a collection of proteins including those designated C1–C9, which participate in an amplifying cascade of enzymes, resulting in large numbers of downstream complement factors. The complement system participates in antigen–antibody reactions when outside the brain. Within the brain, however, complement protein C1q binds to Aβ fibrils, which are then phagocytosed by microglia. This may explain the 10- to 80-fold increase in C1q expression levels found in AD brain regions highly affected by AD pathology, such as the entorhinal cortex, hippocampus, and mid-temporal gyrus (compared to non-AD brains) [41]. These fibrils then may remain largely un-degraded by the microglia, resulting in a 'frustrated phagocytosis' that could lead to a worsened condition due to heightened microglia activation, if the toxic elements of the phagolysosome are released into the cell environment [42]. *In vitro* fibrillar amyloid activates both the classical and alternative complement cascades [43] which could lead to further degeneration as a result of this possible frustrated phagocytosis. In line with this postulation, chronic treatment with a C5a antagonist, PMX205: hydrocinnamate-[Om-Pro-D-cyclohezylalanine-Trp-Arg], decreases AD pathology in two mouse models [44]. C1q has also been shown to bind to NFT, though possibly to a lesser extent [45, 46].

Studies of AD cerebral spinal fluid (CSF) have shown higher levels of C1q, C3d, and C4d in the early stages of AD, and levels show a positive correlation with plaque number from mild to severe cases; furthermore, the patterns of complement-factor expression change over time, indicating a temporal pattern of complement-protein expression in relation to Aβ plaque deposition or other AD pathology [47–49], and possibly providing biomarkers for the disease.

As mentioned above C3 levels increase in AD over the course of the disease, in both clinical cases and AD transgenic mice, and experimentally reduced levels of C3 cause an increase in Aβ deposition in AD transgenic mice. C3 products are thought to attract microglial cells to help clear Aβ deposits, thus C3 is seen as beneficial in AD. In contrast, the increase in components of the terminal pathway are seen as pathogenic, for example increases in levels of C5a and its receptor occur in AD and AD-model transgenic mice; and the specific inhibition of C5a reduces amyloid build-up in transgenic AD mice. A recent cell culture study confirmed that C5a increases the damage to primary neurons caused by Aβ fibrils via the C5a receptor, with the conclusion being that C5aR1 antagonists may provide benefit as AD therapeutics [50]. Interestingly, another study has found that a deficiency in the C5a receptor leads to lower body weight, lower plasma triglyceride, and non-esterified fatty acids levels in C5a receptor knock-out mice fed a high-sucrose diet, indicating C5a receptors also have a role in fat storage and metabolism [51], abnormalities of which have been linked to AD.

8.3.3 Involvement of Cytokines and Chemokines in Inflammation

Aβ activation of microglia causes them to produce inflammatory cytokines, including IL-1β and TNF-α. Aβ also activates the transcription factor nuclear factor-κB (NF-κB), which increases cytokine production by neurons and microglia. Neuronal NF-κB effectors include calcium and inflammatory cytokines, yet NF-κB has also recently been implicated in synaptic plasticity, learning, and memory, and the dysregulation of NF-κB in AD, as well as the many gene targets of NF-κB, needs further study to uncover its role and changes in AD [52]. Microglia also induce enzymes such as nitric oxide synthase, and cause oxidative stress by generating nitric oxide, leading to peroxynitrite [53]. The protein cross-linking enzyme transglutaminase 2 is also overexpressed in AD, and can be induced in microglial, astroglial, and monocyte cell models following inflammation. This overexpression maintains NF-κB, possibly exacerbating inflammation and, as such, transglutaminase 2 and its involvement in neuroinflammation warrants further research (for a review see [54]).

Increases in IL-1β further aggravate the immune/inflammatory response by promoting more amyloid-β precursor protein (APP) synthesis and by promoting the production of more Aβ-binding proteins by astrocytes. The overexpression of IL-1 near amyloid plaques may promote the phosphorylation of tau protein, leading to the formation of NFT and neuron death [55]. Nearly all the cytokines and chemokines that have been studied in reference to AD, including IL-1β, IL-6, TNF-α, IL-8, tumour growth-factor-β (TGF-β), and macrophage inflammatory protein-1α (MIP-1α), seem to be upregulated in individuals with AD when compared to control individuals [56]. Animal models of AD, such as the Tg2576 model (overexpressing APP carrying the Swedish mutation), also show enhanced levels of TNF-α, IL-1α, IL-1β, chemoattractant protein-1, COX-2, and the complement component mentioned above, C1q [57]. In addition, it has also been reported that mice overexpressing the mutant human P301 tau protein have an increased immunoreactivity to IL-1 and COX-2 [58]. The production of interleukins and other cytokines and chemokines, for example by interaction of AGE and Aβ amyloid with receptors for AGE, may also lead to microglial activation, astrogliosis (reactive astrocytes), and further secretion of pro-inflammatory molecules and amyloid, thus perpetuating the pathological cascade of AD [59]. It has been proposed that pro-inflammatory cytokines could affect Aβ formation by raising susceptibility to Aβ deposition or aggregation, or transcriptional upregulation of β-secretase and APP, as will be explained in sections to follow.

Genetic and pharmaco-epidemiological studies have also indicated the central role of inflammation in AD. For example, genome-wide association studies have identified three immune-relevant genes that are associated with an increased risk of developing AD: CLU (clusterin), CR1 (complement receptor 1), and TREM2 (triggering receptor expressed on myeloid cells 2) [60, 61]. More recent meta-analyses found other AD linkages to immune system proteins, including HLA-DRB5-DRB1 (HLA class II histocompatibility antigen, DRB5 beta, allelic variant DRB1) and INPP5D (inositol polyphosphate-5-phosphatase D, linked to cancers of the immune system) [62], as well as MS4A4A (a cell-surface protein found on monocytes) [63].

All the above data suggest that the progression of many neurodegenerative diseases, including AD [64], arise from a cycle of self-perpetuating *inflammatory* neurotoxicity. Stages that may occur include:

a) Multiple inflammatory triggers can lead to initial microglial activation. These triggers can be peripheral (e.g. systemic infections or peripheral chronic inflammation) or central (e.g. degenerating/dying neurons or amyloid deposits). In one widely investigated mouse model, the GFAP-IL-6 mouse, the trigger is the cytokine interleukin-6 (IL-6) [65].
b) Activated microglia release neurotoxic factors such as cytotoxic cytokines like TNF-α and reactive oxygen/nitrogen species, which in turn cause damage to neighbouring neurons. This process can be inhibited by cytokine-suppressive anti-inflammatory drugs (CSAID) [66].
c) These damaged or dying neurons release microglia activators, such as damage-associated molecular pattern molecules (DAMP), resulting in further microglial activation and thus maintain the self-perpetuating cycle of neurotoxicity.

Consequently, targeting chronic neuroinflammation has been suggested as a promising disease-modifying treatment for many neurodegenerative diseases including AD [67].

8.3.4 Inflammation – Susceptibility to Aβ Deposition or Aggregation

Studies performed with a transgenic amyloidosis animal model showed that plaques did not develop unless inflammation was induced: under non-inflammatory conditions, transgenic mice did not develop reactive amyloid or Amyloid A (AA) deposits in the brain. This suggests that cerebral amyloid deposition increases under inflammatory conditions [68]. When a systemic acute-phase response was induced in transgenic mice, however, there was enhanced amyloid deposition. The deposition was preceded by an increase in cytokine levels in the brain, suggesting that systemic inflammation may be a contributing factor in the development of cerebral amyloid. Guo et al. showed that the non-steroidal anti-inflammatory agent, indomethacin, reduces inflammation and cytokine expression and protects against the deposition of AA in the brain [69].

In the case of AD, it has been suggested that the disease may start with abnormally high levels of extracellular Aβ oligomers (due to excessive production or a reduction in clearance of the peptide) triggering inflammation, an effect which is later enhanced by aggregates of tau. The inflammatory response, which is driven by activated microglia, increases over time as the disease progresses [70]. It has also been suggested that Aβ amyloidogenesis results from an IL-1/IL-6 mediated acute phase reaction in the brain [71].

Other studies suggest that metabolic disturbances caused by obesity, insulin resistance, hypertension, and type 2 diabetes lead to oxidative stress and chronic inflammation, which in turn lead to abnormal Aβ metabolism, Aβ aggregation, and then a vicious self-perpetuating cycle of toxic Aβ inducing further inflammation, and vice versa [72]. Nevertheless, all studies indicate that inflammation plays an important role in the process of amyloid deposition, and inhibition of inflammatory cascades may attenuate amyloidogenic processes, such as AD.

8.3.5 Inflammation Can Influence APP Metabolism and Aβ Clearance Directly

Many aspects of inflammation appear to influence the metabolism of APP directly, raising the likelihood of increased Aβ production, or affecting the clearance and breakdown of Aβ. For example, cytokines are able to upregulate β-secretase (BACE1) mRNA, protein and enzymatic activity [73]. In fact, oxidative stress, inflammation, calcium homeostasis disturbance, hypoxia, and the ischaemia that can occur in AD are all capable of activating BACE1 [74].This falls in line with data showing increased expression and activity of BACE1 in NT2 cells exposed to oxidative stress, in experimental traumatic brain injury and in reactive astrocytes in chronic models of gliosis [74]. Interestingly, BACE1 antisense mRNA (BACE1-AS mRNA) has been shown to increase BACE1 levels by stabilising BACE1 mRNA (thus increasing BACE1 translation and most likely Aβ production) [75]. In heart failure, it has been shown recently that levels of Aβ, BACE1 mRNA as well as BACE1-AS mRNA are all upregulated [76], and as heart failure is an acute event in cardiovascular disease (a risk factor for AD), it would be interesting to see whether such BACE1 mRNA changes also occur in earlier stages of cardiovascular disease, and whether they are systemic. BACE1-AS mRNA is markedly upregulated in AD brain, and in a mouse model of AD, it has been shown that BACE1-AS mRNA is higher at very early stages of the disease, disrupting adult neurogenesis [77].

Astrocytes have been shown to clear Aβ by endosomal/lysosomal pathways, yet some enzymes involved in breakdown such as insulin-degrading enzyme and neprilysin can only degrade monomers. The uptake of Aβ by astrocytes can also be carried out, by the low-density lipoprotein receptor-related protein (LRP1), scavenger receptor class B member 1 (SCARB1), and the receptor for AGE (RAGE), yet some receptors such as LRP1 are again only capable of monomer uptake, thus an increasing amount of oligomers and fibrils will eventually reduce the effectiveness of astrocyte-mediated Aβ clearance (for a review see [78]).

It has also been shown that TGF-β treatment of human astrocytes can markedly elevate APP mRNA levels and also increase the half-life of the APP message by at least 5-fold [79]. Rogers et al. also demonstrated that IL-1α and IL-1β increase APP synthesis by up to 6-fold in primary human astrocytes and by 15-fold in human astrocytoma cells without changing the steady-state levels of APP mRNA [80].

The enzyme ADAM17, which is thought to be the regulated APP α-secretase enzyme that precludes Aβ production by cleaving APP within the Aβ region, is also involved in the shedding of extracellular domains of at least 40 other transmembrane proteins, including cytokines, growth factors, and receptors. However, changes in ADAM17 have been shown to play a role in atherosclerosis, in adipose tissue metabolism, insulin resistance, and diabetes – some of which are known risk factors for AD. Furthermore, in inflammation, the pro-inflammatory activity of TNFα is mostly mediated by TNFα receptor type 1 (TNFR1) and to some extent by TNF receptor type 2 (TNFR2), both of which have been found to undergo shedding via ADAM17 [81–83]. ADAM17 and TNFα have been shown to be involved in stress-induced activation of NFκB, a central regulator of inflammation and responses to free radicals etc. All the above evidence indicates ADAM17 will influence APP metabolism on many levels [81]. This is not an exhaustive list, just examples of the many changes to APP-regulating enzymes that are linked to inflammation.

8.4 Current Medications for AD

There are several medications currently used to treat AD, however these do not provide a cure, or halt the disease, they merely provide some temporary improvement in intellectual function, or alleviate associated symptoms such as depression, anxiety, and behavioural difficulties. Many researchers have shifted focus to preventative or disease-slowing therapies, and many such therapies are under development. One potential avenue of treatment is to significantly increase antioxidant levels in the diet, to counteract the age-associated increase in oxidative stress, and to try to reduce some of the inflammation associated with the common age-related (and diet-related) increases in cardiovascular disease, obesity, insulin resistance, and type 2 diabetes. As oxidative stress and inflammation are believed to be involved in the very early stages of AD pathogenesis, it is hoped that reducing these factors will prevent or slow onset of the disease. Current medications and their limits, as well as anti-inflammatory and antioxidant drugs, factors, and supplements which may have the potential to reduce AD pathogenesis, are discussed below.

8.4.1 Current Medications – Acetylcholinesterase Inhibitors and Memantine

The pathogenesis of AD has been linked to a deficiency in the brain neurotransmitter acetylcholine, based on observations that there is a correlation between cholinergic system abnormalities and intellectual impairment. Therefore, acetylcholinesterase inhibitors (AChEI) were developed many years ago to augment acetylcholine-mediated neurotransmission. As a result, the best current treatment for mild to moderate AD is to improve cognitive function by treatment with AChEI. Examples include donepezil, rivastigmine, and galantamine, and these are licensed as medications for symptomatic treatment of AD, despite the fact that the benefit of these agents is modest. However, apart from their use in stabilisation of cognitive decline, there is also evidence linking these agents with improvements in behavioural and psychological symptoms of dementia.

Tacrine (an acridine) was the prototype AChEI, yet produced hepatotoxicity and is no longer marketed. Tacrine derivatives have been examined for efficacy and safety as possible alternatives. Velnacrine, one of these derivatives, was examined in a Cochrane review and, due to a similar side-effect profile to tacrine, was not recommended for use in AD [84].

Donepezil (a piperidine) has a very low incidence of nausea and diarrhoea at the 10 mg dose (the higher of the two available doses), is widely used now, and is administered once daily [85]. Trials suggest that the incidence of nausea and diarrhoea is greater with the other AChEI, rivastigmine (a carbamate) and galantamine (a phenanthrene alkaloid), than with donepezil, especially at the higher doses; both of these are administered twice daily. Studies have suggested that rivastigmine may be a suitable alternative for patients who are unresponsive to donepezil or galantamine [86]. Transdermal patches of rivastigmine are also available [87, 88], and rivastigmine has the benefit of influencing praxis and language as well [87].

Another AChEI that has shown some promise in AD treatment research is physostigmine [89]. Physostigmine was shown to have some benefit in memory improvement more than two decades ago [90], however a Cochrane review concluded that physostigmine shows no benefit over other AChEI drugs and therefore should not be recommended for AD [89].

The glutamatergic inhibitor memantine is also used to treat AD, although usually in the moderate to severe stages of the disease. Memantine blocks N-Methyl-D-aspartate (NMDA) receptors and is sometimes used in conjunction with AChEI in the moderate AD stages, to improve symptoms and slow progression of the disease. However, again, the improvements are always temporary, lasting approximately 6–18 months [91, 92].

8.5 Disease Modification and Treatment Approaches

The drugs mentioned above improve some symptoms temporarily, but do not have any profound disease-modifying effects as they do not address the underlying pathology, so they are of limited benefit to most patients. Similarly, other drugs that are used to manage mood disorder, agitation, and psychosis in later stages of the disease have no disease-modifying effect. Treatments that may influence the pathogenesis, pathology, or progress of the disease are discussed below – and one class of drugs investigated includes the non-steroidal anti-inflammatory drugs (NSAID).

8.5.1 Non-Steroidal Anti-Inflammatory Drugs (NSAID)

Interest in the use of NSAID for AD prevention was sparked by a study that indicated that indomethacin, in doses of 100–150 mg d^{-1}, appeared to protect mild-to-moderately impaired AD patients from the degree of cognitive decline exhibited by well-matched controls. The pathology of AD clearly involves an inflammatory component, and epidemiological evidence indicated that the use of a subset of NSAID appeared to be associated with a reduced risk of AD. However, many studies have been conducted to try to verify this potential utility of NSAID, and reviews and meta-analyses concluded there was no clear evidence of any benefit of NSAID in preventing or treating AD [93–95], although these analyses also concluded that the variability between studies, types of NSAID, and lack of controlled trials made comparisons difficult, and that further studies were needed, particularly with the aim of AD prevention. Nevertheless, some observational studies and other reviews suggest NSAID given for longer terms (for example 2–3 years on one study) are associated with lower AD incidence [91, 96–98]. Furthermore, AD-model animal studies give strong supporting evidence, and also suggest mechanisms may not be via changes to amyloid or NFT deposition. For example, one study found ibuprofen modulated hippocampal gene expression in pathways involved in neuronal plasticity, and increased levels of norepinephrine and dopamine [99–101].

Other putative targets of NSAID actions are thought to be the microglia associated with senile plaques, for example patients receiving long-term NSAID therapy have been shown to exhibit a 65% reduction in plaque-associated reactive microglia. One clinical trial showed reduced risk of AD in NSAID users, but only in association with patients with an apolipoprotein E (*APOE*) ε4 allele (genetic risk factor for AD), and there was no advantage for NSAID that were reported to reduce Aβ_{42} levels [102]. Other studies have suggested NSAID work via COX-2 inhibition or PPARγ activation; some studies also do suggest protection against Aβ aggregation and changes to APP processing; however, overall, the precise mechanisms remain unclear.

However, the prolonged use of NSAID can cause serious gastrointestinal toxicity. Some NSAID have also been linked to increased blood pressure, greatly increased risk of congestive heart failure, and the occurrence of thrombosis. NSAID are specifically designed as inhibitors of cyclooxygenase (COX) enzymes, and, in contrast to CSAID, do not influence the production of pro-inflammatory cytokines such as TNF-α or free radicals such as nitric oxide [103].

These findings illustrate the need to develop novel and safe anti-inflammatory medicines with a broader range of anti-inflammatory effects than conventional NSAID. CSAID have emerged as a new class of anti-inflammatory drugs as they have a broader range of action than NSAID in the treatment of chronic neuroinflammation. CSAID such as curcumin and apigenin specifically target the p38 mitogen-activated protein kinase (MAPK) and NF-κB signalling pathways to inhibit cytokine-mediated events with demonstrated efficacy in a range of animal models [104].

8.6 Some Anti-inflammatory Foods, Supplements, and Newly Developed Drugs for the Treatment of AD

8.6.1 Cinnamon/Cinnamaldehyde

Cinnamaldehyde is a flavonoid that is largely responsible for the flavour and aroma in the spice commonly known as cinnamon. In one of our own studies, we showed that Sri Lankan cinnamon (*C. zeylanicum*) was one of the most potent anti-inflammatory foods out of 115 foods tested [105]. We measured the anti-inflammatory activity of *C. zeylanicum* and *C. cassia* and determined their main phytochemical compounds. When extracts were tested in lipopolysaccharide (LPS) and IFN-γ activated RAW 264.7 macrophages, most of the anti-inflammatory activity, measured by downregulation of nitric oxide and TNF-α production, was observed in the organic extracts. The most abundant compounds in these extracts were *E*-cinnamaldehyde and *o*-methoxycinnamaldehyde. The highest concentration of *E*-cinnamaldehyde was found in the DCM (Dichloromethane) extract of *C. zeylanicum* or *C. cassia* (31 and 34 mg g^{-1} of cinnamon, respectively). When these and other constituents were tested for their anti-inflammatory activity in RAW 264.7 and J774.1 macrophages, the most potent compounds were *E*-cinnamaldehyde and *o*-methoxycinnamaldehyde, which exhibited IC$_{50}$ values for NO with RAW 264.7 cells of $55 \pm 9\,\mu M$ ($7.5 \pm 1.2\,\mu g\,ml^{-1}$) and $35 \pm 9\,\mu M$ ($5.7 \pm 1.5\,\mu g\,ml^{-1}$), respectively; and IC$_{50}$ values for TNF-α of $63 \pm 9\,\mu M$ ($8.6 \pm 1.2\,\mu g\,ml^{-1}$) and $78 \pm 16\,\mu M$ ($12.6 \pm 2.6\,\mu g\,ml^{-1}$), respectively. If therapeutic concentrations can be achieved in target tissues, cinnamon and its components may be useful in the treatment of age-related inflammatory conditions [106].

Cinnamaldehyde's neuroprotective effects were validated in an animal model of ischaemia/reperfusion (I/R)-induced brain injury. These results showed that administration of the compound (10–30 mg kg^{-1}, p.o.) significantly reduced the infarction area, neurological deficit score, and decreased inducible nitric oxide synthase (iNOS) and COX-2 protein expression level in I/R-induced injury brain tissue. Cinnamaldehyde has a potential neuroprotective effect against ischaemic stroke, which may be via the inhibition of neuroinflammation through attenuating iNOS, COX-2 expression, and NF-κB signalling pathway [107].

Previously it was reported that an aqueous extract of cinnamon has the ability to inhibit tau aggregation *in vitro* and can even induce dissociation of tangles isolated from AD brain [108]. In investigations with cinnamaldehyde (CA) and epicatechin (EC), two components of active cinnamon extract, it was found that CA and the oxidised form of EC (ECox) inhibited tau aggregation *in vitro* and the activity was due to their interaction with the two cysteine residues in tau. Mass spectrometry of a synthetic peptide, SKCGS, representing the actual tau sequence, identified the thiol as reacting with CA and ECox. The use of a cysteine double mutant of tau showed that cysteines were necessary for aggregation inhibition by CA. The interaction of CA with tau cysteines was reversible, and the presence of CA did not impair the biological function of tau in tubulin assembly *in vitro*. Further, these compounds protected tau from oxidation caused by the ROS H_2O_2, and prevented subsequent formation of high molecular weight species that are considered to stimulate tangle formation. It was also observed that EC can sequester highly reactive and toxic byproducts of oxidation such as acrolein. These results suggest that small molecules that form a reversible interaction with cysteines have the potential to protect tau from abnormal modifications [109].

Recent studies of a mouse model of cerebral ischaemia have added further evidence of CA inhibiting inflammation, partly mediated by reduced expression of signal transduction molecules such as toll-like receptor 4 (TLR4) and tumour necrosis receptor factor 6, and by reducing the nuclear translocation of NF-κB, resulting in an attenuated increase in TNF-α and IL-1β, amongst others [110]. The inhibition of TLR4/NOX4 signalling is known to reduce oxidative stress/nitrative stress in neuronal damage and apoptosis pathways, and a recent study of LPS-induced cardiac dysfunction in rats found that cinnamaldehyde reduced the intracellular ROS production, and reduced the levels of TNF-α, IL-1β, and IL-6 in the LPS stimulated rats, by blocking the TLR4, NOX4, MAPK, and autophagy signals [111]. Cinnamaldehyde has also been shown to reduce inflammation in high-fat-diet-fed mice [112], and in other mouse and microglial studies involving LPS-induced inflammation, trans-cinnamaldehyde (another anti-inflammatory compound isolated from *cinnamomum cassia*) was shown to improve synaptic plasticity in the mice. It also reduced NO production by accelerating the degradation of iNOS mRNA (in turn thought to occur due to trans-cinnamaldehyde inhibiting the MEK1/2-ERK1/2 signalling pathway) and reduced IL-1β release from primary microglia [113].

8.6.2 (−)Epigallocatechin-3-Gallate (EGCG) and Other Green Tea Polyphenols

Green tea is derived from the steamed and dried leaves of the *Camellia sinensis* plant. Polyphenols from green tea have been shown to be powerful hydrogen-donating antioxidants, free-radical scavengers of ROS and RNS *in vitro* [114]. Many studies have now shown that raising the dietary intake of polyphenols can reduce oxidative stress and reduce the risk for oxidative stress-related diseases including AD, Parkinson's disease, stroke, and Huntington's disease [115]. Among the green tea polyphenols, a subclass termed catechins has received the greatest attention, of which green tea is one of the best-known dietary sources. Of the four major tea catechins, (−)epigallocatechin-3-gallate (EGCG) is the major constituent (∼60%) of the catechins, and 10% of total tea extract dry weight, followed by (−)-epigallocatechin (EGC), then (−)-epicatechin (EC), and then lastly (−)-epicatechin-3-gallate (ECG) [114]. EGCG has previously been shown to prevent neuronal cell death caused by Aβ neurotoxicity in cell cultures [116, 117]. A study by Rezai-Zadeh et al. [118] reported that EGCG also reduced Aβ generation *in vitro* in neuronal-like cells and primary neuronal cultures and promoted the non-amyloidogenic α-secretase proteolytic pathway. Furthermore, when 12-month-old Tg2576 mice were treated with 20 mg kg^{-1} EGCG via intra-peritoneal injections for 60 days, decreased brain levels of Aβ and Aβ plaque load were detected, along with promotion of the α-secretase pathway [118], and it has been shown that EGCG promotes the APP α-secretase pathway via protein kinase C (PKC)-dependent activation [114, 117]. These results indicate EGCG may provide a potential preventative treatment for AD.

Studies of green tea have shown that acetylcholinesterase can be inhibited by green (and white) tea, with EGCG being the most potent [119], suggesting that green tea can act to some extent like the main treatment drugs currently available for AD that were mentioned above and recent studies have indicated that the polyphenols do bind directly to acetylcholinesterase (and butyrylcholinesterase) [120]. Furthermore, primary neuronal cultures exposed to glutamate to induce neurotoxicity were found to be protected by green tea polyphenols, as they inhibited the glutamate-induced ROS release, and the reduction in SOC (Store-operated calcium channels) activity. The green tea polyphenols improved mitochondrial function in the cells, and reduced the changes in Bax, caspase-3, and Bcl-2 that were caused by the glutamate [121], suggesting the polyphenols provided protection via antioxidative and anti-apoptotic pathways. Interestingly, these antioxidative properties are also thought to be the reason green tea polyphenols together with tai chi have been found to reduce oxidative stress and reduce signs of osteoporosis in post-menopausal women [122].

Similar results have been obtained in studies of AD-model (*APP/PSEN1*) transgenic mice given green tea polyphenols in their drinking water along with treadmill exercises for four months. The intervention reduced deficits in spatial learning and memory, and lowered soluble Aβ1-40 and Aβ1-42 levels as well as oxidative stress levels in the brain. The treatment also raised brain-derived neurotrophic factor (BDNF) levels, and activated Akt/GSK-3 (Glycogen Synthase Kinase)/CREB signalling [123]. Other AD-model mouse studies have shown that EGCG could prevent LPS-induced memory impairment, as well as the LPS-induced activation of astrocytes and increased cytokine expression (TNF-α, IL-1β, IL-6), suggesting that EGCG can reduce the inflammation associated with AD [124]. Overall, the ester of epigallocatechin and gallic acid, EGCG, appears to be the most bioactive polyphenol found in green tea extracts. The compound has important anti-inflammatory and anti-atherogenic properties, as well as protective effects against neuronal damage and brain oedema. Other recent studies have shown that EGCG can suppress the expression of TNFα, IL-1β, IL-6, and iNOS and restore the levels of intracellular antioxidants against Aβ-induced and free-radical-induced pro-inflammatory effects in microglia. EGCG could also restore levels of nuclear erythroid-2 related factor 2 (Nrf2; transcription factor that regulates expression of antioxidant proteins) and the haem oxygenase-1 (HO-1; enzyme that degrades haem into CO (Carbon Monoxide), biliverdin, and free iron, all of which have anti-inflammatory and anti-apoptotic properties) [125]. EGCG could also reduce the Aβ-induced toxicity by reducing ROS-induced NF-κB activation and MAPK signalling, including c-Jun N-terminal kinase (JNK) and p38 signalling [125, 126].

Despite the many *in vitro* and animal studies which have indicated many positive effects of green tea extracts, studies suggest EGCG cannot cross the blood–brain barrier in humans. Thus, the positive effects seen in cell culture and particularly in AD-model mice may not occur in humans, or not to the same extent. It has been suggested this may be due to differences in dose and time of administration, or possibly differences in metabolism between mice and humans (reviewed in [126]). However, many dietary and preventative studies are currently suggesting that a healthy diet high in antioxidant polyphenols (such as EGCG) combined with exercise and other physical activity can help reduce the risk of AD, at least partly by reducing oxidative stress and chronic inflammation-associated conditions such as obesity, cardiovascular disease, insulin resistance, and type 2 diabetes [127]. Therefore, benefits may be obtained systemically that may translate to reduced oxidative stress and inflammation in the brain, and further research including epidemiological studies and clinical trials of green tea extracts should be carried out.

8.6.3 Curcumin

Curcumin is a component of the Indian curry spice turmeric (*Curcuma longa Linn*) [128]. Turmeric is derived from the rhizome, or root of the plant and is used for flavour, colour, and as a food preservative, in addition to being long used to treat a variety of ailments in traditional Indian medicine [129, 130]. Curcumin in various experimental preparations has been shown to have antioxidant [131, 132], anti-inflammatory [133, 134], and cholesterol lowering properties [135, 136]. Curcumin has been reported to be several times more potent than vitamin E as a free-radical scavenger [137], and there is also increasing evidence showing that curcumin can inhibit Aβ aggregation [138]. Curcumin inhibits IL-6-mediated signalling via inhibition of IL-6-induced STAT3 phosphorylation and consequent STAT3 nuclear translocation [139], and interferes with the first signalling steps downstream of the IL-6 receptor ('the inflammatory trigger') in microglial activation [140]. Furthermore, curcumin has a broad cytokine-suppressive anti-inflammatory action, downregulating the expression of cyclooxygenase-2 (COX-2), iNOS, TNF-α, IL-1, -2, -6, -8, and -12 [66, 141, 142]. A recent cell culture study using nanoplasmonic fibre-tip probe technology showed that curcumin could reduce intracellular Aβ oligomer levels considerably, and also lower levels of TNF-α to some extent [143], in cells stably overexpressing APP and Aβ.

In a study by Lim et al. [144] curcumin was tested for its ability to inhibit the combined inflammatory and oxidative damage in Tg2576 transgenic mice. In this study, Tg2576 mice aged 10 months old were fed a curcumin diet (160 ppm) for 6 months. Their results showed that the curcumin diet significantly lowered the levels of oxidised proteins, IL-1β, the astrocyte marker glial fibrillary acidic protein (GFAP), soluble and insoluble Aβ, and also plaque burden. The researchers found that the reduction in GFAP was localised, such that increased activity was shown in areas around plaques, suggesting a stimulatory effect of curcumin on the phagocytosis of plaques by microglia. Following on from this work, Yang et al. [138] evaluated the effect of feeding a curcumin diet (500 ppm) to 17-month-old Tg2576 mice for 6 months. When fed to the aged Tg2576 mice with advanced amyloid accumulation, curcumin resulted in reduced soluble amyloid levels and plaque burden. Yang et al. [138] also demonstrated that when curcumin is injected peripherally (via *the carotid artery*), it can enter the brain and bind amyloid plaques. Curcumin's ability to bind amyloid is thought to be due to its structural similarity to the water-soluble dye Congo red, which binds strongly to amyloid fibrils. In addition, curcumin has been shown to inhibit $A\beta_{42}$ oligomer formation, to a similar extent or better than Congo red, without any toxic effects [138]. Curcuminoids may also reduce Aβ levels as the component bisdemethoxycurcumin (BDMC) can reduce BACE1 mRNA and protein levels, while demethoxycurcumin (DMC) can reduce BACE1 mRNA expression [145]. More recently it has been shown that aged female rats supplemented with curcumin for 12 days have improved spatial memory (Morris water-maze test) and again show signs of reduced oxidative damage [146].

These data raise the possibility that dietary supplementation with curcumin may provide a potential preventative treatment for AD, by decreasing Aβ levels and plaque load via inhibition of Aβ oligomer formation and fibrillisation, along with decreasing oxidative stress and inflammation. Formulations of curcumin that can cross the blood–brain barrier have been investigated, as it is not thought to reach the brain in high concentrations. As a result, highly bioavailable curcumin preparations such as 'Longvida' (VS Corp) have been produced, and these can achieve micromolar concentrations in the brain [147, 148]. In humans, 'Longvida' curcumin (400 mg) has been shown to significantly improve working memory and mood after four weeks' treatment in a randomised, double-blind, placebo-controlled human trial [149]. Additionally, the pharmacokinetic properties of curcumin (encapsulated in liposomes or micelles) are favourable for use as a therapeutic.

Overall though, the few clinical trials which have been conducted have produced mixed results, with most not showing significant cognitive benefits (for a review see [150]), however this is thought to be because the stage of AD at the time of administration may have been too late, once pathological damage is considerable. Epidemiological data support the concept that curcumin can reduce AD risk if taken/eaten regularly at much younger ages, and clinical studies need to be carried out at pre-clinical stages, to slow or prevent AD pathogenesis [150]. Furthermore, as with green tea polyphenolic antioxidants, reducing oxidative stress and chronic inflammation with polyphenolic compounds such as the curcuminoids will help reduce AD by lowering the risk of conditions that are themselves risk factors for AD.

8.6.4 Other Polyphenolic Antioxidants

Many other food-derived polyphenolic antioxidants have been investigated. For example, the polyphenols from Oriental plums have been shown to improve cognitive function, lower cholesterol levels, and lower the diet-induced overexpression of BACE1, Aβ, and 24-hydroxycholesterol in mice fed a high-cholesterol diet [151]. Furthermore, polyphenol stilbenes, which can be found in grapes and berries, have demonstrated positive effects on Nrf2 in oxidative stress [152]; certain flavonoids such as scutellarin, daidzein, genistein, and fisetin are thought to increase neurotrophic factor expression, and apigenin and ferulic acid increase cAMP response element-binding (CREB) phosphorylation (for a review see [153]). Cinnamon extracts and derivatives have also been shown to provide anti-inflammatory and cardio-protective actions, as discussed earlier [154].

The importance of olive oil in the traditional Mediterranean diet, a diet that epidemiological studies have indicated can lead to good health and longevity, has led to studies of the polyphenols in olive oil and its byproducts. For example, recent studies have found that oleuropein aglycone, or a mix of polyphenols obtained from olive mill waste-water, can improve cognitive function in transgenic AD-model mice, as well as reduce Aβ1-42 levels and deposition in certain brain regions [155]. Other studies have shown similar neuroprotective effects such as reduced oxidative stress, improved cell signalling, and reduced Aβ1-42 aggregation, through diets high in olive oil or diets that include olive oil polyphenol supplements (for a review see [156]). Further studies of olive oil and olive extracts are needed to show how valuable these products may be in preventing neurodegeneration.

8.6.5 Omega-3 (n-3) Essential Fatty Acids

Docosahexaenoic acid (DHA) is an essential omega-3 (n-3) polyunsaturated fatty acid (PUFA) that is found abundantly in marine fish. DHA is known to be the most important n-3 PUFA in the brain, accounting for roughly 15% of total fatty acids in grey matter, where it is enriched at synapses [157]. The interest in dietary DHA supplementation has arisen from the view of helping to protect from neuronal degeneration and therefore prevent neurological diseases such as AD. Converging epidemiological data suggest that a low dietary intake of n-3 PUFA is a candidate risk factor for AD [158]. In the AD brain DHA is known to be decreased [159, 160], while people who ingest higher levels of DHA are less likely to develop AD [161–163]. A study by Florent et al. [164] demonstrated that DHA provided cortical neurons *in vitro* a higher level of resistance to the cytotoxic effects induced by soluble Aβ oligomers. Lukiw et al. [165] also demonstrated that DHA decreased $Aβ_{40}$ and $Aβ_{42}$ secretion from ageing human neuronal cells. A study by Calon et al. showed that a reduction of dietary n-3 PUFA in Tg2576 transgenic mice resulted in a loss of post-synaptic proteins and behavioural deficits, while a DHA-enriched diet prevented these effects [166]. Other studies have shown that DHA protects neurons from Aβ accumulation and toxicity and ameliorates cognitive impairment in rodent models of AD [167, 168]. A study by Cole and Frautschy showed that DHA supplementation in Tg2576 transgenic mice aged 17 months markedly reduced Aβ accumulation and oxidative damage and also improved cognitive function [169].

Several recent studies concerning the influence of *APOE* alleles on omega-3 fatty acids have been carried out. For example, *APOE* ε4 mice, compared to mice carrying other *APOE* alleles, suffered greater cognitive impairments and anxiety as well as a greater omega-3 fatty acid depletion in organs and tissues when fed a diet deficient in omega-3 fatty acids, yet these levels could be restored by switching to a diet rich in omega-3 fatty acids [170]. This suggests that long-term omega-3 fatty-acid supplementation in middle-aged to elderly people should be encouraged, especially in *APOE* ε4 carriers. However, a study of macrophages from MCI (Mild Cognitive Impairment) patients who have taken fish-derived omega-3 fatty-acid supplements found that expression of cytoprotective genes increased, whereas pro-apoptotic gene expression decreased; Aβ clearance by macrophage phagocytosis was improved, and the Mini-Mental State Examination (MMSE) scores of the patients also improved – though these positive changes were only found in *APOE* ε3/ε3 patients: the other subgroup – *APOE* ε3/ε4 patients, had a high variability in responses [171]. This may reflect other vulnerabilities to AD pathogenesis caused by ε4 alleles that cannot be overcome with omega-3 fatty-acid supplements. In support of this, other differences seen in *APOE* ε4 carriers have been detected, for example ε4-carriers converting to MCI/AD had high arachidonic acid (AA)/DHA ratios in blood phospholipids, compared to cognitively normal ε4 carriers, as well as non-ε4 carriers [172]. There are also many studies which have shown ApoE ε4 is less efficient than other ApoE forms in some other aspects of lipid metabolism, receptor binding, and Aβ clearance [173], and these differences may also influence the potential benefits of DHA supplementation. The topics of ApoE and omega-3/omega-6 fatty acids are also covered in Chapter 7 of this book.

A recent placebo-controlled three-year clinical trial of omega-3 fatty-acid supplementation (+/− a multi-domain lifestyle intervention) did not find any benefits from the treatments [174]. However, the cohort included people over 70 who already had memory complaints and it may be that intervention at this age (and stage of developing AD) is too late. A review of DHA supplementation with respect to AD pathogenesis stage supports this concept, indicating that high-dose DHA supplementation in *APOE* ε4 carriers before the onset of AD dementia may decrease the incidence of AD, yet does not appear to have any benefits once dementia is established [175].

Other studies of the distribution of unsaturated fatty acids in AD brain have shown alterations in the metabolism of unsaturated fatty acids, indicating both global metabolic perturbations in AD, as well as changes related to specific features of AD pathology [176]. Another mechanism whereby the omega-3 fatty acids DHA and eicosapentaenoic acid (EPA) may influence AD pathogenesis is by affecting insulin-degrading enzyme (IDE), a major Aβ-degrading enzyme in the brain. EPA has been shown to increases IDE enzyme activity and to elevate IDE gene expression [177]. DHA also directly stimulates IDE enzyme activity and increases exosome release of IDE, resulting in enhanced Aβ-degradation in the extracellular space [177].

In summary, many studies indicate that dietary supplementation with DHA, or improving the diet to improve the omega-3 : omega-6 fatty-acid ratio – a ratio that ideally would be between 1 : 1 and 1 : 4 (yet that western diets typically cause this ratio to be from 1 : 8–1 : 25) – may decrease Aβ accumulation, inflammation, and oxidative stress, and consequently reduce the risk of AD, or slow its pathogenesis. However, studies would suggest that such supplementation or dietary change need to be lifelong, or at least started around mid-life, to be effective in reducing AD risk.

8.6.6 Lipoic Acid

In vitro and *in vivo* studies suggest that lipoic acid (LA) acts as a powerful micronutrient with diverse pharmacologic and antioxidant properties [178]. LA naturally occurs only as the R-form (RLA), but pharmacological formulations in the past have extensively used a racemic mixture of RLA and S-lipoic acid (SLA), as stereoselective synthesis methods have not been available. LA has been suggested to have the following properties relevant to AD:

a) Increases acetylcholine production by activation of choline acetyltransferase (ChAT) [179].
b) Chelates redox-active transition metals, thereby inhibiting the formation of hydrogen peroxide and hydroxyl radicals [180].
c) Scavenges ROS (thus sparing glutathione) and downregulates redox-sensitive inflammatory signals [181].

d) Scavenges reactive carbonyl compounds including lipid peroxidation products [182].
e) Increases glucose uptake and utilisation [183].
f) Induces enzymes involved in GSH (Glutathione) synthesis and other antioxidant protective enzymes [184].

Dihydrolipoic acid (DHLA), the reduced form of LA, is formed by reduction of LA by the pyruvate dehydrogenase (PDH) complex. Haugaard et al. demonstrated that DHLA strongly increases the activity of a purified preparation of ChAT [185], that removal of DHLA by dialysis from purified ChAT (from rabbit bladder, rat brain, and heart extracts) causes complete disappearance of enzyme activity, and that the addition of DHLA restored activity towards normal levels [186]. The authors concluded that DHLA serves an essential function in the action of this enzyme and that the ratio of reduced : oxidised LA plays an important role in ACh synthesis. From these data it was suggested that DHLA (i) may act as a coenzyme in the ChAT reaction or (ii) is able to reduce an essential functional cysteine residue in ChAT, which cannot be reduced by any other physiological antioxidant, including reduced GSH [186].

There is now compelling evidence that Aβ, the main component of amyloid plaques in the AD-affected brain, combines with excess metal ions in the brain (copper, iron, and zinc), which induces the peptide to precipitate and form plaques. Furthermore, the abnormal combination of Aβ with copper or iron ions induces the production of hydrogen peroxide from molecular oxygen [187], which subsequently produces neurotoxic hydroxyl radicals by the Fenton or Haber-Weiss reactions. Because LA is a potent chelator of divalent metal ions *in vitro*, the effect of a RLA-inclusive diet on cortical iron levels and antioxidant status was investigated in aged rats [188]. It was found that cerebral iron levels in LA-fed older animals were lower when compared to controls, and were similar to levels seen in younger rats. These results thus show that chronic LA supplementation may be a means to modulate the age-related accumulation of cortical iron, thereby lowering oxidative stress associated with ageing [188]. Since amyloid aggregates have been shown to be stabilised by transition metals such as iron and copper, it was also speculated that LA could inhibit aggregate formation or potentially dissolve existing amyloid deposits. Fonte et al. successfully re-solubilised Aβ with transition metal ion chelators, and showed that LA enhanced the extraction of Aβ from the frontal cortex in a mouse model of AD, suggesting that, like other metal chelators, it could reduce amyloid burden in AD patients [189].

A potential side effect of a long-term therapy with high doses of a metal chelator such as LA could be the inhibition of enzymes that require metals as cofactors, such as IDE or SOD (Superoxide dismutase). Suh et al. investigated whether LA and DHLA remove copper or iron from the active sites of Cu,Zn superoxide dismutase and aconitase. They found that even at millimolar concentrations, neither LA nor DHLA altered the activity of these enzymes [190], providing promising results for the long-term use of LA in AD.

As mentioned earlier, AD pathology includes a chronic inflammatory process around amyloid plaques, characterised by the activation of microglia and astrocytes and increased levels of radicals and pro-inflammatory molecules such as iNOS, IL-1β, IL-6, and TNF-α [191]. AD patients also show increased cytokine levels (e.g. IL-1β and TNF-α) in the CSF, with TNF-α being a good predictor for the progression from mild cognitive impairment to AD. Recently, much attention has been paid to ROS as mediators in signalling processes, termed 'redox-sensitive signal transduction'. ROS modulate the activity of cytoplasmic signal transducing enzymes by at least two different mechanisms: oxidation of cysteine residues or reaction with iron-sulphur clusters. One widely investigated sensor protein is the p21Ras protein [192]. Activation of Ras by oxidants is caused by oxidative modification of a specific cysteine residue (Cys118). Ras interacts with PI3-kinase, protein kinase C, diacylglycerol kinase, and MAP-kinase-kinase-kinase, regulating expression of IL-1β, IL-6, and iNOS. LA can scavenge intracellular free radicals (acting as second messengers), downregulate pro-inflammatory redox-sensitive signal transduction processes including NF-κB translocation, and thus attenuate the release of more free radicals and cytotoxic cytokines [181, 193].

Cellular and mitochondrial membranes contain a significant amount of arachidonic acid and linoleic acid, precursors of lipid peroxidation products 4-hydroxynonenal (HNE) and acrolein. Acrolein decreases PDH and α-ketoglutarate dehydrogenase (KGDH) activities by covalently binding to the enzyme cofactor LA, an important component in both the PDH and KGDH complexes. Acrolein may be partially responsible for the dysfunction of mitochondria and loss of energy found in the AD-affected brain through its inhibition of PDH and KGDH activities, potentially contributing to neurodegeneration [194]. In other studies, levels of lipid peroxidation, oxidised glutathione (GSSG), non-enzymatic antioxidants, and the activities of mitochondrial enzymes were measured in liver and kidney mitochondria of young and aged rats before and after LA supplementation. In both the liver and the kidney, a decrease in the activities of mitochondrial enzymes was observed in aged rats. Supplementing the diet of aged rats with LA resulted in a decrease in the levels of lipid peroxidation and inhibition of the activities of mitochondrial enzymes, including isocitrate dehydrogenase, KGDH, succinate dehydrogenase, NADH dehydrogenase, and cytochrome C oxidase. The authors concluded that LA could help to reverse the age-associated decline in mitochondrial enzymes, and therefore may lower the increased risk of oxidative damage that occurs during ageing [195].

Recent studies have suggested new mechanisms whereby lipoic acid influences AD pathogenesis. For example, cell culture studies have found that an increase in BACE1 activity can diminish glucose oxidation by inhibiting key mitochondrial decarboxylation reactions which in turn diminishes substrate delivery to mitochondria. Lipoic acid (or beta-hydroxybutyrate) was found to alleviate this effect of BACE1 [196]. Furthermore, studies of high-fat-diet-fed rats showed that lipoic acid could reduce the diet-induced damage to neuronal insulin signalling and cognitive deficits in the rats [197]. Hippocampus expression levels of the vesicular glutamate transporter (VGlut1), required for release of glutamate, were also reduced by the high-fat diet, and lipoic acid was found to reverse this change, leading the authors to suggest lipoic acid might reduce the glutamatergic deficit seen in AD. Similarly, C57BL/6J mice on a high-fat diet developed insulin resistance, and demonstrated lower brain-glucose uptake, lower levels of glucose transporters, changes to glucose metabolism, and ultimately synaptic loss. Lipoic-acid treatment was again found to prevent many of these metabolic changes and preserve synaptic plasticity [198]. This was attributed to the insulin-like effect of lipoic acid [198], which the researchers had previously demonstrated in AD-model transgenic mice, where lipoic acid was found to prevent the transgene-associated decrease in glucose uptake, to reduce the decrease in IRS activation, and to mediate greater downstream Akt signalling [199].

All these positive effects of lipoic acid suggest lipoic acid supplements or foods high in lipoic acid (broccoli, spinach, red meat, tomatoes, for example) should be encouraged, and innovative drugs based on lipoic acid effects are being developed [200].

8.7 Conclusion

This chapter aimed to provide an overview of inflammation in AD, as well as the antioxidant, anti-inflammatory, anti-amyloidogenic, and neuroprotective effects of a number of phenolic and antioxidant compounds. These compounds have been examined in numerous *in vitro* and *in vivo* studies and a large body of epidemiological data also suggests a beneficial effect on cognition. These compounds have been demonstrated to have varying mechanisms of action, relating to decreasing cognitive deficits, oxidative stress, inflammation, and Aβ levels. However, despite encouraging results from animal studies, the percentage of positive results from AD clinical trials is surprisingly low (as with many other drugs tested in AD prevention or treatment studies, such as the anti-amyloid immunotherapy). The effectiveness of these identified compounds appears enhanced when treatment is initiated early in the disease process, for example, in the case of omega-3 fatty acids which slowed down the progression of the disease, yet only in very mild stages of AD [175, 201]. Future work is required to evaluate the value of these compounds and foods, as well as the efficacy of using combinations of such compounds, which has become common in complementary medicine.

Epidemiological studies have linked the traditional Mediterranean and Okinawa-style diets to longevity and good health [202, 203], diets which themselves already have a high antioxidant content and low levels of foods known to lead to cardiovascular disease and dysregulation of lipid and sugar metabolism. For maximum effectiveness, it would be ideal to combine such polyphenolic antioxidant supplements with a Mediterranean or Okinawa-style diet, to prevent or slow the onset of this devastating disease.

References

1 Gotz, J., Xia, D., Leinenga, G. et al. (2013). What renders TAU toxic. *Front. Neurol.* 4: 72.
2 Gandy, S., Martins, R.N., and Buxbaum, J. (2003). Molecular and cellular basis for anti-amyloid therapy in Alzheimer disease. *Alzheimer Dis. Assoc. Disord.* 17: 259–266.
3 von Bernhardi, R. and Ramirez, G. (2001). Microglia-astrocyte interaction in Alzheimer's disease: friends or foes for the nervous system? *Biol. Res.* 34: 123–128.
4 Wang, W.Y., Tan, M.S., Yu, J.T., and Tan, L. (2015). Role of pro-inflammatory cytokines released from microglia in Alzheimer's disease. *Ann. Transl. Med.* 3: 136.
5 Morales, I., Guzman-Martinez, L., Cerda-Troncoso, C. et al. (2014). Neuroinflammation in the pathogenesis of Alzheimer's disease. A rational framework for the search of novel therapeutic approaches. *Front. Cell. Neurosci.* 8: 112.

6 Francos-Quijorna, I., Amo-Aparicio, J., Martinez-Muriana, A., and Lopez-Vales, R. (2016). IL-4 drives microglia and macrophages toward a phenotype conducive for tissue repair and functional recovery after spinal cord injury. *Glia* 64: 2079–2092.

7 Lee, J.H., Wei, Z.Z., Cao, W. et al. (2016). Regulation of therapeutic hypothermia on inflammatory cytokines, microglia polarization, migration and functional recovery after ischemic stroke in mice. *Neurobiol. Dis.* 96: 248–260.

8 Doens, D. and Fernandez, P.L. (2014). Microglia receptors and their implications in the response to amyloid beta for Alzheimer's disease pathogenesis. *J. Neuroinflammation* 11: 48.

9 Gertig, U. and Hanisch, U.K. (2014). Microglial diversity by responses and responders. *Front. Cell. Neurosci.* 8: 101.

10 Tremblay, M.E., Lecours, C., Samson, L. et al. (2015). From the Cajal alumni Achucarro and Rio-Hortega to the rediscovery of never-resting microglia. *Front. Neuroanat.* 9: 45.

11 Sierra, A., Abiega, O., Shahraz, A., and Neumann, H. (2013). Janus-faced microglia: beneficial and detrimental consequences of microglial phagocytosis. *Front. Cell. Neurosci.* 7: 6.

12 Daria, A., Colombo, A., Llovera, G. et al. (2017). Young microglia restore amyloid plaque clearance of aged microglia. *EMBO J.* 36: 583–603.

13 Raj, D., Yin, Z., Breur, M. et al. (2017). Increased white matter inflammation in aging- and Alzheimer's disease brain. *Front. Mol. Neurosci.* 10: 206.

14 Lopez Gonzalez, I., Garcia-Esparcia, P., Llorens, F., and Ferrer, I. (2016). Genetic and transcriptomic profiles of inflammation in neurodegenerative diseases: Alzheimer, Parkinson, Creutzfeldt-Jakob and Tauopathies. *Int. J. Mol. Sci.* 17: 206.

15 Malik, M., Parikh, I., Vasquez, J.B. et al. (2015). Genetics ignite focus on microglial inflammation in Alzheimer's disease. *Mol. Neurodegener.* 10: 52.

16 Leyns, C.E.G. and Holtzman, D.M. (2017). Glial contributions to neurodegeneration in tauopathies. *Mol. Neurodegener.* 12: 50.

17 Lozano, D., Gonzales-Portillo, G.S., Acosta, S. et al. (2015). Neuroinflammatory responses to traumatic brain injury: etiology, clinical consequences, and therapeutic opportunities. *Neuropsychiatr. Dis. Treat.* 11: 97–106.

18 Liddelow, S.A., Guttenplan, K.A., Clarke, L.E. et al. (2017). Neurotoxic reactive astrocytes are induced by activated microglia. *Nature* 541: 481–487.

19 Su, C.W., Lin, C.C., Kao, C.H., and Chen, H.Y. (2016). Association between glaucoma and the risk of dementia. *Medicine (Baltimore)* 95: e2833.

20 Ramirez, A.I., de Hoz, R., Salobrar-Garcia, E. et al. (2017). The role of microglia in retinal Neurodegeneration: Alzheimer's disease, Parkinson, and glaucoma. *Front. Aging Neurosci.* 9: 214.

21 Lin, I.C., Wang, Y.H., Wang, T.J. et al. (2014). Glaucoma, Alzheimer's disease, and Parkinson's disease: an 8-year population-based follow-up study. *PLoS One* 9: e108938.

22 Ng, R.C. and Chan, K.H. (2017). Potential Neuroprotective effects of adiponectin in Alzheimer's disease. *Int. J. Mol. Sci.* 18 (3): 592. http://doi.org/10.3390/ijms18030592.

23 Khemka, V.K., Bagchi, D., Bandyopadhyay, K. et al. (2014). Altered serum levels of adipokines and insulin in probable Alzheimer's disease. *J. Alzheimers Dis.* 41: 525–533.

24 van Himbergen, T.M., Beiser, A.S., Ai, M. et al. (2012). Biomarkers for insulin resistance and inflammation and the risk for all-cause dementia and alzheimer disease: results from the Framingham Heart Study. *Arch. Neurol.* 69: 594–600.
25 Teixeira, A.L., Diniz, B.S., Campos, A.C. et al. (2013). Decreased levels of circulating adiponectin in mild cognitive impairment and Alzheimer's disease. *Neuromolecular Med.* 15: 115–121.
26 Ng, R.C., Cheng, O.Y., Jian, M. et al. (2016). Chronic adiponectin deficiency leads to Alzheimer's disease-like cognitive impairments and pathologies through AMPK inactivation and cerebral insulin resistance in aged mice. *Mol. Neurodegener.* 11: 71.
27 Song, J., Choi, S.M., and Kim, B.C. (2017). Adiponectin regulates the polarization and function of microglia via PPAR-gamma signaling under amyloid beta toxicity. *Front. Cell Neurosci.* 11: 64.
28 Achari, A.E. and Jain, S.K. (2017). Adiponectin, a therapeutic target for obesity, diabetes, and endothelial dysfunction. *Int. J. Mol. Sci.* 18.
29 Retz, W., Gsell, W., Münch, G. et al. (1998). Free radicals in Alzheimer's disease. *J. Neural. Transm. Suppl.* 54: 221–236.
30 Picklo, M.J., Montine, T.J., Amarnath, V., and Neely, M.D. (2002). Carbonyl toxicology and Alzheimer's disease. *Toxicol. Appl. Pharmacol.* 184: 187–197.
31 Dizdaroglu, M., Jaruga, P., Birincioglu, M., and Rodriguez, H. (2002). Free radical-induced damage to DNA: mechanisms and measurement. *Free Radic. Biol. Med.* 32: 1102–1115.
32 Cochrane, C.G. (1991). Cellular injury by oxidants. *Am. J. Med.* 91: 23s–30s.
33 Requena, J.R., Levine, R.L., and Stadtman, E.R. (2003). Recent advances in the analysis of oxidized proteins. *Amino Acids* 25: 221–226.
34 Guo, L., Tian, J., and Du, H. (2017). Mitochondrial dysfunction and synaptic transmission failure in Alzheimer's disease. *J. Alzheimers Dis.* 57: 1071–1086.
35 Zhu, X., Perry, G., Moreira, P.I. et al. (2006). Mitochondrial abnormalities and oxidative imbalance in Alzheimer disease. *J. Alzheimers Dis.* 9: 147–153.
36 Tonnies, E. and Trushina, E. (2017). Oxidative stress, synaptic dysfunction, and Alzheimer's disease. *J. Alzheimers Dis.* 57: 1105–1121.
37 Abate, G., Marziano, M., Rungratanawanich, W. et al. (2017). Nutrition and AGE-ing: focusing on Alzheimer's disease. *Oxid. Med. Cell. Longev.* 2017: 7039816.
38 Choi, B.R., Cho, W.H., Kim, J. et al. (2014). Increased expression of the receptor for advanced glycation end products in neurons and astrocytes in a triple transgenic mouse model of Alzheimer's disease. *Exp. Mol. Med.* 46: e75.
39 Matrone, C., Djelloul, M., Taglialatela, G., and Perrone, L. (2015). Inflammatory risk factors and pathologies promoting Alzheimer's disease progression: is RAGE the key? *Histol. Histopathol.* 30: 125–139.
40 Yan, S.S., Chen, D., Yan, S. et al. (2012). RAGE is a key cellular target for Abeta-induced perturbation in Alzheimer's disease. *Front. Biosci. (Schol. Ed.)* 4: 240–250.
41 Yasojima, K., Schwab, C., McGeer, E.G., and McGeer, P.L. (1999). Up-regulated production and activation of the complement system in Alzheimer's disease brain. *Am. J. Pathol.* 154: 927–936.
42 Rogers, J. and Lue, L.-F. (2001). Microglial chemotaxis, activation, and phagocytosis of amyloid β-peptide as linked phenomena in Alzheimer's disease. *Neurochem. Int.* 39: 333–340.

43 Fonseca, M.I., Ager, R.R., Woodruff, T.M. et al. (2008). Chronic treatment with C5a antagonist decreases pathology in two mouse models of Alzheimer's disease. *Alzheimers Dement.* 4: T188–T188.

44 Fonseca, M.I., Ager, R.R., Chu, S.H. et al. (2009). Treatment with a C5aR antagonist decreases pathology and enhances behavioral performance in murine models of Alzheimer's disease. *J. Immunol.* 183: 1375–1383.

45 Shen, Y., Lue, L., Yang, L. et al. (2001). Complement activation by neurofibrillary tangles in Alzheimer's disease. *Neurosci. Lett.* 305: 165–168.

46 Rogers, J., Cooper, N.R., Webster, S. et al. (1992). Complement activation by beta-amyloid in Alzheimer disease. *Proc. Natl. Acad. Sci. U S A* 89: 10016–10020.

47 Daborg, J., Andreasson, U., Pekna, M. et al. (2012). Cerebrospinal fluid levels of complement proteins C3, C4 and CR1 in Alzheimer's disease. *J. Neural. Transm. (Vienna)* 119: 789–797.

48 Finehout, E.J., Franck, Z., and Lee, K.H. (2005). Complement protein isoforms in CSF as possible biomarkers for neurodegenerative disease. *Dis. Markers* 21: 93–101.

49 Orsini, F., De Blasio, D., Zangari, R. et al. (2014). Versatility of the complement system in neuroinflammation, neurodegeneration and brain homeostasis. *Front. Cell. Neurosci.* 8: 380.

50 Hernandez, M.X., Namiranian, P., Nguyen, E. et al. (2017). C5a increases the injury to primary neurons elicited by fibrillar amyloid beta. *ASN Neuro* 9 (1): http://doi.org/10.1177/1759091416687871.

51 Roy, C., Gupta, A., Fisette, A. et al. (2013). C5a receptor deficiency alters energy utilization and fat storage. *PLoS One* 8: e62531.

52 Snow, W.M. and Albensi, B.C. (2016). Neuronal gene targets of NF-kappaB and their dysregulation in Alzheimer's disease. *Front. Mol. Neurosci.* 9: 118.

53 Gasic-Milenkovic, J., Dukic-Stefanovic, S., Deuther-Conrad, W. et al. (2003). Beta-amyloid peptide potentiates inflammatory responses induced by lipopolysaccharide, interferon-gamma and 'advanced glycation endproducts' in a murine microglia cell line. *Eur. J. Neurosci.* 17: 813–821.

54 Ientile, R., Curro, M., and Caccamo, D. (2015). Transglutaminase 2 and neuroinflammation. *Amino Acids* 47: 19–26.

55 Tanji, K., Mori, F., Imaizumi, T. et al. (2003). Interleukin-1 induces tau phosphorylation and morphological changes in cultured human astrocytes. *Neuroreport* 14: 413–417.

56 Akiyama, H., Barger, S., Barnum, S. et al. (2000). Inflammation and Alzheimer's disease. *Neurobiol. Aging* 21: 383–421.

57 Münch, G., Apelt, J., Rosemarie Kientsch, E. et al. (2003). Advanced glycation endproducts and pro-inflammatory cytokines in transgenic Tg2576 mice with amyloid plaque pathology. *J. Neurochem.* 86: 283–289.

58 Khandelwal, P.J., Dumanis, S.B., Herman, A.M. et al. (2012). Wild type and P301L mutant tau promote neuro-inflammation and alpha-Synuclein accumulation in lentiviral gene delivery models. *Mol. Cell. Neurosci.* 49: 44–53.

59 Srikanth, V., Maczurek, A., Phan, T. et al. (2011). Advanced glycation endproducts and their receptor RAGE in Alzheimer's disease. *Neurobiol. Aging* 32: 763–777.

60 Patel, A., Rees, S.D., Kelly, M.A. et al. (2014). Genetic variants conferring susceptibility to Alzheimer's disease in the general population; do they also predispose to dementia in Down's syndrome. *BMC Res. Notes* 7: 42.

61 Jun, G., Naj, A.C., Beecham, G.W. et al. (2010). Meta-analysis confirms CR1, CLU, and PICALM as alzheimer disease risk loci and reveals interactions with APOE genotypes. *Arch. Neurol.* 67: 1473–1484.

62 Lambert, J.C., Ibrahim-Verbaas, C.A., Harold, D. et al. (2013). Meta-analysis of 74,046 individuals identifies 11 new susceptibility loci for Alzheimer's disease. *Nat. Genet.* 45: 1452–1458.

63 Naj, A.C., Jun, G., Beecham, G.W. et al. (2011). Common variants at MS4A4/MS4A6E, CD2AP, CD33 and EPHA1 are associated with late-onset Alzheimer's disease. *Nat. Genet.* 43: 436–441.

64 Block, M.L., Zecca, L., and Hong, J.S. (2007). Microglia-mediated neurotoxicity: uncovering the molecular mechanisms. *Nat. Rev. Neurosci.* 8: 57–69.

65 Millington, C., Sonego, S., Karunaweera, N. et al. (2014). Chronic neuroinflammation in Alzheimer's disease: new perspectives on animal models and promising candidate drugs. *Biomed Res. Int.* 2014: 309129.

66 Hansen, E., Krautwald, M., Maczurek, A.E. et al. (2010). A versatile high throughput screening system for the simultaneous identification of anti-inflammatory and neuroprotective compounds. *J. Alzheimers Dis.* 19: 451–464.

67 Heneka, M.T., Golenbock, D.T., and Latz, E. (2015). Innate immunity in Alzheimer's disease. *Nat. Immunol.* 16: 229–236.

68 Games, D., Adams, D., Alessandrini, R. et al. (1995). Alzheimer-type neuropathology in transgenic mice overexpressing V717F beta-amyloid precursor protein. *Nature* 373: 523–527.

69 Guo, J.T., Yu, J., Grass, D. et al. (2002). Inflammation-dependent cerebral deposition of serum amyloid a protein in a mouse model of amyloidosis. *J. Neurosci.* 22: 5900–5909.

70 McGeer, P.L. and McGeer, E.G. (2013). The amyloid cascade-inflammatory hypothesis of Alzheimer disease: implications for therapy. *Acta Neuropathol.* 126: 479–497.

71 Vandenabeele, P. and Fiers, W. (1991). Is amyloidogenesis during Alzheimer's disease due to an IL-1-/IL-6-mediated 'acute phase response' in the brain? *Immunol. Today* 12: 217–219.

72 Verdile, G., Keane, K.N., Cruzat, V.F. et al. (2015). Inflammation and oxidative stress: the molecular connectivity between insulin resistance, obesity, and Alzheimer's disease. *Mediators Inflamm.* 2015: 105828.

73 Sastre, M., Dewachter, I., Rossner, S. et al. (2006). Nonsteroidal anti-inflammatory drugs repress beta-secretase gene promoter activity by the activation of PPARgamma. *Proc. Natl. Acad. Sci. U S A* 103: 443–448.

74 Chami, L. and Checler, F. (2012). BACE1 is at the crossroad of a toxic vicious cycle involving cellular stress and beta-amyloid production in Alzheimer's disease. *Mol. Neurodegener.* 7: 52.

75 Liu, T., Huang, Y., Chen, J. et al. (2014). Attenuated ability of BACE1 to cleave the amyloid precursor protein via silencing long noncoding RNA BACE1AS expression. *Mol. Med. Rep.* 10: 1275–1281.

76 Greco, S., Zaccagnini, G., Fuschi, P. et al. (2017). Increased BACE1-AS long noncoding RNA and beta-amyloid levels in heart failure. *Cardiovasc. Res.* 113: 453–463.

77 Modarresi, F., Faghihi, M.A., Patel, N.S. et al. (2011). Knockdown of BACE1-AS nonprotein-coding transcript modulates beta-amyloid-related hippocampal neurogenesis. *Int. J. Alzheimers Dis.* 2011: 929042.

78 Batarseh, Y.S., Duong, Q.V., Mousa, Y.M. et al. (2016). Amyloid-beta and Astrocytes interplay in amyloid-beta related disorders. *Int. J. Mol. Sci.* 17: 338.

79 Amara, F.M., Junaid, A., Clough, R.R., and Liang, B. (1999). TGF-beta(1), regulation of alzheimer amyloid precursor protein mRNA expression in a normal human astrocyte cell line: mRNA stabilization. *Brain Res. Mol. Brain Res.* 71: 42–49.

80 Rogers, J.T., Leiter, L.M., McPhee, J. et al. (1999). Translation of the alzheimer amyloid precursor protein mRNA is up-regulated by interleukin-1 through 5′-untranslated region sequences. *J. Biol. Chem.* 274: 6421–6431.

81 Xu, J., Mukerjee, S., Silva-Alves, C.R. et al. (2016). A disintegrin and metalloprotease 17 in the cardiovascular and central nervous systems. *Front. Physiol.* 7: 469.

82 Chanthaphavong, R.S., Loughran, P.A., Lee, T.Y. et al. (2012). A role for cGMP in inducible nitric-oxide synthase (iNOS)-induced tumor necrosis factor (TNF) alpha-converting enzyme (TACE/ADAM17) activation, translocation, and TNF receptor 1 (TNFR1) shedding in hepatocytes. *J. Biol. Chem.* 287: 35887–35898.

83 Wang, J., Al-Lamki, R.S., Zhang, H. et al. (2003). Histamine antagonizes tumor necrosis factor (TNF) signaling by stimulating TNF receptor shedding from the cell surface and Golgi storage pool. *J. Biol. Chemi.* 278: 21751–21760.

84 Birks, J. and Wilcock, G.G. (2004). Velnacrine for Alzheimer's disease. *Cochrane Database Syst. Rev.* (2): (Art. No.: CD004748).

85 Birks, J.S. and Harvey, R. (2018). Donepezil for dementia due to Alzheimer's disease. *Cochrane Database Syst. Rev.* (6): CD001190. https://doi.org/10.1002/14651858.CD001190.pub3.

86 Birks, J., Grimley Evans, J., Iakovidou, V. et al. (2009). Rivastigmine for Alzheimer's disease. *Cochrane Database Syst. Rev.* 15 (2): CD001191. https://doi.org/10.1002/14651858.CD001191.pub2. Review. Update in: Cochrane Database Syst Rev. 2015;4:CD001191.

87 Alva, G., Grossberg, G.T., Schmitt, F.A. et al. (2011). Efficacy of rivastigmine transdermal patch on activities of daily living: item responder analyses. *Int J. Geriatr. Psychiatry* 26 (4): 356–363. https://doi.org/10.1002/gps.2534.

88 Sadowsky, C.H., Farlow, M.R., Atkinson, L. et al. (2005). Switching from donepezil to rivastigmine is well tolerated: results of an open-label safety and Tolerability Study. *Prim. Care Companion J. Clin. Psychiatry* 7: 43–48.

89 Coelho, F. and Birks, J. (2001). Physostigmine for Alzheimer's disease. *Cochrane Database Syst. Rev.* (2): CD001499. https://doi.org/10.1002/14651858.CD001499.

90 Marta, M., Castellano, C., Oliverio, A. et al. (1988). New analogs of physostigmine: alternative drugs for Alzheimer's disease? *Life Sci.* 43: 1921–1928.

91 Wang, C.H., Wang, L.S., and Zhu, N. (2016). Cholinesterase inhibitors and non-steroidal anti-inflammatory drugs as Alzheimer's disease therapies: an updated umbrella review of systematic reviews and meta-analyses. *Eur. Rev. Med. Pharmacol. Sci.* 20: 4801–4817.

92 Bond, M., Rogers, G., Peters, J. et al. (2012). The effectiveness and cost-effectiveness of donepezil, galantamine, rivastigmine and memantine for the treatment of Alzheimer's disease (review of technology appraisal no. 111): a systematic review and economic model. *Health Technol. Assess.* 16: 1–470.

93 Miguel-Alvarez, M., Santos-Lozano, A., Sanchis-Gomar, F. et al. (2015). Non-steroidal anti-inflammatory drugs as a treatment for Alzheimer's disease: a systematic review and meta-analysis of treatment effect. *Drugs Aging* 32: 139–147.

94 Jaturapatporn, D., Isaac, M.G., McCleery, J., and Tabet, N. (2012). Aspirin, steroidal and non-steroidal anti-inflammatory drugs for the treatment of Alzheimer's disease. *Cochrane Database Syst. Rev.* 15 (2): CD006378. https://doi.org/10.1002/14651858.CD006378.pub2.

95 Gupta, P.P., Pandey, R.D., Jha, D. et al. (2015). Role of traditional nonsteroidal anti-inflammatory drugs in Alzheimer's disease: a meta-analysis of randomized clinical trials. *Am. J. Alzheimers Dis. Other Demen.* 30: 178–182.

96 Breitner, J.C., Baker, L.D., Montine, T.J. et al. (2011). Extended results of the Alzheimer's disease anti-inflammatory prevention trial. *Alzheimers Dement.* 7: 402–411.

97 Wang, J., Tan, L., Wang, H.F. et al. (2015). Anti-inflammatory drugs and risk of Alzheimer's disease: an updated systematic review and meta-analysis. *J. Alzheimers Dis.* 44: 385–396.

98 Imbimbo, B.P., Solfrizzi, V., and Panza, F. (2010). Are NSAIDs useful to treat Alzheimer's disease or mild cognitive impairment? *Front. Aging Neurosci.* 2 (19): http://doi.org/10.3389/fnagi.2010.00019.

99 Daniels, M.J., Rivers-Auty, J., Schilling, T. et al. (2016). Fenamate NSAIDs inhibit the NLRP3 inflammasome and protect against Alzheimer's disease in rodent models. *Nat. Commun.* 7: 12504.

100 Kotilinek, L.A., Westerman, M.A., Wang, Q. et al. (2008). Cyclooxygenase-2 inhibition improves amyloid-beta-mediated suppression of memory and synaptic plasticity. *Brain* 131: 651–664.

101 Woodling, N.S., Colas, D., Wang, Q. et al. (2016). Cyclooxygenase inhibition targets neurons to prevent early behavioural decline in Alzheimer's disease model mice. *Brain* 139: 2063–2081.

102 Szekely, C.A., Breitner, J.C., Fitzpatrick, A.L. et al. (2008). NSAID use and dementia risk in the Cardiovascular Health Study: role of APOE and NSAID type. *Neurology* 70: 17–24.

103 Steiner, N., Balez, R., Karunaweera, N. et al. (2015). Neuroprotection of Neuro2a cells and the cytokine suppressive and anti-inflammatory mode of action of resveratrol in activated RAW264.7 macrophages and C8-B4 microglia. *Neurochem. Int.*

104 Venigalla, M., Gyengesi, E., and Münch, G. (2015). Curcumin and Apigenin – novel and promising therapeutics against chronic neuroinflammation in Alzheimer's disease. *Neural Regen. Res.* 10: 1181–1185.

105 Gunawardena, D., Shanmugam, K., Low, M. et al. (2013). Determination of anti-inflammatory activities of standardised preparations of plant- and mushroom-based foods. *Eur. J. Nutr.* 2013: 335–343.

106 Gunawardena, D., Karunaweera, N., Lee, S. et al. (2015). Anti-inflammatory activity of cinnamon (C. zeylanicum and C. cassia) extracts – identification of E-cinnamaldehyde and o-methoxy cinnamaldehyde as the most potent bioactive compounds. *Food Funct.* 6: 910–919.

107 Chen, Y.F., Wang, Y.W., Huang, W.S. et al. (2016). Trans-cinnamaldehyde, an essential oil in cinnamon powder, ameliorates cerebral ischemia-induced brain injury via inhibition of Neuroinflammation through attenuation of iNOS, COX-2 expression and NFkappa-B signaling pathway. *Neuromolecular Med.* 18 (3): 322–333. https://doi.org/10.1007/s12017-016-8395-9.

108 Peterson, D.W., George, R.C., Scaramozzino, F. et al. (2009). Cinnamon extract inhibits tau aggregation associated with Alzheimer's disease in vitro. *J. Alzheimers Dis.* 17: 585–597.

109 George, R.C., Lew, J., and Graves, D.J. (2013). Interaction of cinnamaldehyde and epicatechin with tau: implications of beneficial effects in modulating Alzheimer's disease pathogenesis. *J. Alzheimers Dis.* 36: 21–40.

110 Zhao, J., Zhang, X., Dong, L. et al. (2015). Cinnamaldehyde inhibits inflammation and brain damage in a mouse model of permanent cerebral ischaemia. *Br. J. Pharmacol.* 172: 5009–5023.

111 Zhao, H., Zhang, M., Zhou, F. et al. (2016). Cinnamaldehyde ameliorates LPS-induced cardiac dysfunction via TLR4-NOX4 pathway: the regulation of autophagy and ROS production. *J. Mol. Cell. Cardiol.* 101: 11–24.

112 Khare, P., Jagtap, S., Jain, Y. et al. (2016). Cinnamaldehyde supplementation prevents fasting-induced hyperphagia, lipid accumulation, and inflammation in high-fat diet-fed mice. *Biofactors* 42: 201–211.

113 Zhang, L., Zhang, Z., Fu, Y. et al. (2016). Trans-cinnamaldehyde improves memory impairment by blocking microglial activation through the destabilization of iNOS mRNA in mice challenged with lipopolysaccharide. *Neuropharmacology* 110: 503–518.

114 Mandel, S., Weinreb, O., Amit, T., and Youdim, M.B. (2004). Cell signaling pathways in the neuroprotective actions of the green tea polyphenol (-)-epigallocatechin-3-gallate: implications for neurodegenerative diseases. *J. Neurochem.* 88: 1555–1569.

115 Bhullar, K.S. and Rupasinghe, H.P. (2013). Polyphenols: multipotent therapeutic agents in neurodegenerative diseases. *Oxid. Med. Cell. Longev.* 2013: 891748.

116 Choi, Y.T., Jung, C.H., Lee, S.R. et al. (2001). The green tea polyphenol (-)-epigallocatechin gallate attenuates beta-amyloid-induced neurotoxicity in cultured hippocampal neurons. *Life Sci.* 70: 603–614.

117 Levites, Y., Amit, T., Mandel, S., and Youdim, M.B. (2003). Neuroprotection and neurorescue against Abeta toxicity and PKC-dependent release of nonamyloidogenic soluble precursor protein by green tea polyphenol (-)-epigallocatechin-3-gallate. *FASEB. J.* 17: 952–954.

118 Rezai-Zadeh, K., Shytle, D., Sun, N. et al. (2005). Green tea epigallocatechin-3-gallate (EGCG) modulates amyloid precursor protein cleavage and reduces cerebral amyloidosis in Alzheimer transgenic mice. *J. Neurosci.* 25: 8807–8814.

119 Okello, E.J., Leylabi, R., and McDougall, G.J. (2012). Inhibition of acetylcholinesterase by green and white tea and their simulated intestinal metabolites. *Food Funct.* 3: 651–661.

120 Ali, B., Jamal, Q.M., Shams, S. et al. (2016). In silico analysis of green tea polyphenols as inhibitors of AChE and BChE enzymes in Alzheimer's disease treatment. *CNS Neurol. Disord. Drug Targets* 15: 624–628.

121 Cong, L., Cao, C., Cheng, Y., and Qin, X.Y. (2016). Green tea polyphenols attenuated glutamate excitotoxicity via antioxidative and antiapoptotic pathway in the primary cultured cortical neurons. *Oxid. Med. Cell. Longev.* 2016: 2050435.

122 Qian, G., Xue, K., Tang, L. et al. (2012). Mitigation of oxidative damage by green tea polyphenols and tai chi exercise in postmenopausal women with osteopenia. *PLoS One* 7: e48090.

123 Zhang, Z., Wu, H., and Huang, H. (2016). Epicatechin plus treadmill exercise are neuroprotective against moderate-stage amyloid precursor protein/Presenilin 1 mice. *Pharmacogn. Mag.* 12: S139–S146.

124 Lee, Y.J., Choi, D.Y., Yun, Y.P. et al. (2013). Epigallocatechin-3-gallate prevents systemic inflammation-induced memory deficiency and amyloidogenesis via its anti-neuroinflammatory properties. *J. Nutr. Biochem.* 24: 298–310.

125 Cheng-Chung Wei, J., Huang, H.C., Chen, W.J. et al. (2016). Epigallocatechin gallate attenuates amyloid beta-induced inflammation and neurotoxicity in EOC 13.31 microglia. *Eur. J. Pharmacol.* 770: 16–24.

126 Cascella, M., Bimonte, S., Muzio, M.R. et al. (2017). The efficacy of Epigallocatechin-3-gallate (green tea) in the treatment of Alzheimer's disease: an overview of pre-clinical studies and translational perspectives in clinical practice. *Infect. Agent Cancer* 12: 36.

127 Rege, S.D., Geetha, T., Broderick, T.L., and Babu, J.R. (2017). Can diet and physical activity limit Alzheimer's disease risk? *Curr. Alzheimer Res.* 14: 76–93.

128 Ringman, J.M., Frautschy, S.A., Cole, G.M. et al. (2005). A potential role of the curry spice curcumin in Alzheimer's disease. *Curr. Alzheimer Res.* 2: 131–136.

129 Kirby, L., Lehmann, P., and Majeed, A. (1998). Dementia in people aged 65 years and older: a growing problem. *Popul. Trends* 23–28.

130 Kelloff, G.J., Crowell, J.A., Steele, V.E. et al. (1999). Progress in cancer chemoprevention. *Ann. N.Y. Acad. Sci.* 889: 1–13.

131 Sreejayan, R.M.N. (1994). Curcuminoids as potent inhibitors of lipid peroxidation. *J. Pharm. Pharmacol.* 46: 1013–1016.

132 Sreejayan, N. and Rao, M.N. (1996). Free radical scavenging activity of curcuminoids. *Arzneimittelforschung* 46: 169–171.

133 Xu, Y.X., Pindolia, K.R., Janakiraman, N. et al. (1997). Curcumin inhibits IL1 alpha and TNF-alpha induction of AP-1 and NF-kB DNA-binding activity in bone marrow stromal cells. *Hematopathol. Mol. Hematol.* 11: 49–62.

134 Pan, M.H., Lin-Shiau, S.Y., and Lin, J.K. (2000). Comparative studies on the suppression of nitric oxide synthase by curcumin and its hydrogenated metabolites through down-regulation of IkappaB kinase and NFkappaB activation in macrophages. *Biochem. Pharmacol.* 60: 1665–1676.

135 Soni, K.B., Rajan, A., and Kuttan, R. (1992). Reversal of aflatoxin induced liver damage by turmeric and curcumin. *Cancer Letters* 66: 115–121.

136 Soudamini, K.K., Unnikrishnan, M.C., Soni, K.B., and Kuttan, R. (1992). Inhibition of lipid peroxidation and cholesterol levels in mice by curcumin. *Indian J. Physiol. Pharmacol.* 36: 239–243.

137 Zhao, B.L., Li, X.J., He, R.G. et al. (1989). Scavenging effect of extracts of green tea and natural antioxidants on active oxygen radicals. *Cell Biophys.* 14: 175–185.

138 Yang, F., Lim, G.P., Begum, A.N. et al. (2005). Curcumin inhibits formation of amyloid beta oligomers and fibrils, binds plaques, and reduces amyloid in vivo. *J. Biol. Chem.* 280: 5892–5901.

139 Bharti, A.C., Donato, N., and Aggarwal, B.B. (2003). Curcumin (diferuloylmethane) inhibits constitutive and IL-6-inducible STAT3 phosphorylation in human multiple myeloma cells. *J. Immunol.* 171: 3863–3871.

140 Ray, B. and Lahiri, D.K. (2009). Neuroinflammation in Alzheimer's disease: different molecular targets and potential therapeutic agents including curcumin. *Curr. Opin. Pharmacol.* 9: 434–444.

141 Abe, Y., Hashimoto, S., and Horie, T. (1999). Curcumin inhibition of inflammatory cytokine production by human peripheral blood monocytes and alveolar macrophages. *Pharmacol Res.* 39: 41–47.

142 Venigalla, M., Sonego, S., Gyengesi, E. et al. (2015). Novel promising therapeutics against chronic neuroinflammation and neurodegeneration in Alzheimer's disease. *Neurochem. Int.*

143 Liang, F., Wan, Y., Schaak, D. et al. (2017). Nanoplasmonic fiber tip probe detects significant reduction of intracellular Alzheimer's disease-related oligomers by curcumin. *Sci. Rep.* 7: 5722.

144 Lim, G.P., Chu, T., Yang, F. et al. (2001). The curry spice curcumin reduces oxidative damage and amyloid pathology in an Alzheimer transgenic mouse. *J. Neurosci.* 21: 8370–8377.

145 Liu, H., Li, Z., Qiu, D. et al. (2010). The inhibitory effects of different curcuminoids on beta-amyloid protein, beta-amyloid precursor protein and beta-site amyloid precursor protein cleaving enzyme 1 in swAPP HEK293 cells. *Neurosci. Lett.* 485: 83–88.

146 Belviranli, M., Okudan, N., Atalik, K.E., and Oz, M. (2013). Curcumin improves spatial memory and decreases oxidative damage in aged female rats. *Biogerontology* 14: 187–196.

147 Begum, A.N., Jones, M.R., Lim, G.P. et al. (2008). Curcumin structure-function, bioavailability, and efficacy in models of neuroinflammation and Alzheimer's disease. *J. Pharmacol Exp. Ther.* 326: 196–208.

148 Ma, Q.L., Zuo, X., Yang, F. et al. (2013). Curcumin suppresses soluble tau dimers and corrects molecular chaperone, synaptic, and behavioral deficits in aged human tau transgenic mice. *J. Biol. Chem.* 288: 4056–4065.

149 Cox, K.H., Pipingas, A., and Scholey, A.B. (2015). Investigation of the effects of solid lipid curcumin on cognition and mood in a healthy older population. *J. Psychopharmacol.* 29 (5): 642–651. https://doi.org/10.1177/0269881114552744.

150 Goozee, K.G., Shah, T.M., Sohrabi, H.R. et al. (2016). Examining the potential clinical value of curcumin in the prevention and diagnosis of Alzheimer's disease. *Br. J. Nutr.* 115: 449–465.

151 Kuo, P.H., Lin, C.I., Chen, Y.H. et al. (2015). A high-cholesterol diet enriched with polyphenols from oriental plums (Prunus salicina) improves cognitive function and lowers brain cholesterol levels and neurodegenerative-related protein expression in mice. *Br. J. Nutr.* 113: 1550–1557.

152 Reinisalo, M., Karlund, A., Koskela, A. et al. (2015). Polyphenol stilbenes: molecular mechanisms of defence against oxidative stress and aging-related diseases. *Oxid. Med. Cell. Longev.* 2015: 340520.

153 Moosavi, F., Hosseini, R., Saso, L., and Firuzi, O. (2016). Modulation of neurotrophic signaling pathways by polyphenols. *Drug Des. Devel. Ther.* 10: 23–42.

154 Hariri, M. and Ghiasvand, R. (2016). Cinnamon and chronic diseases. *Adv. Exp. Med. Biol.* 929: 1–24.

155 Pantano, D., Luccarini, I., Nardiello, P. et al. (2017). Oleuropein aglycone and polyphenols from olive mill waste water ameliorate cognitive deficits and neuropathology. *Br. J. Clin. Pharmacol.* 83: 54–62.

156 Casamenti, F. and Stefani, M. (2017). Olive polyphenols: new promising agents to combat aging-associated neurodegeneration. *Expert. Rev. Neurother.* 17: 345–358.

157 Salem, N. Jr., Litman, B., Kim, H.Y., and Gawrisch, K. (2001). Mechanisms of action of docosahexaenoic acid in the nervous system. *Lipids* 36: 945–959.

158 Calon, F., Lim, G.P., Morihara, T. et al. (2005). Dietary n-3 polyunsaturated fatty acid depletion activates caspases and decreases NMDA receptors in the brain of a transgenic mouse model of Alzheimer's disease. *Eur. J. Neurosci.* 22: 617–626.

159 Soderberg, M., Edlund, C., Kristensson, K., and Dallner, G. (1991). Fatty acid composition of brain phospholipids in aging and in Alzheimer's disease. *Lipids* 26: 421–425.

160 Prasad, M.R., Lovell, M.A., Yatin, M. et al. (1998). Regional membrane phospholipid alterations in Alzheimer's disease. *Neurochem. Res.* 23: 81–88.

161 Barberger-Gateau, P., Letenneur, L., Deschamps, V. et al. (2002). Fish, meat, and risk of dementia: cohort study. *BMJ* 325: 932–933.

162 Conquer, J.A., Tierney, M.C., Zecevic, J. et al. (2000). Fatty acid analysis of blood plasma of patients with Alzheimer's disease, other types of dementia, and cognitive impairment. *Lipids* 35: 1305–1312.

163 Morris, M.C., Evans, D.A., Bienias, J.L. et al. (2003). Consumption of fish and n-3 fatty acids and risk of incident Alzheimer disease. *Arch. Neurol.* 60: 940–946.

164 Florent, S., Malaplate-Armand, C., Youssef, I. et al. (2006). Docosahexaenoic acid prevents neuronal apoptosis induced by soluble amyloid-beta oligomers. *J. Neurochem.* 96: 385–395.

165 Lukiw, W.J., Cui, J.G., Marcheselli, V.L. et al. (2005). A role for docosahexaenoic acid-derived neuroprotectin D1 in neural cell survival and Alzheimer disease. *J. Clin. Invest.* 115: 2774–2783.

166 Calon, F., Lim, G.P., Yang, F. et al. (2004). Docosahexaenoic acid protects from dendritic pathology in an Alzheimer's disease mouse model. *Neuron* 43: 633–645.

167 Hashimoto, M., Tanabe, Y., Fujii, Y. et al. (2005). Chronic administration of docosahexaenoic acid ameliorates the impairment of spatial cognition learning ability in amyloid beta-infused rats. *J. Nutr.* 135: 549–555.

168 Lim, G.P., Calon, F., Morihara, T. et al. (2005). A diet enriched with the omega-3 fatty acid docosahexaenoic acid reduces amyloid burden in an aged Alzheimer mouse model. *J. Neurosci.* 25: 3032–3040.

169 Cole, G.M. and Frautschy, S.A. (2006). Docosahexaenoic acid protects from amyloid and dendritic pathology in an Alzheimer's disease mouse model. *Nutr. Health* 18: 249–259.

170 Nock, T.G., Chouinard-Watkins, R., and Plourde, M. (2017). Carriers of an apolipoprotein E epsilon 4 allele are more vulnerable to a dietary deficiency in omega-3 fatty acids and cognitive decline. *Biochim. Biophys. Acta* 1862: 1068–1078.

171 Olivera-Perez, H.M., Lam, L., Dang, J. et al. (2017). Omega-3 fatty acids increase the unfolded protein response and improve amyloid-beta phagocytosis by macrophages of patients with mild cognitive impairment. *FASEB J* 31: 4359–4369.

172 Abdullah, L., Evans, J.E., Emmerich, T. et al. (2017). APOE epsilon4 specific imbalance of arachidonic acid and docosahexaenoic acid in serum phospholipids identifies individuals with preclinical mild cognitive impairment/Alzheimer's disease. *Aging (Albany NY)* 9: 964–985.

173 Hauser, P.S. and Ryan, R.O. (2013). Impact of apolipoprotein E on Alzheimer's disease. *Curr. Alzheimer Res.* 10: 809–817.

174 Andrieu, S., Guyonnet, S., Coley, N. et al. (2017). Effect of long-term omega 3 polyunsaturated fatty acid supplementation with or without multidomain intervention on cognitive function in elderly adults with memory complaints (MAPT): a randomised, placebo-controlled trial. *Lancet Neurol.* 16: 377–389.

175 Yassine, H.N., Braskie, M.N., Mack, W.J. et al. (2017). Association of docosahexaenoic acid supplementation with Alzheimer disease stage in Apolipoprotein E epsilon4 carriers: a review. *JAMA Neurol.* 74: 339–347.

176 Snowden, S.G., Ebshiana, A.A., Hye, A. et al. (2017). Association between fatty acid metabolism in the brain and Alzheimer disease neuropathology and cognitive performance: a nontargeted metabolomic study. *PLoS Med.* 14: e1002266.

177 Grimm, M.O., Mett, J., Stahlmann, C.P. et al. (2016). Eicosapentaenoic acid and docosahexaenoic acid increase the degradation of amyloid-beta by affecting insulin-degrading enzyme. *Biochem. Cell Biol.* 94: 534–542.

178 Packer, L., Witt, E.H., and Tritschler, H.J. (1995). Alpha-lipoic acid as a biological antioxidant. *Free Radic. Biol. Med.* 19: 227–250.

179 Münch, G., Maczurek, A., Hager, K. et al. (2008). Lipoic acid as an anti-inflammatory and neuroprotective treatment for Alzheimer's disease. *Adv. Drug Deliv. Rev.* 60: 1463–1470.

180 Holmquist, L., Stuchbury, G., Berbaum, K. et al. (2007). Lipoic acid as a novel treatment for Alzheimer's disease and related dementias. *Pharmacol. Ther.* 113: 154–164.

181 Wong, A., Dukic-Stefanovic, S., Gasic-Milenkovic, J. et al. (2001). Anti-inflammatory antioxidants attenuate the expression of inducible nitric oxide synthase mediated by advanced glycation endproducts in murine microglia. *Eur. J. Neurosci.* 14: 1961–1967.

182 Gasic-Milenkovic, J., Loske, C., and Münch, G. (2003). Advanced glycation endproducts cause lipid peroxidation in the human neuronal cell line SH-SY5Y. *J. Alzheimers Dis.* 5: 25–30.

183 de Arriba, S.G., Loske, C., Meiners, I. et al. (2003). Advanced glycation endproducts induce changes in glucose consumption, lactate production, and ATP levels in SH-SY5Y neuroblastoma cells by a redox-sensitive mechanism. *J. Cereb. Blood Flow Metab.* 23: 1307–1313.

184 Steele, M.L., Fuller, S., Patel, M. et al. (2013). Effect of Nrf2 activators on release of glutathione, cysteinylglycine and homocysteine by human U373 astroglial cells. *Redox Biol.* 1: 441–445.

185 Haugaard, N. and Levin, R.M. (2000). Regulation of the activity of choline acetyl transferase by lipoic acid. *Mol. Cell. Biochem.* 213: 61–63.

186 Haugaard, N. and Levin, R.M. (2002). Activation of choline acetyl transferase by dihydrolipoic acid. *Mol. Cell. Biochem.* 229: 103–106.

187 Huang, X., Atwood, C.S., Hartshorn, M.A. et al. (1999). The A beta peptide of Alzheimer's disease directly produces hydrogen peroxide through metal ion reduction. *Biochemistry* 38: 7609–7616.

188 Suh, J.H., Moreau, R., Heath, S.H., and Hagen, T.M. (2005). Dietary supplementation with (R)-alpha-lipoic acid reverses the age-related accumulation of iron and depletion of antioxidants in the rat cerebral cortex. *Redox Rep.* 10: 52–60.

189 Fonte, J., Miklossy, J., Atwood, C., and Martins, R. (2001). The severity of cortical Alzheimer's type changes is positively correlated with increased amyloid-beta levels: Resolubilization of amyloid-beta with transition metal ion chelators. *J. Alzheimers Dis.* 3: 209–219.

190 Suh, J.H., Zhu, B.Z., deSzoeke, E. et al. (2004). Dihydrolipoic acid lowers the redox activity of transition metal ions but does not remove them from the active site of enzymes. *Redox Rep.* 9: 57–61.

191 Griffin, W.S., Sheng, J.G., Roberts, G.W., and Mrak, R.E. (1995). Interleukin-1 expression in different plaque types in Alzheimer's disease: significance in plaque evolution. *J. Neuropathol. Exp. Neurol.* 54: 276–281.

192 Lander, H.M., Tauras, J.M., Ogiste, J.S. et al. (1997). Activation of the receptor for advanced glycation end products triggers a p21(ras)-dependent mitogen-activated protein kinase pathway regulated by oxidant stress. *J. Biol. Chem.* 272: 17810–17814.

193 Bierhaus, A., Chevion, S., Chevion, M. et al. (1997). Advanced glycation end product-induced activation of NF-kappaB is suppressed by alpha-lipoic acid in cultured endothelial cells. *Diabetes* 46: 1481–1490.

194 Pocernich, C.B. and Butterfield, D.A. (2003). Acrolein inhibits NADH-linked mitochondrial enzyme activity: implications for Alzheimer's disease. *Neurotox. Res.* 5: 515–520.

195 Arivazhagan, P., Ramanathan, K., and Panneerselvam, C. (2001). Effect of DL-alpha-lipoic acid on mitochondrial enzymes in aged rats. *Chem. Biol. Interact.* 138: 189–198.

196 Findlay, J.A., Hamilton, D.L., and Ashford, M.L. (2015). BACE1 activity impairs neuronal glucose oxidation: rescue by beta-hydroxybutyrate and lipoic acid. *Front. Cell. Neurosci.* 9: 382.

197 Rodriguez-Perdigon, M., Solas, M., Moreno-Aliaga, M.J., and Ramirez, M.J. (2016). Lipoic acid improves neuronal insulin signalling and rescues cognitive function regulating VGlut1 expression in high-fat-fed rats: implications for Alzheimer's disease. *Biochim. Biophys. Acta* 1862: 511–517.

198 Liu, Z., Patil, I., Sancheti, H. et al. (2017). Effects of lipoic acid on high-fat diet-induced alteration of synaptic plasticity and brain glucose metabolism: a PET/CT and (13)C-NMR study. *Sci. Rep.* 7: 5391.

199 Sancheti, H., Akopian, G., Yin, F. et al. (2013). Age-dependent modulation of synaptic plasticity and insulin mimetic effect of lipoic acid on a mouse model of Alzheimer's disease. *PLoS One* 8: e69830.

200 Estrada, M., Perez, C., Soriano, E. et al. (2016). New neurogenic lipoic-based hybrids as innovative Alzheimer's drugs with sigma-1 agonism and beta-secretase inhibition. *Future Med. Chem.* 8: 1191–1207.

201 Freund-Levi, Y., Eriksdotter-Jonhagen, M., Cederholm, T. et al. (2006). Omega-3 fatty acid treatment in 174 patients with mild to moderate Alzheimer disease: OmegAD study: a randomized double-blind trial. *Arch. Neurol.* 63: 1402–1408.

202 Willcox, D.C., Willcox, B.J., Todoriki, H., and Suzuki, M. (2009). The Okinawan diet: health implications of a low-calorie, nutrient-dense, antioxidant-rich dietary pattern low in glycemic load. *J. Am. Coll. Nutr.* 28 (Suppl): 500s–516s.

203 Giugliano, D. and Esposito, K. (2008). Mediterranean diet and metabolic diseases. *Curr. Opin. Lipidol* 19: 63–68.

9

Cognitive Impairments in Alzheimer's Disease and Other Neurodegenerative Diseases

Hamid R. Sohrabi[1,2,3,4,5,6] and Michael Weinborn[1,6,7]

[1] Centre of Excellence for Alzheimer's Disease Research and Care, School of Medical and Health Sciences, Edith Cowan University, Joondalup, WA, Australia
[2] Department of Biomedical Sciences, Macquarie University, Sydney, NSW, Australia
[3] School of Psychiatry and Clinical Neurosciences, University of Western Australia, Perth,, WA, Australia
[4] Cooperative Research Centre for Mental Health, Carlton, VIC, Australia
[5] KaRa Institute of Neurological Diseases, Sydney, NSW, Australia
[6] Australian Alzheimer's Research Foundation, Ralph and Patricia Sarich Neuroscience Research Institute, Nedlands, WA, Australia
[7] School of Psychology, University of Western Australia, Crawley, WA, Australia

> 'Soon she developed a rapid loss of memory. She was disoriented in her home, carried things from one place to another and hid them, sometimes she thought somebody was trying to kill her and started to cry loudly.'
>
> Extracted from Alois Alzheimer's notes on Auguste Deter, the first documented case of Alzheimer's disease [1].

9.1 Introduction

Dementia is primarily characterised by progressive impairment in cognition, behaviour, and functional faculties in the absence of a decline in consciousness. Dementia, or as it has been defined in the Diagnostic and Statistical Manual of Mental Disorders (DSM-V) [2]: major neurocognitive disorder, encompasses heterogeneous cognitive disorders resulting from various neurodegenerative causes. Dementia causes are not mutually exclusive and one may be diagnosed with two or more types simultaneously. However, the exact type and cause of dementia can currently be established only by post-mortem brain autopsy. Dementia due to Alzheimer's disease (AD) is the most common form of dementia syndrome, known for its characteristic and progressive memory loss, combined with extensive extracellular amyloid deposition in the brain. AD usually begins with impairments in episodic memory, but other manifestations have also been reported including visual and language difficulties, as well as behavioural and personality changes. Other types of dementias commonly seen in older adults include dementia with Lewy bodies (DLB), frontotemporal dementia (FTD), and vascular dementia (VaD). This chapter will discuss some of the neurocognitive deficits experienced in these conditions, with the primary focus on different stages of dementia due to AD.

Neurodegeneration and Alzheimer's Disease: The Role of Diabetes, Genetics, Hormones, and Lifestyle,
First Edition. Edited by Ralph N. Martins, Charles S. Brennan, W.M.A.D. Binosha Fernando, Margaret A. Brennan and Stephanie J. Fuller.
© 2019 John Wiley & Sons Ltd. Published 2019 by John Wiley & Sons Ltd.

9.2 Dementia due to Alzheimer's Disease

Dementia due to AD is best described as progressive and irreversible changes in cognition in the absence of any impairment in consciousness. Amongst the affected cognitive functions, memory decline is considered as a primary manifestation of the dementia syndrome in AD. Interestingly, Aloysius (Alois) Alzheimer's clinical notes and hospital records on the very well-known case of AD, Auguste Deter, and on the lesser known case of Johann Feigl, provide considerable details of the amnestic, yet progressive nature of the disease [3]. Alzheimer noted such deficits as reduced ability in comprehension and memory, aphasia, disorientation, unpredictable behaviour, paranoia, auditory hallucinations, and pervasive psychosocial impairment in addition to agraphia, or as Alzheimer coined it, 'amnestic writing disorder' [3]. Since then, much work has been done to establish the cognitive and clinical features that can be reliably used for diagnostic purposes as well as screening individuals at higher risk of AD. This is still an ongoing quest for which various measures and assessment tools have been developed.

9.2.1 Subjective Cognitive Decline [4] and Mild Cognitive Impairment (MCI)

There is a consensus that the classic AD neuropathological features, i.e. the deposition of Aβ-amyloid (senile) plaques and neurofibrillary tangles of tau, start 10 to 20 years prior to cognitive and clinical manifestations of the disease. Clifford Jack Jr. et al. have published a hypothetical model, suggesting that changes resulting in AD commence with Aβ aggregation and amyloid accumulation, synaptic dysfunction, tau-mediated neuronal injury, and brain structural changes that are finally accompanied by cognitive decline, behavioural changes, and functional impairments, respectively [5]. The neuropathological changes commence in cognitively normal people, who later proceed to mild cognitive impairment (MCI) and finally progress to full-blown dementia. However, research suggests that subtle changes in some aspects of cognition accompany the slow progression of neuropathological changes, and that these changes may be detectable long before the more standard clinical signs and symptoms. For example, subtle difficulties in cognitive functions have been reported up to 18 years prior to clinical diagnosis [6]. Currently, dementia due to AD is defined as a spectrum that includes clusters of biological, cognitive, and clinical features. The earliest cognitive change detectable in the AD spectrum is perhaps subjective cognitive decline (SCD) [4], also known as subjective memory complaints (SMC) or subjective cognitive/memory impairments. The working group of the Subjective Cognitive Decline Initiative (SCD-I) has characterised SCD as persistent self-experienced reports or reports by others of decline in cognitive abilities as compared to one's normal abilities [4]. However, this personal account of cognitive decline is not accompanied by objective decline measured using standard neuropsychological assessment. In addition, individuals with SCD preserve their abilities to personal, societal, and career-related responsibilities. The SCD by itself is not necessarily a diagnostic pre-clinical AD condition, nor is it required for progression to AD [4]. That is, the course and prognosis of SCD as a pre-clinical condition is not yet completely understood. Epidemiological studies indicate that SMC are common [7] and can be seen in different age groups including young, middle-aged, and older adults [8]. It has been estimated that about 27–32% of individuals aged 60 and above report significant concerns with their memory [9–11]. The exact number of SCD individuals who will develop MCI or AD is unknown. However, accumulating evidence indicates that, (i) SCD is associated with an increased risk of dementia due to AD [12, 13]; (ii) a wide range of biomarkers associated with AD are commonly seen amongst SCD individuals [14–17]; and (iii) SCD individuals positive for apolipoprotein E ε4 allele show an additive effect concerning increased risk for AD [18–20]. A recent publication has reported a 20% higher risk of converting to MCI, in a subgroup of SCD individuals; specifically those who were *worried* about the cognitive changes they reported to be experiencing [21]. As Figure 9.1 indicates, the prevalence and the potential relationship between SCD, MCI, and AD are intertwined, and that, in the case of the first two conditions, they may reverse to normal situation or remain stable and show no further decline. However, research indicates that SCD, specifically when accompanied by minimal depressive symptoms, is significantly associated with delayed recall abilities, a sensitive measure for diagnosis and prediction of future AD [22]. A study of 559 older adults has shown that SCD is accompanied by a fourfold risk of progression to MCI (Hazard ratio = 4.1, $p < 0.0001$) [23]. Another definition of SCD known as SCD-plus has been formulated to clarify features of SCD that increase the likelihood of a correct pre-clinical AD diagnosis. These include: (i) a subjective decline in memory, rather than declines in other domains of cognition; (ii) SCD onset within the last five years; (iii) age of onset ≥ 60 years; (iv) the expression of concerns and worries about developing SCD; and (v) the expression of concerns of performing worse than others in the same age group [4]. Another study has shown that in addition to increased rate of progression to dementia, SCD is associated with a shorter dementia-free survival period [24]. A recent study, compared several early cognitive decline classification methods, including SCD, SCD-plus, and National Institute on Aging-Alzheimer's Association (NIA-AA) stages 1–3, and found that NIA-AA stage 2 (low cerebrospinal fluid [CSF] Aβ and increased CSF tau) classification was the most successful at predicting objective cognitive decline or dementia. Interestingly, their results also suggested that SCD which triggered help-seeking was most likely concurrent with NIA-AA stage 2 [25], in agreement with a previous study [26]. Other recent studies have shown that some level of impairment in semantic verbal fluency can be detected in patients with SCD [27], with differences being found to be in storage ability (i.e. retaining information over time), rather than a retrieval problem [28]. In addition, naturalistic measures of prospective memory (PM) have detected problems of PM (i.e. memory for future and upcoming events) in SCD [29]. Disruptions to functional connectivity (as measured by magnetic resonance imaging [MRI]) have also been reported in SCD and to a greater extent in MCI [30]. In other studies, more detailed research into changes in CSF Aβ42 levels has shown that lower 'normal' levels were associated with faster cognitive decline, and this also depended on baseline cognitive status, such as SCD or MCI [31]. Further studies are required to clarify characteristics of SCD, to help to develop tools for detecting early AD, and to enable differential diagnosis, all of which are critical in preventive and ameliorative clinical trials.

The diagnosis of MCI requires the presence of SCD as well as objective evidence of declines in cognitive function, in the absence of impairment in daily living activities and functional capabilities [32, 33]. Individuals with MCI may present with difficulties in single or multiple cognitive domains. As a result, MCI may or may not include a measurable decline in memory, which is a primary symptom of dementia due to AD. Interestingly, the new research criteria introduced by the NIA-AA is relying more on biomarkers for the differential diagnosis of MCI due to AD [34]. This is

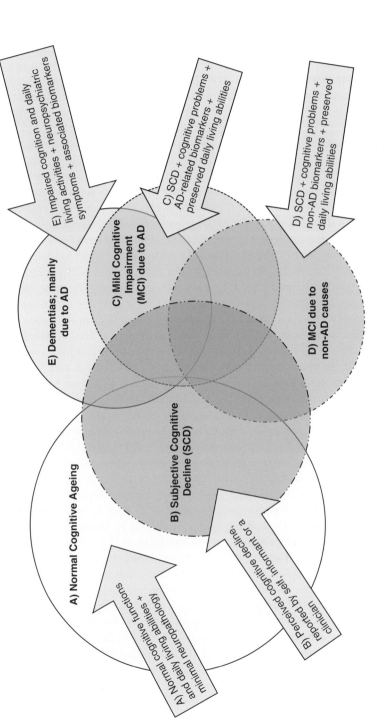

Figure 9.1 The relationships between normal cognitive ageing, subjective cognitive decline, and neuropathological conditions. The Figure shows five potential scenarios of cognitive ageing. Some individuals live long without significant pathological cognitive impairment or concerns affecting their independent lifestyle and daily living activities (A). A group of older adults may report noticeable decline in cognition (SCD), (B) [48]. In fact up to 27% of older adults aged 60 years old and over may report serious concerns about their cognitive changes [11]. Individuals reporting SMC are twice as likely to develop dementia as compared to those without such complaints [48]. A group of individuals with SCD will develop cognitive decline that can be detected by objective measures (MCI; C and D). The prevalence of MCI [49] amongst older adults is about 16% and it is considered as a prodromal condition with increased risk of developing dementia [34]. Dementia due to AD (E) is very common [50] and can be seen in up to 50% of older adults, depending on age, genetic risk factors, sex, ethno-racial group, and education level. Each arrow corresponds to a brief description of the core criteria for diagnosing each stage of the cognitive decline progression. The dashed barriers emphasise the permeability between conditions while the solid line indicates the irreversibility of the AD neuropathological changes based on our current knowledge. Source: This figure was inspired and modified from: [51]. (*See color plate section for the color representation of this figure.*)

important because MCI as a pre-clinical condition is heterogeneous [35] and may appear unstable [36]. For example, current evidence suggests a strong link between amnestic, multi-domain MCI and future dementia due to AD, whereas non-amnestic MCI appears to be more likely to progress to dementia due to Lewy bodies [37].

Preliminary evidence noted that around 17–40% of individuals diagnosed with MCI experience an improvement in cognitive function [38], i.e. they return to their pre-MCI cognitive functioning state. In African Americans, this reversal happens in about 18% of cases (95% CI: 16.7–20.4%), and was reported more in younger MCI patients (below age 80 years old) when compared to older MCI patients (above 80 years old) [39]. Although in most cases, as mentioned above, cognitive abilities of SCD and MCI patients often deteriorate over time, reverting to normal is most likely due to differences in the causes of cognitive impairment, incorrect diagnosis, or low sensitivity of assessment tools.

In summary, MCI is a heterogeneous, pre-clinical condition presenting with difficulties in a variety of cognitive domains including memory, language, working memory, executive functioning, praxis (i.e. ability to plan and act), abstract thinking, and so on [35]. Therefore, cognitive impairments seen in dementia due to AD are to a lesser degree present in MCI due to AD as well. This is the case with the cognitive deficits discussed below.

In the next section, the cognitive functions affected during the natural course of AD and other neurodegenerative diseases are briefly examined. It should be noted that this Chapter is not an exhaustive review of the literature, and as such we have deliberately decided to discuss the most common neurocognitive features of AD as well as other common types of dementias.

9.2.2 Memory Impairments in AD

9.2.2.1 Episodic Memory

A decline in memory is one of the earliest and most notable features of AD dementia. While various aspects of memory may in fact be affected, a decline in episodic memory is a commonly replicated finding in this field. Episodic memory and semantic memory are considered as the two main components of declarative or explicit, conscious memory, as opposed to non-declarative, procedural, or implicit memory. Endel Tulving, who coined the term episodic memory, describes it as the ability to retain and recollect a piece of information with a relatively subjective sense of when, where, what, and who [40]. Episodic memory in AD patients has been extensively studied over the last 40 years. The primary deficit of episodic memory in AD patients appears to be in encoding and storage of information as compared to retrieval-related processes, i.e. recall and recognition [41, 42]. Interestingly, AD patients do not seem to benefit from information that may improve encoding, such as the semantic or sequential relationships [43]. Forgetfulness in AD patients occurs within the first few minutes of learning, but seems to reach a plateau afterwards [44]. The rate of forgetting in AD patients is very steep and similar to those with Korsakkof's syndrome [45]. Rapid decay of information storage and forgetting has been proposed as a possible reason for the episodic memory failure seen in AD patients [44, 46], however this has not been seen in some studies [41]. For example, if memory tasks are properly selected and the level of learning is matched with controls, the rate or speed of forgetting in AD patients does not seem to exceed that of controls [47].

9.2.2.2 Semantic Memory

In addition to autobiographical information, we learn, store, and retrieve information without its reference to us – i.e. semantic memory [52]. Semantic memory is usually assessed on measures such as category fluency (i.e. naming vegetables), pictures/objects naming (recognition), picture-picture matching, true–false sentences, and semantic priming. Research on semantic memory in AD patients indicates that this type of memory is commonly affected in clinical stages of the disease [53], although the impairment in semantic memory is usually less severe in AD patients as compared to other degenerative diseases [54]. Early researchers argued that if the semantic memory measure did not demand a very effortful retrieval, AD patients, in fact, performed as well as normal elderly people [55]. However, more recent research indicates that semantic memory deficits are prominent in AD [56] and can be detected in MCI patients as well [57]. The underlying mechanism(s) of semantic memory failure in AD is still under investigation. Some evidence points to storage degradation as the cause of semantic problems in AD [58]. In addition, impairment in the structural description and phonological output systems has been proposed as another underlying cognitive mechanism [59]. Other studies have suggested the breakdown in the organisation and structure of semantic knowledge as the cognitive mechanism which leads to the semantic memory deficits commonly seen in AD [60]. Recent MRI evidence has shown that medial perirhinal cortex (mPRC) atrophy plays an important role in the semantic deficits of AD patients [61]. Further research has shown that neurofibrillary pathology is associated with the cognitive impairments associated with these brain regions. Furthermore, differences in semantic memory (tested with an animal fluency test) can detect MCI at around four years prior to clinical diagnosis [62, 63], and semantic object memory impairments as an indication of mPRC pathology can be detected up to 12 years before an AD diagnosis [64].

9.2.2.3 Prospective Memory (PM)

This is a more newly described type of memory as compared to episodic and semantic memory. It refers to the ability to plan and enact specific intentions or activities in a specific time/place in the future. The PM can be examined on event- or time-based assessment modules or a combination of these two tasks. In a large population study, PM was found to be inversely associated with age, male gender, less education, and lower social status [65]. One of the very first studies examined the distinctive pattern of PM impairment as compared to retrospective memory (RM) in mild to severe dementia patients. In this study, Huppert and Beardsall [66] reported that impairment in PM was as prominent in mild dementia as it was in severe dementia, while impairment in RM was not so severe. Thus, while some studies reported a more severe decline in PM with normal ageing, other studies reported that RM tasks were more impaired than PM tasks in AD patients [67]. Furthermore, in another study of non-demented elderly individuals, RM was found to be more impaired than PM [68], highlighting the inconsistent findings on PM and RM abilities, in relation to ageing and dementia.

More recent studies have shown that deficits in PM could be an early sign of MCI due to AD [69]. In a comparison of participants with MCI and AD, it was found that while both groups were impaired in terms of PM, the AD group was more severely impaired and PM difficulties were more uniquely present in this group as compared to other cognitively impaired groups [70]. In more recent studies, in a naturalistic PM task, it was found that older adults (average ~73 years), who reported high levels of subjective memory decline, performed more poorly than other older adults who did not report such significant memory decline [29]. Again, this is a little different to what was found in previous studies reporting that in both amnestic and non-amnestic MCI, the focal PM accuracy was significantly lower than in healthy controls whereas non-focal PM showed little difference between the groups [72, 73].

In conclusion, while PM research is still in relatively early stages and proper measures are yet to be developed, the findings are promising and may prove very useful in patients' assessments and in screening of individuals at risk of developing AD. So far, it has been suggested that deficits seen in PM indicate that the patient's spontaneous retrieval processes are compromised in the very early stages of AD [71].

9.2.3 Attention and Executive Dysfunction in AD

Attention and working memory deficits are also commonly seen in AD patients [74, 75]. Following the amnestic phase of AD, attention is the second cognitive function to be affected, long before difficulties with other cognitive functions including language and praxis [76].

Attention is composed of at least three broad subtypes including sustained, selective, and divided attentional abilities [For a review see [77]]. In AD patients, the ability to sustain attention (i.e. the ability to maintain attention over time) may remain preserved for longer periods of time, as compared to selective and divided attentions (i.e. ability to focus on one task in spite of distracting stimuli and the ability of allocating cognitive resources to two or more tasks, respectively). In fact, research on maintaining focus over time, and divided attention, has indicated that distractibility, and losing the ability to do two tasks at the same time (e.g. listening to radio while driving or talking while walking), are amongst the earlier signs of dementia [78–80]. This could be because of the problems in the central executive component of working memory that is involved in dual tasks capacity [74]. Executive functions (EF) include higher cognitive processes enabling one to decide, plan, and deploy, and ultimately achieve a goal [81]. From an experimental psychology point of view, the EF abilities include updating (working memory), shifting (ability to switch attention between multiple tasks), and inhibition (ability to postpone and delay a response for a more appropriate or correct response), as well as accessing the long-term memory [82, 83]. It has been known for a while that impairment in EF is common in AD patients [84]. For example, a study reported that AD patients performed poorly on four different EF tests (i.e. the Self-Ordering, the Hukok Logical Thinking Matrices, Trail Making Tests A and B, and Controlled Oral Word Association Test [COWAT; letters FAS-version]) when compared to cognitively normal individuals [85]. Others reported that, in AD patients, the primary EF deficits include inhibition and concurrent coordination of information storage and processing [86]. More recently, research has shown that EF deficits are also seen in amnestic MCI. For example, MCI patients have difficulties with response inhibition, switching, and cognitive flexibility [87]. Furthermore, other recent studies suggest EF deficits in normal elderly people may also predict future risk of dementia [88].

Earlier researchers argued that EF dysfunction could be seen only in a subgroup of AD patients and that this impairment did not appear to be associated with the severity or duration of disease [89]. There was also the suggestion that EF problems may independently coexist in AD patients, and be largely associated with the development of neuropsychiatric symptoms and functional impairment, rather than other and more prominent cognitive difficulties (e.g. episodic memory) [90].

More recent literature indicates that impairments in episodic memory and executive deficits occur in the very early stages of AD, and precede other cognitive defects including praxis, language, and attention [91]. In one study where MCI patients were divided into four subgroups (amnestic versus non-amnestic, single versus multiple domain, on the basis of common neuropsychological tests), it was found the EF components planning/problem solving and working memory (but not judgement) were more impaired in multi-domain patients as compared to other groups, resulting in the conclusion that this group had the poorest prognosis and was most likely to convert to AD dementia [92]. Later studies by the same group on MCI patients over a four-year period showed measures of EF (i.e. inhibitory control) were associated with MCI outcome, but that age and global measures of cognitive and functional decline were better at predicting incident dementia [93]. A very rare form of AD, the behavioural/dysexecutive variant, has been described recently, with primary symptoms being more often behavioural changes than cognition. Patients with behavioural AD performed similarly to more standard AD patients, but worse than the behavioural variant of FTD on memory measures; however, the EF composite scores of the behavioural AD patients were significantly lower compared to AD and the other patients groups [94].

In summary, impairments in EF and attention/working memory need further characterisation. While it appears that attention deficits should be present in the early stages of the disease, at least following the early amnestic phase, they have not always been reported. One retrospective study reported no decline in working memory/attention of post-mortem autopsy-confirmed AD patients who developed dementia later in life, as compared to those with confirmed pathology without dementia syndrome during their lifetime [95]. The current inconsistency indicates that even the less complicated cognitive functions such as attention may in fact need more rigorous assessment measures than once believed. This line of research is worth pursuing further, as problems in behaviour and EF could be very informative for diagnostic purposes, even though they are less commonly presented compared to other AD signs and symptoms. Patients with the recently described frontal variant of AD or behavioural/dysexecutive variant [94, 96] demonstrate such symptoms as significant problems in EF [e.g. as evident in the Trail Making Tests and COWAT; [96]], apathy, disinhibition, and compulsiveness [94]. These changes are in addition to the AD-related cognitive problems (e.g. episodic memory) but are more pronounced.

9.2.4 Language

Language examination as part of the neuropsychological assessment of AD often includes such skills as spontaneous speech, expressive and receptive skills, naming abilities, repetition, reading and writing, and so on. Language difficulties such as finding the right word (experiencing the tip of the tongue phenomenon) and names of objects can usually be seen in the very early stages of the disease. Research is slightly more conclusive about language difficulties associated with AD. For example, in a recent study, participants who progressed to dementia due to AD, confirmed by post-mortem examination, showed difficulties in language, while such difficulties were not reported for non-progressors, or those with autopsy-confirmed AD brain pathology without dementia syndrome [95].

Research into language difficulties in AD has been more concerned with the complex aspects of language (e.g. word finding, semantics/category fluency) rather that the mechanics of speech (e.g. articulation) [97]. It is clear that language difficulties will increase with disease severity. For example, impairments in fluency, animal naming, and confrontational naming are commonly present in earlier stages, but in later stages abnormal articulation and repetition of words also occur [98]. However, in late stages of AD, language difficulties gradually increase in a manner similar to the stages of language loss in aphasia disorders including anomic, transcortical sensory, Wernicke's, and global aphasias [99]. Automatic Spontaneous Speech Analysis and Emotional Response Analysis as well as Automatic Speech Analysis and Recognition (ASR) tests are currently being carried out to investigate such speech features in AD and MCI patients, and some studies are indicating an 80% diagnostic accuracy rate in diagnosing AD from non-AD patients [100]. Specific temporal characteristics of spontaneous speech (e.g. speech tempo, frequency and duration of pauses in speech) are now considered as early markers for AD [101]. As mentioned earlier, lexico-semantic variables appear to be the most useful for AD diagnosis, at the prodromal or amnestic mild cognitive impairment (aMCI) stages, particularly when looking at semantic fluency. Discourse and pragmatic level analysis may also be useful for AD diagnosis at aMCI stages, as may be data from naming pictures of unique/famous people, buildings, and events. On the other hand, object-naming tasks and connected speech analysis appear to be less reliable in diagnosis (for a review see [102]).

In relation to language difficulties, similar to what was first described by Alzheimer [3], a significant impairment in writing abilities, agraphia, is increasingly considered as a clinical feature of AD [103]. Agraphia in AD includes such problems as shorter sentences, less informative and simpler sentences, using fewer words, misspelling, intrusions, semantic substitutions, and so on [104]. While the underlying mechanism of agraphia in AD is as yet unknown, it seems that such cognitive domains as languages, graphomotor and visuo-spatial abilities are central to writing problems of AD patients [103, 105]. However, more recently, specific spelling difficulties have been shown to occur in AD, indicating lexical-semantic (words and their meanings), as opposed to sublexical (spelling according to the sound of a word) spelling deficits [106]. These studies suggested that areas in the posterior inferior temporal lobe and the superior region of the parietal cortex, as well as the putamen, are responsible for agraphia.

A rare form of AD, the language variant, has been recently described, with atypical presentation including early onset (before age 65 years old), significant impairment in language abilities (e.g. difficulties in sentence repetition and word finding, anomia) and, to a lesser degree, memory difficulties. This rare presentation of AD has been previously best described as the logopenic variant of Primary Progressive Aphasia, also known as Logopenic Progressive Aphasia (LPA) [107]. However, the presence of AD-related neuropathology in autopsy cases [108] as well as cerebral amyloid burden and brain glucose hypometabolism [109, 110] indicate the need for appropriate neuroimaging methods (e.g. amyloid phosphatidylethanolamine [PE]) for differential and diagnostic purposes. Such atypical cases indicate that, in diagnosis and clinical management of AD patients, clinicians should utilise clinical and neuropsychological results in combination with biomarkers to accurately diagnose such a complex syndrome, and to provide appropriate treatment plans, should such treatment become available.

9.2.5 Visuospatial Abilities

Visuospatial construction (VSC) or visuo-constructional abilities refer to one's ability to replicate, rebuild, or reassemble a previously encountered, visually perceived design or object [111]. Problems in VSC are very common amongst AD patients [112] and can be seen in the early stages of the disease [113]. While significant impairment in this ability is reported to occur in the later stages of sporadic AD, such impairments are reported as major early features of some forms of early onset AD [114, 115]; and interestingly, problems in VSC tasks are commonly found in patients with DLB [115]. Impairments in VSC can be used for screening those at higher risk of AD. It has been shown that in the pre-clinical stages, a steep decline in various cognitive domains including VSC can been seen in the performance of those who will be clinically diagnosed with dementia in the next two to three years [116].

The rare visual variant of AD [117], or posterior cortical atrophy (PCA) also known as Benson's disease [118], is usually accompanied by problems in higher order visual functions and in visuo-constructional abilities [119]. However, it should be noted that this rare variant of AD is not always caused by the neuropathological changes due to AD, as other neurodegenerative diseases may result in PCA as well. Again, assessing such atypical patients should include both neuropsychological and radiological measures as complementary information for differential diagnosis, yet even with molecular biomarkers to help with differential diagnosis, the process still poses challenges [120]. Recent MRI studies have shown that the asymmetric visual field deficits of PCA patients reflect the pattern of degeneration of both white and grey matter in the occipital lobe, with damage also seen in the corpus callosum [121]. Compared to more typical AD patients, PCA patients show significant hypometabolism in bilateral parietal and occipital lobes, particularly the right occipitotemporal junction, with spatial attention and shape discrimination scores being positively associated with regional glucose metabolism in these lobes [122]. In addition, compared to typical AD patients, PCA patients have been found to display better recognition and recall scores, and these differences were shown to correlate with larger hippocampal volumes [122].

9.2.6 Dementia with Lewy Bodies and Parkinson's Disease with Dementia

Dementia with Lewy Bodies (DLB) accounts for approximately 10–20% of dementia diagnoses, although some estimates suggest higher ranges (e.g. up to 35% of cases [123, 124]). Lewy bodies are neuronal inclusion bodies commonly found in subcortical regions amongst individuals with Parkinson's disease (PD) without dementia. However, amongst individuals with DLB and PD with dementia, these inclusion bodies are present in neocortical regions, producing a progressive dementia. DLB was identified as a potentially distinct disorder beginning in the 1960s through the 1980s [125, 126], but more formal diagnostic criteria for this condition were not published until the 1990s [127–129].

The neuro-behavioural presentation of DLB is characterised by fluctuations in attention and alertness (seen in up to 80% of patients), recurrent visual hallucinations (up to 50%), and an onset of parkinsonism, seen after or temporally close to the onset of cognitive decline (up to 70%). Indeed, the dementia seen in PD can appear quite similar to that of DLB, and is most reliably distinguished by the relative timing of the onset of cognitive and behavioural symptoms versus that of the movement disorder symptoms – with DLB diagnosed when cognitive and behavioural symptoms emerge first, or in close proximity to the onset of motor symptoms, whereas PD dementia is diagnosed when motor symptoms precede cognitive symptoms by a substantial period of time.

In DLB, syncope and repeated falls, sensitivity to neuroleptic medications, unexplained loss of consciousness, rapid eye movement (REM) sleep disorders, systemised delusions, and non-visual hallucinations are also common [130]. Importantly, fluctuating attention and alertness is evident early in DLB and may affect an individual's performance on a variety of cognitive measures [note: fluctuations in attention may be assessed formally with the Mayo Clinic Fluctuations Scale [131] completed by an informant]. However, the typical neuropsychological profile seen in DLB reflects the mixed cortical-subcortical neuropathology [37]. There are usually also significant deficits in most aspects of visuospatial functioning, including deficits in higher order visual reasoning and visuo-constructional abilities, and greater visuospatial deficits appear to be associated with a higher risk of visual hallucinations [132]. When visual hallucination occurs within the first five years of dementia, this is usually DLB, and it is usually associated with limbic Lewy body pathology [133]. Language functions (e.g. confrontational naming and comprehension) are usually relatively spared, although performance on formal measures of verbal fluency may be reduced due to executive impairments. Episodic memory is also usually relatively spared early in DLB, and when it does occur, typically presents as difficulty with efficient encoding and retrieval, rather than rapid forgetting [e.g. [134]]. Executive dysfunction is seen across multiple domains, including working memory, set-shifting, and as described above, verbal production [135].

DLB has an average age of onset in the late 60s, roughly similar to AD [136]. As described above, many cognitive abilities including language and aspects of memory are relatively spared early in the course of the disease. However, as DLB progresses, memory impairments become common and eventually global, and severe cognitive impairment is seen. It has previously been thought that disease progression may be more rapid in DLB compared to AD, but this pattern has not been consistently reported [137]. The average survival post-diagnosis is approximately six years, but there is substantial variability.

9.2.7 Vascular Dementia

Vascular Dementia (VaD) is often considered the second most common subtype of dementia after AD, accounting for 10–30% of cases [e.g. [138–140]]. However, the prevalence rates have been the subject of some debate. It has been argued that 'pure' cases of VaD are relatively uncommon [141], as VaD pathology is more commonly seen in 'mixed' dementias, with the brains of many affected individuals showing DLB or, more commonly, AD pathology in addition to vascular changes [e.g. [142]]. Regardless of additional comorbid neuropathologies, VaD is itself a diverse diagnostic entity with many potential etiological contributors to vascular damage that may be either confined to one or more strategic focal regions, or diffusely distributed throughout cortical and subcortical regions.

Historically, the focus in VaD had been limited to one discreet cerebrovascular accident (CVA) or a series of CVA over time ('multi-infarct dementia'), which tend to produce focal neurocognitive deficits that worsen in a stepwise manner as additional vascular events occur. Haemorrhagic strokes (caused by ruptured aneurysms or other brain blood-vessel wall breaches) are less common than ischaemic strokes (caused by a thrombus or embolism blocking a vessel and preventing blood from reaching downstream cerebral structures) – but both may cause significant cerebral injury through a series of direct effects (e.g. anoxic injury, mass effect, and herniation) and after-effects (e.g. ischaemic cascade, increased intracranial pressure, oedema). A single stroke may affect a 'strategic' region and produce 'focal' cognitive deficits – that is, deficits in cognitive domains primarily mediated by the affected neural regions (e.g. an expressive aphasia following a stroke affecting substantial portions of Broca's area). Notably, even micro-infarcts in the hippocampus, for example, may produce significant, but relatively isolated, memory impairments that still result in dementia [143]. Larger infarcts, that may involve multiple regions and/or greater neural volume, typically result in more severe impairment.

Multi-infarct dementia may have a similar initial presentation to a single strategic infarct, but since by definition it involves additional strokes, additive and dynamic effects usually occur, depending on the total amount of brain tissue involved. The type and severity of cognitive impairments may develop over the course of these multiple strokes, producing a 'stepwise' decline – that is, a course characterised by periods of recovery and stability between strokes, only to present additional significant decline with each additional vascular injury, often resulting in significant cognitive impairment and disability.

However, there is now a general consensus that the construct of VaD has differing clinical presentations, and focal and multi-infarct VaD represent only two of these possible manifestations. For example, Bowler et al. [144] found only 40% of his clinical VaD sample showed traditional focal signs or clear evidence of a discreet CVA. Subsequently, VaD now requires *either* clinical evidence (e.g. brain imaging or focal neurological signs) of stroke, *or* other subclinical vascular injury that is associated with impairment in at least one neurocognitive domain [145]. Subsequently three primary subtypes of VaD presentation have been proposed: (i) *Strategic infarct VaD* involving cortical or subcortical regions and (ii) *Multi-infarct VaD* as described above, but also, (iii) *VaD due to subcortical vascular encephalopathy* [146]. However, the frequent comorbidity of VaD and AD means that the pathophysiology of cerebrovascular disease including clarification of typical findings from *in vivo* imaging, as well as interactions between the combined pathologies, need further research, in order to improve diagnosis and our understanding of contributions of both conditions to symptomatology and disease outcomes [147].

Subclinical vascular pathology often involves subcortical small vessel disease, including arteriosclerosis, atherosclerosis, lipohyalinosis, and arteriolosclerosis [143], and therefore the course of this subtype of VaD usually differs in that it does not typically show an acute precipitous decline in function, as is normally associated with a clinically obvious stroke. Rather, this subtype shows a slower, more insidious decline in cognition and daily function, which develops over months or years.

While the nature of the neurocognitive impairments seen in the first two subtypes of VaD mentioned above are often highly dependent on the neural region(s) affected and may differ somewhat across individuals (e.g. severe memory disturbance if the memory structures are affected vs. significant expressive or receptive aphasia if Broca's or Wernicke's area are involved), there are some commonalities seen in VaD, particularly those with subcortical involvement including the subcortical vascular subtype [139]. These changes most commonly include psychomotor slowing, cognitive inefficiencies, and attentional deficits. Disconnection syndromes are also common, particularly when white-matter circuits connecting prefrontal cortex and subcortical structures are interrupted, which can result in significant executive dysfunction, including impairments in working memory, cognitive flexibility, spontaneous initiation of behaviour, and self-regulation. There may be apathy, decreased speech complexity, and flat speech tone. Psychiatric symptoms, including depression, irritability, and agitation may also be seen. True amnestic memory impairments are less common in subcortical VaD, but inefficient encoding due to executive impairments is common, as is efficient retrieval of learned information. With such individuals, cognitive rehabilitation focusing on learning strategies and use of retrieval cues may be useful.

9.2.8 Frontotemporal Dementia

Frontotemporal lobar degeneration (FTLD) or frontotemporal dementia (FTD), is also a heterogeneous group of disorders, but as a group they all involve focal atrophy of the frontal and/or temporal lobes with relative sparing of other regions of the brain, at least until the more advanced stages of the disease. Affected individuals typically show significant dysexecutive function (e.g. impulsivity, poor judgement, stereotypical or repetitive behaviours), personality change (changes in comportment, poor social awareness, loss of typical emotional responses), and/or language impairment (reduction in speech production or comprehension, word-finding difficulties). Also discussed in Chapter 2, it is the fourth most common type of dementia amongst older adults, but is the second most common cause of dementia in adults under age 65 [148]. This is because the average age of onset is about 60, considerably younger than that of AD. Historically, FTD has been thought to be caused by, or at least associated with, the presence of Pick bodies, argentophillic neuronal inclusion bodies which were found post-mortem in the brains of some of the earliest patients identified with focal lobar atrophy. These individuals were described by Arnold Pick, a neurologist practicing in Prague around the turn of the twentieth century, as having severe language disturbance and focal atrophy in the left temporal and frontal lobes, and would meet the criteria for the disease initially named after him – Pick's disease [149]. However, over time it became clear that only some individuals presenting with focal lobar atrophy may have these neural inclusion bodies. That is, Pick's disease is just one of a number of neuropathologies associated with the development of FTD syndrome, and it is now seen as one of several tau-related dementias [150].

In addition to the neuropathological heterogeneity seen in FTD, there has been a recent general consensus [150] of at least two subtypes of FTD, (i) the primarily Frontal lobe (or Behavioural) Variant, and (ii) the primary Temporal lobe (or Language) Variant. The language variant has been further subdivided into progressive nonfluent aphasia (PNFA) and semantic dementia (SD).

The Frontal/Behavioural Variant usually presents initially with gradual changes in personality, social comportment, and executive functions. These changes include an increase in problematic behaviours such as disinhibition/impulsiveness, risk-taking, and lack of social awareness (i.e. rude or inappropriate remarks). Conversely, individuals with this variant may display decreases in adaptive spontaneous behaviours, e.g. loss of interest in previously enjoyed activities or relationships, apathy or abulia (lack of decision/willpower), decreased initiation, and lack of empathy. Affected individuals may also show a variety of symptoms often seen amongst individuals with frontal lobe injury, including perseveration, stimulus-bound and/or repetitive compulsive behaviours, and changes in eating (e.g. increased consumption) and sexual (e.g. inappropriate sexual comments or increased fixation on sex) behaviours. Deficits in neuropsychological measures are primarily seen in EFs, including cognitive flexibility (e.g. seen as impaired set-shifting on the Trail Making Test B or Wisconsin Card Sorting Tests), inhibition of prepotent responses (e.g. on the Stoop or go-no go tasks), working memory (e.g. the digit span backwards or serial 7s tasks), and novel problem-solving (e.g. the Iowa Gambling Task or Six Elements tasks). Language skills (i.e. comprehension, conversational fluency, confrontational naming) may be affected, but not to the extent seen in the Temporal/Language Variant of FTD. Episodic memory may be spared early in the disease (but cf. [151]), as are visual spatial skills, but performance on aspects of these domains that require significant executive components (e.g. strategic encoding of word lists) may be impaired. The affected individual usually has poor awareness of changes in personality, behaviour, and cognition, even early in the disease course. As the dementia worsens, extreme apathy/abulia predominate, and affected individuals may have very limited spontaneous behaviour. While neuroimaging may be unremarkable in very early stages, focal atrophy or hypofunction involving the frontal and temporal lobes emerge (esp. right hemisphere; [150]), and increase as the disease progresses.

The temporal lobe/language variant of FTD is usually divided into two subtypes: PNFA and SD as mentioned above. PNFA usually involves focal atrophy/hypofunction of the posterior inferior dominant-hemisphere frontal lobe, and is primarily defined by an aphasia syndrome characterised by non-fluent, agrammatic speech similar to that seen in CVA-related Broca's Aphasia. That is, hesitant effortful speech with reduced detail, richness, elaboration and spontaneity is observed. Further, the speech that is produced is marked by poor articulation, grammatical errors, paraphasias, and word-finding difficulties. Agraphia and alexia may also be seen. Speech comprehension may be subtly affected, but often remains relatively spared. Similarly, episodic memory and visuo-spatial skills are usually spared, but formal neuropsychological assessment of non-language cognitive domains may be adversely affected by the expressive language deficits, and results must be interpreted with caution. As the non-fluent aphasia syndrome progresses, the result is usually mutism, but communication through assistive language devices may be possible [139].

SD usually involves focal atrophy/hypofunction of the anterior temporal regions of the dominant cerebral hemisphere early in the course of the disease, but spreads to these same regions in the non-dominant hemisphere as the disease progresses [150]. Again, similarity to a CVA-related Wernicke's aphasia is notable, with generally fluent but vague or 'empty' speech that maintains grammatical rules, but lacks meaningful content, and is marked by semantic paraphasic errors and anomia [139]. Comprehension of even single word meaning is impaired, and conversation with affected individuals can be marked by reliance on jargon or overlearned phrases that may initially mask the severity of the comprehension deficit. In addition to the fluent aphasia syndrome, other deficits include visual agnosia for faces and objects, and surface dyslexia (inability to read words that do not follow typical grapheme–phoneme rules and relationships). Impaired comprehension and language production errors make formal neuropsychological assessment challenging, but individuals with SD usually show relatively spared arithmetic skills, visuospatial skills, episodic memory, ability to read words that follow typical grapheme–phoneme rules, and single word repetition.

9.3 Conclusions

Our understanding of the neurocognitive changes that occur over the many years of pre-clinical and later stages of dementia is still inconclusive, as is our understanding of the specific pathology underlying the changes. Specifically, the pre-clinical and early stages of dementia are yet to be objectively defined. Cognitive changes due to neurodegenerative processes appear to start at the very early stages of such diseases. Whilst these changes may not be detected by the currently available brief neuropsychological measures used in research, they could be objectified in more detailed assessments. For example, Schmid et al. [152] investigated 115 neuropsychological variables that could discriminate baseline matched controls from participants who developed dementia 8 years later, with 11 variables that optimally discriminated between the two groups. These included intrusions; response bias in verbal learning and memory tasks; delayed figure recall; three variables from the Wechsler Adult Intelligence Scale (WAIS) Block Design subtest; number of errors and repetitions on letter fluency; and self-report of memory problems, a feeling of sadness, and cardiac problems [152]. In addition, self-reports and informants' observations of the changes in cognitive abilities of the patients can provide significant information. These observed or reported changes in cognitive abilities are multifaceted, and one should be aware that the prominent presentation may not be the result of a single neurodegenerative disease. In fact, most neurodegenerative diseases, specifically in their advanced stages, share impairments in various cognitive domains. For example, while the neuropathological changes in AD start some 20 years prior to clinical diagnosis, the manifestation of the disease in the pre-clinical stages may include amnestic and/or non-amnestic MCI as well as behavioural changes that may also be seen in other conditions, as discussed earlier.

Neuropsychological assessment in degenerative diseases is still in the early stages. Appropriate assessment tools are gradually being developed, and we may need more psychometrically driven measures to be able to accommodate proper screening needs for preventive and ameliorative intervention, both in research and in clinical settings. There is a critical need for such measures that can accurately assess subjective, self- or other-reported decline. Increased longevity is accompanied by higher rates of problems in various sensory and perceptual abilities. However, this has not been properly addressed in the neuropsychological assessment of the elderly. For example, appropriate assessment measures for vision- and hearing-impaired older adults have yet to be developed, and as a future direction we should develop measures accommodating these cases, using appropriate normative scores that may or may not be necessarily similar to what we currently use.

The use of computerised neuropsychological assessment is gradually increasing. Given the continued surge in electronic devise usage and online assessments as part of research and clinical assessment, we should develop cost-effective, valid, and reliable computerised measures that are ecologically valid, automatically scored against age, education, and gender stratified norms, and of course are user friendly. The availability of such digital measures is a major shift and a potential advantage for future clinical and research practice, yet such measures should be properly examined prior to becoming widely available. In conclusion, both research and clinical work in cognitive assessment of dementia, while slowly growing, is still far from what is needed for accurate screening of those at risk, and for diagnosing those individuals with this syndrome.

There is a gradual major shift in cognitive and clinical examination, using online and computerised measures. The traditional neuropsychological approach of 'in-person' testing should adapt and make use of such an unprecedented approach that can bring big-data available for clinical practice, establishing psychometric basis of the available measures, and providing an avenue to develop new measures.

References

1 Stelzmann, R.A., Norman Schnitzlein, H., and Reed Murtagh, F. (1995). An English translation of Alzheimer's 1907 paper,"Über eine eigenartige Erkankung der Hirnrinde". *Clinical Anatomy* 8 (6): 429–431.

2 American, Psychiatric Association (ed.), Ed.(2013). *Diagnostic and Statistical Manual of Mental Disorders-Fifth Edition (DSM-5)*. Arlington, VA, USA: American Psychiatric Association.

3 Maurer, K., Volk, S., and Gerbaldo, H. (1997). Auguste D and Alzheimer's disease. *Lancet* 349 (9064): 1546–1549.

4 Jessen, F., Amariglio, R.E., van Boxtel, M. et al. (2014). A conceptual framework for research on subjective cognitive decline in preclinical Alzheimer's disease. *Alzheimers & Dementia* 10 (6): 844–852.

5 Jack, C.R. Jr., Knopman, D.S., Jagust, W.J. et al. (2013). Update on hypothetical model of Alzheimer's disease biomarkers. *Lancet Neurology* 12 (2): 207–216.

6 Rajan, K.B., Wilson, R.S., Weuve, J. et al. (2015). Cognitive impairment 18 years before clinical diagnosis of Alzheimer disease dementia. *Neurology* 85 (10): 898–904.

7 Brown, F.H., Dodrill, C.B., Clark, T. et al. (1991). An investigation of the relationship between self-report of memory functioning and memory test-performance. *Journal of Clinical Psychology* 47 (6): 772–777.

8 Commissaris, C.J.A.M., Ponds, R.W.H.M., and Jolles, J. (1998). Subjective forgetfulness in a normal Dutch population: possibilities for health education and other interventions. *Patient Education and Counseling* 34 (1): 25–32.

9 Montejo, P., Montenegro, M., Fernandez, M.A. et al. (2011). Subjective memory complaints in the elderly: prevalence and influence of temporal orientation, depression and quality of life in a population-based study in the city of Madrid. *Aging and Mental Health* 15 (1): 85–96.

10 Begum, A., Morgan, C., Chiu, C.C. et al. (2012). Subjective memory impairment in older adults: aetiology, salience and help seeking. *International Journal of Geriatric Psychiatry* 27 (6): 612–620.

11 Fritsch, T., MJ, M.C., Wallendal, M.S. et al. (2014). Prevalence and cognitive bases of subjective memory complaints in older adults: evidence from a community sample. *Journal of Neurodegenerative Diseases*; 2014: 176843.

12 van Oijen, M., de Jong, F.J., Hofman, A. et al. (2007). Subjective memory complaints, education, and risk of Alzheimer's disease. *Alzheimers & Dementia* 3 (2): 92–97.

13 Reisberg, B., Shulman, M.B., Torossian, C. et al. (2010). Outcome over seven years of healthy adults with and without subjective cognitive impairment. *Alzheimers & Dementia* 6 (1): 11–24.

14 Perrotin, A., Mormino, E.C., Madison, C.M. et al. (2012). Subjective cognition and amyloid deposition imaging: a Pittsburgh Compound B Positron Emission

Tomography Study in normal elderly individuals. *Archives of Neurology* 69 (2): 223–229.

15 Sohrabi, H.R., Bates, K.A., Rodrigues, M. et al. (2009). Olfactory dysfunction is associated with subjective memory complaints in community-dwelling elderly individuals. *Journal of Alzheimer's Disease* 17 (1): 135–142.

16 Bates, K.A., Sohrabi, H.R., Rodrigues, M. et al. (2009). Association of cardiovascular factors and Alzheimer's disease plasma amyloid-beta protein in subjective memory complainers. *Journal of Alzheimer's Disease* 17 (2): 305–318.

17 Wang, Y., West, J.D., Flashman, L.A. et al. (2012). Selective changes in white matter integrity in MCI and older adults with cognitive complaints. *Biochimica et Biophysica Acta* (BBA)-Molecular Basis of Disease 1822 (3): 423–430.

18 van Harten, A.C., Visser, P.J., Pijnenburg, Y.A. et al. (2013). Cerebrospinal fluid Aβ42 is the best predictor of clinical progression in patients with subjective complaints. *Alzheimer's & Dementia: The Journal of the Alzheimer's Association* 9 (5): 481–487.

19 Prichep, L.S., John, E.R., Ferris, S.H. et al. (2006). Prediction of longitudinal cognitive decline in normal elderly with subjective complaints using electrophysiological imaging. *Neurobiology of Aging* 27 (3): 471–481.

20 Dik, M.G., Jonker, C., Comijs, H.C. et al. (2001). Memory complaints and APOE-epsilon4 accelerate cognitive decline in cognitively normal elderly. *Neurology* 57 (12): 2217–2222.

21 Fernandez-Blazquez, M.A., Avila-Villanueva, M., Maestu, F. et al. (2016). Specific features of subjective cognitive decline predict faster conversion to mild cognitive impairment. *Journal of Alzheimer's Disease* 52 (1): 271–281.

22 Jessen, F., Wiese, B., Cvetanovska, G. et al. (2007). Patterns of subjective memory impairment in the elderly: association with memory performance. *Psychological Medicine* 37 (12): 1753–1762.

23 Donovan, N.J., Amariglio, R.E., Zoller, A.S. et al. (2014). Subjective cognitive concerns and neuropsychiatric predictors of progression to the early clinical stages of Alzheimer disease. *American Journal of Geriatric Psychiatry* 22 (12): 1642–1651.

24 Luck, T., Luppa, M., Matschinger, H. et al. (2015). Incident subjective memory complaints and the risk of subsequent dementia. *Acta Psychiatrica Scandinavica* 131 (4): 290–296.

25 Eckerstrom, M., Gothlin, M., Rolstad, S. et al. (2017). Longitudinal evaluation of criteria for subjective cognitive decline and preclinical Alzheimer's disease in a memory clinic sample. *Alzheimers & Dementia (Amst)* 8: 96–107.

26 Amariglio, R.E., Mormino, E.C., Pietras, A.C. et al. (2015). Subjective cognitive concerns, amyloid-beta, and neurodegeneration in clinically normal elderly. *Neurology* 85 (1): 56–62.

27 Nikolai, T., Bezdicek, O., Markova, H. et al. (2017). Semantic verbal fluency impairment is detectable in patients with subjective cognitive decline. *Applied Neuropsychology Adult* 1–10.

28 Lehrner, J., Coutinho, G., Mattos, P. et al. (2017). Semantic memory and depressive symptoms in patients with subjective cognitive decline, mild cognitive impairment, and Alzheimer's disease. *International Psychogeriatrics* 29 (7): 1123–1135.

29 Lee, S.D., Ong, B., Pike, K.E. et al. (2017). Prospective memory and subjective memory decline: a neuropsychological indicator of memory difficulties in community-dwelling older people. *Journal of Clinical and Experimental Neuropsychology* 1–15.

30 Lopez-Sanz, D., Bruna, R., Garces, P. et al. (2017). Functional connectivity disruption in subjective cognitive decline and mild cognitive impairment: a common pattern of alterations. *Frontiers in Aging Neuroscience* 9: 109.

31 Tijms, B.M., Bertens, D., Slot, R.E. et al. (2017). Low normal cerebrospinal fluid Abeta42 levels predict clinical progression in nondemented subjects. *Annals of Neurology* 81 (5): 749–753.

32 Petersen, R.C., Smith, G.E., Waring, S.C. et al. (1997). Aging, memory, and mild cognitive impairment. *International Psychogeriatrics* 9 (S1): 65–69.

33 Petersen, R.C., Smith, G.E., Waring, S.C. et al. (1999). Mild cognitive impairment: clinical characterization and outcome. *Archives of Neurology* 56 (3): 303–308.

34 Albert, M.S., ST, D.K., Dickson, D. et al. (2011). The diagnosis of mild cognitive impairment due to Alzheimer's disease: recommendations from the National Institute on Aging-Alzheimer's Association workgroups on diagnostic guidelines for Alzheimer's disease. *Alzheimers & Dementia* 7 (3): 270–279.

35 Nordlund, A., Rolstad, S., Hellstrom, P. et al. (2005). The Goteborg MCI study: mild cognitive impairment is a heterogeneous condition. *Journal of Neurology Neurosurgery and Psychiatry* 76 (11): 1485–1490.

36 Larrieu, S., Letenneur, L., Orgogozo, J.M. et al. (2002). Incidence and outcome of mild cognitive impairment in a population-based prospective cohort. *Neurology* 59 (10): 1594–1599.

37 Ferman, T.J., Smith, G.E., Kantarci, K. et al. (2013). Nonamnestic mild cognitive impairment progresses to dementia with Lewy bodies. *Neurology* 81 (23): 2032–2038.

38 Maioli, F., Coveri, M., Pagni, P. et al. (2007). Conversion of mild cognitive impairment to dementia in elderly subjects: a preliminary study in a memory and cognitive disorder unit. *Archives of Gerontology and Geriatrics* 44: 233–241.

39 Gao, S., Unverzagt, F.W., Hall, K.S. et al. (2014). Mild cognitive impairment, incidence, progression, and reversion: findings from a community-based cohort of elderly African Americans. *American Journal of Geriatric Psychiatry* 22 (7): 670–681.

40 Tulving, E. (2002). Episodic memory: from mind to brain. *Annual Review of Psychology* 53: 1–25.

41 Greene, J.D., Baddeley, A.D., and Hodges, J.R. (1996). Analysis of the episodic memory deficit in early Alzheimer's disease: evidence from the doors and people test. *Neuropsychologia* 34 (6): 537–551.

42 Weingartner, H., Kaye, W., Smallberg, S.A. et al. (1981). Memory failures in progressive idiopathic dementia. *Journal of Abnormal Psychology* 90 (3): 187–196.

43 Granholm, E. and Butters, N. (1988). Associative encoding and retrieval in Alzheimer's and Huntington's disease. *Brain and Cognition* 7 (3): 335–347.

44 Hart, R.P., Kwentus, J.A., Harkins, S.W. et al. (1988). Rate of forgetting in mild Alzheimer's-type dementia. *Brain and Cognition* 7 (1): 31–38.

45 Kopelman, M.D. (1985). Rates of forgetting in Alzheimer-type dementia and Korsakoff's syndrome. *Neuropsychologia* 23 (5): 623–638.

46 Butters, N., Salmon, D.P., Cullum, C.M. et al. (1988). Differentiation of amnesic and demented patients with the Wechsler memory scale-revised. *The Clinical Neuropsychologist* 2 (2): 133–148.

47 Christensen, H., Kopelman, M., Stanhope, N. et al. (1998). Rates of forgetting in Alzheimer dementia. *Neuropsychologia* 36 (6): 547–557.

48 Mitchell, A., Beaumont, H., Ferguson, D. et al. (2014). Risk of dementia and mild cognitive impairment in older people with subjective memory complaints: meta-analysis. *Acta Psychiatrica Scandinavica* 130 (6): 439–451.

49 Petersen, R.C., Roberts, R.O., Knopman, D.S. et al. (2010). Prevalence of mild cognitive impairment is higher in men the Mayo Clinic study of aging. *Neurology* 75 (10): 889–897.

50 Duthey, B. (2013). *Background Paper 6.11: Alzheimer Disease and Other Dementias*, 1–74. A Public Health Approach to Innovation. World Health Organisation (WHO).

51 Unverzagt, F.W., Gao, S., Lane, K.A. et al. (2007). Mild cognitive dysfunction: an epidemiological perspective with an emphasis on African Americans. *Journal of Geriatric Psychiatry and Neurology* 20 (4): 215–226.

52 Tulving, E. (1972). Episodic and semantic memory 1. In: *Organization of Memory* (ed. E. Tulving and W. Donaldson), 381–403. London: Academic Press.

53 Hodges, J.R. and Patterson, K. (1995). Is semantic memory consistently impaired early in the course of Alzheimer's disease? Neuroanatomical and diagnostic implications. *Neuropsychologia* 33 (4): 441–459.

54 Rogers, T.T., Ivanoiu, A., Patterson, K. et al. (2006). Semantic memory in Alzheimer's disease and the frontotemporal dementias: a longitudinal study of 236 patients. *Neuropsychology* 20 (3): 319–335.

55 Nebes, R.D., Martin, D.C., and Horn, L.C. (1984). Sparing of semantic memory in Alzheimer's disease. *Journal of Abnormal Psychology* 93 (3): 321–330.

56 Giffard, B., Desgranges, B., Nore-Mary, F. et al. (2001). The nature of semantic memory deficits in Alzheimer's disease. *Brain* 124 (8): 1522–1532.

57 Joubert, S., Felician, O., Barbeau, E.J. et al. (2008). Patterns of semantic memory impairment in mild cognitive impairment. *Behavioural Neurology* 19 (1–2): 35–40.

58 Hodges, J.R., Salmon, D.P., and Butters, N. (1992). Semantic memory impairment in Alzheimer's disease: failure of access or degraded knowledge? *Neuropsychologia* 30 (4): 301–314.

59 Daum, I., Riesch, G., Sartori, G. et al. (1996). Semantic memory impairment in Alzheimer's disease. *Journal of Clinical and Experimental Neuropsychology* 18 (5): 648–665.

60 Salmon, D.P., Butters, N., and Chan, A.S. (1999). The deterioration of semantic memory in Alzheimer's disease. *Canadian Journal of Experimental Psychology/Revue Canadienne de Psychologie Expérimentale* 53 (1): 108.

61 Hirni, D.I., Kivisaari, S.L., Monsch, A.U. et al. (2013). Distinct neuroanatomical bases of episodic and semantic memory performance in Alzheimer's disease. *Neuropsychologia* 51 (5): 930–937.

62 Mistridis, P., Krumm, S., Monsch, A.U. et al. (2015). The 12 years preceding mild cognitive impairment due to Alzheimer's disease: the temporal emergence of cognitive decline. *Journal of Alzheimer's Disease* 48 (4): 1095–1107.

63 Sugarman, M.A., Woodard, J.L., Nielson, K.A. et al. (2012). Functional magnetic resonance imaging of semantic memory as a presymptomatic biomarker of Alzheimer's disease risk. *Biochimica et Biophysica Acta* 1822 (3): 442–456.

64 Hirni, D.I., Kivisaari, S.L., Krumm, S. et al. (2016). Neuropsychological markers of medial Perirhinal and Entorhinal cortex functioning are impaired twelve years preceding diagnosis of Alzheimer's dementia. *Journal of Alzheimer's Disease* 52 (2): 573–580.

65 Huppert, F.A., Johnson, T., Nickson, J. et al. (2000). High prevalence of prospective memory impairment in the elderly and in early-stage dementia: findings from a population-based study. *Applied Cognitive Psychology* 14: S63–S81.

66 Huppert, F.A. and Beardsall, L. (1993). Prospective memory impairment as an early indicator of dementia. *Journal of Clinical and Experimental Neuropsychology* 15 (5): 805–821.

67 Maylor, E.A., Smith, G., Della Sala, S. et al. (2002). Prospective and retrospective memory in normal aging and dementia: an experimental study. *Memory & Cognition* 30 (6): 871–884.

68 Henry, J.D., MS, M.L., Phillips, L.H. et al. (2004). A meta-analytic review of prospective memory and aging. *Psychology and Aging* 19 (1): 27–39.

69 Blanco-Campal, A., Coen, R.F., Lawlor, B.A. et al. (2009). Detection of prospective memory deficits in mild cognitive impairment of suspected Alzheimer's disease etiology using a novel event-based prospective memory task. *Journal of the International Neuropsychological Society* 15 (1): 154–159.

70 Thompson, C., Henry, J.D., Rendell, P.G. et al. (2010). Prospective memory function in mild cognitive impairment and early dementia. *Journal of the International Neuropsychological Society* 16 (2): 318–325.

71 McDaniel, M.A., Shelton, J.T., Breneiser, J.E. et al. (2011). Focal and nonfocal prospective memory performance in very mild dementia: a signature decline. *Neuropsychology* 25 (3): 387–396.

72 Chi, S.Y., Rabin, L.A., Aronov, A. et al. (2014). Differential focal and nonfocal prospective memory accuracy in a demographically diverse group of nondemented community-dwelling older adults. *Journal of the International Neuropsychological Society* 20 (10): 1015–1027.

73 Niedzwienska, A., Kvavilashvili, L., Ashaye, K. et al. (2017). Spontaneous retrieval deficits in amnestic mild cognitive impairment: a case of focal event-based prospective memory. *Neuropsychology* 31 (7): 735.

74 Baddeley, A., Logie, R., Bressi, S. et al. (1986). Dementia and working memory. *Quarterly Journal of Experimental Psychology A* 38 (4): 603–618.

75 Stopford, C.L., Thompson, J.C., Neary, D. et al. (2012). Working memory, attention, and executive function in Alzheimer's disease and frontotemporal dementia. *Cortex* 48 (4): 429–446.

76 Grady, C.L., Haxby, J.V., Horwitz, B. et al. (1988). Longitudinal study of the early neuropsychological and cerebral metabolic changes in dementia of the Alzheimer type. *Journal of Clinical and Experimental Neuropsychology* 10 (5): 576–596.

77 Perry, R.J. and Hodges, J.R. (1999). Attention and executive deficits in Alzheimer's disease. A critical review. *Brain* 122 (Pt 3): 383–404.

78 Perry, R.J., Watson, P., and Hodges, J.R. (2000). The nature and staging of attention dysfunction in early (minimal and mild) Alzheimer's disease: relationship to episodic and semantic memory impairment. *Neuropsychologia* 38 (3): 252–271.

79 Calderon, J., Perry, R.J., Erzinclioglu, S.W. et al. (2001). Perception, attention, and working memory are disproportionately impaired in dementia with Lewy bodies compared with Alzheimer's disease. *Journal of Neurology, Neurosurgery, and Psychiatry* 70 (2): 157–164.

80 Greenwood, P.M., Parasuraman, R., and Alexander, G.E. (1997). Controlling the focus of spatial attention during visual search: effects of advanced aging and Alzheimer disease. *Neuropsychology* 11 (1): 3–12.

81 Elliott, R. (2003). Executive functions and their disorders imaging in clinical neuroscience. *British Medical Bulletin* 65 (1): 49–59.

82 Miyake, A., Friedman, N.P., Emerson, M.J. et al. (2000). The unity and diversity of executive functions and their contributions to complex "frontal lobe" tasks: a latent variable analysis. *Cognitive Psychology* 41 (1): 49–100.

83 Fisk, J.E. and Sharp, C.A. (2004). Age-related impairment in executive functioning: updating, inhibition, shifting, and access. *Journal of Clinical and Experimental Neuropsychology* 26 (7): 874–890.

84 Swanberg, M.M., Tractenberg, R.E., Mohs, R. et al. (2004). Executive dysfunction in Alzheimer disease. *Archives of Neurology* 61 (4): 556–560.

85 Lafleche, G. and Albert, M.S. (1995). Executive function deficits in mild Alzheimer's disease. *Neuropsychology* 9 (3): 313.

86 Collette, F., Van der Linden, M., and Salmon, E. (1999). Executive dysfunction in Alzheimer's disease. *Cortex* 35 (1): 57–72.

87 Traykov, L., Raoux, N., Latour, F. et al. (2007). Executive functions deficit in mild cognitive impairment. *Cognitive and Behavioral Neurology* 20 (4): 219–224.

88 Hazlett, K.E., Figueroa, C.M., and Nielson, K.A. (2015). Executive functioning and risk for Alzheimer's disease in the cognitively intact: family history predicts Wisconsin Card Sorting Test performance. *Neuropsychology* 29 (4): 582–591.

89 Binetti, G., Magni, E., Padovani, A. et al. (1996). Executive dysfunction in early Alzheimer's disease. *Journal of Neurology, Neurosurgery and Psychiatry* 60 (1): 91–93.

90 Chen, S.T., Sultzer, D.L., Hinkin, C.H. et al. (1998). Executive dysfunction in Alzheimer's disease: association with neuropsychiatric symptoms and functional impairment. *Journal of Neuropsychiatry and Clinical Neurosciences* 10 (4): 426–432.

91 Baudic, S., Dalla Barba, G., Thibaudet, M.C. et al. (2006). Executive function deficits in early Alzheimer's disease and their relations with episodic memory. *Archives of Clinical Neuropsychology* 21 (1): 15–21.

92 Brandt, J., Aretouli, E., Neijstrom, E. et al. (2009). Selectivity of executive function deficits in mild cognitive impairment. *Neuropsychology* 23 (5): 607.

93 Aretouli, E., Tsilidis, K.K., and Brandt, J. (2013). Four-year outcome of mild cognitive impairment: the contribution of executive dysfunction. *Neuropsychology* 27 (1): 95–106.

94 Ossenkoppele, R., Pijnenburg, Y.A., Perry, D.C. et al. (2015). The behavioural/dysexecutive variant of Alzheimer's disease: clinical, neuroimaging and pathological features. *Brain* 138 (Pt 9): 2732–2749.

95 Hassenstab, J., Monsell, S.E., Mock, C. et al. (2015). Neuropsychological markers of cognitive decline in persons with Alzheimer disease neuropathology. *Journal of Neuropathology and Experimental Neurology* 74 (11): 1086–1092.

96 Johnson, J.K., Head, E., Kim, R. et al. (1999). Clinical and pathological evidence for a frontal variant of Alzheimer disease. *Archives of Neurology* 56 (10): 1233–1239.

97 Murdoch, B.E., Chenery, H.J., Wilks, V. et al. (1987). Language disorders in dementia of the Alzheimer type. *Brain and Language* 31 (1): 122–137.

98 Weiner, M.F., Neubecker, K.E., Bret, M.E. et al. (2008). Language in Alzheimer's disease. *Journal of Clinical Psychiatry* 69 (8): 1223–1227.

99 Kertesz, A., Appell, J., and Fisman, M. (1986). The dissolution of language in Alzheimer's disease. *Canadian Journal of Neurological Sciences* 13 (4 Suppl): 415–418.

100 Laske, C., Sohrabi, H.R., Frost, S.M. et al. (2015). Innovative diagnostic tools for early detection of Alzheimer's disease. *Alzheimers & Dementia* 11 (5): 561–578.
101 Szatloczki, G., Hoffmann, I., Vincze, V. et al. (2015). Speaking in Alzheimer's disease, is that an early sign? Importance of changes in language abilities in Alzheimer's disease. *Frontiers in Aging Neuroscience* 7: 195.
102 Boschi, V., Catricala, E., Consonni, M. et al. (2017). Connected speech in neurodegenerative language disorders: a review. *Frontiers in Psychology* 8: 269.
103 Croisile, B. (1999). Agraphia in Alzheimer's disease. *Dementia and Geriatric Cognitive Disorders* 10 (3): 226–230.
104 Henderson, V.W., Buckwalter, J., Sobel, E. et al. (1992). The agraphia of Alzheimer's disease. *Neurology* 42 (4): 776–776.
105 Lambert, J., Giffard, B., Nore, F. et al. (2007). Central and peripheral agraphia in Alzheimer's disease: from the case of Auguste D. to a cognitive neuropsychology approach. *Cortex* 43 (7): 935–951.
106 Rodriguez-Ferreiro, J., Martinez, C., Perez-Carbajal, A.J. et al. (2014). Neural correlates of spelling difficulties in Alzheimer's disease. *Neuropsychologia* 65: 12–17.
107 Gorno-Tempini, M., Brambati, S., Ginex, V. et al. (2008). The logopenic/phonological variant of primary progressive aphasia. *Neurology* 71 (16): 1227–1234.
108 Rohrer, J.D., Rossor, M.N., and Warren, J.D. (2012). Alzheimer's pathology in primary progressive aphasia. *Neurobiology of Aging* 33 (4): 744–752.
109 Mendez, M.F. and Sabodash, V. (2015). Clinical amyloid imaging in logopenic progressive aphasia. *Alzheimer Disease and Associated Disorders* 29 (1): 94–96.
110 Rabinovici, G.D., Jagust, W.J., Furst, A.J. et al. (2008). Aβ amyloid and glucose metabolism in three variants of primary progressive aphasia. *Annals of Neurology* 64 (4): 388–401.
111 Mervis, C.B., Robinson, B.F., and Pani, J.R. (1999). Visuospatial construction. *The American Journal of Human Genetics* 65 (5): 1222–1229.
112 Weintraub, S., Wicklund, A.H., and Salmon, D.P. (2012). The neuropsychological profile of Alzheimer disease. *Cold Spring Harbor Perspectives in Medicine* 2 (4): a006171.
113 Karantzoulis, S. and Galvin, J.E. (2011). Distinguishing Alzheimer's disease from other major forms of dementia. *Expert Review of Neurotherapeutics* 11 (11): 1579–1591.
114 Mendez, M.F., Lee, A.S., Joshi, A. et al. (2012). Nonamnestic presentations of early-onset Alzheimer's disease. *American Journal of Alzheimer's Disease & Other Dementias* 27 (6): 413–420.
115 Johnson, D.K., Morris, J.C., and Galvin, J.E. (2005). Verbal and visuospatial deficits in dementia with Lewy bodies. *Neurology* 65 (8): 1232–1238.
116 Johnson, D.K., Storandt, M., Morris, J.C. et al. (2009). Longitudinal study of the transition from healthy aging to Alzheimer disease. *Archives of Neurology* 66 (10): 1254–1259.
117 Levine, D.N., Lee, J.M., and Fisher, C. (1993). The visual variant of Alzheimer's disease a clinicopathologic case study. *Neurology* 43 (2): 305–305.
118 Benson, D.F., Davis, R.J., and Snyder, B.D. (1988). Posterior cortical atrophy. *Archives of Neurology* 45 (7): 789–793.
119 Crutch, S.J., Lehmann, M., Schott, J.M. et al. (2012). Posterior cortical atrophy. *The Lancet Neurology* 11 (2): 170–178.

120 Dickerson, B.C., SM, M.G., Xia, C. et al. (2017). Approach to atypical Alzheimer's disease and case studies of the major subtypes. *CNS Spectrums* 1–11.

121 Millington, R.S., James-Galton, M., Maia Da Silva, M.N. et al. (2017). Lateralized occipital degeneration in posterior cortical atrophy predicts visual field deficits. *Neuroimage Clinical* 14: 242–249.

122 Peng, G., Wang, J., Feng, Z. et al. (2016). Clinical and neuroimaging differences between posterior cortical atrophy and typical amnestic Alzheimer's disease patients at an early disease stage. *Scientific Reports* 6: 29372.

123 Aarsland, D., Rongve, A., Piepenstock Nore, S. et al. (2008). Frequency and case identification of dementia with Lewy bodies using the revised consensus criteria. *Dementia and Geriatric Cognitive Disorders* 26 (5): 445–452.

124 Geser, F., Wenning, G.K., Poewe, W. et al. (2005). How to diagnose dementia with Lewy bodies: state of the art. *Movement Disorders* 20 (S12): S11–S20.

125 Kosaka, K., Yoshimura, M., Ikeda, K. et al. (1983). Diffuse type of Lewy body disease: progressive dementia with abundant cortical Lewy bodies and senile changes of varying degree--a new disease? *Clinical Neuropathology* 3 (5): 185–192.

126 Okazaki, H., Lipkin, L.E., and Aronson, S.M. (1961). Diffuse intracytoplasmic ganglionic inclusions (Lewy type) associated with progressive dementia and quadriparesis in flexion. *Journal of Neuropathology & Experimental Neurology* 20 (2): 237–244.

127 Byrne, E., Lennox, G., Godwin-Austen, R. et al. (1991). Dementia associated with cortical Lewy bodies: proposed clinical diagnostic criteria. *Dementia and Geriatric Cognitive Disorders* 2 (5): 283–284.

128 McKeith, I.G., Galasko, D., Kosaka, K. et al. (1996). Consensus guidelines for the clinical and pathologic diagnosis of dementia with Lewy bodies (DLB) Report of the consortium on DLB international workshop. *Neurology* 47 (5): 1113–1124.

129 McKeith, I.G., Perry, R., Fairbairn, A. et al. (1992). Operational criteria for senile dementia of Lewy body type (SDLT). *Psychological Medicine* 22 (04): 911–922.

130 McKeith, I., Dickson, D.W., Lowe, J. et al. (2005). Diagnosis and management of dementia with Lewy bodies third report of the DLB consortium. *Neurology* 65 (12): 1863–1872.

131 Ferman, T., Smith, G., Boeve, B. et al. (2004). DLB fluctuations specific features that reliably differentiate DLB from AD and normal aging. *Neurology* 62 (2): 181–187.

132 Perri, R., Monaco, M., Fadda, L. et al. (2014). Neuropsychological correlates of behavioral symptoms in Alzheimer's disease, frontal variant of frontotemporal, subcortical vascular, and lewy body dementias: a comparative study. *Journal of Alzheimer's Disease* 39 (3): 669–677.

133 Ferman, T.J., Arvanitakis, Z., Fujishiro, H. et al. (2013). Pathology and temporal onset of visual hallucinations, misperceptions and family misidentification distinguishes dementia with Lewy bodies from Alzheimer's disease. *Parkinsonism & Related Disorders* 19 (2): 227–231.

134 Hamilton, J.M., Salmon, D.P., Galasko, D. et al. (2004). A comparison of episodic memory deficits in neuropathologically-confirmed dementia with Lewy bodies and Alzheimer's disease. *Journal of the International Neuropsychological Society* 10 (05): 689–697.

135 Salmon, D.P., Galasko, D., Hansen, L.A. et al. (1996). Neuropsychological deficits associated with diffuse Lewy body disease. *Brain and Cognition* 31 (2): 148–165.

136 Jellinger, K.A., Wenning, G.K., and Seppi, K. (2007). Predictors of survival in dementia with lewy bodies and Parkinson dementia. *Neurodegenerative Diseases* 4 (6): 428–430.

137 Breitve, M., Chwiszczuk, L., Hynninen, M. et al. (2014). Is there a faster rate of cognitive decline in dementia with Lewy bodies than in Alzheimer's disease? A systematic review. *Alzheimer's Research & Therapy* 6 (5): 53.

138 Lobo, A., Launer, L., Fratiglioni, L. et al. (2000). Prevalence of dementia and major subtypes in Europe: a collaborative study of population-based cohorts. *Neurology (Minneapolis)* 54 (11 Suppl. 5): S4–S9.

139 Reilly, J., Rodriguez, A.D., Lamy, M. et al. (2010). Cognition, language, and clinical pathological features of non-Alzheimer's dementias: an overview. *Journal of Communication Disorders* 43 (5): 438–452.

140 O'Brien, J.T., Erkinjuntti, T., Reisberg, B. et al. (2003). Vascular cognitive impairment. *The Lancet Neurology* 2 (2): 89–98.

141 Jellinger, K.A. and Attems, J. (2010). Is there pure vascular dementia in old age? *Journal of the Neurological Sciences* 299 (1): 150–154.

142 Xuereb, J., Brayne, C., Dufouil, C. et al. (2000). Neuropathological findings in the very old: results from the first 101 brains of a population-based longitudinal study of dementing disorders. *Annals of the New York Academy of Sciences* 903 (1): 490–496.

143 Grinberg, L.T. and Thal, D.R. (2010). Vascular pathology in the aged human brain. *Acta Neuropathologica* 119 (3): 277–290.

144 Bowler, J.V. (2002). The concept of vascular cognitive impairment. *Journal of the Neurological Sciences* 203: 11–15.

145 Gorelick, P.B., Scuteri, A., Black, S.E. et al. (2011). Vascular contributions to cognitive impairment and dementia a statement for healthcare professionals from the American Heart Association/American Stroke Association. *Stroke* 42 (9): 2672–2713.

146 Ferrer, I. (2010). Cognitive impairment of vascular origin: neuropathology of cognitive impairment of vascular origin. *Journal of the Neurological Sciences* 299 (1): 139–149.

147 McAleese, K.E., Alafuzoff, I., Charidimou, A. et al. (2016). Post-mortem assessment in vascular dementia: advances and aspirations. *BMC Medicine* 14 (1): 129.

148 Neary, D., Snowden, J., and Mann, D. (2005). Frontotemporal dementia. *The Lancet Neurology* 4 (11): 771–780.

149 Mendez, M.F. and Cummings, J.L. (2003). *Dementia: A Clinical Approach*. Butterworth-Heinemann.

150 Finger, E.C. (2016). Frontotemporal dementias. *Continuum: Lifelong Learning in Neurology* 22 (2 Dementia): 464–489.

151 Hornberger, M. and Piguet, O. (2012). Episodic memory in frontotemporal dementia: a critical review. *Brain* 135 (3): 678–692.

152 Schmid, N.S., Taylor, K.I., Foldi, N.S. et al. (2013). Neuropsychological signs of Alzheimer's disease 8 years prior to diagnosis. *Journal of Alzheimer's Disease* 34 (2): 537–546.

10

Animal Models of Alzheimer's Disease

Prashant Bharadwaj

Centre of Excellence for Alzheimer's Disease Research and Care, School of Medical Sciences, Edith Cowan University, Sarich Neuroscience Research Institute, Nedlands, Australia
School of Pharmacy and Biomedical Sciences, Curtin Health and Innovation Research Institute (CHIRI), Faculty of Health Sciences, Curtin University, Perth, WA, Australia
Australian Alzheimer's Research Foundation, Ralph and Patricia Sarich Neuroscience Research Institute, Nedlands, Australia

10.1 Introduction

Alzheimer's disease (AD), the most common cause of dementia, accounts for approximately two-thirds of all dementia cases and affects more than 35 million individuals worldwide, including more than 350,000 people in Australia. Based on the age at onset, the major types of AD are differentiated into the early-onset forms (lesser than age of 65), and late-onset forms (greater than age of 65). Neuropathologically, AD is characterised by the accumulation of amyloidβ (Aβ) plaques in addition to synaptic loss, inflammation, oxidative damage, and eventually widespread neuronal death. The early-onset Alzheimer's disease (EOAD) cases account for about 5% of all AD cases, often have a clear family history of AD, and are caused by autosomal dominant mutations in the genes encoding amyloid precursor protein (APP), presenilin-1 (PS1), or presenilin-2 (PS 2) [1–3]. The other important hallmark of AD is the formation of intraneuronal neurofibrillary tangles (NFT). The NFT comprise hyperphosphorylated tau (MAPT, microtubule associated protein tau), a protein involved in microtubule assembly and stabilisation [4–7]. Notably, mutations in the tau gene are associated with frontotemporal dementia (FTD), but not with AD. A more complete breakdown and description of the various forms of AD can be found in a later chapter on the genetics of AD.

Animal models have played a major role in assessing disease-related proteins and have been leading the development of novel therapeutic approaches for AD. Over the last several decades, an abundance of research has been carried out, mainly in transgenic rodents, in an attempt to characterise the onset and course of AD. Transgenic mouse models of AD have been engineered to manifest different aspects of the condition including abnormal Aβ and tau expression, neurodegeneration, and neurobehavioural deficits [8, 9]. The main phenotypes that are looked for in an AD model include Aβ amyloid plaques, NFT, neuronal loss, astrogliosis and/or microgliosis, changes in long-term potentiation (LTP)/long-term depression (LTD), and cognitive impairment. Such animal models have helped to characterise the onset and course of AD, and provided experimental settings to test interventions for the likelihood of clinical efficacy.

Neurodegeneration and Alzheimer's Disease: The Role of Diabetes, Genetics, Hormones, and Lifestyle,
First Edition. Edited by Ralph N. Martins, Charles S. Brennan, W.M.A.D. Binosha Fernando, Margaret A. Brennan and Stephanie J. Fuller.
© 2019 John Wiley & Sons Ltd. Published 2019 by John Wiley & Sons Ltd.

Numerous animal models have been used to develop diverse potential therapeutics targeting different aspects of AD pathology. This chapter details various mice models of AD (as well as some other models of AD) and also discusses disparities between pre-clinical animal studies and human AD.

10.2   Transgenic Mouse Models

The neuropathology and clinical phenotype are generally indistinguishable in the early-onset familial versus the sporadic forms of the disease, although it can be said that EOAD cases develop more rapidly, and have a shorter time course from diagnosis to the eventual death of a patient. While EOAD accounts for only a small fraction of AD cases, it has provided essential information when considering the fundamental aspects of the disorder. The existence of early-onset familial forms of AD allowed the identification of causative mutations and key proteins, the elucidation of pathogenic mechanisms, and the development of transgenic animal models. A total of 143 AD mouse models expressing a wide range of disease-relevant mutated human genes were identified from the Alzforum database. The transgenes (most with AD-associated mutations) which have been used for these mouse models include one or more of the genes for the proteins APP, PS1, PS2, beta-site APP cleaving enzyme 1 (BACE1), BACE2, apolipoprotein E (ApoE), amyloid precursor-like protein-2 (APLP2), a type II membrane protein BRI2, C9ORF72, the RNA-binding protein fused- in sarcoma (FUS), MAPT, nitrogen oxide synthase-2 (NOS2), platelet derived growth factor receptor-β (PDGFRB), the receptor for advanced glycation end-products (RAGE), superoxide dismutase-1 (SOD1), and transactive response (TAR) DNA binding protein (TARDBP) [10].

The most commonly used transgenes are based on the EOAD mutations in *APP*, *PSEN1*, and *PSEN2*. These include a total of 77 transgenic mouse models as identified from the Alzforum database [10]. Some of these most commonly used models including their transgenic mutations and neurological phenotype have been listed here (Table 10.1). These transgenic mouse lines express (usually over-produce) human APP proteins and PS1/2 with one or more of these EOAD mutations. Some of the commonly used mutations in transgenic models include *APP*: Swedish (K670N/M671L), London (V717I) and Indiana (V717F) [25–27], and *PSEN1*: M146L and M146V.

Mice expressing mutated PS1 or PS2 alone do not develop Aβ plaques [28–30]. However, doubly transgenic mice expressing both mutated APP and PS1 develop Aβ plaques at a much earlier age than mice expressing mutated APP alone, with increased Aβ deposition, inflammation, and cognitive decline [19, 31–34]. The combined expression of five genetic mutations associated with Familial AD (*APP* K670N/M671L (Swedish), I716V (Florida), V717I (London), *PSEN1* M146L and L286V) in the 5XFAD mouse line results in significant aggravation of Aβ accumulation [11]. Mice expressing both BACE1 and human APP exhibit neurodegeneration despite reduced Aβ levels [35].

Generally speaking, the extracellular deposits of Aβ and other AD neuropathological symptoms develop at various time points during the course of the animal's life, depending on transgenic type, or combination of transgenes (see Figure 10.1). Moreover, the animals often display cognitive and behavioural deficits, when compared to wild-type animals [12, 18, 23, 36]. The use of transgenic mouse models of amyloid pathology has led to new insights regarding the processing of Aβ and the role of Aβ in the pathogenesis

Table 10.1 Commonly used AD mouse models.

Name	Genes	Mutations	Neurological/behavioural phenotype	Reference
3xTg	APP, PSEN1, MAPT	APP KM670/671NL (Swedish), MAPT P301L, PSEN1 M146V	4 months. Impairments occur prior to plaques and tangles. Deficits in both spatial and contextual based paradigms	Oddo et al. [8]
5xFAD	APP, PSEN1	APP KM670/671NL (Swedish), APP I716V (Florida), APP V717I (London), PSEN1 M146L, PSEN1 L286V	Age-dependent memory deficits including spatial memory, stress-related memory, and memory stabilisation	Oakley et al. [11]
APP23	APP	APP KM670/671NL (Swedish)	Spatial memory defects at 3 months that progress with age	Sturchler-Pierrat et al. [12]
APPPS1	APP, PSEN1	APP KM670/671NL (Swedish), PSEN1 L166P	Cognitive deficits in spatial learning and memory at 7 months	[13]
APPSwDI/NOS2-/-	APP, NOS2	APP KM670/671NL (Swedish), APP E693Q (Dutch), APP D694N (Iowa)	Severe learning and memory deficits. Impaired spatial memory at 52–56 weeks	[14, 15]
ARTE10	APP, PSEN1	APP KM670/671NL (Swedish), PSEN1 M146V	Age-related learning and memory deficits, in select paradigm-specific tasks by 12 months	[16]
hTau.P301S	MAPT	MAPT P301S	Early motor impairment at 4–5 months. Deficits progress to severe paraparesis	Allen et al. [17]
J20 (PDGF-APPSw,Ind)	APP	APP KM670/671NL (Swedish), APP V717F (Indiana)	Learning and memory deficits are age-dependent and may appear as early as 16 weeks	Mucke et al. [18]
PSEN/APP	APP, PSEN1	APP KM670/671NL (Swedish), PSEN1 M146L	Progressive impairment between 5–7 and 15–17 months in some tests of cognitive performance	Holcomb et al. [19]

(Continued)

Table 10.1 (Continued)

Name	Genes	Mutations	Neurological/behavioural phenotype	Reference
Tau P301L	*MAPT*	MAPT P301L	Age-associated deficits starting at 5 months. Progressive motor impairment and reduced activity, accompanied by increased clasping of hind and then forelimbs around 7 months	[20]
Tau P301S	*MAPT*	MAPT P301S	Impairments in spatial memory and learning ability. Paralysis at 7–10 months associated with a hunched-back posture and feeding difficulties	[21]
Tg2576	*APP*	APP KM670/671NL (Swedish)	Impaired spatial learning, working memory, and contextual fear conditioning reported at <6 months	[22]
TgCRND8	*APP*	APP KM670/671NL (Swedish), APP V717F (Indiana)	Early impairment in memory and learning by 3 months. Cognitive deficits in at 7 months but not at 2 months	Chishti et al. [23]
APP-NL-F Knock-in	*APP*	APP KM670/671NL (Swedish), APP I716F (Iberian)	Memory impairment in homozygous mice at 18 months as measured by the Y maze test. No significant deficit was seen in the Morris water maze at 18 months	Saito et al. [24]

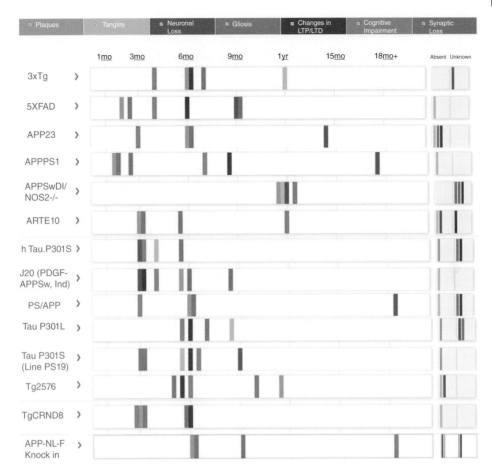

Figure 10.1 Phenotypes of commonly used AD mouse models generated from Alzforum. (*See color plate section for the color representation of this figure.*)

of AD [37]. However, while many of these transgenic mice develop Aβ plaque pathology and cognitive impairment, they do not develop NFT (Figure 10.1).

To address the role of tau protein hyperphosphorylation and NFT in the pathogenesis of AD, several other mouse models have been developed that overexpress either wild-type or mutated human MAPT protein. A total of 30 transgenic mouse models based on mutations in MAPT can be identified from the Alzforum database [10]. The introduction of human tau proteins containing FTD mutations does result in NFT formation [17, 38, 39]. However, if the introduced tau protein contains G272V, P301L, and P301S this results in both NFT formation and severe cognitive deficits [40]. Although they develop motor and learning deficits, mice expressing only mutant tau do not develop Aβ plaques.

Transgenic mice expressing human APP Swedish (K670N/M671L) and PS1 (M146V) as well as tau protein (P301L) develop both Aβ plaques and NFT pathology. Additionally, the mice develop other pathological and behavioural characteristics similar to AD including gliosis, synaptic damage, and memory impairment [8]. As described in Table 10.1 and Figure 10.1, different transgenic models show significant differences in the onset and development of neuropathological and behavioural phenotypes.

10.3 Knock-in AD Mice Models

There are certain limitations and drawbacks to APP/PS over-expressing AD mouse models. The over-expression of proteins, whether normal or mutant forms of proteins, may cause stress on protein processing within cells, thus introducing pathology or changes that do not reflect what happens in AD. In addition, the proteins are often expressed in a distribution pattern that does not resemble normal expression in a human brain. Other drawbacks of these models include the overproduction of all the other APP/PS1/PS2 protein fragments, which, again, does not reflect what is found in the human AD brain, and furthermore, the genes inserted lack non-coding regions, such that any mRNA splicing or post-transcriptional regulation cannot be examined. The Aβ fragments that are found accumulating in these mice do not have the same sequence lengths as those in human AD, for example the Aβ fragments extracted from a human brain have a considerable number of fragments truncated at the N-terminal end, frequently modified (isomerisation, oxidation, N-terminal degradation, racemisation, and pyroglutamyl formation), and the ratios of the main forms; Aβ1-40 to Aβ1-42 are also different [41].

To address some of these differences, *APP* knock-in mice were developed recently, where the murine Aβ sequence was changed to that of human Aβ, and two EOAD mutations were introduced, the KM670/671NL (Swedish) and I716F (Beyreuther/Iberian) mutations [24]. These APP^{NL-F} mice do not over-express APP but produce high levels of Aβ1-42 in the cerebral cortex and hippocampus, as well as neuroinflammation, including infiltration of astrocytes and microglia around plaques, starting at about six months of age. The APP^{NL-F} mice show functional deficits at 18 months, including spatial memory and flexible learning dysfunction, reduced attention, as well as compulsive behaviour [42]. Although these APP^{NL-F} mice also produce an abnormally large amount of C-terminal fragments and soluble APP fragments cleaved at the BACE-1 cleavage site, this has been shown in some other studies not to affect the AD-like pathology that develops [24, 42]. The mice do not develop tauopathies or neurodegeneration; although signs of neurodegeneration have been detected, as studies of these mice have shown that synaptic 'mushroom' spines are reduced in these mice [43]. In cultures of APP^{NL-F} mice neurons, extracellular Aβ1-42 has been shown to overactivate mGluR5 receptors, leading to elevated Ca^{2+} levels in endoplasmic reticulum, compensatory downregulation of stromal interaction molecule-2 (STIM2) expression, impaired synaptic neuronal store-operated calcium entry (nSOC), and reduced Ca2+/calmodulin-dependent protein kinase II (CaMKII) activity.

Other researchers have produced *APP* knock-in mice that carry the Swedish double mutation (KM670/671NL), Dutch (E693Q, linked to cerebral amyloid angiopathy) and London (V717I) mutations, also with the human Aβ sequence. Interestingly, these mutations did not result in much deposition of Aβ, but when cross-bred with *PSEN1* (containing the M146V mutation) mice, the mice gradually developed deposits of Aβ in the parenchyma and vasculature of the cerebral cortex, thus although not models of AD, they may be good models of human cerebral amyloid angiopathy [44]. It has been suggested that previous results obtained using the most common transgenic mouse models of AD should probably be verified in these 'second-generation' mouse models, as they more closely reflect the human APP metabolism [41]. Some of the pathological changes in the over-expressing transgenic mice are thought to be artefacts of protein over-expression.

There are also other aspects of human AD that are most likely too difficult to replicate. The majority of elderly people who develop AD have co-morbidities, including cardiovascular disease, hypertension, stroke, insulin resistance, type 2 diabetes, and even other neuropathologies. The two to three decades that the pathology has been developing in humans also results in different Aβ modifications, as mentioned earlier. The majority of AD cases also do not have mutations in their *APP* or *PSEN* genes either, therefore testing drugs that may influence APP cleavage may have little relevance in sporadic AD, since the Familial AD-associated mutations often cause AD by altering APP cleavage sites and/or enzyme activities. Even in the knock-in mice, apart from the humanised Aβ sequence, the rest of the sequence is still that of the mouse. All of these differences impact the validity of using these mouse models to some extent, however these models are still considered valuable for studying molecular mechanisms, biomarker evaluation, and pre-clinical drug development.

10.4 Non-Transgenic and Other Mammalian Animal Models

While the transgenic mice described above have been very widely used in AD research, a number of other non-transgenic and higher-order mammalian animal models have been developed as well. The senescence-accelerated mouse strain (SAM) is an accelerated ageing model established through phenotypic selection, that is a commonly used model for ageing [45]. SAMP8, a sub-strain of SAM has been shown to exhibit learning and memory deficits and also to develop Aβ deposits in the brain [46]. Unlike mice, guinea pigs and rabbits share an identical Aβ peptide sequence with humans; however, they do not spontaneously develop any AD-like disease [47]. High-cholesterol diets in rabbits and guinea pigs have been shown to cause the development of AD-like pathology and symptoms including Aβ deposition, tau pathology, neuronal loss, and cognitive impairment [48, 49]. Although some debate the importance of cholesterol and dyslipidaemia in the pathogenesis of AD [50], further evidence has been recently provided as a result of genetic studies of mild cognitive impairment (MCI) patients, and studies of cholesterol-fed rabbits which showed endolysosome dysfunction (which occurs in AD) features in skeletal muscle. The muscles had abnormally large endolysosomes, a decrease in lysosomal enzymes, and an accumulation of free cholesterol, Aβ, phosphorylated tau, and ubiquitin [51]. Other recent studies showed rabbits on a high-cholesterol diet had increased levels of 27-hydroxycholesterol in the circulation, which can (and does) cross the blood–brain barrier and influence oestrogen receptors in the brain. Oestrogen receptor expression was found to be altered, and some neurodegeneration of the hippocampus was detected, along with a decrease in hippocampal mitochondria [52]. This is of importance as mitochondrial dysfunction is believed to be one of the earliest stages in AD-related neurodegeneration [52, 53]. These studies showed that diet-induced neurodegenerative models can provide useful information concerning the involvement of dietary and lifestyle factors in AD.

Dogs are considered a useful model of AD due to their highly developed social and communicative behaviour [54]. In addition to homology between canine and human APP-related proteins [47], ageing canines have been shown to develop cognitive symptoms similar to AD in humans [55–58]. Aged dogs have also been shown to develop Aβ pathology and neuronal degeneration in their brains, although they do not develop NFT [59].

Non-human primates (NHP) are long-lived species and are the genetically and physiologically closest relatives to humans. The cognitive abilities and brain anatomy of NHP is similar to that of humans, and the sequence of NHP APP is identical to that of humans. Several species of NHP develop age-related cognitive deficits associated with brain atrophy, Aβ plaques, and neuronal loss [60–63]. A few species also develop tau pathology in addition to Aβ plaques [59].

Animal studies and other research has indicated that oxidative stress, mitochondrial dysfunction, chronic and disrupted inflammation, dyslipidemia, disruptions to energy metabolism, and brain ischaemia may have a part to play in the complex aetiology of late-onset sporadic AD. However, the relevance of each of these and any other changes is still being determined. This is because pathogenesis is thought to start up to 30 years before symptoms are apparent, with various pathogenic stages occurring, and this long time-course, the complexity of the disease, and the frequency of overlap with other conditions in the elderly has made the aetiology difficult to study. Animal models have relied on the utilisation of genetic mutations associated with EOAD, with the underlying principle that, once the pathogenic steps have started, the pathogenic processes leading to the clinical symptoms are likely to be similar. Although no single mouse model recapitulates all of the aspects of the disease, each model has provided insight into specific components of the disease, and has been invaluable in determining the molecular mechanisms of disease progression and for testing potential therapeutics.

10.5 Drug Development and Translational Issues

Current AD treatments mostly target cognitive decline by trying to improve neurotransmission, and provide only minor benefits across the array of clinical symptoms [64, 65]. Approved AD drugs such as acetylcholinesterase (AChE) inhibitors (aricept, namenda, exelon, etc.) and N-methyl-D-aspartate (NMDA) receptor antagonists (memantine) are generally prescribed in monotherapy or in combination. However, they are expensive and, most importantly, do not prevent disease progression and are of limited benefit to most patients [66, 67]. Other drugs are used to manage mood disorder, anxiety, and neurosis in later stages of the disease, but no treatment with a disease-modifying effect is currently available.

Animal models are indispensable to drug discovery and development. In particular, animal models have a key role in target discovery and validation. Ideally, the key aetiological and symptomatic features of AD would be replicated in an animal model of the disease. However, as mentioned earlier, most AD animal models are incomplete, and focus only on specific aspects of a complex multifactorial disease process. Unfortunately, the lack of a reliable model for pre-clinical validation has significantly impacted drug development in AD. It is estimated that several hundred interventions have been tested in AD transgenic mice, including ~300 in the Tg2576 mouse model alone [68]. A brief non-exhaustive list of some of drugs tested in animal models is provided here (Table 10.2). Despite a number of these interventions improving Aβ pathology and cognitive loss in mice, they have failed to produce similar benefits in human clinical trials. During the 2002–2012 observation period, 413 AD trials were performed: 124 Phase I

Table 10.2 AD drug development in transgenic mouse models.

Compound	Proposed mechanism of action	Animal model	Study outcome	Reference
Donepezil	Cholinesterase inhibitor	APP23 mice	Treatment significantly enhanced cognitive performance	[69]
Galantamine	Cholinesterase inhibitor	5 x FAD	Treatment improved performance in behavioural tests and lowered plaque density in the brain	[70]
Phenserine	Cholinesterase inhibitor	Tg2576	Treatment improved cognition in rodent models of AD	[71]
Memantine	NMDA antagonist	3 x Tg	Treatment improved visual-spatial learning deficit and reduced Aβ, tau and glycogen synthase kinase-3β (GSK-3β) levels	[72]
Semagacestat	γ-secretase inhibitor	PDAPP	Treatment induced a dose-dependent reduction in Aβ levels in plasma, cerebrospinal fluid, and brain	[73]
DAPT	γ-secretase inhibitor	PDAPP Tg2576	Inconsistencies in cognitive outcome, with the drug reducing Aβ levels in young mice and having no effect in older mice	[74, 75]
CHF5074	γ-secretase modulator	Tg2576	Treatment increased hippocampal neurogenesis and reduced cortical plaque burden and contextual memory deficit	[76]
Scyllo-inositol	Aβ aggregation inhibitor	TgCRND8	Treatment reduced visual-spatial learning deficit, brain Aβ levels, synaptic loss, and inflammation.	[77]
Homotaurine (tramiprosate)	Aβ intercalators	TgCRND8	Treatment reduced soluble and insoluble brain Aβ40 and Aβ42 levels	[78]
PBT-2	Metal-protein attenuating compound	Tg2576	Improvement of visual-spatial learning deficit and reduced insoluble Aβ and phosphorylated tau levels in the brain	[79]
Bapineuzumab	Promote Aβ clearance (immunotherapy)	PDAPP mice	Reduction in Aβ aggregates and synaptic pathology; fewer cognitive deficits in mice	[80]
Solanezumab	Promote Aβ clearance (immunotherapy)	PDAPP mice	Reduction in Aβ aggregates and synaptic pathology; fewer cognitive deficits in mice	[81]
Ponezumab	Promote Aβ clearance (immunotherapy)	Tg2576	Reduction in Aβ aggregates and synaptic pathology; fewer cognitive deficits in mice	[82]
Gammagard	Promote Aβ clearance (immunotherapy)	APP/PS1 transgenic mice	Reduced Aβ deposition, modulated inflammatory response in mice	[83]
Lithium	Inhibition GSK-3β linked to tau hyperphosphorylation	Tau P301S	Treatment reduced tau phosphorylation and aggregated tau, but no rescue of motor and working memory deficits	[84]

trials, 206 Phase II trials, and 83 Phase III trials. A very high attrition rate with an overall success rate during the 2002–2012 period of 0.4% (99.6% failure) was shown [85]. The reasons for clinical trial failure are often complex and multifactorial. However, this translational road block observed in AD has raised fundamental biological questions about pre-clinical models and their validity in the field.

10.6 Correlations Between Animal Models of AD and Human AD

As mentioned above, a variety of intrinsic differences exist between the aetiology of AD in animal models and the sporadic disease in humans. First, the transgenic animals developed for AD research express human genes containing mutations associated with EOAD. However, a majority of AD cases are sporadic and not associated with any particular genetic risk factor. As a result, the transgenic animal models with EOAD-related mutations that have been developed to model AD are not relevant to sporadic AD, or at least not to the early stages [86, 87]. Second, the available transgenic mouse models have used a variety of promoters, contributing to the discrepancies in results among animal studies. As mentioned above, the overexpression of human genes in rodent models may itself lead to artefacts and confound interpretation of results [26, 88].

Other discrepancies between rodent and human AD pathology also mentioned earlier are the lack of neuronal loss and the altered nature of Aβ plaques. Single-transgenic rodent models exhibit very little neuronal loss during the course of disease, whereas human AD is characterised by progressive loss of cholinergic neurons [26, 89]. Moreover, human AD exhibits significant atrophy of the brain, particularly in the hippocampus, entorhinal cortex, and amygdala [26]. While brain atrophy is observed in double/triple transgenic mice, it occurs very early in life and prior to the accumulation of Aβ [90–93]. In humans, Aβ deposits begin in the neocortex, extending into allocortical brain regions, and finally in the regions of brain stem and cerebellum. However, in mouse models of AD, the spatial distribution of pathology depends largely on the promoter used to drive expression of the transgenes [26]. Even with ubiquitous neuronal expression in some mouse models, there is still a remarkable regional specificity. One example is the APP23 mice. These mice have a seven-fold higher expression of mutant human APP bearing the pathogenic Swedish mutation, and plaques are primarily found in the hippocampus and cortex. Furthermore, the plaques generated in these animals have a greater solubility in comparison with those formed in the human brain, thought to be due to species differences in other proteins, as well as the much shorter time frame for plaque formation, which doesn't allow as much time for post-translational modifications as mentioned earlier, such as isomerisation, oxidation, N-terminal degradation, racemisation, and pyroglutamyl formation [88, 89], many of which increase Aβ hydrophobicity and resistance to degradation.

Rodent Aβ is much less prone to aggregation compared to human Aβ, which is the main reason human sequences are needed in transgenic constructs, although over-production is also necessary due to the much shorter time available to develop amyloid plaques. In comparison with human Aβ, mouse Aβ has three amino acid substitutions in the N-terminal region, Arg5Gly, Tyr10Phe, and His13Arg [94]. In humans, Aβ peptides are the primary components of so-called senile plaques [95, 96], and several different lengths of Aβ are present in these plaques, including Aβ1-40, Aβ1-42, and numerous N-truncated peptides [95], with these various lengths being present in different amounts. AD transgenic mice have different ratios of the different forms of Aβ; for example, in the APP23 mice, there are almost no Aβ molecules shortened at the N-terminus, whereas these can account for over 50% of the plaque amyloid in humans.

One of the biggest differences between most of the mouse AD models is the lack of NFT. In addition to the presence of Aβ plaques, the hyperphosphorylation of tau protein, followed by the development of NFT is an important hallmark of AD. Several of the Aβ transgenic mouse lines develop hyperphosphorylation of tau protein, but they do not develop NFT [97–99]. Furthermore, transgenic mice expressing normal human tau protein isoforms also exhibit hyperphosphorylation of tau protein, but no NFT formation [100–103]. NFT formation has only been observed in transgenic mouse models in which a mutated human tau protein has been introduced [38–40, 104]. However, it is important to note that mutations in tau protein are not associated with human AD [105].

10.7 Experimental Design and Reporting

While there are fundamental differences between the pathology and clinical presentation of AD when compared to the many phenotypes and pathological changes seen in the various transgenic AD mice models, there are also several validity issues that are within the scope of experimental design including overall study design, sample size calculation, the reporting of blinded assessment of outcome, and the reporting of random allocation to group. Numerous pathological outcomes have often been assessed in transgenic mouse studies, including plaque burden, levels of Aβ40 and Aβ42, tau, and inflammation markers alongside neurodegeneration. Transgenic studies differ from clinical studies in the respect that pathological outcome measures are much more commonly reported than neurobehavioural outcomes. While there have been some studies in transgenic models investigating the association between pathological outcomes and cognition [106], there is no definitive data to demonstrate a direct relationship between a specific pathology and behaviour.

It is also important to consider the appropriate age at which animal models best reflect human disease, and due to differences in disease course, mutation, and promoter used in the different mouse models, different models reflect different aspects of the disease to a greater or lesser extent than other models. Despite these complications, the data from mouse studies (as well as clinical studies) is making it clear that developing treatments for established disease will be substantially more challenging and potential treatments are more likely to be effective when administered at an early stage. Interventions in transgenic mouse models are designed to ascertain whether a given drug is likely to improve clinical outcomes in people with AD and a key determinant of this is to demonstrate statistical significance. Previous studies have suggested that many animal studies of neurological disorders are underpowered [107, 108]. It is suggested from a systematically collated data set in the Collaborative Approach to Meta-Analysis and Review of Animal Data from Experimental Studies (CAMARADES database that many publications were identified where a sample size calculation had not been conducted. This finding is consistent with experience across the animal modelling of many neurological disorders [109]. Systematic review work also suggests that one of the most influential factors that has contributed to translational failure in the amyotrophic lateral sclerosis (ALS) field is the fact that *in vivo* studies were underpowered [110].

Blinded outcomes are a method of improving experimental rigour by masking the identity of the control and treatment groups from those who measure the outcome, handle the data, or analyse the data. Across experimental neuroscience, the reporting of blinded assessment of outcome is relatively uncommon. Vesterinen and colleagues were able to demonstrate that the reporting of blinding was associated with smaller estimates of neurobehavioural effect size in multiple sclerosis models [108]. Similar findings have been identified in pre-clinical studies of stroke and Parkinson's disease [109]. It is likely that some outcome measures are more susceptible to influence from this bias than others.

10.8 The Future of Animal Models in AD

Although animal models used to investigate AD have largely failed to yield successful treatments, they have had a profound influence on gaining an understanding of the mechanisms underlying AD pathology. For the next generation of animal models, there may be advantages in genetically modifying other animal species, particularly those in which the endogenous Aβ sequence is identical to humans and those in which the processing of tau is more closely aligned to that in humans. Ideally, it would also be advantageous to have aged animal models for sporadic AD. Such models would enable us to study the various aspects of the ageing process that drive the pathology so that we can target them for prevention. However, developing such models will be challenging, and may require novel approaches in recombinant technology and animal breeding. Depending on the animal species investigated, this may extend studies to many more years than a mouse life-span, and raise ethical issues. These two considerations have probably been the main reasons little has been done so far on other animal AD models.

Once potential AD drugs or treatments prove to be promising in *in vitro* investigations, the standard next step is to test the drugs or interventions in transgenic mouse models for AD. To circumvent future clinical trial failures, it will be vital to evaluate more carefully the utility of existing data from both clinical and pre-clinical studies. Evidence synthesis techniques such as meta-analyses must be used to identify the gaps in the use of animal models for disease interventions. This will enable the development of better guidelines for future conduct in all the animal studies and early clinical studies, and to help assess if there is enough significant evidence in favour of an intervention before embarking on more substantial clinical trials. In addition to using transgenic models, post-mortem studies, investigations of human patient samples, advances in the technology of induced pluripotent stem cells from AD patients [111, 112], the use of clinical imaging techniques that can monitor brain pathology development well before clinical symptoms start [113, 114], and the development of pre-clinical biomarkers (blood-based), will all help us to understand the pathological changes occurring in AD. This variety of scientific resources, combined with epidemiological studies, observational research with AD patients, and clinical trials will provide further data to address the gaps in AD research.

References

1 Levy-Lahad, E., Wasco, W., Poorkaj, P. et al. (1995). Candidate gene for the chromosome 1 familial Alzheimer's disease locus. *Science* 269: 973–977.
2 Rogaev, E.I., Sherrington, R., Rogaeva, E.A. et al. (1995). Familial Alzheimer's disease in kindreds with missense mutations in a gene on chromosome 1 related to the Alzheimer's disease type 3 gene. *Nature* 376: 775–778.
3 Sherrington, R., Rogaev, E.I., Liang, Y. et al. (1995). Cloning of a gene bearing missense mutations in early-onset familial Alzheimer's disease. *Nature* 375: 754–760.
4 Brion, J.P., Couck, A.M., Passareiro, E., and Flament-Durand, J. (1985). Neurofibrillary tangles of Alzheimer's disease: an immunohistochemical study. *J. Submicrosc. Cytol.* 17: 89–96.
5 Ihara, Y., Nukina, N., Miura, R., and Ogawara, M. (1986). Phosphorylated tau protein is integrated into paired helical filaments in Alzheimer's disease. *J. Biochem.* 99: 1807–1810.
6 Iqbal, K., Grundke-Iqbal, I., Zaidi, T. et al. (1986). Defective brain microtubule assembly in Alzheimer's disease. *Lancet* 2: 421–426.
7 Delacourte, A. and Defossez, A. (1986). Alzheimer's disease: tau proteins, the promoting factors of microtubule assembly, are major components of paired helical filaments. *J. Neurol. Sci.* 76: 173–186.
8 Oddo, S., Caccamo, A., Shepherd, J.D. et al. (2003). Triple-transgenic model of Alzheimer's disease with plaques and tangles: intracellular Abeta and synaptic dysfunction. *Neuron* 39: 409–421.
9 Hochgrafe, K., Sydow, A., and Mandelkow, E.M. (2013). Regulatable transgenic mouse models of Alzheimer disease: onset, reversibility and spreading of tau pathology. *FEBS J.* 280: 4371–4381.
10 Alzforum, Research Models, http://www.alzforum.org/research-models. Accessed 16 May.
11 Oakley, H., Cole, S.L., Logan, S. et al. (2006). Intraneuronal beta-amyloid aggregates, neurodegeneration, and neuron loss in transgenic mice with five familial Alzheimer's disease mutations: potential factors in amyloid plaque formation. *J. Neurosci.* 26: 10129–10140.
12 Sturchler-Pierrat, C., Abramowski, D., Duke, M. et al. (1997). Two amyloid precursor protein transgenic mouse models with Alzheimer disease-like pathology. *Proc. Natl. Acad. Sci. U.S.A.* 94: 13287–13292.
13 Radde, R., Bolmont, T., Kaeser, S.A. et al. (2006). Abeta42-driven cerebral amyloidosis in transgenic mice reveals early and robust pathology. *EMBO Rep.* 7 (9): 940–946.
14 Colton, C.A., Wilcock, D.M., Wink, D.A. et al. (2008). The effects of NOS2 gene deletion on mice expressing mutated human AbetaPP. *J. Alzheimers. Dis.* 15 (4): 571–587.
15 Wilcock, D.M., Lewis, M.R., Van Nostrand, W.E. et al. (2008). Progression of amyloid pathology to Alzheimer's disease pathology in an amyloid precursor protein transgenic mouse model by removal of nitric oxide synthase 2. *J Neurosci.* 28 (7): 1537–1545.

16 Willuweit, A., Velden, J., Godemann, R. et al. (2009). Early-onset and robust amyloid pathology in a new homozygous mouse model of Alzheimer's disease. *PLoS One* 4 (11).

17 Allen, B., Ingram, E., Takao, M. et al. (2002). Abundant tau filaments and nonapoptotic neurodegeneration in transgenic mice expressing human P301S tau protein. *J. Neurosci.* 22: 9340–9351.

18 Mucke, L., Masliah, E., Yu, G.Q. et al. (2000). High-level neuronal expression of abeta 1-42 in wild-type human amyloid protein precursor transgenic mice: synaptotoxicity without plaque formation. *J. Neurosci.* 20: 4050–4058.

19 Holcomb, L., Gordon, M.N., McGowan, E. et al. (1998). Accelerated Alzheimer-type phenotype in transgenic mice carrying both mutant amyloid precursor protein and presenilin 1 transgenes. *Nat. Med.* 4: 97–100.

20 Terwel, D., Lasrado, R., Snauwaert, J. et al. (2005). Changed conformation of mutant Tau-P301L underlies the moribund tauopathy, absent in progressive, non-lethal axonopathy of Tau-4R/2N transgenic mice. *J. Biol. Chem.* 280 (5): 3963–3973.

21 Yl, Y., Higuchi, M., Zhang, B. et al. (2007). Synapse loss and microglial activation precede tangles in a P301S tauopathy mouse model. *Neuron.* 53 (3): 337–351.

22 Hsiao, K., Chapman, P., Nilsen, S. et al. (1996). Correlative memory deficits, Abeta elevation, and amyloid plaques in transgenic mice. *Science* 274: 99–102.

23 Chishti, M.A., Yang, D.S., Janus, C. et al. (2001). Early-onset amyloid deposition and cognitive deficits in transgenic mice expressing a double mutant form of amyloid precursor protein 695. *J. Biol. Chem.* 276: 21562–21570.

24 Saito, T., Matsuba, Y., Mihira, N. et al. (2014). Single App knock-in mouse models of Alzheimer's disease. *Nat. Neurosci.* 17: 661–663.

25 Chartier-Harlin, M., Crawford, F., Houlden, H. et al. (1991). Early-onset Alzheimer's disease caused by mutations at codon 717 of the b-amyloid precursor protein gene. *Nature* 353: 844–846.

26 Duyckaerts, C., Potier, M.C., and Delatour, B. (2008). Alzheimer disease models and human neuropathology: similarities and differences. *Acta Neuropathol.* 115: 5–38.

27 Goate, A., Chartier-Harlin, M.C., Mullan, M. et al. (1991). Segregation of a missense mutation in the amyloid precursor protein gene with familial Alzheimer's disease. *Nature* 349: 704–706.

28 Mattson, M.P. and Chan, S.L. (2001). Dysregulation of cellular calcium homeostasis in Alzheimer's disease: bad genes and bad habits. *J. Mol. Neurosci.* 17: 205–224.

29 Oyama, F., Sawamura, N., Kobayashi, K. et al. (1998). Mutant presenilin 2 transgenic mouse: effect on an age-dependent increase of amyloid beta-protein 42 in the brain. *J. Neurochem.* 71: 313–322.

30 Sawamura, N., Morishima-Kawashima, M., Waki, H. et al. (2000). Mutant presenilin 2 transgenic mice. A large increase in the levels of Abeta 42 is presumably associated with the low density membrane domain that contains decreased levels of glycerophospholipids and sphingomyelin. *J. Biol. Chem.* 275: 27901–27908.

31 Casas, C., Sergeant, N., Itier, J.M. et al. (2004). Massive CA1/2 neuronal loss with intraneuronal and N-terminal truncated Abeta42 accumulation in a novel Alzheimer transgenic model. *Am. J. Pathol.* 165: 1289–1300.

32 Borchelt, D.R., Ratovitski, T., van Lare, J. et al. (1997). Accelerated amyloid deposition in the brains of transgenic mice coexpressing mutant presenilin 1 and amyloid precursor proteins. *Neuron* 19: 939–945.

33 Blanchard, V., Moussaoui, S., Czech, C. et al. (2003). Time sequence of maturation of dystrophic neurites associated with Abeta deposits in APP/PS1 transgenic mice. *Exp. Neurol.* 184: 247–263.

34 McGowan, E., Sanders, S., Iwatsubo, T. et al. (1999). Amyloid phenotype characterization of transgenic mice overexpressing both mutant amyloid precursor protein and mutant presenilin 1 transgenes. *Neurobiol. Dis.* 6: 231–244.

35 Rockenstein, E., Mante, M., Alford, M. et al. (2005). High beta-secretase activity elicits neurodegeneration in transgenic mice despite reductions in amyloid-beta levels: implications for the treatment of Alzheimer disease. *J. Biol. Chem.* 280: 32957–32967.

36 Games, D., Adams, D., Alessandrini, R. et al. (1995). Alzheimer-type neuropathology in transgenic mice overexpressing V717F beta-amyloid precursor protein. *Nature* 373: 523–527.

37 Schaeffer, E.L., Figueiro, M., and Gattaz, W.F. (2011). Insights into Alzheimer disease pathogenesis from studies in transgenic animal models. *Clinics (Sao Paulo)* 66 (Suppl 1): 45–54.

38 Gotz, J., Chen, F., van Dorpe, J., and Nitsch, R.M. (2001). Formation of neurofibrillary tangles in P301l tau transgenic mice induced by Abeta 42 fibrils. *Science* 293: 1491–1495.

39 Lewis, J., McGowan, E., Rockwood, J. et al. (2000). Neurofibrillary tangles, amyotrophy and progressive motor disturbance in mice expressing mutant (P301L) tau protein. *Nat. Genet.* 25: 402–405.

40 Schindowski, K., Bretteville, A., Leroy, K. et al. (2006). Alzheimer's disease-like tau neuropathology leads to memory deficits and loss of functional synapses in a novel mutated tau transgenic mouse without any motor deficits. *Am. J. Pathol.* 169: 599–616.

41 Sasaguri, H., Nilsson, P., Hashimoto, S. et al. (2017). APP mouse models for Alzheimer's disease preclinical studies. *EMBO J.* 36: 2473–2487.

42 Masuda, A., Kobayashi, Y., Kogo, N. et al. (2016). Cognitive deficits in single App knock-in mouse models. *Neurobiol. Learn. Mem.* 135: 73–82.

43 Zhang, H., Wu, L., Pchitskaya, E. et al. (2015). Neuronal store-operated calcium entry and mushroom spine loss in amyloid precursor protein knock-in mouse model of Alzheimer's disease. *J. Neurosci.* 35: 13275–13286.

44 Li, H., Guo, Q., Inoue, T. et al. (2014). Vascular and parenchymal amyloid pathology in an Alzheimer disease knock-in mouse model: interplay with cerebral blood flow. *Mol. Neurodegener.* 9: 28.

45 Del Valle, J., Duran-Vilaregut, J., Manich, G. et al. (2010). Early amyloid accumulation in the hippocampus of SAMP8 mice. *J. Alzheimers Dis.* 19: 1303–1315.

46 Butterfield, D.A. and Poon, H.F. (2005). The senescence-accelerated prone mouse (SAMP8): a model of age-related cognitive decline with relevance to alterations of the gene expression and protein abnormalities in Alzheimer's disease. *Exp. Gerontol.* 40: 774–783.

47 Johnstone, E.M., Chaney, M.O., Norris, F.H. et al. (1991). Conservation of the sequence of the Alzheimer's disease amyloid peptide in dog, polar bear and five other mammals by cross-species polymerase chain reaction analysis. *Brain Res. Mol. Brain Res.* 10: 299–305.

48 Sharman, M.J., Moussavi Nik, S.H., Chen, M.M. et al. (2013). The guinea pig as a model for sporadic Alzheimer's disease (AD): the impact of cholesterol intake on expression of AD-related genes. *PLoS One* 8: e66235.

49 Sparks, D.L. (2008). The early and ongoing experience with the cholesterol-fed rabbit as a model of Alzheimer's disease: the old, the new and the pilot. *J. Alzheimers Dis.* 15: 641–656.

50 Wood, W.G., Li, L., Muller, W.E., and Eckert, G.P. (2014). Cholesterol as a causative factor in Alzheimer's disease: a debatable hypothesis. *J. Neurochem.* 129: 559–572.

51 Chen, X., Wagener, J.F., Ghribi, O., and Geiger, J.D. (2016). Role of endolysosomes in skeletal muscle pathology observed in a cholesterol-fed rabbit model of Alzheimer's disease. *Front. Aging Neurosci.* 8: 129.

52 Brooks, S.W., Dykes, A.C., and Schreurs, B.G. (2017). A high-cholesterol diet increases 27-hydroxycholesterol and modifies estrogen receptor expression and neurodegeneration in rabbit hippocampus. *J. Alzheimers Dis.* 56: 185–196.

53 Zhu, X., Perry, G., Smith, M.A., and Wang, X. (2013). Abnormal mitochondrial dynamics in the pathogenesis of Alzheimer's disease. *J. Alzheimers Dis.* 33 (Suppl 1): S253–S262.

54 Hare, B. and Tomasello, M. (2005). Human-like social skills in dogs? *Trends Cogn. Sci.* 9: 439–444.

55 Landsberg, G. (2005). Therapeutic agents for the treatment of cognitive dysfunction syndrome in senior dogs. *Prog. Neuropsychopharmacol. Biol. Psychiatry* 29: 471–479.

56 Opii, W.O., Joshi, G., Head, E. et al. (2008). Proteomic identification of brain proteins in the canine model of human aging following a long-term treatment with antioxidants and a program of behavioral enrichment: relevance to Alzheimer's disease. *Neurobiol. Aging* 29: 51–70.

57 Tapp, P.D., Siwak, C.T., Estrada, J. et al. (2003). Effects of age on measures of complex working memory span in the beagle dog (*Canis familiaris*) using two versions of a spatial list learning paradigm. *Learn. Mem.* 10: 148–160.

58 Cummings, B.J., Head, E., Afagh, A.J. et al. (1996). Beta-amyloid accumulation correlates with cognitive dysfunction in the aged canine. *Neurobiol. Learn. Mem.* 66: 11–23.

59 Sarasa, M. and Pesini, P. (2009). Natural non-trasgenic animal models for research in Alzheimer's disease. *Curr. Alzheimer Res.* 6: 171–178.

60 Lemere, C.A., Oh, J., Stanish, H.A. et al. (2008). Cerebral amyloid-beta protein accumulation with aging in cotton-top tamarins: a model of early Alzheimer's disease? *Rejuvenation Res.* 11: 321–332.

61 Gearing, M., Tigges, J., Mori, H., and Mirra, S.S. (1997). Beta-amyloid (A beta) deposition in the brains of aged orangutans. *Neurobiol. Aging* 18: 139–146.

62 Schultz, C., Hubbard, G.B., Rub, U. et al. (2000). Age-related progression of tau pathology in brains of baboons. *Neurobiol. Aging* 21: 905–912.

63 Bons, N., Rieger, F., Prudhomme, D. et al. (2006). Microcebus murinus: a useful primate model for human cerebral aging and Alzheimer's disease? *Genes Brain Behav.* 5: 120–130.

64 Omerovic, M., Teipel, S.J., and Hampel, T. (2007). Dementia with Lewy bodies: clinical improvement under treatment with an acetylcholinesterase inhibitor. *Nervenarzt* 78: 1052–1057.

65 Tariot, P.N. (2006). Contemporary issues in the treatment of Alzheimer's disease: tangible benefits of current therapies. *J. Clin. Psychiatry* 67 (Suppl 3): 15–22; quiz 23.

66 Jelic, V., Kivipelto, M., and Winblad, B. (2006). Clinical trials in mild cognitive impairment: lessons for the future. *J. Neurol. Neurosurg. Psychiatry* 77: 429–438.

67 Raschetti, R., Albanese, E., Vanacore, N., and Maggini, M. (2007). Cholinesterase inhibitors in mild cognitive impairment: a systematic review of randomised trials. *PLoS Med.* 4: e338.

68 Zahs, K.R. and Ashe, K.H. (2010). 'Too much good news' - are Alzheimer mouse models trying to tell us how to prevent, not cure, Alzheimer's disease? *Trends Neurosci.* 33: 381–389.

69 Van Dam, D., Coen, K., and De Deyn, P.P. (2008). Cognitive evaluation of disease-modifying efficacy of donepezil in the APP23 mouse model for Alzheimer's disease. *Psychopharmacology (Berl).* 197 (1): 37–43.

70 Bhattacharya, S., Haertel, C., Maelicke, A., and Montag, D. (2014). Galantamine slows down plaque formation and behavioral decline in the 5XFAD mouse model of Alzheimer's disease. *PLoS One* 21: 9(2).

71 Lilja, A.M., Luo, Y., Yu, Q.S. et al. (2013). Neurotrophic and neuroprotective actions of (-)- and (+)-phenserine, candidate drugs for Alzheimer's disease. *PLoS One* 8: e54887.

72 Martinez-Coria, H., Green, K.N., Billings, L.M. et al. (2010). Memantine improves cognition and reduces Alzheimer's-like neuropathology in transgenic mice. *Am J Pathol* 176: 870–880.

73 Henley, D.B., May, P.C., Dean, R.A., and Siemers, E.R. (2009). Development of semagacestat (LY450139), a functional gamma-secretase inhibitor, for the treatment of Alzheimer's disease. *Expert Opin. Pharmacother.* 10: 1657–1664.

74 Dovey, H.F., John, V., Anderson, J.P. et al. (2001). Functional gamma-secretase inhibitors reduce beta-amyloid peptide levels in brain. *J. Neurochem.* 76: 173–181.

75 Lanz, T.A., Himes, C.S., Pallante, G. et al. (2003). The gamma-secretase inhibitor N-[N-(3,5-difluorophenacetyl)-L-alanyl]-S-phenylglycine t-butyl ester reduces A beta levels in vivo in plasma and cerebrospinal fluid in young (plaque-free) and aged (plaque-bearing) Tg2576 mice. *J. Pharmacol. Exp. Ther.* 305: 864–871.

76 Imbimbo, B.P., Del Giudice, E., Colavito, D. et al. (2007). 1-(3′,4′-Dichloro-2-fluoro[1,1′-biphenyl]-4-yl)-cyclopropanecarboxylic acid (CHF5074), a novel gamma-secretase modulator, reduces brain beta-amyloid pathology in a transgenic mouse model of Alzheimer's disease without causing peripheral toxicity. *J. Pharmacol. Exp. Ther.* 323 (3): 822–830.

77 J1, M.L., Kierstead, M.E., Brown, M.E. et al. (2006). Cyclohexanehexol inhibitors of Abeta aggregation prevent and reverse Alzheimer phenotype in a mouse model. *Nat. Med.* 12: 801–808.

78 F, G., Paquette, J., Morissette, C. et al. (2007). Targeting soluble Abeta peptide with Tramiprosate for the treatment of brain amyloidosis. *Neurobiol. Aging.* 28: 537–547.

79 Adlard, P.A., Cherny, R.A., Finkelstein, D.I. et al. (2008). Rapid restoration of cognition in Alzheimer's transgenic mice with 8-hydroxy quinoline analogs is associated with decreased interstitial Abeta. *Neuron.* 59: 43–55.

80 Fl, B., Fox, M., Friedrich, S. et al. (2012). Sustained levels of antibodies against Abeta in amyloid-rich regions of the CNS following intravenous dosing in human APP transgenic mice. *Exp. Neurol.* 238: 38–43.

81 Imbimbo, B.P., Ottonello, S., Frisardi, V. et al. (2012). Solanezumab for the treatment of mild-to-moderate Alzheimer's disease. *Expert. Rev. Clin. Immunol.* 8: 135–149.

82 La Porte, S.L., Bollini, S.S., Lanz, T.A. et al. (2012). Structural basis of C-terminal beta-amyloid peptide binding by the antibody ponezumab for the treatment of Alzheimer's disease. *J. Mol. Biol.* 421: 525–536.

83 Sudduth, T.L., Greenstein, A., and Wilcock, D.M. (2013). Intracranial injection of Gammagard, a human IVIg, modulates the inflammatory response of the brain and lowers Abeta in APP/PS1 mice along a different time course than anti-Abeta antibodies. *J. Neurosci.* 33: 9684–9692.

84 Leroy, K., Ando, K., Héraud, C. et al. (2010). Lithium treatment arrests the development of neurofibrillary tangles in mutant tau transgenic mice with advanced neurofibrillary pathology. *J Alzheimers Dis.* 19 (2): 705–719.

85 Cummings, J.L., Morstorf, T., and Zhong, K. (2014). Alzheimer's disease drug-development pipeline: few candidates, frequent failures. *Alzheimers Res. Ther.* 6: 37.

86 Chai, C.K. (2007). The genetics of Alzheimer's disease. *Am. J. Alzheimers Dis. Other Demen.* 22: 37–41.

87 Rossor, M.N., Fox, N.C., Freeborough, P.A., and Harvey, R.J. (1996). Clinical features of sporadic and familial Alzheimer's disease. *Neurodegeneration* 5: 393–397.

88 Thyagarajan, T., Totey, S., Danton, M.J., and Kulkarni, A.B. (2003). Genetically altered mouse models: the good, the bad, and the ugly. *Crit. Rev. Oral Biol. Med.* 14: 154–174.

89 Calhoun, M.E., Wiederhold, K.H., Abramowski, D. et al. (1998). Neuron loss in APP transgenic mice. *Nature* 395: 755–756.

90 Dodart, J.C., Mathis, C., Saura, J. et al. (2000). Neuroanatomical abnormalities in behaviorally characterized APP(V717F) transgenic mice. *Neurobiol. Dis.* 7: 71–85.

91 Gonzalez-Lima, F., Berndt, J.D., Valla, J.E. et al. (2001). Reduced corpus callosum, fornix and hippocampus in PDAPP transgenic mouse model of Alzheimer's disease. *Neuroreport* 12: 2375–2379.

92 Valla, J., Schneider, L.E., Gonzalez-Lima, F., and Reiman, E.M. (2006). Nonprogressive transgene-related callosal and hippocampal changes in PDAPP mice. *Neuroreport* 17: 829–832.

93 Redwine, J.M., Kosofsky, B., Jacobs, R.E. et al. (2003). Dentate gyrus volume is reduced before onset of plaque formation in PDAPP mice: a magnetic resonance microscopy and stereologic analysis. *Proc. Natl. Acad. Sci. U.S.A.* 100: 1381–1386.

94 Yamada, T., Sasaki, H., Furuya, H. et al. (1987). Complementary DNA for the mouse homolog of the human amyloid beta protein precursor. *Biochem. Biophys. Res. Commun.* 149: 665–671.

95 Sergeant, N., Bombois, S., Ghestem, A. et al. (2003). Truncated beta-amyloid peptide species in pre-clinical Alzheimer's disease as new targets for the vaccination approach. *J. Neurochem.* 85: 1581–1591.

96 Roher, A.E., Palmer, K.C., Yurewicz, E.C. et al. (1993). Morphological and biochemical analyses of amyloid plaque core proteins purified from Alzheimer disease brain tissue. *J. Neurochem.* 61: 1916–1926.

97 Blanchard, V., Czech, C., Bonici, B. et al. (1997). Immunohistochemical analysis of presenilin 2 expression in the mouse brain: distribution pattern and co-localization with presenilin 1 protein. *Brain Res.* 758: 209–217.

98 Lazarov, O., Morfini, G.A., Pigino, G. et al. (2007). Impairments in fast axonal transport and motor neuron deficits in transgenic mice expressing familial Alzheimer's disease-linked mutant presenilin 1. *J. Neurosci.* 27: 7011–7020.

99 Shukkur, E.A., Shimohata, A., Akagi, T. et al. (2006). Mitochondrial dysfunction and tau hyperphosphorylation in Ts1Cje, a mouse model for down syndrome. *Hum. Mol. Genet.* 15: 2752–2762.

100 Brion, J.P., Tremp, G., and Octave, J.N. (1999). Transgenic expression of the shortest human tau affects its compartmentalization and its phosphorylation as in the pretangle stage of Alzheimer's disease. *Am. J. Pathol.* 154: 255–270.

101 Duff, K. and Suleman, F. (2004). Transgenic mouse models of Alzheimer's disease: how useful have they been for therapeutic development? *Brief Funct. Genomic. Proteomic.* 3: 47–59.

102 Probst, A., Gotz, J., Wiederhold, K.H. et al. (2000). Axonopathy and amyotrophy in mice transgenic for human four-repeat tau protein. *Acta Neuropathol.* 99: 469–481.

103 Ishihara, T., Hong, M., Zhang, B. et al. (1999). Age-dependent emergence and progression of a tauopathy in transgenic mice overexpressing the shortest human tau isoform. *Neuron* 24: 751–762.

104 Tanemura, K., Murayama, M., Akagi, T. et al. (2002). Neurodegeneration with tau accumulation in a transgenic mouse expressing V337M human tau. *J. Neurosci.* 22: 133–141.

105 Spillantini, M.G., Murrell, J.R., Goedert, M. et al. (1998). Mutation in the tau gene in familial multiple system tauopathy with presenile dementia. *Proc. Natl. Acad. Sci. U.S.A.* 95: 7737–7741.

106 Westerman, M.A., Cooper-Blacketer, D., Mariash, A. et al. (2002). The relationship between Abeta and memory in the Tg2576 mouse model of Alzheimer's disease. *J. Neurosci.* 22: 1858–1867.

107 Shineman, D.W., Basi, G.S., Bizon, J.L. et al. (2011). Accelerating drug discovery for Alzheimer's disease: best practices for preclinical animal studies. *Alzheimers Res. Ther.* 3: 28.

108 Vesterinen, H.M., Sena, E.S., ffrench-Constant, C. et al. (2010). Improving the translational hit of experimental treatments in multiple sclerosis. *Mult. Scler.* 16: 1044–1055.

109 van der Worp, H.B., Howells, D.W., Sena, E.S. et al. (2010). Can animal models of disease reliably inform human studies? *PLoS Med.* 7: e1000245.

110 Scott, S., Kranz, J.E., Cole, J. et al. (2008). Design, power, and interpretation of studies in the standard murine model of ALS. *Amyotroph. Lateral Scler.* 9: 4–15.

111 Mungenast, A.E., Siegert, S., and Tsai, L.H. (2016). Modeling Alzheimer's disease with human induced pluripotent stem (iPS) cells. *Mol. Cell. Neurosci.* 73: 13–31.

112 Sullivan, S.E. and Young-Pearse, T.L. (2017). Induced pluripotent stem cells as a discovery tool for Alzheimers disease. *Brain Res.* 1656: 98–106.
113 Anand, K. and Sabbagh, M. (2017). Amyloid imaging: poised for integration into medical practice. *Neurotherapeutics* 14: 54–61.
114 Zhang, S., Smailagic, N., Hyde, C. et al. (2014). (11)C-PiB-PET for the early diagnosis of Alzheimer's disease dementia and other dementias in people with mild cognitive impairment (MCI). *Cochrane Database Syst. Rev.* (7): CD010386. https://doi.org/10.1002/14651858.CD010386.pub2.

11

The Products of Fermentation and Their Effects on Metabolism, Alzheimer's Disease, and Other Neurodegenerative Diseases: Role of Short-Chain Fatty Acids (SCFA)

W.M.A.D Binosha Fernando[1,2], *Charles S. Brennan*[3,4,5,6] *and Ralph N. Martins*[1,2,7,8,9]

[1] *Centre of Excellence for Alzheimer's Disease Research and Care, School of Medical and Health Sciences, Edith Cowan University, Joondalup, WA, Australia*
[2] *Australian Alzheimer's Research Foundation, Ralph and Patricia Sarich Neuroscience Research Institute, Nedlands, WA, Australia*
[3] *Department of Wine, Food and Molecular Biosciences, Lincoln University, Lincoln, New Zealand*
[4] *School of Food Science, South China University of Technology, Guangzhou, China*
[5] *Riddet Institute, Palmerston North, New Zealand*
[6] *School of Food Science, Tianjin University of Commerce, Tianjin, China*
[7] *Department of Biomedical Sciences, Macquarie University, Sydney, NSW, Australia*
[8] *School of Psychiatry and Clinical Neurosciences, University of Western Australia, Perth,, WA, Australia*
[9] *KaRa Institute of Neurological Diseases, Sydney, NSW, Australia*

11.1 Introduction

Fermentation is a process whereby anaerobic bacteria break down carbohydrate and protein to obtain energy for their growth and for the maintenance of cellular functions. This is also an important process which occurs as part of our digestion in the large bowel and is indispensable for the healthy functioning of the gut as well as other tissues such as the brain. It also helps reduce the risk of a number of chronic diseases including heart disease, certain cancers, and diabetes. The major end-products of fermentation are short-chain fatty acids (SCFA), found in the highest concentration in colonic contents and in portal blood.

The importance of fermentation in the human digestive process lies primarily in the end-products and their influence on the human body. SCFA are different from medium chain (6–12 carbons) and long-chain free fatty acids, due to their shorter hydrophobic chains attached to the hydrophilic carboxyl group. SCFA are rapidly absorbed, principally from the large bowel, and passed to the portal vein and then to the liver. SCFA have a direct impact on colonic epithelial cells as they are a major energy source, and they also act as tumour suppressor agents and as modulators of the enteric neuroendocrine system. More recently, neuroprotective properties of SCFA have been discovered and these are receiving considerable attention. For instance, it has been found that SCFA can cross the blood–brain barrier and can influence brain regions through two G protein-coupled receptors (GPCR, also known as GPR): free fatty-acid receptor 2 (FFAR2) and free fatty-acid receptor 3 (FFAR3).

Other products of fermentation include branched-chain fatty acids (from the breakdown of branched-chain amino acids), gases including H_2, CO_2 and ammonia, phenols, and energy. The fate of many of these products is largely unknown.

Neurodegeneration and Alzheimer's Disease: The Role of Diabetes, Genetics, Hormones, and Lifestyle,
First Edition. Edited by Ralph N. Martins, Charles S. Brennan, W.M.A.D. Binosha Fernando,
Margaret A. Brennan and Stephanie J. Fuller.
© 2019 John Wiley & Sons Ltd. Published 2019 by John Wiley & Sons Ltd.

Fermentation is vital in human metabolism, and the regulation of fermentation is mainly through bacteria. This is because the enzymes required to ferment substrates such as dietary fibre and undigested proteins are lacking in humans, yet are present in bacteria. Although we humans cannot control fermentation to a great extent, we can clearly control our diet, which is the substrate source for the colonic flora.

SCFA exert beneficial effects on many aspects of health and metabolism such as body weight, food intake, glucose homeostasis, and insulin sensitivity; SCFA also reduce the risk of inflammatory bowel disease, cardiovascular disease, colon cancer, obesity, and diabetes, which are all known metabolic risk factors of neurodegenerative diseases [1]. This chapter will discuss the influence of SCFA on energy metabolism and the immune system, as well as on metabolic and neurogenerative diseases.

11.2 Fermentable Substrates and Short-Chain Fatty Acids

SCFA, which have a 2–6 carbon chain length, are the major metabolic end-products of the fermentation of dietary carbohydrates- mainly polysaccharides, resistant starches and dietary fibre- by the anaerobic intestinal microbiota. Oligosaccharides, proteins, glycoprotein precursors, unabsorbed sugars, raffinose, stachyose, polydextrose and modified cellulose are also all considered as fermentable substrates in the colon [2]. Fermentable carbohydrates pass the upper gastrointestinal (GI) tract unaffected and are fermented in the caecum and the large intestine by the anaerobic caecal and colonic microbiota, resulting in multiple groups of metabolites, in which SCFA are the major products [2]. Among the substrates, soluble fibres such as pectins, gums, mucilages, and some hemicelluloses are easily fermented by colonic microflora. However, 5–20% of dietary-resistant starch which are insoluble fibres such as lignins, cellulose, and some hemicelluloses are not fermented in the human colon. Although insoluble fibres are resistant to fermentation by colonic microflora, they are nevertheless important in faecal bulking (Figure 11.1).

The three major SCFA produced by fermentation include acetate (two carbons), propionate (three carbons), and butyrate (four carbons). Experimental data show that SCFA production is in the order of acetate > propionate > butyrate in a molar ratio of approximately 3 : 1 : 1, respectively, in the proximal and distal colon [2]. Concentrations of SCFA are approximately 13 mM in the terminal ileum, ~130 mM in the caecum, and ~80 mM in the descending colon [2]. SCFA are readily absorbed and used as energy sources by colonocytes, liver, and muscle (5–10% of human colonocytes' basal energy requirements are provided by SCFA) [2]. Although most of the SCFA are absorbed in the colon, 10–20% are excreted in the faeces. The rate, extent, and molar ratio of products formed are dependent upon the nature of the substrate, the gut microbiota, source, and gut transit time. For example, Bridges et al. identified that an intake of oat bran increased 14-hour mean serum acetate concentrations by 45%, compared with wheat bran [3].

Substrate $\longrightarrow$ **SCFA** + H_2O + CO_2 + NH_3 (ammonia) + energy
Anaerobic fermentation

Figure 11.1 Fermentation in a simple format.

11.2.1 Colonic Microflora and Fermentation

The human gut is inhabited by a vast number of bacteria: archaea, viruses, and unicellular eukaryotes [4, 5], altogether as many as 10^{14} bacterial cells [6, 7]. Most of the bacteria in the human gut are anaerobic bacteria, dominated by facultative bacteria (bacteria that make adenosine triphosphate (ATP) by aerobic respiration if oxygen is present, and fermentation when oxygen is absent) [8]. The most common types are Bacteroidetes, Bifidobacterium, Eubacterium, Fusobacterium, Clostridium, Lactobacillus, and Enterococcus. The intestinal flora retrieves energy through fermentation of substrates, mainly carbohydrates, not digested in the upper gut. Colonic bacteria use hydrolysing enzymes in the human gut to digest substrates which have not (or cannot) be digested by humans, to generate hydrogen, methane, carbon dioxide, SCFA, and lactate.

11.2.1.1 Probiotics and Prebiotics

Probiotics are defined as 'live microorganisms administered in adequate amounts to confer a beneficial health effect on the host' [9], and they produce significant quantities of SCFA following fermentation of dietary fibre. The most commonly used probiotics are the lactic acid bacteria (Lactobacillus sp., Bifidobacterium sp., Enterococcus sp., and Streptococcus sp.). The oral administration of probiotic therapies may be helpful in diseases both inside and outside the gastrointestinal (GI) tract, as shown in Table 11.1. The effects of probiotics include the upregulation of immunoglobulins such as IgA, the downregulation of inflammatory cytokines, and the enhancement of gut-barrier function, all of which are believed to be important for slowing down the progression of neurodegenerative diseases. Currently, probiotics are mainly consumed as fermented dairy products such as yoghurt or freeze-dried cultures.

Dietary components that stimulate selectively the growth and activity of specific species of bacteria in the gut, usually bifidobacteria and lactobacilli, with benefits to health, are known as prebiotics. SCFA formation varies with different prebiotics, as shown in Figure 11.2, and Tables 11.2 and 11.3.

Table 11.1 Functions of probiotic bacteria.

Increase	Decrease
Allergen-specific IgG	Bacterial translocation
Mucosal IgA	
Epithelial barrier	
Tight junction protein expression	Th2 cytokines IL-4, IL-5, IL-13
Pathogen exclusion/killing	
Bacteriocin production	Adherence to epithelia, mucus
SCFA	
Anti-inflammatory	Inflammatory infiltrate
Regulatory T-cell (Treg) numbers and function, IL 10, TGF-β	
Th1 cytokines	

Th1/2 cytokines (cytokines released by T-helper cells), IL (interleukin), TGF-β (transforming growth factor-β).
Source: Toh et al. [10].

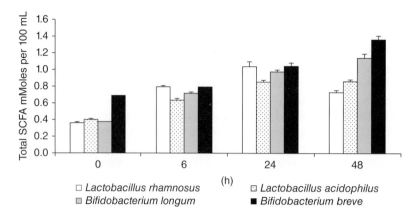

Figure 11.2 Total SCFA formation during the fermentation of two different varieties of rice over 48 hours using four different probiotic micro-organisms. Results are expressed as the mean value of two trials ± SE. Source: Fernando et al. [11].

Table 11.2 SCFA produced by a mixed population of human faecal bacteria after 48 h growth on different polysaccharide substrates in mMoles per 100 ml.

Polysaccharide	Acetate	Propionate	Butyrate	Total
Starch	0.25 (50)	0.13 (22)	0.21 (29)	0.59
Arabinogalactan	0.19 (50)	0.20 (42)	0.04 (8)	0.43
Xylan	0.42 (82)	0.10 (15)	0.02 (3)	0.54
Pectin	0.27 (84)	0.06 (14)	0.01 (2)	0.35

Bacteria were grown anaerobically in batch culture at 37 °C. Values in parentheses are molar ratios of SCFA.
Source: Englyst et al. [12].

Table 11.3 Molar ratios of major fermentation products from various carbohydrates.

Substrate	Acetate	Propionate	Butyrate
Starch	62	15	23
Arabinogalactan	50	42	8
Guar	58	29	13
Pectin	84	14	2
Gum arabic	66	25	8
Oatbran	57	21	22

Source: Cummings [13].

11.2.2 Propionic Acid (PPA)

Propionic acid (PPA), a weak organic acid, which exists in ionised (propionate) and non-ionised forms, is the main metabolic product of ruminant cellulose digestion. This is considered as a sex pheromone, and is involved in lactation. It is commonly used as a preservative in many processed foods and it is also found naturally in refined wheat and dairy products. In humans, PPA is mainly found in the human gut, and this is then principally metabolised in the liver. If there are genetic and/or acquired aberrations in metabolism, higher than normal levels of PPA can sometimes be detected in the circulation. Importantly, it has been shown that PPA and other SCFA can cross lipid membranes including gut–blood and blood–brain barrier membranes, both passively and/or actively via high–affinity transporters. For example, PPA and related SCFA use monocarboxylate receptors in the gut lumen and cerebrovascular endothelium, as well as in neurons and glia, to supply energy for brain metabolism, particularly during early brain development [14–17]. Such aspects of PPA metabolism are important because several lines of evidence point towards PPA contributing to the behavioural, neuropathological, and biochemical abnormalities observed in neurodegenerative diseases.

11.2.3 Acetic Acid

Acetic acid, more commonly found as acetate, is the most abundant SCFA in the colon and a key metabolic substrate; it is mainly metabolised in the liver. Acetic acid is usually absorbed by tissues and converted to acetyl-CoA; this acetyl-CoA can then react with oxaloacetate to form citrate, which in turn can undergo metabolism via the Krebs (citric acid) cycle. Acetate is pivotal in the synthesis of the short- and medium-length fatty acids in the mammary gland, and acetate is also the main precursor in the synthesis of body fat in ruminants. However, unlike longer-chain carboxylic acids, acetic acid does not occur in natural triglycerides. In human studies, since acetate is the main SCFA in the blood, it is often tested to help diagnose colonic events. At physiological pH, acetic acid is usually fully ionised to acetate [18–20].

11.2.4 Butyric Acid

Butyric acid is known to be the preferred fuel source of the colonocytes, explaining to some extent how butyric acid contributes to the maintenance of intestinal health. Butyric acid also plays an important role in balancing electrolyte levels in the body via enhancing transportation of sodium chloride and water from the lumen into the blood stream. Moreover, butyric acid is an important regulator of colonocyte proliferation and apoptosis, and it is a major energy source for colonocytes. Butyric acid/butyrate is also involved in gastrointestinal tract motility and bacterial microflora composition, immune regulation, and anti-inflammatory activity [21, 22]. Clostridium spp., Eubacterium spp., Fusobacterium spp., Butyrivibrio spp., Megasphaera elsdenii, Mitsuokella multiacida, Roseburia intestinalis, Faecalibacterium prausnitzii, and Eubacterium hallii are the most common species that produce butyrate in the human gut [23]. However, western diets, which often include a high intake of highly processed, low-fibre food products rich in simple sugars, can result in low (unhealthy) concentrations of butyrate in the intestinal lumen [21].

11.2.5 Short-Chain Fatty Acids and Free Fatty-Acid Receptor Signalling

Obesity and type 2 diabetes (T2D) are two major risk factors for neurodegenerative diseases, especially Alzheimer's disease (AD). T2D is a metabolic syndrome that involves insulin resistance, inflammation, and pancreatic beta-cell toxicity, as well as aberrations in glucose homeostasis, lipid metabolism, and mitochondrial function. Although dysfunctional insulin signalling is the main cause of T2D, many other metabolic activities are impaired due to poor cellular response. However, research indicates most of the impaired cellular functions can be restored by activation of GPCR ([24]. GPCR, membrane-bound proteins, are members of a large family that share common structural motifs, and are important signalling molecules for many aspects of cellular function [25]. They are targets for a diverse range of hormones, neurotransmitters, environmental cues (light and odours), and drugs. Interestingly, several recent studies have observed that unbound free fatty acids including SCFA activate GPCR such as GPR40, GPR41, GPR43, GPR84, and GPR120 [25]. Among the SCFA-activated GPCR, certain SCFA activate specifically GPR41 (also known as FFAR3) and GPR43 (FFAR2) [26, 27]. The most effective activators for FFAR2 are acetate and propionate, whereas FFAR3 is mostly activated by propionate and butyrate.

GPCR play a major role in neurotransmitter systems in the brain that are disrupted in AD [28]. GPCR also modulate α-, β-, and γ-secretases, thus are involved in the proteolysis of the amyloid-β precursor protein (APP), which leads to the production of the AD-related amyloid-β (Aβ) peptide, the major constituent of AD plaques. GPCR can also regulate Aβ degradation: binding to the GPCR-somatostatin receptor increases the expression of Aβ-degrading enzymes such as neprilysin in the brain, thus enhancing Aβ degradation in the brain [28]. Such research suggests that the combination of memory enhancement, neuroprotection, and anti-Aβ activity of GPCR could be used as a therapeutic target for AD [28]. Other research evidence indicates SCFA can also influence the expression of the GPCRs, FFAR2 and FFAR3 in the colon, small intestine, tissues, and organs beyond the gut [29, 30]. For instance, FFAR2 mRNA has been observed to increase in immune cells, skeletal muscle, heart, spleen, and adipose tissue [27], and FFAR3 mRNA levels increase in adipose tissue, peripheral blood mononuclear cells, pancreas, spleen, bone marrow, and lymph nodes, as a result of stimulation by SCFA [26]. A recent study has also detected FFAR3 expression in postganglionic sympathetic and sensory neurons in both the autonomic and somatic peripheral nervous system [31], suggesting that SCFA can influence the entero-endocrine system as well as influence communication between the gastro-intestinal tract and the peripheral nervous system.

11.2.6 Short-Chain Fatty Acids and Energy Intake

Many studies indicate strong links between obesity and brain atrophy, white matter changes, disturbances in blood–brain barrier integrity, and an increased risk of late-onset dementia and AD. Thus, the maintenance of healthy energy homeostasis would be highly desirable, not only to avoid a variety of metabolic disorders, but also AD (Figure 11.3).

A large number of studies indicate that a diet with a high proportion of vegetables, fruit, whole grains, and seeds (and low in saturated fat), which would therefore be rich in dietary fibre, can help considerably in the fight against obesity. Diets rich

Figure 11.3 Beneficial effects of colonic SCFA production on appetite regulation and energy homeostasis.

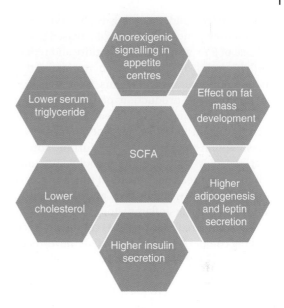

in fibre increase the formation of SCFA in the gut and the evidence suggests that propionate may lead to this partly by causing a reduction in food intake. Interestingly however, butyrate and acetate can protect against diet-induced obesity without causing hypophagia (lower feeding behaviour and food intake) [32, 33]. However, the underlying mechanisms accountable for decreasing food intake and body-weight normalisation are still unclear. It has been proposed that SCFA may regulate gut hormones via their endogenous receptors FFAR2 and FFAR3, but the current evidence is incomplete and sometimes contradictory [34]. For example, some experiments investigating FFAR3 KO(knockout) mice found the KO mice to be leaner than control mice, and suggested that FFAR3 inhibition might result in decreased extraction of energy from the diet and thus lower weight gain [35, 36], whereas more recent studies of SCFA activating these receptors suggest the opposite [37] (for a review see Spreckley and Murphy). The main hormones that are stimulated by SCFA are anorectic gut hormones such as glucagon-like peptide-1 (GLP-1) and peptide YY (PYY). Among the SCFA, butyrate and propionate have been found to be more effective in stimulating the hormones than acetate: evidence from studies of FFAR2 and FFAR3 showed that release of GLP-1 and PYY is due to the presence of SCFA, either butyrate or propionate, in the colon [36, 38, 39]. Conversely, more recent work by Lin et al. using FFAR3 knockout mice showed that FFAR3 is pivotal for maximal GLP-1 induction by butyrate; however, they also found that FFAR3 is not required for butyrate- and propionate-dependent effects on body weight, or for the butyrate- and propionate-induced stimulation of glucose-dependent insulinotropic polypeptide (GIP) [33]. Other recent studies by Psichas et al. indicate that propionate can stimulate the secretion of both GLP-1 and PYY, via FFAR2 [40]. A study of mice using positron-emission tomography-computed tomography scanning noted that 3% of ^{11}C-acetate tracer could be transported to the brain by crossing the blood–brain barrier and it indicated that acetate itself could be considered as an anorectic signal [38, 41, 42], which had not been reported previously. However, the role of FFAR3 in mediating these effects remains controversial [39, 43].

The current understanding is that the release of GLP-1 leads to the secretion of insulin from pancreatic β-cells, decreased gastric emptying, and increased satiation; the release of PYY also slows GI motility and reduces food intake. As GLP-1 and PYY have both been shown to influence energy intake, they have been given serious consideration as potential therapeutic agents for reducing obesity [37, 41, 44, 45]. Altering diets to increase the production of GLP-1 and PYY have already been attempted. For example, replacing fat in a meal with inulin (a natural carbohydrate) or lupin-kernel fibre results in lower fat and energy intake, a greater level of satiety, and lower food consumption the next day [46]; furthermore, eating a meal of Swedish brown beans that provides ≤35 g starchy carbohydrate, and comparing to an equivalent meal of white wheat bread [47] results in lower energy intake the next day, appetite suppression with significantly higher PYY and lower ghrelin (hunger hormone), and significantly lower levels of the inflammatory markers interleukin (IL-6) and IL-18. However, such studies compare foods that also contain different levels of proteins and other nutrients, making comparisons a little difficult; nevertheless, test subjects are often shown to have significantly higher levels of SCFA following the test meals compared to the control meals. Similarly, results from long-term investigations propose that supplementation with oligofructose (16–30 g d^{-1}) [48, 49] and wheat fibre [50] significantly increases feelings of satiety, reduces feelings of hunger, reduces energy intake, increases PYY production, and reduces ghrelin levels, at the same time as increasing production of SCFA. However, authors are not in agreement concerning the time period required for gut microbiota to adapt to the extra fermentable content of the diet introduced in all the experiments, and to produce high quantities of SCFA [51].

Another group [38] reported that acetate could increase oxygen consumption, while butyric acid and propionate could enhance cold-induced adaptive thermogenesis and increase heart rate, respectively, to reduce weight [21, 22]. SCFA have also been reported to regulate leptin secretion from the adipose tissue: propionate and butyrate have been shown to increase the expression of the leptin gene in adipose tissue, and oral administration of propionate increases circulating levels of leptin in mice [43]. It should be remembered that leptin, an anorectic hormone, is an adipose-derived hormone that regulates a wide variety of physiological processes, including feeding behaviour, metabolic rate, sympathetic nerve activity, reproduction, and immune responses.

Other studies have suggested that the transfer of gut microbiota alone may influence body weight and adiposity, the theory being that the transfer of gut microbiota will change the levels of SCFA in the colon, and that SCFA may inhibit fat accumulation. Ridaura et al. identified that co-housing mice harbouring an obese twin's microbiota with mice containing the lean co-twin's microbiota could prevent the development of increased body mass and obesity-associated metabolic phenotypes in obese mice [52, 53]. Furthermore, Liou et al. observed that transfer of the gut microbiota from RYGB-treated (Roux-en-Y gastric bypass mice) to un-operated, germ-free mice could result in weight loss and decreased fat mass in the recipient animals relative to recipients of microbiota induced by sham surgery, potentially due to altered microbiota producing an increased level of SCFA [54]. Similar studies also noticed low levels of acetate and higher levels of propionate being formed in the colon, changes thought to be important in decreasing lipogenesis [55]. These studies also found that the changes in microbiota induced some alterations in the epigenetic regulation of genes such as the FFAR3 gene. Due to studies such as these, which have shown that changes in the colon microbial composition appear to be capable of influencing appetite regulation and energy homeostasis [56], dietary interventions influencing gut microbial composition are being considered as an option in the prevention of metabolic syndrome in humans.

However, although research indicates that obesity and metabolic disorders are associated with SCFA, the mechanism(s) by which SCFA influence metabolism are still not well understood. Although, SCFA have been shown to alter gut-hormone secretion in animal studies, clinical evidence of this effect is inadequate, and the downstream signalling pathways are still being defined. There is no doubt that future studies to determine the SCFA signalling mechanisms and their influence on metabolism and obesity will aid the development of novel therapies for T2D and obesity.

11.2.7 Short-Chain Fatty Acids and Energy Expenditure

Not only have higher levels of SCFA been linked to a reduction in energy intake, as described above, there is also evidence (for example from rodent studies) that SCFA may increase energy expenditure via increasing the rates of oxygen consumption, enhancing both adaptive thermogenesis and fat oxidation and increasing mitochondrial function [57]. For example, Marsman and McBurney reported a disparity in substrate oxidation and product formation in rats fed an elemental diet, when compared with rats fed an elemental diet supplemented with 30% mixed dietary fibre for 14 days [58]. The study reported higher levels of SCFA and glucose oxidation rates in colonocytes when compared to enterocytes, whereas there was greater glutamate formation in enterocytes, when compared to colonocytes. This study also observed that dietary fibre consumption, which enhanced the formation of SCFA, increased substrate oxidation by isolated colonocytes, but not distal small intestinal enterocytes. However, it was unclear whether the higher oxidation was due to the higher luminal SCFA supply, or was due to cellular changes associated with increased colonocyte proliferation. Thus, more studies are needed to understand the underlying mechanism. In other studies, Gao et al. [38] found that butyrate added to a mouse high-fat diet (5% wt/wt) can avert and treat the high-fat-diet-induced insulin resistance, and that the potential mechanism of action caused by the butyrate was associated with higher energy expenditure and enhanced mitochondrial function. This study also found that a diet enriched with whole grains resulted in a decrease in urinary excretion of markers of protein catabolism, tricarboxylic acid (TCA) cycle intermediates, which positively correlated with SCFA formation. The whole-grain diet appeared to influence a variety of metabolic pathways involved in protein and lipid metabolism. The authors also suggested that the lower excretion of TCA-cycle intermediates indicates a reduction in energy flux through the TCA cycle from glycolysis, supported by the observations of lower concentrations of pyruvate, which indicates lower conversion of pyruvate to acetyl-CoA [38].

Other studies indicate that FFAR2 and FFAR3 may be important in energy expenditure and homeostasis in other ways. For example, FFAR3 KO mice show reduced energy expenditure, compared with wild-type (WT) mice [59], and FFAR2 KO mice show a lower energy expenditure when fed a high-fat diet, compared with WT mice. In contrast, mice with adipose-specific over-expression of FFAR2 exhibit an increase in energy expenditure [60]. The authors propose that FFAR2 may be increasing the energy expenditure and the oxidation of fat via the suppression of fat accumulation, following lower adipose tissue insulin signalling.

To balance energy intake, dietary excess and starvation trigger an increase or a decrease in energy usage, respectively, by regulating the function of the sympathetic nervous system. In other mouse studies [56, 57], higher intakes of propionate have resulted in higher rates of oxygen consumption. It was hypothesised that the propionate binds to FFAR3 in the periportal afferent system, which then induces intestinal gluconeogenesis (IGN) via a gut–brain neural circuit, to gain higher oxygen utilisation [56]. This is discussed in greater detail in the section on SCFA and glucose regulation.

Other animal studies have shown that SCFA can be a useful energy source for protein production. When pigs were fed a diet which provided less than their daily energy requirements with low levels of protein, yet with high quantities of fibre, the pigs were found to gain protein. It was suggested that this may be due to better retention of nitrogen after the consumption of SCFA [61].

11.2.8 Regulation of Fatty-Acid Metabolism by SCFA

It has been found that SCFA play a role in regulating fatty-acid synthesis and fatty-acid oxidation, and can cause a reduction in free fatty acids levels in plasma. The receptors involved again include FFAR2 and FFAR3 (as described above), as well as AMP-activated protein kinase (AMPK). AMPK is known to be a major regulator of energy homeostasis. Its activation positively regulates signalling pathways that replenish cellular ATP levels, including fatty-acid oxidation and autophagy. AMPK can also negatively regulate ATP-consuming biosynthetic processes such as gluconeogenesis, and lipid and protein synthesis. The role of AMPK in this SCFA-linked regulation is believed to involve triggering the expression of peroxisome proliferator activated receptor gamma co-activator (PGC)-1α, which controls the transcriptional activity of several transcription factors such as peroxisome proliferator activated receptor (PPAR)α, PPARδ, PPARγ, liver X receptor (LXR), and farnesoid X receptor (FXR) [38, 62]. These receptors are of key importance in the regulation of cholesterol, lipid, and glucose metabolism [63], which in turn means they can have significant effects on metabolic risk factors for AD.

AMPK also exerts influence through direct phosphorylation of enzymes, and there is evidence that increasing the levels of SCFA produced in the colon enhances the activity of AMPK, thus the oxidation of fatty acids in tissues as well as in liver. SCFA also contribute to increased expression of PGC-1α protein, and uncoupling protein from (UCP)-1 in brown adipose tissues, thereby enhancing thermogenesis and fatty-acid oxidation. Though the mechanism involved in SCFA activating AMPK is still unclear, *in vitro* studies suggest that SCFA either affects the AMP/ATP ratio directly and/or influences AMPK indirectly via the FFAR2/FFAR3 receptors, influencing lipid metabolism for example via the FFAR2-leptin pathway. In support of this, a recent mouse study showed that SCFA induced a PPARγ-dependent switch from lipid synthesis to utilisation; this caused an increase in the expression of mitochondrial UCP 2 and raised the AMP/ATP ratio, thereby stimulating oxidative metabolism in liver and adipose tissue via AMPK [64–66].

11.2.9 Effect of Short-Chain Fatty Acids on Glucose Regulation

As SCFA influence so many aspects of energy metabolism, it is not surprising that FFAR2, AMPK, and the gut hormones PYY and GLP-1 are believed to play an important role in the regulation of glucose metabolism. Some studies have reported that propionate can increase blood glucose concentration in humans in a dose-dependent manner [67–69]. Another study showed that the oral administration of acetate and propionate can reduce glycaemia in diabetic hyperglycaemic KK-A(y) mice as well as in normal rats [70]. The authors suggested that the mechanism may involve AMPK decreasing gene expression of the gluconeogenic enzymes, glucose 6-phosphatase (G6Pase), and phosphoenolpyruvate carboxykinase (PEPCK) [70], thus reducing glycaemia in diabetics. More recent studies have shown that IGN, which was discovered in studies of diabetes [71], can be influenced by butyrate and propionate. Delaere et al. [72] demonstrated that propionate acts as a substrate for IGN, it is also an agonist of FFAR3 in the periportal afferent neural system to induce IGN via a gut–brain neural circuit [73]. Butyrate on the other hand triggers the expression of genes required for IGN in enterocytes through an increase in cAMP (not via FFAR2), and further studies have revealed that these functions of SCFA are important in lowering weight gain, reducing adiposity, improving glucose control, and reducing hepatic glucose production [73].

This last study also investigated the gut–brain communication, and revealed the importance of propionate in this process. Firstly, propionate was shown to be necessary for the activation of FFAR3, which itself was found to be localised in the nerve fibres of the portal vein. It was then shown (via measurement of c-fos induction) that the propionate was responsible for activation of regions of the central nervous system (CNS) implicated in signalling from the portal area – the dorsal vagal complex, which receives inputs from the vagal pathway, the C1 segment of the spinal cord and the parabrachial nucleus, which receive inputs from the spinal pathway, and the hypothalamus [73].

We mentioned earlier that SCFA increase levels of the gut hormones PYY and GLP-1 [74], and this is also likely to influence plasma glucose levels. GLP-1 increases the secretion of insulin and decreases the secretion of glucagon by the pancreas. This was demonstrated in mice lacking FFAR2 or FFAR3, which exhibited reduced SCFA triggered GLP-1 secretion, along with impairment of glucose tolerance [74].

11.2.10 Regulation of Cholesterol Metabolism by Short-Chain Fatty Acids

Cholesterol is required in the body for the formation of cell membranes as well as hormone production; however, it is also well known that an excess of cholesterol, particularly cholesterol attached to low-density lipoproteins (LDL), can lead to dyslipidemia and atherosclerosis, and increases the risk of cardiovascular disease and ischaemic stroke. On the other hand, cholesterol in high-density lipoprotein (HDL), or lowering the LDL/HDL ratio, are considered beneficial, as HDL reduces the risk of cardiovascular disease, since it carries cholesterol away from the blood stream. As mentioned earlier, dyslipidemia and cardiovascular disease are considered major risk factors for AD.

Cholesterol is obtained from the diet, and is absorbed from the intestine with the help of bile salts. Alternatively it is synthesised from its precursor unit, acetyl-CoA, via a complex metabolic pathway in which 3-hydroxy-3-methylglutaryl-CoA reductase (HMGCR) behaves as the rate-limiting enzyme.

SCFA have been shown to influence cholesterol synthesis, as *in vitro* and *in vivo* studies have demonstrated that propionate can lower the cholesterol synthesis rate by decreasing the enzyme activity of hepatic 3-hydroxy-3-methylglutaryl-CoA synthase

(HMGCS) as well as HMGCR [75]. Fushimi et al. [76] showed that rats receiving a diet containing 1% (w/w) cholesterol with 0.3% (w/w) of acetate had lower plasma cholesterol levels compared to those fed cholesterol without the acetate, and they also had higher HMGCoA levels and sterol regulatory element binding protein-1 mRNA in the liver. Interestingly, the addition of 15–30 ml d^{-1} vinegar (which contains acetate) to the diet, has been shown to reduce body weight and serum triglyceride levels in obese Japanese subjects [77]. Several authors have suggested that the cholesterol-lowering effect of SCFA is mediated mainly through the activation of AMPK by SCFA [77, 78].

However, unlike the above studies, most studies indicate that acetate also acts as a substrate for cholesterol and lipid synthesis, thus is more obesogenic than the other SCFA. Propionate has been shown to decrease cholesterol synthesis by inhibiting the activity of the enzyme acetyl-CoA synthetase (converts acetate to acetyl-CoA, an early step in cholesterol synthesis), thereby antagonising the cholesterol-increasing action of acetate, and, as mentioned previously, propionate (as well as butyrate) also stimulates the production of leptin, the anorectic hormone produced in adipose tissue. Animal studies have found that feeding animals acetate causes higher serum cholesterol levels, yet when acetate and propionate are administered together, serum cholesterol does not rise. This is thought to be due to increased gluconeogenesis caused by propionate – the gluconeogenesis consumes more fatty acids and thus diverts them from being available for synthesis of cholesterol [79].

11.2.11 Regulation of Inflammation by Short-Chain Fatty Acids

Brain inflammation is a pathological hallmark of AD. Microglia, astrocytes, and neurons are all involved in the inflammatory reaction in the brain. Once activated, these cells produce inflammatory mediators such as pro-inflammatory cytokines, chemokines, macrophage inflammatory proteins, monocyte chemo-attractant proteins, prostaglandins, leukotrienes, thromboxanes, coagulation factors, reactive oxygen species (ROS) (and other radicals), nitric oxide, complement factors, proteases, protease inhibitors, pentraxins, and C-reactive protein, with increased expression of proteins and pro-inflammatory cytokines which are barely observed in healthy brains [80] (see Table 11.4).

In the periphery, leucocytes, including lymphocytes, monocytes, granulocytes and neutrophils, are white blood cells which protect the body against foreign particles. Evidence suggests that SCFA regulate inflammation by modifying the direction of circulating leukocytes, specifically neutrophils, to inflammatory sites; for example, *in vitro* studies have shown that SCFA induce chemotaxis of neutrophils by activation of FFAR2 (GPR43) [90]. GPR43/FFAR2 couples to Gi/o and Gq proteins and is expressed in neutrophils and monocytes, as well as cells of the distal ileum, colon, and adipose tissue – all tissues exposed to high concentrations of SCFA. As mentioned previously, FFAR2 activates several intracellular pathways including mitogen-activated protein kinase (MAPK), protein kinase C, and transcriptional factors [91]. SCFA also controls the formation and discharge of chemokines and expression of adhesion molecules in neutrophils. Thus the SCFA activation of FFAR2 and FFAR3 on intestinal epithelial cells leads to MAPK signalling and rapid production of chemokines and cytokines, and such pathways have been shown to mediate protective immunity and regulate tissue inflammation in mice [92].

Table 11.4 Effect of SCFA on the production of inflammatory mediators by isolated cells.

Cell type	Effect observed	Effective fatty acid
Raw 264.7 cells [81]	↓ TNF-α, IL-6, NO, ↑ IL-10	Butyrate
Mononuclear cells of the blood [82]	↓ TNF-α, ↑ PGE$_2$	Butyrate
Monocytes and macrophages [83]	↓ TNF-α	Butyrate
Monocytes [84]	↓ TNF-α, IL-12, IFN-γ,	Butyrate
	↑ IL-10	Butyrate
	↓ MCP-1, IL-10, ↑ PGE$_2$	Acetate, propionate Butyrate
Microglial cells- N9 cells [85]	↑ IL-6, NO	Propionate, butyrate
Rat primary microglia [85]	↓ TNF-α, IL-6, NO	Butyrate
Murine BV2 cell [86]	↓ NO	Butyrate
Mesencephalic, neuron-glia cultures [87]	↓ TNF-α, NO	Butyrate
Kupffer cells [88]	↓ TNF-α, ↑ PGE$_2$	Butyrate

IFN-γ (interferon-γ), IL-6 (interleukin-6), IL-10 (interleukin-10), IL-12 (interleukin-12), MCP (macrophage chemoattractant protein), NO (nitric oxide) PGE$_2$ (prostaglandin E$_2$), TNF-α (tumour necrosis factor-α) (↑) increase and (↓) reduction.
Source: Marco et al. [89].

Cox et al. demonstrated that SCFA can induce PGE2 production, either alone or in synergy with lipopolysaccharides, in human monocytes and peripheral blood monocuclear cells (PBMC); they also identified the inhibitory effect of SCFA on the production of macrophage chemoattractant protein-1 (MCP-1/CCL2) [84]. Butyrate was found to be a more effective inhibitor than propionate or acetate [84], and this study also noted that SCFA, mainly butyrate, could suppress the lipopolysaccharide- and cytokine-stimulated production of pro-inflammatory mediators including TNF-α, IL-6 and NO [84]. However, this 2009 study (and another 2009 study) did not observe all the SCFA-induced changes that have been previously documented, suggesting further work is necessary (Table 11.4) [84, 91]. Furthermore, the effects of SCFA on ROS production by neutrophils remain controversial. Some groups have found that SCFA induce ROS production [91], whereas others have shown inhibition [93]. The discrepancy in the results also indicates more research is necessary to understand the mechanisms better.

In other recent studies, it has been found that SCFA can directly promote T-cell differentiation into T cells (either regulatory or effector) producing IL-17, interferon (IFN-γ), and/or IL10, depending on cytokine milieu. This effect does not require FFAR2 or FFAR3, but depends on histone deacetylase (HDAC; removes the acetyl group from histone proteins on DNA, making the DNA less accessible to transcription factors) inhibitor activity, which eventually leads to regulation of the mTOR pathway. This suggests SCFA, depending on the immunological setting, can help promote either immunity or immune tolerance [94]. Although HDAC involvement in SCFA effects are still not well understood, it is becoming evident that both FFAR and HDAC play important roles in SCFA effects, which now are known to include altering chemotaxis and phagocytosis, inducing ROS, influencing cell proliferation and function, as well as anti-inflammatory, anti-tumorigenic, and antimicrobial effects [95].

11.2.12 Short-Chain Fatty Acids and Neuroprotection

Research indicates that perturbations in histone acetylation are associated with the onset of age-related memory impairment and the pathogenesis of neurodegenerative diseases [96]. The acetylation of histones is regulated by the antagonistic activities of histone acetyltransferases (HAT) and HDAC. The positively charged amine groups on lysines and arginines of histone tails normally bind to the negatively charged phosphates of DNA. When the amines are acetylated, this reduces binding to the DNA. Thus histone acetylation increases the DNA accessible to transcription machinery and enhances gene expression. On the other hand, HDAC activity decreases the likelihood of gene expression by reducing the chromatin structure. Changes to DNA methylation can also influence gene expression, and although many methylation changes have been identified in AD brains as well as in one mouse model, the results of studies have been far from conclusive [97]. Overall, AD has been associated with DNA hyper-methylation and histone deacetylation, suggesting a general repressed chromatin state, with epigenetically dysregulated genes and reduced plasticity in AD. In fact, it has been shown that a mouse model of learning and memory impairment can reduce such impairments by environmental enrichment, which was shown to correlate with increased histone acetylation [96, 97]. Fischer et al. [98] also showed that HDAC inhibitors could have neuroprotective and neuroregenerative effects in the mice, inducing dendrite sprouting and synapse formation. Furthermore, other studies have found that treatment with pan-HDAC inhibitors such as sodium butyrate (SB), trichostatin A (TSA), suberoylanilide hydroxamic acid (SAHA), or sodium phenyl butyrate improves memory function in mouse models for ageing and brain injury. These findings suggest that HDAC inhibitors are potential therapeutic agents for reducing cognitive impairment in AD [98]. However, potential effects of HDAC inhibitors are still not clear, and the majority of epigenetic alterations observed in AD are based on correlations, and do not identify whether the alterations are cause or effect [97, 99]. Furthermore, it has been suggested that every subtype of neuron, or possibly every cell, may have its own specific epigenetics-regulated expression profile, thus considerably complicating analysis.

Nevertheless, studies of midbrain neuron-glia mixed cultures have discovered effects of HDAC activity that may provide therapeutic potential; for example, valproic acid (mood stabiliser, anticonvulsant, and HDAC inhibitor), sodium butyrate, and TSA (both also HDAC inhibitors) increase the expression of brain-derived neurotrophic factor (BDNF) and glial cell line-derived neurotrophic factor (GDNF) in astrocytes, which provide protection for dopaminergic neurons [99, 100]. In a rat-brain ischaemic injury model, sodium butyrate was found to increase the ischaemia-induced neurogenesis via HDAC inhibition, and sodium butyrate also increased the number of cells expressing polysialic acid-neural cell adhesion molecule, nestin, glial fibrillary acidic protein (GFAP), and phospho-cAMP response element-binding protein (CREB). These changes coincided with cognitive improvements in the rat model [101] and activation of BDNF-TrkB signalling appeared crucial for these effects. In other rat studies, sodium butyrate combined with behavioural therapy was found to improve learning and memory in brain-injured mice [102] and stroke studies in mice found sodium butyrate could induce oligodendrogenesis, increase levels of vascular endothelial growth factor (VEGF), reduce inflammation by blocking caspase-3, inhibit microglial activation, and ameliorate ageing-related memory decline in rats [103]; and recent studies of normal-aged rats found that systemic injection of sodium butyrate enhanced memory consolidation which persisted for the 14 days of testing [104]. Such behavioural studies support the concept that the cellular and biochemical changes reported earlier are likely to benefit brain function, and give further evidence of the therapeutic potential of SCFA, particularly butyrate.

Other studies have indicated effects of SCFA on the sympathetic nervous system, for example propionate has been shown to promote sympathetic outflow via FFAR3, whereas the ketone body β-hydroxybutyrate (produced during starvation or diabetes) suppressed sympathetic nervous system activity, leading to the concept that SCFA and ketones exert some control over metabolic homeostasis via FFAR2 [105]. SCFA have been shown to increase firing and norepinephrine release from sympathetic neurons; however, these results have been contradicted in other studies which showed that activation of FFAR3 by SCFA impairs N-type calcium channel activity [106]. It has been suggested that this contradiction is due to the effects being in different ganglia; further studies of SCFA effects on different parts of the nervous system will help to clarify these uncertainties [106].

Other changes in the brain that would influence neuronal health are SCFA-induced changes to microglia in the CNS. Recent studies have shown that host microbiota regulate microglial maturation and function in the CNS, and that this occurs via SCFA [107]. However, it needs to be remembered that many such studies have used germ-free mice, and thus one could argue that the mice may have nutritional deficiencies that may also contribute to such effects; nevertheless, mice deficient for the FFAR2 receptor also had similar microglial defects [107].

Although possibly not directly relevant to neurodegeneration, many studies have demonstrated SCFA and microbiota change during pregnancy, at times which coincide with periods of foetal brain 'growth spurts' [108], such that gut microbiota from the third trimester exhibited a distinct metabolic phenotype capable of promoting greater energy storage compared with first trimester microbiota. Furthermore, studies have shown that after birth the gut microbiota of infants change considerably, and this is also a critical time for brain development. It is thought that perturbations in early-life developing gut microbiota can impact on the CNS and potentially lead to adverse mental health outcomes [109]. The concept that there are critical developmental times for microbial-neural-metabolic interactions implies that there may be opportunities for developing novel microbiota-modulating-based therapeutic interventions for early life stages, to combat or prevent neurodevelopmental deficits and brain disorders [110].

11.3 Conclusions

Our understanding of the roles of SCFA in metabolism has grown rapidly in recent years, as scientists have produced an abundance of information about their mechanisms of action in the last decade. The number of recent reviews is testament to the fact that researchers have had a lot of new data to collate and summarise [56, 79, 111, 112]. SCFA have been shown to exert multiple beneficial effects on various aspects of mammalian metabolism. However, some of the results are still contradictory. This is partly caused by a lack of human study data: many of the conclusions have been obtained from animal work, and may not translate directly to humans. Recent advances have nevertheless indicated that SCFA exert considerable influence on the central and peripheral nervous systems, as well as on immune responses (microglia) in the CNS [113]. SCFA have also been shown to influence aspects of brain function; for example, they improve behavioural symptoms in a subset of people with autism spectrum disorders [114]. Furthermore, animal model studies suggest SCFA can influence anxiety and depression, possibly by disturbing the hypothalamic–pituitary–adrenal axis [115]; however, this research is relatively young, as is the research into the relevance of SCFA biology in AD pathogenesis and neurodegeneration.

Concerning the pathogenesis of AD, SCFA have been shown to influence the regulation of fatty acid, glucose, and cholesterol metabolism. Abnormalities in the metabolism of glucose and lipids are central aspects of insulin resistance, T2D, cardiovascular disease, metabolic syndrome, and hypertension, all of which have been shown to be risk factors for AD. Thus, it would appear that improvements in dietary fibre quantity and quality could help reduce the risk of AD. Also of considerable interest and relevance to AD is the influence of SCFA on the function of leukocytes, for instance in the production of inflammatory mediators and the induction of apoptosis in lymphocytes, macrophages, and neutrophils.

With SCFA displaying multiple effects on different cells involved in the inflammatory and immune responses, a lot more research is required to elucidate the role of SCFA in mammalian energy metabolism as well as in neuroprotection.

References

1 Slavin, J. (2013). Fiber and prebiotics: mechanisms and health benefits. *Nutrients* 5: 1417–1435.
2 Cummings, J.H., Pomare, E.W., Branch, W.J. et al. (1987). Short chain fatty acids in human large intestine, portal, hepatic and venous blood. *Gut* 28: 1221–1227.
3 Bridges, S.R., Anderson, J.W., Deakins, D.A. et al. (1992). Oat bran increases serum acetate of hypercholesterolemic men. *Am. J. Clin. Nutr.* 56: 455–459.
4 Kunz, C., Kuntz, S., and Rudloff, S. (2009). Intestinal flora. *Adv. Exp. Med. Biol.* 639: 67–79.
5 Ley, R.E., Peterson, D.A., and Gordon, J.I. (2006). Ecological and evolutionary forces shaping microbial diversity in the human intestine. *Cell* 124: 837–848.
6 Morelli, L. (2008). Postnatal development of intestinal microflora as influenced by infant nutrition. *J. Nutr.* 138: S1791–S1795.
7 Whitman, W.B., Coleman, D.C., and Wiebe, W.J. (1998). Prokaryotes: the unseen majority. *Proc. Natl. Acad. Sci. U.S.A.* 95: 6578–6583.
8 Harris, M.A., Reddy, C.A., and Carter, G.R. (1976). Anaerobic bacteria from the large intestine of mice. *Appl. Environ. Microbiol.* 31: 907–912.
9 FAO/WHO (2002). *Guidelines for the Evaluation of Probiotics in Food*. Ontario, Canada: Report of a Joint FAO/WHO Working Group on Drafting Guidelines for the Evaluation of Probiotics in Food.

10 Toh, Z.Q., Anzela, A., Tang, M.L., and Licciardi, P.V. (2012). Probiotic therapy as a novel approach for allergic disease. *Front. Pharmacol.* 21 (3): 171. https://doi.org/10.3389/fphar.2012.00171. eCollection 2012.

11 Fernando, W.M.A.D.B., Brennan, C.S., Flint, S. et al. (2010). Enhancement of short chain fatty acid formation by pure cultures of probiotics on rice fibre. *Int. J. Food Sci. Technol.* 45: 690–696.

12 Englyst, H.N., Hay, S., and Macfarlane, G.T. (1987). Polysaccharide breakdown by mixed populations of human faecal bacteria. *FEMS Microbiol. Lett.* 45: 163–171.

13 Cummings, J.H., Rombeau, J.L., and Sakata, T. (1995). *Physiological and Clinical Spects of Short Chain Fatty Acids*. Cambridge: Cambridge University Press.

14 Nakao, S., Moriya, Y., Furuyama, S. et al. (1998). Propionic acid stimulates superoxide generation in human neutrophils. *Cell. Biol. Int.* 22: 331–337.

15 Brock, M. and Buckel, W. (2004). On the mechanism of action of the antifungal agent propionate. *Eur. J. Biochem.* 271: 3227–3241.

16 Tamai, I., Takanaga, H., Maeda, H. et al. (1995). Participation of a proton-cotransporter, MCT1, in the intestinal transport of monocarboxylic acids. *Biochem. Biophys. Res. Commun.* 214: 482–489.

17 Karuri, A.R., Dobrowsky, E., and Tannock, I.F. (1993). Selective cellular acidification and toxicity of weak organic acids in an acidic microenvironment. *Br. J. Cancer* 68: 1080–1087.

18 Sim, J.H., Kamaruddin, A.H., Long, W.S., and Najafpour, G. (2007). Clostridium aceticum – a potential organism in catalyzing carbon monoxide to acetic acid: application of response surface methodology. *Enzyme Microb. Technol.* 40: 1234–1243.

19 Fiume, M.Z. (2003). Final report on the safety assessment of triacetin. *Int. J. Toxicol.* 22 (Suppl 2): 1–10.

20 MacFabe, D.F. (2012). Short-chain fatty acid fermentation products of the gut microbiome: implications in autism spectrum disorders. *Microb. Ecol. Health Dis.* 23: https://doi.org/10.3402/mehd.v3423i3400.19260.

21 Bird, A.R., Conlon, M.A., Christophersen, C.T., and Topping, D.L. (2010). Resistant starch, large bowel fermentation and a broader perspective of prebiotics and probiotics. *Benef. Microbes* 1: 423–431.

22 Roy, C.C., Kien, C.L., Bouthillier, L., and Levy, E. (2006). Short-chain fatty acids: ready for prime time? *Nutr. Clin. Pract.* 21: 351–366.

23 Hold, G.L., Schwiertz, A., Aminov, R.I. et al. (2003). Oligonucleotide probes that detect quantitatively significant groups of butyrate-producing bacteria in human feces. *Appl. Environ. Microbiol.* 69: 4320–4324.

24 Bowden, D.W., Cox, A.J., Freedman, B.I. et al. (2010). Review of the diabetes heart study (DHS) family of studies: a comprehensively examined sample for genetic and epidemiological studies of type 2 diabetes and its complications. *Rev. Diabet. Stud.* 7: 188–201.

25 Oh, D.Y., Talukdar, S., Bae, E.J. et al. (2010). GPR120 is an omega-3 fatty acid receptor mediating potent anti-inflammatory and insulin-sensitizing effects. *Cell* 142: 687–698.

26 Brown, A.J., Goldsworthy, S.M., Barnes, A.A. et al. (2003). The orphan G protein-coupled receptors GPR41 and GPR43 are activated by propionate and other short chain carboxylic acids. *J. Biol. Chem.* 278: 11312–11319.

27 Le Poul, E., Loison, C., Struyf, S. et al. (2003). Functional characterization of human receptors for short chain fatty acids and their role in polymorphonuclear cell activation. *J. Biol. Chem.* 278: 25481–25489.
28 Slack, B.E. and Wurtman, R.J. (2007). Regulation of Synthesis and Metabolism of the Amyloid Precursor Protein by Extracellular Signals. In: *Research Progress in Alzheimer's Disease and Dementia. Hauppauge: Nova Publishers*, vol. 2 (ed. M.-K. Sun), 1–25.
29 Li, G., Su, H., Zhou, Z., and Yao, W. (2014). Identification of the porcine G protein-coupled receptor 41 and 43 genes and their expression pattern in different tissues and development stages. *PLoS One* 9: e97342.
30 Nohr, M.K., Pedersen, M.H., Gille, A. et al. (2013). GPR41/FFAR3 and GPR43/FFAR2 as cosensors for short-chain fatty acids in enteroendocrine cells vs FFAR3 in enteric neurons and FFAR2 in enteric leukocytes. *Endocrinology* 154: 3552–3564.
31 Nohr, M.K., Egerod, K.L., Christiansen, S.H. et al. (2015). Expression of the short chain fatty acid receptor GPR41/FFAR3 in autonomic and somatic sensory ganglia. *Neuroscience* 290: 126–137.
32 Cherbut, C., Ferrier, L., Roze, C. et al. (1998). Short-chain fatty acids modify colonic motility through nerves and polypeptide YY release in the rat. *Am. J. Physiol.* 275: G1415–G1422.
33 Lin, H.V., Frassetto, A., Kowalik, E.J. Jr. et al. (2012). Butyrate and propionate protect against diet-induced obesity and regulate gut hormones via free fatty acid receptor 3-independent mechanisms. *PLoS One* 7: e35240.
34 Eaton, S.B. (2006). The ancestral human diet: what was it and should it be a paradigm for contemporary nutrition? *Proc. Nutr. Soc.* 65: 1–6.
35 Samuel, B.S., Shaito, A., Motoike, T. et al. (2008). Effects of the gut microbiota on host adiposity are modulated by the short-chain fatty-acid binding G protein-coupled receptor, Gpr41. *Proc. Natl. Acad. Sci. U. S. A.* 105: 16767–16772.
36 Kaji, I., Karaki, S., Tanaka, R., and Kuwahara, A. (2011). Density distribution of free fatty acid receptor 2 (FFA2)-expressing and GLP-1-producing enteroendocrine L cells in human and rat lower intestine, and increased cell numbers after ingestion of fructo-oligosaccharide. *J. Mol. Histol.* 42: 27–38.
37 Spreckley, E. and Murphy, K.G. (2015). The L-cell in nutritional sensing and the regulation of appetite. *Front. Nutr.* 2: 23.
38 Gao, Z., Yin, J., Zhang, J. et al. (2009). Butyrate improves insulin sensitivity and increases energy expenditure in mice. *Diabetes* 58: 1509–1517.
39 Hong, Y.H., Nishimura, Y., Hishikawa, D. et al. (2005). Acetate and propionate short chain fatty acids stimulate adipogenesis via GPCR43. *Endocrinology* 146: 5092–5099.
40 Psichas, A., Sleeth, M.L., Murphy, K.G. et al. (2015). The short chain fatty acid propionate stimulates GLP-1 and PYY secretion via free fatty acid receptor 2 in rodents. *Int. J. Obes. (Lond.)* 39: 424–429.
41 Cani, P.D., Neyrinck, A.M., Maton, N., and Delzenne, N.M. (2005). Oligofructose promotes satiety in rats fed a high-fat diet: involvement of glucagon-like peptide-1. *Obes. Res.* 13: 1000–1007.

42 Isken, F., Klaus, S., Osterhoff, M. et al. (2010). Effects of long-term soluble vs. insoluble dietary fiber intake on high-fat diet-induced obesity in C57BL/6J mice. *J. Nutr. Biochem.* 21: 278–284.

43 Xiong, Y., Miyamoto, N., Shibata, K. et al. (2004). Short-chain fatty acids stimulate leptin production in adipocytes through the G protein-coupled receptor GPR41. *Proc. Natl. Acad. Sci. U. S. A.* 101: 1045–1050.

44 Delmee, E., Cani, P.D., Gual, G. et al. (2006). Relation between colonic proglucagon expression and metabolic response to oligofructose in high fat diet-fed mice. *Life Sci.* 79: 1007–1013.

45 Reimer, R.A., Maurer, A.D., Eller, L.K. et al. (2012). Satiety hormone and metabolomic response to an intermittent high energy diet differs in rats consuming long-term diets high in protein or prebiotic fiber. *J. Proteome Res.* 11: 4065–4074.

46 Archer, B.J., Johnson, S.K., Devereux, H.M., and Baxter, A.L. (2004). Effect of fat replacement by inulin or lupin-kernel fibre on sausage patty acceptability, post-meal perceptions of satiety and food intake in men. *Br. J. Nutr.* 91: 591–599.

47 Nilsson, A., Johansson, E., Ekstrom, L., and Bjorck, I. (2013). Effects of a brown beans evening meal on metabolic risk markers and appetite regulating hormones at a subsequent standardized breakfast: a randomized cross-over study. *PLoS One* 8: e59985.

48 Cani, P.D., Joly, E., Horsmans, Y., and Delzenne, N.M. (2006). Oligofructose promotes satiety in healthy human: a pilot study. *Eur. J. Clin. Nutr.* 60: 567–572.

49 Parnell, J.A. and Reimer, R.A. (2009). Weight loss during oligofructose supplementation is associated with decreased ghrelin and increased peptide YY in overweight and obese adults. *Am. J. Clin. Nutr.* 89: 1751–1759.

50 Freeland, K.R., Wilson, C., and Wolever, T.M. (2010). Adaptation of colonic fermentation and glucagon-like peptide-1 secretion with increased wheat fibre intake for 1 year in hyperinsulinaemic human subjects. *Br. J. Nutr.* 103: 82–90.

51 David, L.A., Maurice, C.F., Carmody, R.N. et al. (2014). Diet rapidly and reproducibly alters the human gut microbiome. *Nature* 505: 559–563.

52 Ridaura, V.K., Faith, J.J., Rey, F.E. et al. (2013). Gut microbiota from twins discordant for obesity modulate metabolism in mice. *Science* 341: 1241214.

53 Ridaura, V.K., Faith, J.J., Rey, F.E. et al. (2013). Cultured gut microbiota from twins discordant for obesity modulate adiposity and metabolic phenotypes in mice. *Science (New York, N.Y.)* 341: https://doi.org/10.1126/science.1241214.

54 Liou, A.P., Paziuk, M., Luevano, J.M. Jr. et al. (2013). Conserved shifts in the gut microbiota due to gastric bypass reduce host weight and adiposity. *Sci. Transl. Med.* 5: 178ra141.

55 Remely, M., Aumueller, E., Merold, C. et al. (2014). Effects of short chain fatty acid producing bacteria on epigenetic regulation of FFAR3 in type 2 diabetes and obesity. *Gene* 537: 85–92.

56 Byrne, C.S., Chambers, E.S., Morrison, D.J., and Frost, G. (2015). The role of short chain fatty acids in appetite regulation and energy homeostasis. *Int. J. Obes.* 39: 1331–1338.

57 Kimura, I., Inoue, D., Maeda, T. et al. (2011). Short-chain fatty acids and ketones directly regulate sympathetic nervous system via G protein-coupled receptor 41 (GPR41). *Proc. Natl. Acad. Sci. U. S. A.* 108: 8030–8035.

58 Marsman, K.E. and McBurney, M.I. (1995). Dietary fiber increases oxidative metabolism in colonocytes but not in distal small intestinal enterocytes isolated from rats. *J. Nutr.* 125: 273–282.

59 Bellahcene, M., O'Dowd, J.F., Wargent, E.T. et al. (2013). Male mice that lack the G-protein-coupled receptor GPR41 have low energy expenditure and increased body fat content. *Br. J. Nutr.* 109: 1755–1764.

60 Kimura, I., Ozawa, K., Inoue, D. et al. (2013). The gut microbiota suppresses insulin-mediated fat accumulation via the short-chain fatty acid receptor GPR43. *Nat. Commun.* 4: 1829.

61 Jorgensen, H., Larsen, T., Zhao, X.Q., and Eggum, B.O. (1997). The energy value of short-chain fatty acids infused into the caecum of pigs. *Br. J. Nutr.* 77: 745–756.

62 Lin, J., Handschin, C., and Spiegelman, B.M. (2005). Metabolic control through the PGC-1 family of transcription coactivators. *Cell Metab.* 1: 361–370.

63 Jager, S., Handschin, C., St-Pierre, J., and Spiegelman, B.M. (2007). AMP-activated protein kinase (AMPK) action in skeletal muscle via direct phosphorylation of PGC-1alpha. *Proc. Natl. Acad. Sci. U. S. A.* 104: 12017–12022.

64 Friedman, J.M. and Halaas, J.L. (1998). Leptin and the regulation of body weight in mammals. *Nature* 395: 763–770.

65 Robertson, M.D., Bickerton, A.S., Dennis, A.L. et al. (2005). Insulin-sensitizing effects of dietary resistant starch and effects on skeletal muscle and adipose tissue metabolism. *Am. J. Clin. Nutr.* 82: 559–567.

66 den Besten, G., Bleeker, A., Gerding, A. et al. (2015). Short-chain fatty acids protect against high-fat diet-induced obesity via a PPARgamma-dependent switch from Lipogenesis to fat oxidation. *Diabetes* 64: 2398–2408.

67 Wolever, T.M., Spadafora, P., and Eshuis, H. (1991). Interaction between colonic acetate and propionate in humans. *Am. J. Clin. Nutr.* 53: 681–687.

68 den Besten, G., Lange, K., Havinga, R. et al. (2013). Gut-derived short-chain fatty acids are vividly assimilated into host carbohydrates and lipids. *Am. J. Physiol. Gastrointest. Liver Physiol.* 305: G900–G910.

69 Jin, E.S., Szuszkiewicz-Garcia, M., Browning, J.D. et al. (2014). Influence of liver triglycerides on suppression of glucose production by insulin in men. *J. Clin. Endocrinol. Metab.* 100: 235–243.

70 Sakakibara, S., Yamauchi, T., Oshima, Y. et al. (2006). Acetic acid activates hepatic AMPK and reduces hyperglycemia in diabetic KK-A(y) mice. *Biochem. Biophys. Res. Commun.* 344: 597–604.

71 Croset, M., Rajas, F., Zitoun, C. et al. (2001). Rat small intestine is an insulin-sensitive gluconeogenic organ. *Diabetes* 50: 740–746.

72 Delaere, F., Duchampt, A., Mounien, L. et al. (2013). The role of sodium-coupled glucose co-transporter 3 in the satiety effect of portal glucose sensing. *Mol. Metab.* 2: 47–53.

73 De Vadder, F., Kovatcheva-Datchary, P., Goncalves, D. et al. (2014). Microbiota-generated metabolites promote metabolic benefits via gut-brain neural circuits. *Cell* 156: 84–96.

74 Boey, D., Lin, S., Karl, T. et al. (2006). Peptide YY ablation in mice leads to the development of hyperinsulinaemia and obesity. *Diabetologia* 49: 1360–1370.

75 Rodwell, V.W., Nordstrom, J.L., and Mitschelen, J.J. (1976). Regulation of HMG-CoA reductase. *Adv. Lipid Res.* 14: 1–74.
76 Fushimi, T., Suruga, K., Oshima, Y. et al. (2006). Dietary acetic acid reduces serum cholesterol and triacylglycerols in rats fed a cholesterol-rich diet. *Br. J. Nutr.* 95: 916–924.
77 Kondo, T., Kishi, M., Fushimi, T. et al. (2009). Vinegar intake reduces body weight, body fat mass, and serum triglyceride levels in obese Japanese subjects. *Biosci. Biotechnol. Biochem.* 73: 1837–1843.
78 Zydowo, M.M., Smolenski, R.T., and Swierczynski, J. (1993). Acetate-induced changes of adenine nucleotide levels in rat liver. *Metabolism* 42: 644–648.
79 Chakraborti, C.K. (2015). New-found link between microbiota and obesity. *World J. Gastrointest. Pathophysiol.* 6: 110–119.
80 Tuppo, E.E. and Arias, H.R. (2005). The role of inflammation in Alzheimer's disease. *Int. J. Biochem. Cell Biol.* 37: 289–305.
81 Chakravortty, D., Koide, N., Kato, Y. et al. (2000). The inhibitory action of butyrate on lipopolysaccharide-induced nitric oxide production in RAW 264.7 murine macrophage cells. *J. Endotoxin Res.* 6: 243–247.
82 Usami, M., Kishimoto, K., Ohata, A. et al. (2008). Butyrate and trichostatin a attenuate nuclear factor kappaB activation and tumor necrosis factor alpha secretion and increase prostaglandin E2 secretion in human peripheral blood mononuclear cells. *Nutr. Res.* 28: 321–328.
83 Fukae, J., Amasaki, Y., Yamashita, Y. et al. (2005). Butyrate suppresses tumor necrosis factor alpha production by regulating specific messenger RNA degradation mediated through a cis-acting AU-rich element. *Arthritis Rheum.* 52: 2697–2707.
84 Cox, M.A., Jackson, J., Stanton, M. et al. (2009). Short-chain fatty acids act as anti-inflammatory mediators by regulating prostaglandin E(2) and cytokines. *World J. Gastroenterol.* 15: 5549–5557.
85 Huuskonen, J., Suuronen, T., Nuutinen, T. et al. (2004). Regulation of microglial inflammatory response by sodium butyrate and short-chain fatty acids. *Br. J. Pharmacol.* 141: 874–880.
86 Park, J.S., Woo, M.S., Kim, S.Y. et al. (2005). Repression of interferon-gamma-induced inducible nitric oxide synthase (iNOS) gene expression in microglia by sodium butyrate is mediated through specific inhibition of ERK signaling pathways. *J. Neuroimmunol.* 168: 56–64.
87 Chen, P.S., Wang, C.C., Bortner, C.D. et al. (2007). Valproic acid and other histone deacetylase inhibitors induce microglial apoptosis and attenuate lipopolysaccharide-induced dopaminergic neurotoxicity. *Neuroscience* 149: 203–212.
88 Perez, R., Stevenson, F., Johnson, J. et al. (1998). Sodium butyrate upregulates Kupffer cell PGE2 production and modulates immune function. *J. Surg. Res.* 78: 1–6.
89 Vinolo, M.A.R., Rodrigues, H.G., Nachbar, R.T., and Curi, R. (2011). Regulation of inflammation by short chain fatty acids. *Nutrients* 3: 858–876.
90 Sina, C., Gavrilova, O., Forster, M. et al. (2009). G protein-coupled receptor 43 is essential for neutrophil recruitment during intestinal inflammation. *J. Immunol.* 183: 7514–7522.

91 Maslowski, K.M., Vieira, A.T., Ng, A. et al. (2009). Regulation of inflammatory responses by gut microbiota and chemoattractant receptor GPR43. *Nature* 461: 1282–1286.

92 Kim, M.H., Kang, S.G., Park, J.H. et al. (2013). Short-chain fatty acids activate GPR41 and GPR43 on intestinal epithelial cells to promote inflammatory responses in mice. *Gastroenterology* 145: 396–406. e391–310.

93 Sandoval, A., Trivinos, F., Sanhueza, A. et al. (2007). Propionate induces pH(i) changes through calcium flux, ERK1/2, p38, and PKC in bovine neutrophils. *Vet. Immunol. Immunopathol.* 115: 286–298.

94 Park, J., Kim, M., Kang, S.G. et al. (2015). Short-chain fatty acids induce both effector and regulatory T cells by suppression of histone deacetylases and regulation of the mTOR-S6K pathway. *Mucosal Immunol.* 8: 80–93.

95 Tan, J., McKenzie, C., Potamitis, M. et al. (2014). The role of short-chain fatty acids in health and disease. *Adv. Immunol.* 121: 91–119.

96 Fischer, A., Sananbenesi, F., Wang, X. et al. (2007). Recovery of learning and memory is associated with chromatin remodelling. *Nature* 447: 178–182.

97 Sanchez-Mut, J.V. and Graff, J. (2015). Epigenetic alterations in Alzheimer's disease. *Front. Behav. Neurosci.* 9: 347.

98 Kazantsev, A.G. and Thompson, L.M. (2008). Therapeutic application of histone deacetylase inhibitors for central nervous system disorders. *Nat. Rev. Drug Discov.* 7: 854–868.

99 Levenson, J.M., O'Riordan, K.J., Brown, K.D. et al. (2004). Regulation of histone acetylation during memory formation in the hippocampus. *J. Biol. Chem.* 279: 40545–40559.

100 Wu, X., Chen, P.S., Dallas, S. et al. (2008). Histone deacetylase inhibitors up-regulate astrocyte GDNF and BDNF gene transcription and protect dopaminergic neurons. *Int. J. Neuropsychopharmacol.* 11: 1123–1134.

101 Kim, H.J., Leeds, P., and Chuang, D.M. (2009). The HDAC inhibitor, sodium butyrate, stimulates neurogenesis in the ischemic brain. *J. Neurochem.* 110: 1226–1240.

102 Dash, P.K., Orsi, S.A., and Moore, A.N. (2009). Histone deactylase inhibition combined with behavioral therapy enhances learning and memory following traumatic brain injury. *Neuroscience* 163: 1–8.

103 Kim, H.J. and Chuang, D.M. (2014). HDAC inhibitors mitigate ischemia-induced oligodendrocyte damage: potential roles of oligodendrogenesis, VEGF, and anti-inflammation. *Am. J. Transl. Res.* 6: 206–223.

104 Blank, M., Werenicz, A., Velho, L.A. et al. (2015). Enhancement of memory consolidation by the histone deacetylase inhibitor sodium butyrate in aged rats. *Neurosci. Lett.* 594: 76–81.

105 Inoue, D., Tsujimoto, G., and Kimura, I. (2014). Regulation of energy homeostasis by GPR41. *Front. Endocrinol.* 5.

106 Lopez Soto, E.J., Gambino, L.O., and Mustafa, E.R. (2014). Free fatty acid receptor 3 is a key target of short chain fatty acid. What is the impact on the sympathetic nervous system? *Channels (Austin)* 8: 169–171.

107 Erny, D., de Hrabe, A.A.L., Jaitin, D. et al. (2015). Host microbiota constantly control maturation and function of microglia in the CNS. *Nat. Neurosci.* 18: 965–977.

108 Koren, O., Goodrich, J.K., Cullender, T.C. et al. (2012). Host remodeling of the gut microbiome and metabolic changes during pregnancy. *Cell* 150: 470–480.
109 Clarke, G., O'Mahony, S.M., Dinan, T.G., and Cryan, J.F. (2014). Priming for health: gut microbiota acquired in early life regulates physiology, brain and behaviour. *Acta Paediatr.* 103: 812–819.
110 Borre, Y.E., O'Keeffe, G.W., Clarke, G. et al. (2014). Microbiota and neurodevelopmental windows: implications for brain disorders. *Trends Mol. Med.* 20: 509–518.
111 Neves, A.L., Chilloux, J., Sarafian, M.H. et al. (2015). The microbiome and its pharmacological targets: therapeutic avenues in cardiometabolic diseases. *Curr. Opin. Pharmacol.* 25: 36–44.
112 Canfora, E.E., Jocken, J.W., and Blaak, E.E. (2015). Short-chain fatty acids in control of body weight and insulin sensitivity. *Nat. Rev. Endocrinol.* 11: 577–591.
113 Bienenstock, J., Kunze, W., and Forsythe, P. (2015). Microbiota and the gut-brain axis. *Nutr. Rev.* 73 (Suppl 1): 28–31.
114 MacFabe, D.F. (2015). Enteric short-chain fatty acids: microbial messengers of metabolism, mitochondria, and mind: implications in autism spectrum disorders. *Microb. Ecol. Health Dis.* 26: 28177.
115 Selkrig, J., Wong, P., Zhang, X., and Pettersson, S. (2014). Metabolic tinkering by the gut microbiome: implications for brain development and function. *Gut Microbes* 5: 369–380.

12

Hormonal Expression Associated with Alzheimer's Disease and Neurodegenerative Diseases

Giuseppe Verdile[1,2,3]*, Anna M. Barron*[4,5] *and Ralph N. Martins*[2,3,4,6,7]

[1] School of Pharmacy and Biomedical Sciences, Faculty of Health Sciences, Curtin Health Innovation Research Institute, Curtin University of Technology, Bentley, WA, Australia
[2] Centre of Excellence for Alzheimer's Disease Research and Care, School of Medical and Health Sciences, Edith Cowan University, Joondalup, WA, Australia
[3] Australian Alzheimer's Research Foundation, Ralph and Patricia Sarich Neuroscience Research Institute, Nedlands, WA, Australia
[4] School of Psychiatry and Clinical Neurosciences, University of Western Australia, Perth, WA, Australia
[5] Lee Kong Chian School of Medicine, Nanyang Technological University, Singapore
[6] Department of Biomedical Sciences, Macquarie University, Sydney, NSW, Australia
[7] KaRa Institute of Neurological Diseases, Sydney, NSW, Australia

12.1 The Hypothalamic–Pituitary–Gonadal (HPG) Axis

The steroidal sex hormones are predominately synthesised in the gonads, under the control of tightly regulated feedback systems within the hypothalamic–pituitary–gonadal (HPG) axis (see Figure 12.1). The first step in steroidal hormone production is the conversion of cholesterol to pregnenolone, which is the precursor for all steroidogenic hormones. In the gonads, expression of the steroidogenic enzymes and availability of cholesterol for synthesis of pregnenolone is tightly regulated by the gonadotropins. The pituitary gonadotropin hormones, luteinising hormone (LH), and follicle stimulating hormone (FSH) are synthesised and secreted from the gonadotrope cells under the regulation of gonadotropin-releasing hormone (GnRH), pituitary factors, and gonadal hormone feedback. GnRH is secreted from the hypothalamus and acts on the anterior pituitary, where it binds GnRH receptors and stimulates gonadotrope function. In response to GnRH stimulation, LH and FSH are secreted in a pulsatile manner from the pituitary into the peripheral circulation. The gonadotropin hormones, LH and FSH, then act on the gonads to stimulate the production of hormones including testosterone, oestrogen, progesterone, activin, and inhibin.

The oestrogens are made up of three endogenous biologically different compounds: oestrone, oestradiol, and oestriol, with oestradiol being the most active of these three, as it binds with greatest affinity to oestrogen receptors – oestrogen receptor-α or -β. Testosterone and dihydrotestosterone (DHT) act on the androgen receptor (AR); however, DHT is also able to act indirectly through oestrogen receptor-β. Furthermore, since testosterone can be aromatised to oestrogen, it is often difficult to decipher which hormone and associated receptors are involved in its actions. In sex steroid research,

---

Neurodegeneration and Alzheimer's Disease: The Role of Diabetes, Genetics, Hormones, and Lifestyle,
First Edition. Edited by Ralph N. Martins, Charles S. Brennan, W.M.A.D. Binosha Fernando,
Margaret A. Brennan and Stephanie J. Fuller.
© 2019 John Wiley & Sons Ltd. Published 2019 by John Wiley & Sons Ltd.

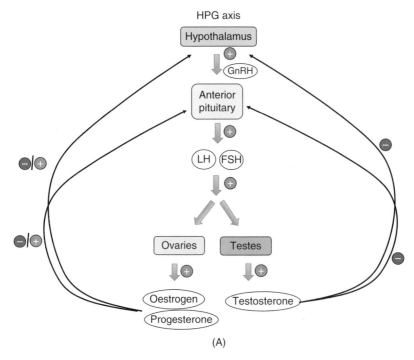

Figure 12.1 The HPG axis and changes in hormone levels that occur with age. The reproductive hormones are under tight regulatory control within the hypothalamic–pituitary–gonadal (HPG) axis. (A): Regulation of the HPG axis during reproductive age: Sex steroid synthesis is regulated by negative/positive feedback mechanisms. Secretion of gonadotropin-releasing hormone (GnRH) by the hypothalamus acts on the pituitary to release luteinising hormone/follicle-stimulating hormone (LH/FSH) which in turn act on the gonads to stimulate sex hormone production. (B) and (C): Synthesis of sex steroids declines with age. With reproductive senescence in women, the normal pulsatile production of gonadotropins and oestrogen/progesterone is disrupted, resulting in a dramatic reduction in sex steroid production. This disrupts the feedback mechanisms to the hypothalamus/pituitary leading to marked and rapid increases in gonadotropin. In ageing men, this process is more subtle, with a gradual decline in testosterone and increase in gonadotropins.

AR antagonists and the non-aromatisable 5αDHT have been used to determine which receptors are involved when studying the effect of androgens on receptors; similarly, selective oestrogen receptor modulators (SERM) are a class of drugs that act on oestrogen receptors, and these have been used to determine effects of binding to either the α- or β-oestrogen receptor [1].

12.1.1 Dysregulation of the HPG Axis During Ageing

Reproductive senescence is characterised by age-related hormonal changes during disruption of the HPG axis. This is particularly evident in post-menopausal women where there is complete loss of reproductive function. With the onset of the menopause (clinically defined as the cessation of menstruation), there are too few follicles remaining to sustain HPG interactions [2]. This results in diminished sex hormone secretion from the ovaries and correspondingly increased gonadotropin secretion. Although

12.1 The Hypothalamic–Pituitary–Gonadal (HPG) Axis

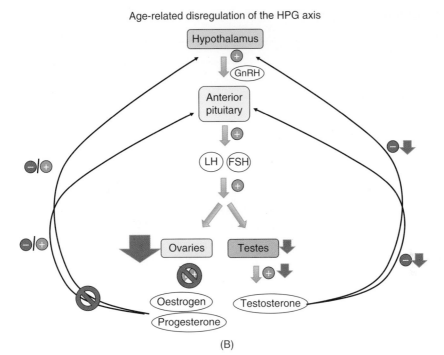

Figure 12.1 (Continued)

there are compensatory increases in oestrogen production from non-gonadal tissues (e.g. subcutaneous fat [3, 4]), peripheral oestrogen levels are not significantly altered [5–7]. Symptoms resulting from the hormonal changes post-menopause can include insomnia, vasomotor disturbances, weight gain or redistribution of body fat, decreased bone density, and mood/behavioural changes [8].

In contrast to menopause, androgen deficiency in ageing males (ADAM) is not necessarily coupled with the loss of reproductive function, and for men, hormonal changes are gradual and occur on average between the ages of 40 and 70 [9]. The major biologically active androgen in men is testosterone, and its action is mediated via binding to the AR, either directly or after 5α-reduction to the more active DHT. Men can experience considerable individual variation in age-related androgen deficiency, which is reflected by correspondingly variable hormonal changes and symptoms [9]. The gradual decline in testosterone levels (~1% per year) in men is accompanied by subtle increases in gonadotropin levels [10, 11]. Ageing men with androgen deficiency (often termed andropause or ADAM) experience symptoms of hypogonadism, including reduced muscle and bone mass, increased fat, lethargy, depression, and reduced libido [9, 12].

Reductions in sex hormone levels result in a failure of negative feedback systems which normally inhibit gonadotropin secretion, therefore central and peripheral post-menopausal and andropausal GnRH, LH, and FSH levels become elevated. Additionally, in post-menopausal women, the HPG axis shows insensitivity to negative feedback, further exacerbating gonadotropin hormone increases [13]. In women, LH

Age-related changes in levels of reproductive hormones

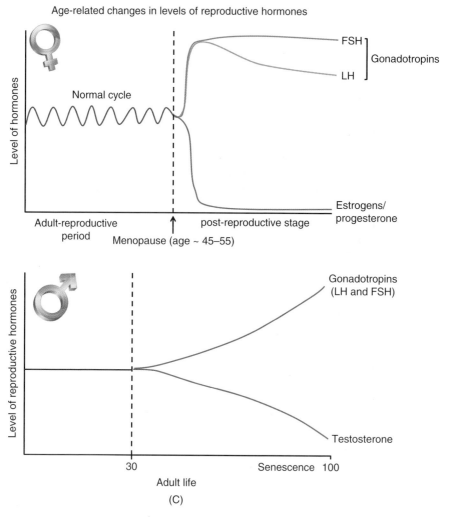

Figure 12.1 (Continued)

levels begin to rise after the age of 35 until post-menopause, where serum levels have been reported to increase up to 18-fold that of levels observed during the reproductive years [14]. Furthermore, post-menopausal FSH serum levels are threefold that usually seen in the reproductive years [14]. Gonadotropin levels peak between one and four years post-menopause, then begin to decline with age [15, 16]. Similar, though less severe changes have been reported in ageing men, with levels of serum LH and FSH in men aged 50–76 being two to three times that seen in men aged 20–48 years old [17]. These reductions in sex steroids and increases in gonadotropins have been associated with cognitive decline and with the risk and pathogenesis of neurodegenerative diseases such as AD.

12.2 Roles for Sex Steroids and Gonadotropins in the Neurodegenerative Process in AD

As discussed in previous chapters, major pathological features of an AD brain include the accumulation of extracellular plaques and fibrils, and intracellular neurofibrillary tangles, as well as chronic inflammation and widespread synaptic and neuronal loss, leading to brain atrophy and dysfunction. The deposition of amyloid plaques is possibly a defining feature of the AD brain, whereas neurofibrillary tangles are featured in other neurodegenerative diseases [18, 19]. Nevertheless, it is believed that the major component of neurofibrillary tangles, the hyperphosphorylated tau protein, also plays a critical role in the progression of AD, as it acts together with the major component of amyloid plaques (Aβ peptides), to drive neurodegeneration [20, 21]. Amyloid deposition is thought to occur early in the disease process [22], and the accumulation of toxic small Aβ aggregates ('oligomers') is thought to play a critical role in other early pathogenic events that include tau hyperphosphorylation and accumulation, oxidative stress and inflammatory processes, that lead to neurodegeneration and the onset of cognitive impairment and symptomatic AD [20, 23, 24].

Reduced levels of sex steroids are observed in AD and have been shown to be associated with AD pathogenesis and cognitive decline [25]. In a study comparing serum levels of oestrogens in women who were clinically diagnosed with AD to non-dementia controls, those individuals with AD had lower serum oestradiol and oestrone levels [26]. In contrast, a subsequent study showed that compared to cognitively normal post-menopausal women, serum levels of oestrone but not oestradiol were significantly higher in AD subjects [27]. In another study, serum levels of oestradiol (but not progesterone or testosterone) were significantly lower in women with AD compared to those with non-AD-type dementia and controls [28], in agreement with the original study by Manly and colleagues [26].

In studies of women without dementia, the majority of studies have failed to show overall cognitive decline during the natural transition of menopause in women (reviewed in [29]), though some studies have shown some minor changes. For example, longitudinal studies which followed women pre-menopause to six months after menopause found some associations with impairment in certain cognitive domains, particularly on verbal fluency [30]. Studies that have investigated correlations between cognitive changes and endogenous serum levels of oestrogens have also produced conflicting results. A review of cohorts from cross-sectional and longitudinal studies undertaken by Henderson and Popat [31], in women without dementia or other cognitive disorders, concluded that endogenous serum levels of oestradiol or oestrone in midlife (<64 years) were not associated with declines in episodic memory. In contrast, the Rotterdam Elderly study reported positive correlations with episodic memory [32]; however, in US studies (Osteoporotic Fractures and the Rancho Bernando retirement community) no [33] or inverse correlations [34] were observed between oestrogen levels and executive functioning. As with many of these studies, age, sample size, sensitivity of measurement of oestrogens, *APOE ε4* genotype (the major genetic risk factor for AD), and the presence of other co-morbidities as risk factors for cognitive decline can influence the interpretation of the results.

Brain levels of oestradiol and other hormones have also been investigated with respect to AD. Initial studies by Twist and colleagues [35] showed no changes in oestradiol levels between female AD cases and healthy female controls. More recently Rosario and colleagues [36] analysed post-mortem brain samples from post-menopausal women aged over 60 and found no changes in levels of sex steroid hormones during normal ageing (oestrone, oestrogen). However, when comparing brain-hormone levels in normal and AD cases, lower levels of oestrogens and androgens were found to be associated with AD pathology, yet only in those over 80 years of age, no difference was seen in the 60–79-year age range.

Reduced levels of testosterone in men have also been associated with cognitive decline and AD. Several studies have reported that compared to controls, men with AD and other dementias have lower serum testosterone levels [37–39]. In addition, studies have reported a reduction in brain levels of testosterone with age, as well as in men neuropathologically diagnosed with AD [36, 40, 41]. Further, longitudinal studies have shown that lower free testosterone levels can be detected 5–10 years prior to the diagnosis of AD [42], suggesting that low testosterone is a risk factor for AD rather than merely as a result of AD. Similarly, we have reported an association between serum testosterone concentrations and cognitive performance in healthy elderly men [43].

Further evidence for a role of testosterone in AD pathology comes from studies that investigated correlations between blood levels of testosterone and the accumulation of Aβ in men. Our own previous small studies have shown that reduced serum testosterone levels are associated with increased blood Aβ levels in men with dementia, or those who have undergone chemical castration as part of treatment for prostate cancer [44–46]. Rosario et al. also recorded an inverse relationship between brain levels of testosterone and soluble Aβ, in males over 60 with mild neuropathological changes [36]. More recently, we have extended these findings in a larger cohort from the Australian Imaging Biomarker and Lifestyle (AIBL) study to show that lower testosterone levels are associated with greater neocortical amyloid load (as assessed by PiB-PET imaging) in men with mild cognitive impairment (MCI) [47]; and in studies of groups of prostate cancer patients, it has been found that those given androgen deprivation therapy have a significantly greater risk of developing AD [48].

Together, these cohort, cross-sectional, and longitudinal studies indicate a potential role for the sex steroids in contributing to disease onset and in promoting disease pathology. *In vitro* and *in vivo* studies have suggested potential mechanisms underlying these associations that have been observed in clinical studies.

12.2.1 Sex Steroids Modulate Aβ Accumulation

The Aβ peptide is generated from its parent molecule, the amyloid precursor protein (APP) via sequential proteolytic processing by the enzymes β-secretase (β-site APP cleaving enzyme-1, BACE-1) and γ-secretase [49], to generate Aβ peptides of varying amino acid lengths (usually within 39–43 amino acids, most commonly 40 or 42 amino acids). When APP is cleaved by the alternative non-amyloidogenic pathway, no Aβ is produced as APP is cleaved in the middle of the Aβ sequence by an enzyme known as α-secretase (the metalloprotease ADAM10) releasing a secreted form of APP (α-APPs), and a much shorter peptide (p3), following γ-secretase cleavage.

Aβ peptides aggregate readily into oligomers and fibrils, and small oligomers of the longer, more easily aggregating 42 amino acid peptide (Aβ1-42) are considered to be the most neurotoxic Aβ species, as they promote oxidative stress, membrane damage, and inflammation, leading to AD pathogenesis. The accumulation of Aβ can occur through over-production via altered APP processing (reviewed in [49]) or impaired removal from the brain through impairments in microglial phagocytosis, clearance to the periphery or enzymatic degradation (reviewed in [50]). Sex steroids can modulate these mechanisms and thus modulate Aβ levels – as explained below.

Increased levels of both oestrogen and testosterone have been shown to modulate APP processing and to lower Aβ production. *In vitro* studies have shown that treatment of neuronal cells with these sex steroids leads to an increased secretion of α-APPs and a reduction in Aβ production [51–54], indicating that non-amyloidogenic processing of APP is favoured in the presence of sex steroids. This pathway is promoted potentially through activating the mitogen-activated protein kinase (MAPK) signalling pathway [55], however testosterone may also mediate these effects though AR signalling [56]. In addition, the aromatisation of testosterone to oestrogen has been shown to be involved in the testosterone-induced secretion of α-APPs, as inhibition of aromatase in the presence of testosterone results in a reduction in α-APPs [54]. There is also evidence that sex steroids can modulate substrate availability for the secretase enzymes, for example oestrogen can alter intracellular tracking of APP to compartments that favour α-APPs secretion [57, 58], and regulate APP over-expression following focal ischaemia [59].

In addition to modulating APP metabolism, sex steroids can enhance Aβ clearance. Oestrogen can stimulate Aβ clearance and degradation by microglial phagocytosis [60], and by increasing the expression of Aβ degrading enzymes, most notably IDE and neprilysin [61–63]. Testosterone has also been shown to enhance the degradation of Aβ by regulating expression levels of neprilysin [64].

Alternative splicing of the APP gene yields three major mRNA species – APP695, APP751, and APP770 mRNAs. Mice studies have shown that oestrogen can regulate alternative splicing of APP in the brain [65], such that APP695 is upregulated in both male and female mice, except for elderly male mice. It has also been found that gonadectomy upregulates APP695 mRNA levels except in adult females, where levels of brain cortex APP695 mRNA decrease. More recent studies by Sivanandam and Thakur [66] investigated total APP mRNA, and found testosterone or oestrogen decreased total APP mRNA in adult and old female mice, whereas testosterone supplementation increased the mRNA levels in both adult and old male mice, and oestrogen supplementation decreased mRNA levels in adult mice but increased them in old male mice. It was also found that, compared to levels found in adult mice, APP mRNA levels were higher in the older mice brains. Such studies of sex steroid effects on brain APP levels, and gender differences in these effects, need to be characterised further.

In vivo studies have generally confirmed effects of sex steroids that have been seen in *in vitro* models, however there have been discrepancies between studies. Oestrogen depletion induced via ovariectomy in mice or guinea pigs has been reported to promote the increase in brain Aβ42 levels, an effect that is partially reversed following oestrogen replacement [58, 67–69]. In contrast, other studies which used a transgenic mouse model of AD reported that oestrogen depletion via ovariectomy had no significant effect on Aβ burden [70–72]. Discrepancies between these effects of ovariectomy on Aβ levels may result from differences in neural oestrogen status, since Yue et al. [73] found that ovariectomy was insufficient to deplete oestrogen levels in the brain, whereas aromatase knockout mice exhibited significantly depleted central and peripheral oestrogen levels. Similarly, although ovariectomy is the commonly used experimental model of oestrogen deficiency, it appears that, at least in some circumstances, ovariectomy does not induce oestrogen depletion in the CNS. In fact, high oestrogen activity has been demonstrated in the brain of ovariectomised mice relative to other body regions, suggesting that CNS and peripheral oestrogen homeostasis may be controlled independently.

The levels and effects of hormone receptors such as the oestrogen receptor, as well as levels of their downstream coregulators will also influence brain function. These receptors and coregulators are implicated in crucial brain functions including neuronal growth and differentiation, migration and synapse formation [74]. Accumulating evidence is indicating that decreases in sex hormone receptors in the brain are linked to cognitive decline, for example AD patient frontal-cortex oestrogen-receptor-α levels correlate with cognitive function, as assessed by the Mini-Mental State Examination (MMSE) [75].

Testosterone and its more potent metabolite, DHT, exhibit Aβ-lowering potential *in vivo*, however by different mechanisms. DHT has been shown to have no effect on α-APPs levels, yet can reduce Aβ levels in rat brain [76], potentially by enhancing its degradation [64]. This suggests that although both testosterone and DHT have neuroprotective effects (that are possibly AR-dependent), they have independent effects on APP processing, with testosterone effects mediated potentially by aromatisation of testosterone to oestrogen [54]. However, in a study of AD mice crossed with aromatase knockout mice, testosterone was shown to reduce amyloid accumulation by downregulating BACE expression and upregulating Aβ degradation, suggesting that testosterone can have direct benefits, independent of its conversion to oestrogen [77].

Studies of AD transgenic mice have provided further evidence that androgens can influence Aβ levels. For example, the depletion of androgens by gonadectomy of the triple transgenic mouse model of AD (3x Tg-AD mouse) led to enhanced Aβ accumulation in the brains of the male transgenic mice, without altering the levels of the APP C-terminal fragment (APP cleavage intermediate product, just prior to Aβ production), suggesting that the effect was independent of the processing of APP [40]. In addition, impairments in hippocampal-dependent behavioural performance were observed in the androgen-depleted animals, whereas if the mice were administered DHT, cerebral Aβ levels were reduced and hippocampal function indicators improved [40]. Studies in our laboratory have demonstrated that androgen depletion in guinea pigs results in a significant increase in both CSF and plasma Aβ levels [78]. Following low dose testosterone treatment, both CSF and plasma Aβ levels decreased. However, at high doses of testosterone, we found that CSF Aβ levels decreased further, yet plasma Aβ levels increased. Further studies are required to determine whether these results are due to tissue-specific actions of testosterone, or alternatively, for example, enhanced clearance of Aβ from the CSF into the periphery.

12.2.2 Sex Steroids and Oxidative Stress

Gender differences in the responses to oxidative stressors suggest that reproductive hormones have the potential to modulate pro-oxidant/antioxidant balances, and thereby modulate the susceptibility to oxidative stress. Women have been found to have lower lipid peroxide levels than men of the same age [79], and animal studies have indicated that the female brain is more resistant to oxidative insults mediated by ischaemic injury [80, 81]. These gender differences in oxidative stress susceptibility have been attributed to reproductive hormones, in particular oestrogen, which exhibits antioxidant properties due to its phenolic structure. However, compared to pre-menopausal women, post-menopausal women exhibit age-independent increases in levels of lipid peroxidation markers coupled with reduced antioxidant levels [79, 82]. Similarly, elevated lipid peroxide levels have been reported in women that have undergone surgically-induced menopause via ovariectomy [83]. In post-menopausal women, hormone replacement therapy (HRT) has been found to decrease lipid oxidation, which has been suggested to provide a cardioprotective effect [84]. Similarly, recent studies of ovariectomised rats showed that HRT could reduce lipid oxidation in arterial walls [85].

The antioxidant properties of oestrogen were originally thought to result from classical oestrogen-receptor-mediated signalling pathways. However, a number of findings argue against this being the sole mode of action. The antioxidant features of oestrogen are still observed in neuronal cells lacking oestrogen receptors [86] and are not diminished by competitive inhibition studies using an oestrogen-receptor antagonist [87–89]. In addition, biologically inactive oestrogen variants that don't bind to and activate receptor signalling (such as 17α-oestradiol), also exhibit antioxidant activity [88, 90]. The phenolic ring of oestrogen is thought to be responsible for oestrogen's antioxidant properties, as it facilitates the direct scavenging of free radicals [89, 91, 92]. Thus, oestrogens have been coined 'natural antioxidants', and they have been demonstrated to inhibit lipid peroxidation in a variety of biological systems. In microsomal lipid preparations, oestrogens have been reported to inhibit iron-induced lipid peroxidation [92]. In neurons, 17β-oestradiol has been found to be a potent inhibitor of oxidative stress, by protecting cells against ROS-mediated oxidative damage [93] and to decrease ROS production by the mitochondria [87]. Furthermore, 17β-oestradiol has been shown to inhibit iron-induced lipid peroxidation in both rat and human brain homogenates [94].

However, apart from its phenolic ring properties and direct chemical effects, oestrogen does also reduce oxidative stress by regulating endogenous antioxidants, as well as enzymes involved in their metabolism [95, 96]. Many cell culture studies have shown such effects; for example, oestrogen dose-dependently increases glutathione levels in glial, hippocampal, and cortical neuron cultures [95], and oestrogen increases catalase activity in glial cells (yet decreases catalase activity in hippocampal cells) [96]. *In vivo*, ovariectomy has been associated with increased catalase levels (yet unchanged glutathione and superoxide dismutase levels) [97]. Compared to women of reproductive age, post-menopausal women have altered levels of antioxidant enzymes [79, 98], and in post-menopausal women who have undergone hormone therapy, the increases in oestrogen levels have been associated with increases in glutathione levels [79], whereas oestrogen + progestin therapy has been shown to result in increased Mn-superoxide dismutase and Cu/Zn superoxide dismutase activity in the plasma [99]. Further, oestrogen replacement therapy (ERT) has been shown to prevent and reverse the effects of oophorectomy on the expression of key antioxidant genes [100]. More recently, treatment using oestrogen in combination with progestin increased superoxidase dismutase activity and total antioxidant capacity in post-menopausal women [99]; and in a model of retinal degeneration, the synthetic progestin norgestrel modulated the signalling of the antioxidant transcription factor- nuclear factor erythroid 2-related factor 2 (Nrf2, causing it to increase levels of superoxide dismutase 2 in photoreceptor cells [101]. Together these studies suggest that ERT may offer benefits by supplementing/promoting antioxidant defences in an AD brain that is undergoing oxidative stress, and that progesterone may also provide some benefit.

Progesterone, however, has generally been found to be far less effective at inhibiting lipid peroxidation and neuronal death than oestradiol. In fact, it has been suggested to antagonise the effects of oestrogens [93, 102], and recent studies have found evidence that progesterone increases macrophage CD36 expression and oxidised LDL accumulation (CD36 is a receptor for oxidised LDL, and oxidised LDL enhances foam-cell formation, a pathological step in atherosclerosis), via the transcription factor peroxisome proliferator-activated receptor γ (PPARγ) [103]. Weak antioxidant properties of progesterone were shown to occur in response to iron-induced oxidative stress in neural cells [93]; on the other hand, progesterone was not found to improve neuronal survival following hydrogen peroxide treatment [86].

Interestingly, testosterone exhibits neuroprotective effects in cerebellar granule cells against the oxidative insults mediated by ROS, hydrogen peroxide, and nitric oxide [104, 105]. These neuroprotective effects of testosterone have been suggested to be mediated via conversion to oestrogen by aromatase [105], however other studies suggest that testosterone effects are mediated by AR signalling, as the antioxidant effects can be reduced by flutamide, an AR antagonist [105]. Testosterone can also upregulate the expression of the antioxidant enzymes superoxide dismutase and catalase in the brain, thus promoting the scavenging of oxygen radicals [104], and testosterone has been implicated in the regulation of glutathione, with increased levels reported in rat-brain homogenate following testosterone treatment [106]. Testosterone treatment has also been shown to reduce levels of lipid peroxidation in both the circulation and the brain in testosterone-deprived rats [107]. This effect was found to be less obvious in obese rats, and the attenuation of hippocampal synaptic plasticity and cognitive function in the testosterone-deprived rats was also not restored by testosterone treatment if the mice were obese. Such findings give further evidence of the additional oxidative stress caused by obesity, which is a risk factor for AD, as discussed in other chapters of this book. Whilst the neuroprotective effects of testosterone are well-established, further assessment of the underlying mechanisms is necessary to determine the degree of neuroprotection that is afforded by its antioxidant properties.

12.2.3 Sex Steroids and Inflammation

Neurosteroids and gonadal sex steroids have been demonstrated to modulate inflammatory responses of astroglia following neural injury. The gonadal hormones, 17β-oestradiol, progesterone, and testosterone decrease reactive gliosis in ovariectomised or castrated rats following penetrating injury to the hippocampus [108]. Similarly, 17β-oestradiol, progesterone, dehydroepiandrosterone (DHEA), and pregnenolone have all been found to decrease reactive gliosis in castrated male rats in response to penetrating brain injury, indicating that the above-mentioned hormone treatment inhibits astrocyte proliferation and/or migration [108]. In this particular study [108], the neuroactive steroid DHEA was found to be the most potent inhibitor of reactive gliosis. There was also evidence that brain injury upregulates the synthesis of oestrogen from testosterone in astrocytes [108], indicating that, in this model, at least some of the effects of testosterone may be due to its conversion to oestrogen.

Neurosteroids and gonadal sex hormones also have the capacity to induce morphological changes in astrocytes [109]. 17β-oestradiol, testosterone, and pregnenolone, but not progesterone, were found to increase the number of GFAP-immnunoreactive astrocyte processes, perhaps indicative of astrocyte arborisation [109]. It is clear that oestrogen not only has the capacity to suppress reactive gliosis following injury, but it can also modulate potential neuroprotective activities of astrocytes.

Oestrogen also has been implicated in the regulation of a wide range of microglial functions including the expression of cytokines and cell-surface molecules, apoptotic signalling pathways, and free-radical generation [110]. Cultured microglial cells exhibit respiratory burst activity, phagocytic activity, iNOS expression, and subsequent NOS production in response to inflammatory stimuli, all of which can be dose-dependently inhibited by oestrogen [111–113]. These studies suggest that *in vivo* production of reactive oxygen and nitrogen species by activated microglia might be inhibited by oestrogen treatment, thereby reducing the oxidative burden caused by chronic inflammatory responses. Similarly, oestrogen has been implicated in the modulation of NO production from peripheral macrophages [114], and furthermore, the pre-incubation of microglial cultures with DHEA also decreased NO secretion (but not iNOS expression) [115]. The inhibitory effects of oestrogen on microglial activation were shown to be dependent on the oestrogen receptor, as microglial responses were not observed following 17α-oestradiol treatment, which is biologically inactive at the levels of this receptor [112]; and in support of this, oestrogen receptor antagonists were found to abolish the inhibitory effects of oestrogen [116]. It has been hypothesised that binding to the oestrogen receptor [116] activates the MAPK to moderate microglial responses, since MAPK inhibitors also attenuate the effects of oestrogen on microglial activation [111, 112]. Interestingly, oestrogen was found to attenuate microglial activation only when oestrogen treatment was given to the cultures prior to the inflammatory insult, indicating oestrogen does not have the capacity to modulate inflammatory reactions once microglial activation has been initiated [116].

Neurodegenerative processes in several CNS disorders including spinal cord injury, multiple sclerosis, and Parkinson's disease (PD) as well as AD, are all associated with the activation of microglia and astrocytes, which drive the neuroinflammatory response. Considering the fact chronic inflammation is thought to be a key and initiating factor in AD pathogenesis, the inhibitory activity of oestrogen receptor agonists on microglial activation has been suggested as a beneficial therapeutic option for delaying the onset or progression of AD and other neurodegenerative diseases [117]. Oestrogens have also been shown to suppress the activation of microglia and recruit the blood-derived monocytes in rat brain after bacterial lipopolysaccharide [118] insults to the brain, and to suppress the expression of pro-inflammatory cytokines such as IL-1β and TNF-α in primary astrocytes following LPS exposure [119]. Other studies have shown that the selective expression of oestrogen receptor-α allowed protection by oestrogen against Aβ peptide-induced toxicity in HT22 cells, indicating the requirement for these receptors in mediating oestrogen's neuroprotective effects [120]. However, the binding of the selective oestrogen receptor-α agonist (propylpyrazole triol, PPT) and the oestrogen receptor-β agonist (diarylpropionitrile; DPN) have both resulted in neuroprotective actions in cell culture studies, indicating that binding to both receptors can provide neuroprotection. For example, PPT and DPN have been shown to provide neuroprotection against glutamate toxicity individually, by increasing the expression of the anti-apoptotic

Bcl-2 protein and by modulating the stress kinase signalling pathways [121, 122]. Several SERM such as tamoxifen, raloxifene, and bazedoxifene have been investigated to establish their neuroprotective strengths, and results show some promise; however, further research is necessary to improve blood–brain barrier permeability of such drugs and to reduce feminising effects [117].

12.2.4 Testosterone and Diabetes

Two major common factors between type 2 diabetes and AD include chronic inflammation and oxidative stress, which, as we have already discussed above, are influenced by hormone levels. Therefore, it should not be a surprise that recent studies have indicated associations between testosterone levels and type 2 diabetes – a known risk factor for AD; in fact there is now much evidence that low testosterone levels are associated with both insulin resistance and type 2 diabetes [123]. Similarly, men with prostate cancer treated with androgen-deprivation therapy appear to be at greater risk for type 2 diabetes and cardiovascular disease [124]. Conversely, testosterone treatment of men with type 2 diabetes has resulted in reduced insulin resistance, improved glycaemic control, and improvements in adiposity and fat distribution [125], as reviewed recently by Asih et al. [126]. Mechanisms for this effect have been explored, and there is now evidence that testosterone levels influence several steps in the insulin-signalling pathway [126]. This influence on insulin signalling and insulin resistance is highly noteworthy, as insulin resistance is thought to be an early common pathogenic event in both type 2 diabetes and AD: it implies testosterone influences the early stages of AD pathogenesis, and underscores the importance of maintaining normal physiological testosterone levels in older men for the prevention of several age-related conditions, though this should be in conjunction with a healthy diet that would also reduce the risk of insulin resistance, adiposity, and type 2 diabetes.

The effect of testosterone on diabetes in women is much less clear, and in fact some studies suggest testosterone, or an androgen excess, has the effect of increasing insulin resistance in women [127], though most studies have concentrated on women with polycystic ovary syndrome. Hormonal differences between men and women would clearly influence the effect of testosterone in women, and studies of testosterone treatment post-menopause have shown some minor improvements in insulin resistance [128], yet more research is needed in this area to characterise potential benefits of testosterone (or testosterone together with oestrogen) therapy in reducing risk of type 2 diabetes and AD.

As mentioned elsewhere in this review, clinical trials of testosterone treatment in men have not always shown positive results that would indicate a reduction in risk of AD, or improvements in cognition, as highlighted by two recent meta-analyses [129, 130]. Conclusions suggested that the levels of serum-hormone binding protein could influence bioavailable testosterone, which was confusing some of the results, and that levels of both serum-hormone binding protein as well as total testosterone should be measured in future studies. Nevertheless, the association between type 2 diabetes and AD, and the fact that type 2 diabetes increases the risk of AD, strengthens the concept that levels of testosterone are likely to influence AD and cognitive decline, and further clinical studies should be carried out to investigate the potential of testosterone therapy.

12.2.5 A Role for Gonadotropins in AD Pathogenesis

The main gonadotropins LH and FSH have also been implicated in the pathogenesis of AD. With respect to LH, there are several lines of evidence supporting this concept. Firstly, serum levels of LH and its homologue human chorionic gonadotropin (hCG) correlate with the incidence of AD: the increase in LH after menopause is greater and occurs earlier in women, and women are known to be more susceptible to AD than men (who have a slower increase in LH as they go through andropause). Early clinical studies using small cohorts found that the serum levels of gonadotropins are higher in AD patients compared to age-matched controls [131, 132]. Later studies of a large cohort of elderly women without dementia (n = 450) indicated that age-related increases in LH serum levels were associated with a reduction in cognition [133]. Similarly, increased serum LH levels have been associated with poor memory recall in cognitively normal men [134]; however, this last study also showed that testosterone was associated with declines in global cognition, indicating different roles for testosterone and LH in cognition. Interestingly, the Rodrigues et al. [135] study showed that in contrast to an increase in LH levels, high serum levels of FSH were associated with improved cognition. The significance of this contrasting effect with FSH requires further investigation and suggests that increases in FSH levels with age may protect against cognitive decline. The role of FSH in cognition and memory has been largely unexplored, and further *in vitro* and *in vivo* work should determine whether this gonadotropin has neuroprotective properties or attenuates Aβ accumulation. It is also known that several brain regions in various species, including humans, express functional LH/hCG receptors; in particular, the hippocampus contains the highest density of LH receptor (LHR), and rat brain studies suggest the hippocampus also expresses FSH receptors [136, 137].

Other studies which have indicated that LH might play a role in AD include our own studies which showed that LH accumulates within pyramidal neurons of AD brains, when compared with age-matched control brains [138]. In subsequent studies, we treated cultured neuronal cells with LH to investigate the role of gonadotropins in promoting amyloidogenesis. We found that intracellular levels of APP did not change [139], however the proteolytic processing of APP was altered, as evidenced by increased secretion and insolubility of Aβ [139]. This report was the first to show that LH could modulate Aβ levels. Animal studies then provided support for this theory, as it was shown that exogenous human LH [140, 141], over-expression of LH [142], or the addition of its more potent analogue, hCG [143, 144] could all increase the accumulation of cerebral Aβ levels and impair hippocampus-associated behaviour.

More recently, we investigated similar associations between LH and Aβ in clinical studies, since there was evidence that LH levels correlated with AD incidence. In an initial study, we investigated whether serum LH levels were associated with plasma Aβ levels in a small group of elderly men [145]. The results showed that the serum levels of LH correlate positively with plasma Aβ levels. No association was shown between free, bio-available levels of testosterone and plasma Aβ levels. However, this was a relatively small study (n = 40) and it could not be ruled out that this effect was due to androgen insensitivity or as a response to changes in the HPG feedback system. Recently, we extended our previous studies with plasma Aβ to investigate whether changes in serum levels of testosterone or LH were associated with amyloid burden in elderly men from the AIBL cohort containing four clinical subgroups: healthy controls, subjective memory complainers (SMC), MCI, and AD. The results from this study showed that in addition to *APOE-ε4* status, increased serum LH levels were significantly associated with cortical PiB retention in the SMC group (PiB-PET imaging measures Aβ levels in the brain). This association was not present in MCI or AD groups [47], instead reduced LH levels were found to be associated with higher PiB retention in these groups. These results suggest that whilst LH may play a more prominent role in promoting amyloid deposition in the brain, prior to onset of clinical symptoms, the impact of lower testosterone on Aβ deposition may be greater when clinical symptoms manifest, or alternatively that the brain cell loss, particularly in the hippocampus, in later stages of AD reduces the strength/function of this association. This relationship is influenced by a number of factors including age and the presence of the *APOE ε4* allele. Longitudinal follow-up studies are required to investigate these relationships further in those participants who convert from control to MCI, or MCI to AD.

The mechanisms by which LH modulates Aβ metabolism in the brain remain to be determined. It is not clear whether LH in the periphery can have effects in the CNS. Early studies in primates and humans demonstrated the presence of gonadotropins in the CSF and synchrony between the CSF and blood gonadotropin levels [146, 147]. Subsequent studies in rodents demonstrated that a small percentage of LH and its more potent analogue, hCG, but not FSH can cross the blood–brain barrier [148]. However, more recent evidence suggests that LH is synthesised within neurons, as the receptor for GnRH has been identified in the brain, including in regions involved in memory and learning that are affected by AD pathology [138, 149, 150]. In addition, LH mRNA has been detected in the brain, and has been found to be reduced in AD brain [150]. However, the extent of production and effects of *de novo* synthesis of LH on normal brain function and in AD pathogenesis are not known.

Evidence for a role of LH in Aβ metabolism in the CNS has also been presented by investigating the LHR. Gonadotropin receptors are found in steroidogenic cells such as the cells of Leydig and granulosa cells, yet, as we have mentioned, they are also found in the brain, indicating that the CNS is a target tissue for LH (reviewed in [151]). Studies have shown that changes in LH signalling can modulate Aβ levels [141], with the strongest evidence coming from the crossing of LHR knockout mice with AD transgenic mice [152]. These mice showed a reduction in AD pathology, namely Aβ amyloid pathology, astrogliosis, and tau phosphorylation. These LHR mice are devoid of sex steroids for the duration of their life and show increased peripheral levels of gonadotropins, which from human, *in vitro* and *in vivo* evidence are known to be associated with AD pathology. Further studies in cell culture models containing mutant or defective LHR binding or signalling steps may address some of the mechanisms associated with LH-mediated modulation of Aβ metabolism [153, 154].

Recent findings by Palm et al. [150], lend further support for LH synthesis in the brain, and also suggest that reducing peripheral LH levels may slow AD pathogenesis and cognitive impairment. Their study found that increases in brain amyloid and tau deposition as a result of ovariectomy in 21-month-old AD mice (3xTg) could not be attenuated by oestrogen replacement or lowering serum LH levels with leuprolide acetate (leuprolide acetate is a GnRH receptor agonist, yet chronic use suppresses LH and FSH secretion, which subsequently suppresses gonadal sex steroid production). However, lowering peripheral LH levels, but not oestrogen replacement, improved spatial memory which was associated with enhanced neuronal plasticity. These findings suggest there may be benefits when AD pathology is already established, but do not rule out the possibility that lowering serum LH could prevent accumulation of Aβ and tau, or slow down progression at a different disease stage in these mice, or in humans. Further, another study [155] showed that leuprolide decreased peripheral LH levels, yet increased brain LH levels in ovariectomised mice in regions associated with spatial memory, and that this increased brain LH correlated with cognitive improvements. Lower peripheral LH was also associated with decreased glycogen synthase kinase-3β (GSK3-β – involved in the formation of paired helical filament-tau), expression of β-catenin (linked to GSK3-β pathway, and levels correlate with cognitive function), and transcription of BDNF (important for neuroplasticity) [150]. The evidence suggests that an inverse relationship exists between peripheral and CNS LH levels. However, these experiments were conducted in ovariectomised AD-model transgenic mice, and further studies are required to establish if these results translate to ageing human females. Interestingly though, it was also shown by Palm and colleagues that transcription of LH was significantly lower in the cortex and hippocampus tissue of human female AD brains in comparison to healthy controls, and since other studies have already suggested AD is associated with higher peripheral LH, these results together support the concept of an inverse relationship between circulating and brain LH. Further studies are required to understand the potentially beneficial effects of modulating LH levels or LHR function in the CNS and periphery, as some studies indicate a reduction in AD pathology, others indicate improvements in cognitive function, and the timing of treatment appears to be crucial.

12.3 Hormone-based Therapies

12.3.1 The Oestrogens

Women who have undergone oophorectomy due to ovarian conditions, before menopause, consistently show an increased risk of cognitive decline and dementia (reviewed in [156]), supporting the concept that hormone replacement therapies might reduce dementia risk. Animal and cell-culture studies have provided support for testosterone and oestrogen having potential therapeutic benefits in AD. However, translations of the experimental findings to clear benefits in clinical trials have not been particularly successful. Early clinical trials of ERT for women overall have not shown benefits in women with mild to moderate AD (reviewed in [157, 158]). Furthermore, despite some retrospective and observational studies reporting improved cognition and reduced risk of AD in female ERT users [159–161], other observational and randomised trials have reported no neuroprotective or cognitive benefit of ERT in post-menopausal women [162, 163], whilst some randomised longitudinal studies have reported negative effects of ERT on cognition and AD risk in post-menopausal women [164, 165]. One issue with these studies is that most of them evaluated ERT in women well past the peri-menopause stage, mostly in cohorts over 60 years of age, which many researchers believe is too late, as discussed further below.

When evaluating the benefits of oestrogen on the brain in human trials, it is important to consider confounding factors such as co-morbidities (diabetes and obesity) and genetic risk factors. The *APOE ε4* genotype has been shown to strongly determine the outcome of oestrogen replacement in women, as studies where the influence of *APOE* genotype was assessed showed oestrogen provided no benefit to *APOE ε4* carriers [166, 167]. Studies have indicated that it is also important to consider age, type of menopause (natural vs induced), or timing of treatment with respect to cognitive impairment. Case-control studies have shown a beneficial effect of oestrogens on cognition if started early post-menopause (most commonly at ages between 50 and 60) [31, 168]. A study from the Cache County, Utah, showed that, compared to women who reported no use of hormone therapy, women who initiated therapy within five years of menopause had 30% lower incidence of AD [169]. No added benefit to lowering risk was apparent if treatment was administered more than five years post-menopause. A recent Cochrane Database review of 22 clinical studies of hormone therapy concluded that ERT or hormone therapy in general was not worthwhile for the primary or secondary prevention of cardiovascular disease or dementia, nor for prevention of cognitive decline [170]; however, all included studies involved cohorts well past menopause. A large Finnish study that comprised over 230 000 women over the period 1995–2011 found that ERT for over 10 years reduced AD risk, yet that similar long-term progesterone-only or combined hormone therapy was not related to AD risk [171]. A smaller study by the same group covering the years 1989–2009 found that long-term self-reported post-menopausal hormone therapy was associated with reduced AD risk [172], and the starting age for cohort inclusion was 47–56 years – which includes peri-menopausal years for most women.

The influence of ERT on gonadotropin homeostasis should also be considered. Ideally physiological concentrations of oestrogen should reduce gonadotropin levels to pre-menopausal levels through feedback mechanisms in the HPG axis. However, an early study examining the effect of continuous oestradiol on gonadotropin homeostasis found both LH and FSH levels were elevated after a six-month treatment period in surgical menopausal women, yet decreased in patients with a natural menopause [173]. Potential beneficial effects of hormone therapy may therefore be counteracted by elevated gonadotropin levels, depending on type of menopause. A small study evaluating the effect of body mass index on hormone changes caused by low-dose combined HRT found that six months of treatment resulted in decreased FSH levels, with smaller decreases seen in overweight women (LH wasn't measured) [174]. Another study of post-menopausal women between 48 and 61 years of age who took HRT for eight weeks to treat a variety of menopause symptoms had significantly lower FSH and LH levels after the eight-week treatment time [175]; and a study of oestriol for ERT found that plasma LH and FSH levels dropped, particularly in those patients for whom the oestriol was markedly effective [176]. More studies are needed to determine how brain LH levels are influenced by HRT or ERT, and to determine and characterise hormonal changes that may lead to beneficial cognitive changes.

12.3.2 Testosterone Therapy

In contrast to ERT, only a handful of small clinical trials have assessed the benefits of testosterone replacement in men on cognition, depression, and quality of life. Results from these studies have been inconclusive with some showing benefits of testosterone replacement on selective cognitive functioning including spatial memory, whilst others have shown minimal effects on cognition but an improvement in quality of life [177]. These studies are discussed further below.

An initial study of nine men with dementia showed that six weeks of treatment with oral testosterone improved the clinical global impression of change in seven men [178].

However, this study was not placebo-controlled or blinded and could be biassed by learning effects. Subsequent small-scale (5–32 participants), double-blinded, placebo-controlled randomised trials have produced contradictory results. A 12-week trial of 32 men with AD or MCI on weekly testosterone injections showed increased spatial and verbal memory compared to placebo [179]. A longer 24-week trial in 16 men with AD, who were administered testosterone transdermally, showed no improvement in verbal or spatial memory [180]. Other very small trials (5/6 men with AD) also showed conflicting results [181, 182]. Results from trials of eugonadal cognitively normal elderly men have shown similar mixed results, and the few trials in hypogonadal men have shown no overall benefit of testosterone on improving cognition (reviewed in [183]).

In more recent studies, in men aged over 65 years with low testosterone and age-associated memory impairment, treatment with testosterone gel for one year did not improve memory or several other cognitive functions such as visual memory and executive function [184]. Another smaller study of men with testosterone deficiency (mean age around 57 years ±12 years) found that testosterone replacement therapy improved cognitive function in those with cognitive impairment at baseline [185]. A larger randomised double-blind, placebo-controlled trial of men aged 60 and over with low-to-normal testosterone levels involved treatment for 29–31 months with testosterone gel or placebo, and it was found that testosterone treatment did not improve cognitive function [186].

A number of factors may account for the discrepancies in the outcomes of these trials, including differences in type and dosage of treatment. For example, studies employing intramuscular injections of testosterone enanthate have shown some benefits in areas of cognition relating to spatial and verbal memory [179, 187–189], compared to others that have administered testosterone orally (capsules containing the testosterone ester, testosterone undecanoate) [190, 191], or transdermally (T-gel/transdermal patches) [180, 181, 192]. There is also evidence from studies that suggest there is an optimal level of testosterone, that if surpassed offers no improvement or no further benefit [193–196]. Other factors may include the age of the patients, the cognitive function of the patients at baseline, and the role of the conversion of testosterone to oestrogen in men, which is poorly understood and has been addressed only by a few studies that have used inhibitors of aromatase in conjunction with testosterone to assess whether there are added benefits [179, 192].

In a similar manner to its influence on ERT in women, the *APOE ε4* allele also appears to modulate the association between testosterone and the risk of developing dementia in men. We have previously reported an association between serum testosterone levels and cognitive performance in healthy elderly men [43]. This study showed that higher levels of free, bio-available testosterone, were associated with better cognitive function, yet only in men who did not possess the *APOE ε4* genotype. However, in animal studies the therapeutic benefit of testosterone therapy was present even in the presence of the ε4 allele. One study showed that inhibiting the effects of testosterone by blocking the AR in male mice expressing *APOE ε4* results in the development of prominent deficits in spatial learning and memory [197]. Interestingly, female *APOE ε4* mice, when compared to female *APOE ε3* mice, exhibit such deficits in learning and memory without AR blockade, yet treatment with either testosterone or DHT attenuates the deficits [197].

To assess the benefits of testosterone in preventing AD, large-scale randomised, placebo-controlled intervention studies to assess cognitive, biochemical, and brain-imaging parameters at early stages are required. We have recently undertaken small pilot studies to assess the effects of testosterone on cognition and some of these parameters, in a non-randomised, open-label, single-group study with topical testosterone cream (Andromen Forte® Cream), administered for four months in cognitively normal elderly (n = 21, average age 57 ± 1 year) men with clinically defined low serum levels of testosterone. Serum testosterone levels increased from baseline levels following a month of administering Andromen, and this was associated with reductions in LH which persisted following four months of treatment (Martins et al., unpublished). These changes were associated with reductions in plasma Aβ and improvements in verbal memory (Martins et al., unpublished). We have recently completed a small (n = 44), double-blinded placebo-controlled cross-over clinical study in Indonesian men with low testosterone and with subjective memory complaints. One group received 24 weeks of testosterone treatment (Andromen Forte Cream), followed by 4 weeks washout, and then 24 weeks of placebo; the second group received the same treatments, in reverse order (placebo, washout, and then testosterone treatment). Compared to baseline, there was a significant improvement in general cognitive functioning following testosterone treatment. Additionally, we found that testosterone treatment improved participants' depression levels [198]. Comprehensive biochemical analysis that included serum LH, PSA (prostate specific antigen) levels, lipid profiles, and plasma Aβ levels revealed significant, marked reductions in LH and that the cream was safe and well-tolerated [199]. However, there were no significant changes to lipid profile (total cholesterol, HDL, LDL), insulin, or plasma Aβ [199]. Larger, longitudinal studies may reveal changes in some of these biochemical parameters. In addition, the measurement of established diseased biomarkers such as CSF Aβ and phosphorylated tau, as well as amyloid deposition assessed by PET imaging (reviewed in [200]), is required to assess the benefits of testosterone interventions. This is particularly relevant considering our recent data in the AIBL study [47], as it would provide an opportunity to determine the impact of testosterone treatment on the associations observed between LH/testosterone and neocortical amyloid load, particularly in those who are at high risk of AD but have yet to develop symptoms (amyloid +ve SMC, for example).

One concern for therapies that increase testosterone levels is the potential risks of such an approach. For many decades it was thought that raising testosterone levels would increase the risk of prostate cancer; however, when physiological doses of testosterone are used, the evidence suggests there is no increased risk [201, 202]. Similarly, some studies have linked testosterone treatment to other important adverse health outcomes such as increased risks in myocardial infarcts, heart attacks, and stroke (reviewed in [203]). However, again, the risks of such events remain uncertain, particularly at physiological doses, and the analysis of the literature surrounding this issue remains inconclusive (see recent meta-analysis [204]).

12.3.3 Selective Oestrogen or Androgen Receptor Modulators (SERM or SARM)

The long-term clinical use of oestrogens is not advised, due to their oncogenic effects on reproductive tissues. Furthermore, the high doses of oestrogen necessary to elicit antioxidant activity have the potential to increase free radical production through catechol oestrogen metabolism when administered long-term. Synthetic oestrogens with greater scavenging activity have been developed for use in cancer treatments, in order to eliminate potential problems arising from increased oestrogenic action through classical receptor signalling pathways [205]. In particular, SERM have been developed for the treatment of hormonal-driven cancer, to antagonise oestrogenic effects on reproductive organs, whilst preserving the beneficial effects on other organs [206]. The majority of SERM have been designed to bind to the oestrogen receptors, either ERα or ERβ, and they may also be selective for cell type, tissue, or species.

Due to the evidence that oestrogen may be protective against AD, SERM have been investigated and have shown benefits. Whether benefits are observed with ERα-specific more than ERβ-specific ligands (or vice versa) is unclear, with studies showing conflicting findings. For example: the SERM PPT, an ERα-binding ligand, has been shown to protect cultured neurons against Aβ-induced toxicity, whilst the ERβ agonist DPN showed minimal protection [207, 208]. PPT was shown to mimic oestradiol in reducing amyloid accumulation and improving memory performance in an AD mouse model, whilst no such benefits were observed for DPN. In contrast, other ERβ agonists such as Genistein have been shown to reduce oxidative stress and improve memory in rats [209], and ERβ are thought to be more relevant in prevention of AD, as described below.

One promising SERM is STX, which does not bind nuclear oestrogen receptors (ERα and ERβ), rather it binds membrane oestrogen receptors. Recent studies of this SERM have shown it prevents Aβ-induced cell death in neuroblastoma lines, possibly by raising mitochondrial gene expression and ATP levels, and enhancing dendritic growth and synaptic differentiation [210]. Protection for mitochondria following activation of the nuclear oestrogen receptors (ERα and ERβ) has also been shown, via regulation of calcium signalling and anti-apoptotic protein-mediated signalling cascades [211]. In other recent studies, the SERM raloxifene was trialled for 12 months in a recent pilot study involving a cohort of 42 women with mild to moderate AD (mean age 76), yet showed no cognitive benefits following the treatment, compared to placebo-treated controls [212]. This may not be that surprising as HRT or ERT have been shown to reduce cognitive decline or reduce risk of AD only when given at early peri-menopause or early menopause stages. In another recent study using a mouse model of amyloidosis, the SERM tamoxifen was shown to enhance spatial and contextual memory, possibly by reducing dopamine metabolism and increasing acetylcholine levels [213]. Tamoxifen has also been shown to protect against neuronal apoptosis, improve synaptic plasticity, as well as improve memory in ovariectomised mice [213, 214]. SERM or oestrogens may also protect against apoptosis via modulation of voltage-dependent anion channels in lipid rafts [215].

Further validation is required to determine the therapeutic benefit of SERM, and they are also an attractive approach as they are blood–brain barrier-permeable. As ERα and ERβ are both expressed in the brain, the development of SERM that selectively bind these receptors in the brain would be of advantage to circumvent any unwanted potential side effects associated with oestradiol. However, the two receptors have different distributions – ERα mRNA is expressed mostly in the amygdala and the hypothalamus, whereas ERβ mRNA expression is abundant in areas such as the hippocampal formation, cerebral cortex, and thalamus [216, 217]. Binding to the two receptors also has different downstream effects, and it is believed that changes to ERβ levels occur in ageing, whereas few changes occur to ERα levels. Downstream effects following binding to the ERβ may also be more relevant in the prevention of AD, as it has been shown that insulin-degrading enzyme (an enzyme that can degrade Aβ) is upregulated by binding to ERβ only. Furthermore, several polymorphisms in the ERβ gene have been linked to AD risk (whereas ERα polymorphisms seem to have little effect), ERβ-specific phytoestrogenic formulations prolong survival, improve spatial recognition memory, and slow amyloid pathology development in female triple transgenic AD-model mice, as well as prevent physical and neurological changes in ovariectomised mice [218], and it has also been shown that both BDNF and TrkB protein levels are significantly reduced in the hippocampus of ERβ but not ERα knockout adult mice (for a review of ER differences see [219]).

Following the concept of SERM, researchers have been motivated to develop tissue-specific AR modulators (SARM) that lack significant androgen action in the prostate yet exert agonist effects in selective androgen-responsive tissues [220]. The SARM that have been developed have been shown to have low androgenic activity in the prostate, yet to have equivalent or greater potency than testosterone in bone and muscle, offering benefits for osteoporosis and sarcopenia [221, 222].

The effects of SARM on the brain are largely unknown, and neuroprotective efficacy is now being explored. For example, the SARM RAD140, has been shown to protect neurons against induced neuronal death *in vitro* and *in vivo* [61]. Another, NEP28, has also been shown to increase activity of the Aβ-degrading enzyme, neprilysin, in brains from gonadectomised rats, although the resulting effects on brain Aβ levels was not explored. In other studies, a SARM ACP-105, alone as well as in combination with a selective ERβ agonist AC-186, was tested in male gonadectomised triple transgenic AD model mice, and it was found that ACP-105 alone decreased anxiety, yet the combination increased neprilysin and IDE levels, decreased brain Aβ levels, and improved cognition [223]. SARM treatment may offer a more selective, minimal-risk approach to androgen-based or combined SERM/SARM therapies.

12.3.4 Gonadotropin-Lowering Agents

As gonadotropins have important roles in AD pathogenesis, they are potential targets for developing appropriate therapeutic strategies for AD. In this regard, leuprolide acetate is one of the most widely studied agents for AD that targets gonadotropins, and it has already shown some promise in clinical trials. As mentioned earlier, leuprolide acetate is a GnRH receptor agonist that initially stimulates the production of LH, but chronic administration results in the downregulation of gonadotropin secretion [224]. Although mostly used for the treatment of hormone-responsive cancers such as prostate and breast cancer, animal and clinical studies have shown leuprolide acetate to have potential as a therapeutic agent for AD. Initial studies in transgenic and non-transgenic mice showed that leuprolide could reduce brain Aβ accumulation and levels of Aβ40 and Aβ42 levels [139, 140]. Some similar studies have not shown positive changes, possibly due to differences in the severity of pathology of the animal model, sex of the animals, or the over-expression of Aβ, which may have masked the potency of leuprolide (it is noted in the Casadesus et al. [140] study that the reduction in amyloid deposition, although significant, is very modest).

Animal studies which showed that leuprolide may improve memory and modulate AD pathology, together with epidemiological data suggesting that treatment may reduce AD risk [155, 225, 226], led to the trial of leuprolide acetate (Lupron Depot) in a clinical setting. A 48-week, double-blind placebo-controlled clinical trial administering Lupron to women over 65 years of age with mild–moderate AD showed promising results [227]. The results showed memory and cognition (assessed by ADAS-Cog) and ability to perform activities of daily living (assessed by ADCS-ADL) improved in a group of women with AD (n = 109) receiving acetylcholine esterase inhibitor (AChEI) and a high dose of leuprolide acetate, compared to those women receiving placebo and AChEI. While the early clinical trials to lower LH as an effective treatment for mild–moderate AD are encouraging, treatment at pre-clinical stages, MCI, or earlier stages of AD should also be carried out to determine if such treatment can slow or stop progression of the disease, to enable independent living for as long as possible.

A recent study of ovariectomised mice showed that leuprolide treatment, both immediately and four months after ovariectomy, lowered serum LH levels, improved cognitive function, and increased dendritic spine density on cortical pyramidal neurons, when compared to untreated (or 17β-oestradiol-treated) ovariectomised mice [228]. Dendritic spine density and plasticity is strongly associated with learning and memory [229], suggesting a possible mechanism whereby lower LH levels may help cognitive function, and indicating such treatment is worth investigating further.

12.4 Conclusions

The regulation of the sex steroids and gonadotropins is tightly linked, and following reproductive senescence, reductions in sex hormone levels are coupled to elevated gonadotropin levels. These changes are associated with an increased risk of cognitive decline and AD, and promote the development of AD pathology. Although mechanism(s) are yet to be fully determined, it is conceivable that the combined effects of sex steroids and gonadotropins can influence not only Aβ accumulation but also neuronal plasticity and other features of neurodegeneration such as oxidative stress and inflammation. Modulation of these hormones in human clinical trials is showing some promising results, though treatment timing, hormone type, stage of disease, and genetic considerations all appear to influence outcome. Given the diverse actions of the reproductive hormones, combinational hormone therapy may also prove to be more efficacious in the prevention of AD. However, this notion requires further validation in appropriate *in vivo* animal studies followed by clinical trials.

References

1 Spence, R.D. and Voskuhl, R.R. (2012). Neuroprotective effects of estrogens and androgens in CNS inflammation and neurodegeneration. *Front Neuroendocrinol.* 33: 105–115.

2 Bornstein, J., Goldschmid, N., and Sabo, E. (2004). Hyperinnervation and mast cell activation may be used as histopathologic diagnostic criteria for vulvar vestibulitis. *Gynecol. Obstet. Invest.* 58: 171–178.

3 Labrie, F., Belanger, A., Cusan, L., and Candas, B. (1997). Physiological changes in dehydroepiandrosterone are not reflected by serum levels of active androgens and estrogens but of their metabolites: intracrinology. *J. Clin. Endocrinol. Metab.* 82: 2403–2409.

4 Simpson, E.R. and Davis, S.R. (2001). Minireview: aromatase and the regulation of estrogen biosynthesis--some new perspectives. *Endocrinology* 142: 4589–4594.

5 Agarwal, S.K. and Judd, H.L. (1997). Menopause. *Curr. Ther. Endocrinol. Metab.* 6: 624–631.

6 Bulun, S.E. and Simpson, E.R. (1994). Breast cancer and expression of aromatase in breast adipose tissue. *Trends Endocrinol. Metab.* 5: 113–120.

7 Misso, M.L., Jang, C., Adams, J. et al. (2005). Differential expression of factors involved in fat metabolism with age and the menopause transition. *Maturitas* 51: 299–306.

8 Guthrie, J.R., Lehert, P., Dennerstein, L. et al. (2004). The relative effect of endogenous estradiol and androgens on menopausal bone loss: a longitudinal study. *Osteoporos. Int.* 15: 881–886.

9 Mastrogiacomo, I., Feghali, G., Foresta, C., and Ruzza, G. (1982). Andropause: incidence and pathogenesis. *Arch. Androl.* 9: 293–296.

10 Feldman, H.A., Longcope, C., Derby, C.A. et al. (2002). Age trends in the level of serum testosterone and other hormones in middle-aged men: longitudinal results from the Massachusetts male aging study. *J. Clin. Endocrinol. Metab.* 87: 589–598.

11 Gray, A., Feldman, H.A., McKinlay, J.B., and Longcope, C. (1991). Age, disease, and changing sex hormone levels in middle-aged men: results of the Massachusetts male aging study. *J. Clin. Endocrinol. Metab.* 73: 1016–1025.

12 Tenover, J.L. (1998). Male hormone replacement therapy including 'andropause'. *Endocrinol. Metab. Clin. North Am.* 27: 969–987, x.

13 Rossmanith, W.G., Handke-Vesely, A., Wirth, U., and Scherbaum, W.A. (1994). Does the gonadotropin pulsatility of postmenopausal women represent the unrestrained hypothalamic-pituitary activity? *Eur. J. Endocrinol.* 130: 485–493.

14 Chakravarti, S., Collins, W.P., Forecast, J.D. et al. (1976). Hormonal profiles after the menopause. *Br. Med. J.* 2: 784–787.

15 Lenton, E.A., Sexton, L., Lee, S., and Cooke, I.D. (1988). Progressive changes in LH and FSH and LH: FSH ratio in women throughout reproductive life. *Maturitas* 10: 35–43.

16 Tungphaisal, S., Chandeying, V., Sutthijumroon, S., and Krisanapan, O. (1992). Symptomatology and hormonal levels among Thai women with natural menopause. *J. Med. Assoc. Thai.* 75: 697–703.

17 Neaves, W.B., Johnson, L., Porter, J.C. et al. (1984). Leydig cell numbers, daily sperm production, and serum gonadotropin levels in aging men. *J. Clin. Endocrinol. Metab.* 59: 756–763.

18 Lee, V.M., Goedert, M., and Trojanowski, J.Q. (2001). Neurodegenerative tauopathies. *Annu. Rev. Neurosci.* 24: 1121–1159.

19 Frost, B., Gotz, J., and Feany, M.B. (2015). Connecting the dots between tau dysfunction and neurodegeneration. *Trends Cell Biol.* 25: 46–53.

20 Ittner, L.M. and Gotz, J. (2011). Amyloid-beta and tau – a toxic *pas de deux* in Alzheimer's disease. *Nat. Rev. Neurosci.* 12: 65–72.

21 Ittner, L.M., Ke, Y.D., Delerue, F. et al. (2010). Dendritic function of tau mediates amyloid-beta toxicity in Alzheimer's disease mouse models. *Cell* 142: 387–397.

22 Villemagne, V.L., Burnham, S., Bourgeat, P. et al. (2013). Amyloid beta deposition, neurodegeneration, and cognitive decline in sporadic Alzheimer's disease: a prospective cohort study. *Lancet. Neurol.* 12: 357–367.

23 Walsh, D.M. and Selkoe, D.J. (2007). A beta oligomers – a decade of discovery. *J. Neurochem.* 101: 1172–1184.

24 O'Malley, T.T., Oktaviani, N.A., Zhang, D. et al. (2014). Abeta dimers differ from monomers in structural propensity, aggregation paths and population of synaptotoxic assemblies. *Biochem. J.* 461: 413–426.

25 Pike, C.J. (2017). Sex and the development of Alzheimer's disease. *J. Neurosci. Res.* 95: 671–680.

26 Manly, J.J., Merchant, C.A., Jacobs, D.M. et al. (2000). Endogenous estrogen levels and Alzheimer's disease among postmenopausal women. *Neurology* 54: 833–837.

27 Cunningham, C.J., Sinnott, M., Denihan, A. et al. (2001). Endogenous sex hormone levels in postmenopausal women with Alzheimer's disease. *J. Clin. Endocrinol. Metab.* 86: 1099–1103.

28 Tsolaki, M., Grammaticos, P., Karanasou, C. et al. (2005). Serum estradiol, progesterone, testosterone, FSH and LH levels in postmenopausal women with Alzheimer's dementia. *Hell. J. Nucl. Med.* 8: 39–42.

29 Hogervorst, E. and Bandelow, S. (2010). Sex steroids to maintain cognitive function in women after the menopause: a meta-analyses of treatment trials. *Maturitas* 66: 56–71.

30 Fuh, J.L., Wang, S.J., Lee, S.J. et al. (2006). A longitudinal study of cognition change during early menopausal transition in a rural community. *Maturitas* 53: 447–453.

31 Henderson, V.W. and Popat, R.A. (2011). Effects of endogenous and exogenous estrogen exposures in midlife and late-life women on episodic memory and executive functions. *Neuroscience* 191: 129–138.

32 den Heijer, T., Geerlings, M.I., Hofman, A. et al. (2003). Higher estrogen levels are not associated with larger hippocampi and better memory performance. *Arch. Neurol.* 60: 213–220.

33 Yaffe, K., Grady, D., Pressman, A., and Cummings, S. (1998). Serum estrogen levels, cognitive performance, and risk of cognitive decline in older community women. *J. Am. Geriatr. Soc.* 46: 816–821.

34 Barrett-Connor, E. and Goodman-Gruen, D. (1999). Cognitive function and endogenous sex hormones in older women. *J. Am. Geriatr. Soc.* 47: 1289–1293.

35 Twist, S.J., Taylor, G.A., Weddell, A. et al. (2000). Brain oestradiol and testosterone levels in Alzheimer's disease. *Neurosci. Lett.* 286: 1–4.

36 Rosario, E.R., Chang, L., Head, E.H. et al. (2011). Brain levels of sex steroid hormones in men and women during normal aging and in Alzheimer's disease. *Neurobiol. Aging* 32: 604–613.

37 Hogervorst, E., Williams, J., Budge, M. et al. (2001). Serum total testosterone is lower in men with Alzheimer's disease. *Neuro. Endocrinol. Lett.* 22: 163–168.

38 Hogervorst, E., Combrinck, M., and Smith, A.D. (2003). Testosterone and gonadotropin levels in men with dementia. *Neuro. Endocrinol. Lett.* 24: 203–208.

39 Hogervorst, E., Bandelow, S., Combrinck, M., and Smith, A.D. (2004). Low free testosterone is an independent risk factor for Alzheimer's disease. *Exp. Gerontol.* 39: 1633–1639.

40 Rosario, E.R., Carroll, J.C., Oddo, S. et al. (2006). Androgens regulate the development of neuropathology in a triple transgenic mouse model of Alzheimer's disease. *J. Neurosci.* 26: 13384–13389.

41 Rosario, E.R., Chang, L., Beckett, T.L. et al. (2009). Age-related changes in serum and brain levels of androgens in male Brown Norway rats. *Neuroreport* 20: 1534–1537.

42 Moffat, S.D., Zonderman, A.B., Metter, E.J. et al. (2004). Free testosterone and risk for Alzheimer disease in older men. *Neurology* 62: 188–193.

43 Burkhardt, M.S., Foster, J.K., Clarnette, R.M. et al. (2006). Interaction between testosterone and apolipoprotein E epsilon4 status on cognition in healthy older men. *J. Clin. Endocrinol. Metab.* 91: 1168–1172.

44 Almeida, O.P., Waterreus, A., Spry, N. et al. (2004). One year follow-up study of the association between chemical castration, sex hormones, beta-amyloid, memory and depression in men. *Psychoneuroendocrinology* 29: 1071–1081.

45 Gillett, M.J., Martins, R.N., Clarnette, R.M. et al. (2003). Relationship between testosterone, sex hormone binding globulin and plasma amyloid beta peptide 40 in older men with subjective memory loss or dementia. *J. Alzheimers Dis.* 5: 267–269.

46 Gandy, S., Almeida, O.P., Fonte, J. et al. (2001). Chemical andropause and amyloid-beta peptide. *Jama* 285: 2195–2196.

47 Verdile, G., Laws, S.M., Henley, D. et al. (2014). Associations between gonadotropins, testosterone and beta amyloid in men at risk of Alzheimer's disease. *Mol. Psychiatry* 19: 69–75.

48 Nead, K.T., Gaskin, G., Chester, C. et al. (2016). Androgen deprivation therapy and future Alzheimer's disease risk. *J. Clin. Oncol.* 34: 566–571.

49 Krishnaswamy, S., Verdile, G., Groth, D. et al. (2009). The structure and function of Alzheimer's gamma secretase enzyme complex. *Crit. Rev. Clin. Lab. Sci.* 46: 282–301.

50 Bates, K.A., Verdile, G., Li, Q.X. et al. (2009). Clearance mechanisms of Alzheimer's amyloid-beta peptide: implications for therapeutic design and diagnostic tests. *Mol. Psychiatry* 14: 469–486.

51 Jaffe, A.B., Toran-Allerand, C.D., Greengard, P., and Gandy, S.E. (1994). Estrogen regulates metabolism of Alzheimer amyloid beta precursor protein. *J. Biol. Chem.* 269: 13065–13068.

52 Xu, H., Gouras, G.K., Greenfield, J.P. et al. (1998). Estrogen reduces neuronal generation of Alzheimer beta-amyloid peptides. *Nat. Med.* 4: 447–451.

53 Gouras, G.K., Xu, H., Gross, R.S. et al. (2000). Testosterone reduces neuronal secretion of Alzheimer's beta-amyloid peptides. *Proc. Natl. Acad. Sci. U. S. A.* 97: 1202–1205.

54 Goodenough, S., Engert, S., and Behl, C. (2000). Testosterone stimulates rapid secretory amyloid precursor protein release from rat hypothalamic cells via the activation of the mitogen-activated protein kinase pathway. *Neurosci. Lett.* 296: 49–52.

55 Manthey, D., Heck, S., Engert, S., and Behl, C. (2001). Estrogen induces a rapid secretion of amyloid beta precursor protein via the mitogen-activated protein kinase pathway. *Eur. J. Biochem.* 268: 4285–4291.

56 Nguyen, T.V., Yao, M., and Pike, C.J. (2005). Androgens activate mitogen-activated protein kinase signaling: role in neuroprotection. *J. Neurochem.* 94: 1639–1651.

57 Greenfield, J.P., Leung, L.W., Cai, D. et al. (2002). Estrogen lowers Alzheimer beta-amyloid generation by stimulating trans-Golgi network vesicle biogenesis. *J. Biol. Chem.* 277: 12128–12136.

58 Xu, H., Wang, R., Zhang, Y.W., and Zhang, X. (2006). Estrogen, beta-amyloid metabolism/trafficking, and Alzheimer's disease. *Ann. N. Y. Acad. Sci.* 1089: 324–342.
59 Shi, J., Panickar, K.S., Yang, S.H. et al. (1998). Estrogen attenuates over-expression of beta-amyloid precursor protein messager RNA in an animal model of focal ischemia. *Brain Res.* 810: 87–92.
60 Li, R., Shen, Y., Yang, L.B. et al. (2000). Estrogen enhances uptake of amyloid beta-protein by microglia derived from the human cortex. *J. Neurochem.* 75: 1447–1454.
61 Jayaraman, A., Carroll, J.C., Morgan, T.E. et al. (2012). 17beta-estradiol and progesterone regulate expression of beta-amyloid clearance factors in primary neuron cultures and female rat brain. *Endocrinology* 153: 5467–5479.
62 Liang, K., Yang, L., Yin, C. et al. (2010). Estrogen stimulates degradation of beta-amyloid peptide by up-regulating neprilysin. *J. Biol. Chem.* 285: 935–942.
63 Zhao, L., Yao, J., Mao, Z. et al. (2011). 17beta-estradiol regulates insulin-degrading enzyme expression via an ERbeta/PI3-K pathway in hippocampus: relevance to Alzheimer's prevention. *Neurobiol. Aging* 32: 1949–1963.
64 Yao, M., Nguyen, T.V., Rosario, E.R. et al. (2008). Androgens regulate neprilysin expression: role in reducing beta-amyloid levels. *J. Neurochem.* 105: 2477–2488.
65 Thakur, M.K. and Mani, S.T. (2005). Estradiol regulates APP mRNA alternative splicing in the mice brain cortex. *Neurosci. Lett.* 381: 154–157.
66 Sivanandam, T.M. and Thakur, M.K. (2011). Amyloid precursor protein (APP) mRNA level is higher in the old mouse cerebral cortex and is regulated by sex steroids. *J. Mol. Neurosci.* 43: 235–240.
67 Levin-Allerhand, J.A., Lominska, C.E., Wang, J., and Smith, J.D. (2002). 17Alpha-estradiol and 17beta-estradiol treatments are effective in lowering cerebral amyloid-beta levels in AbetaPPSWE transgenic mice. *J. Alzheimers Dis.* 4: 449–457.
68 Petanceska, S.S., Nagy, V., Frail, D., and Gandy, S. (2000). Ovariectomy and 17beta-estradiol modulate the levels of Alzheimer's amyloid beta peptides in brain. *Neurology* 54: 2212–2217.
69 Zheng, H., Xu, H., Uljon, S.N. et al. (2002). Modulation of a(beta) peptides by estrogen in mouse models. *J. Neurochem.* 80: 191–196.
70 Golub, M.S., Germann, S.L., Mercer, M. et al. (2008). Behavioral consequences of ovarian atrophy and estrogen replacement in the APPswe mouse. *Neurobiol. Aging* 29: 1512–1523.
71 Green, P.S., Bales, K., Paul, S., and Bu, G. (2005). Estrogen therapy fails to alter amyloid deposition in the PDAPP model of Alzheimer's disease. *Endocrinology* 146: 2774–2781.
72 Heikkinen, T., Kalesnykas, G., Rissanen, A. et al. (2004). Estrogen treatment improves spatial learning in APP + PS1 mice but does not affect beta amyloid accumulation and plaque formation. *Exp. Neurol.* 187: 105–117.
73 Yue, X., Lu, M., Lancaster, T. et al. (2005). Brain estrogen deficiency accelerates Abeta plaque formation in an Alzheimer's disease animal model. *Proc. Natl. Acad. Sci. U. S. A.* 102: 19198–19203.
74 Konar, A., Singh, P., and Thakur, M.K. (2016). Age-associated cognitive decline: insights into molecular switches and recovery avenues. *Aging Dis.* 7: 121–129.

75 Kelly, J.F., Bienias, J.L., Shah, A. et al. (2008). Levels of estrogen receptors alpha and beta in frontal cortex of patients with Alzheimer's disease: relationship to mini-mental state examination scores. *Curr. Alzheimer Res.* 5: 45–51.

76 Ramsden, M., Nyborg, A.C., Murphy, M.P. et al. (2003). Androgens modulate beta-amyloid levels in male rat brain. *J. Neurochem.* 87: 1052–1055.

77 McAllister, C., Long, J., Bowers, A. et al. (2010). Genetic targeting aromatase in male amyloid precursor protein transgenic mice down-regulates beta-secretase (BACE1) and prevents Alzheimer-like pathology and cognitive impairment. *J. Neurosci.* 30: 7326–7334.

78 Wahjoepramono, E.J., Wijaya, L.K., Taddei, K. et al. (2008). Distinct effects of testosterone on plasma and cerebrospinal fluid amyloid-beta levels. *J. Alzheimers Dis.* 15: 129–137.

79 Massafra, C., Gioia, D., De Felice, C. et al. (2002). Gender-related differences in erythrocyte glutathione peroxidase activity in healthy subjects. *Clin. Endocrinol. (Oxf)* 57: 663–667.

80 Hall, E.D., Pazara, K.E., and Linseman, K.L. (1991). Sex differences in postischemic neuronal necrosis in gerbils. *J. Cereb. Blood Flow Metab.* 11: 292–298.

81 Park, K.M., Cho, H.J., and Bonventre, J.V. (2005). Orchiectomy reduces susceptibility to renal ischemic injury: a role for heat shock proteins. *Biochem. Biophys. Res. Commun.* 328: 312–317.

82 Vural, P., Akgul, C., and Canbaz, M. (2005). Effects of menopause and tibolone on antioxidants in postmenopausal women. *Ann. Clin. Biochem.* 42: 220–223.

83 Yagi, K. (1997). Female hormones act as natural antioxidants – a survey of our research. *Acta Biochim. Pol.* 44: 701–709.

84 Escalante Gomez, C. and Quesada Mora, S. (2013). HRT decreases DNA and lipid oxidation in postmenopausal women. *Climacteric.* 16: 104–110.

85 Escalante, C.G., Mora, S.Q., and Bolanos, L.N. (2017). Hormone replacement therapy reduces lipid oxidation directly at the arterial wall: a possible link to estrogens' cardioprotective effect through atherosclerosis prevention. *J. Midlife Health* 8: 11–16.

86 Behl, C., Widmann, M., Trapp, T., and Holsboer, F. (1995). 17-beta estradiol protects neurons from oxidative stress-induced cell death in vitro. *Biochem. Biophys. Res. Commun.* 216: 473–482.

87 Culmsee, C., Vedder, H., Ravati, A. et al. (1999). Neuroprotection by estrogens in a mouse model of focal cerebral ischemia and in cultured neurons: evidence for a receptor-independent antioxidative mechanism. *J. Cereb. Blood Flow Metab.* 19: 1263–1269.

88 Sawada, H., Ibi, M., Kihara, T. et al. (1998). Estradiol protects mesencephalic dopaminergic neurons from oxidative stress-induced neuronal death. *J. Neurosci. Res.* 54: 707–719.

89 Subbiah, M.T., Kessel, B., Agrawal, M. et al. (1993). Antioxidant potential of specific estrogens on lipid peroxidation. *J. Clin. Endocrinol. Metab.* 77: 1095–1097.

90 Behl, C., Skutella, T., Lezoualc'h, F. et al. (1997). Neuroprotection against oxidative stress by estrogens: structure-activity relationship. *Mol. Pharmacol.* 51: 535–541.

91 Ruiz-Larrea, M.B., Mohan, A.R., Paganga, G. et al. (1997). Antioxidant activity of phytoestrogenic isoflavones. *Free Radic. Res.* 26: 63–70.

92 Sugioka, K., Shimosegawa, Y., and Nakano, M. (1987). Estrogens as natural antioxidants of membrane phospholipid peroxidation. *FEBS Lett.* 210: 37–39.
93 Goodman, Y., Bruce, A.J., Cheng, B., and Mattson, M.P. (1996). Estrogens attenuate and corticosterone exacerbates excitotoxicity, oxidative injury, and amyloid beta-peptide toxicity in hippocampal neurons. *J. Neurochem.* 66: 1836–1844.
94 Vedder, H., Anthes, N., Stumm, G. et al. (1999). Estrogen hormones reduce lipid peroxidation in cells and tissues of the central nervous system. *J. Neurochem.* 72: 2531–2538.
95 Schmidt, A.J., Krieg, J., and Vedder, H. (2002). Differential effects of glucocorticoids and gonadal steroids on glutathione levels in neuronal and glial cell systems. *J. Neurosci. Res.* 67: 544–550.
96 Schmidt, A.J., Krieg, J.C., and Vedder, H. (2005). Antioxidative and steroid systems in neurological and psychiatric disorders. *World J. Biol. Psychiatry* 6: 26–35.
97 Ozgonul, M., Oge, A., Sezer, E.D. et al. (2003). The effects of estrogen and raloxifene treatment on antioxidant enzymes in brain and liver of ovarectomized female rats. *Endocr. Res.* 29: 183–189.
98 Vural, F., Vural, B., Yucesoy, I., and Badur, S. (2005). Ovarian aging and bone metabolism in menstruating women aged 35-50 years. *Maturitas* 52: 147–153.
99 Unfer, T.C., Figueiredo, C.G., Zanchi, M.M. et al. (2015). Estrogen plus progestin increase superoxide dismutase and total antioxidant capacity in postmenopausal women. *Climacteric* 18: 379–388.
100 Bellanti, F., Matteo, M., Rollo, T. et al. (2013). Sex hormones modulate circulating antioxidant enzymes: impact of estrogen therapy. *Redox. Biol.* 1: 340–346.
101 Byrne, A.M., Ruiz-Lopez, A.M., Roche, S.L. et al. (2016). The synthetic progestin norgestrel modulates Nrf2 signaling and acts as an antioxidant in a model of retinal degeneration. *Redox. Biol.* 10: 128–139.
102 Wassmann, K., Wassmann, S., and Nickenig, G. (2005). Progesterone antagonizes the vasoprotective effect of estrogen on antioxidant enzyme expression and function. *Circ. Res.* 97: 1046–1054.
103 Yang, X., Zhang, W., Chen, Y. et al. (2016). Activation of peroxisome proliferator-activated receptor gamma (PPARgamma) and CD36 protein expression: the dual pathophysiological roles of progesterone. *J. Biol. Chem.* 291: 15108–15118.
104 Ahlbom, E., Grandison, L., Bonfoco, E. et al. (1999). Androgen treatment of neonatal rats decreases susceptibility of cerebellar granule neurons to oxidative stress in vitro. *Eur. J. Neurosci.* 11: 1285–1291.
105 Ahlbom, E., Prins, G.S., and Ceccatelli, S. (2001). Testosterone protects cerebellar granule cells from oxidative stress-induced cell death through a receptor mediated mechanism. *Brain Res.* 892: 255–262.
106 Atroshi, F., Paulin, L., Paalanen, T., and Westermarck, T. (1990). Glutathione level in mice brain after testosterone administration. *Adv. Exp. Med. Biol.* 264: 199–202.
107 Pintana, H., Pongkan, W., Pratchayasakul, W. et al. (2015). Testosterone replacement attenuates cognitive decline in testosterone-deprived lean rats, but not in obese rats, by mitigating brain oxidative stress. *Age (Dordr)* 37: 84.
108 Garcia-Estrada, J., Luquin, S., Fernandez, A.M., and Garcia-Segura, L.M. (1999). Dehydroepiandrosterone, pregnenolone and sex steroids down-regulate reactive astroglia in the male rat brain after a penetrating brain injury. *Int. J. Dev. Neurosci.* 17: 145–151.

109 Del Cerro, S., Garcia-Estrada, J., and Garcia-Segura, L.M. (1995). Neuroactive steroids regulate astroglia morphology in hippocampal cultures from adult rats. *Glia* 14: 65–71.

110 Dimayuga, F.O., Reed, J.L., Carnero, G.A. et al. (2005). Estrogen and brain inflammation: effects on microglial expression of MHC, costimulatory molecules and cytokines. *J. Neuroimmunol.* 161: 123–136.

111 Bruce-Keller, A.J., Barger, S.W., Moss, N.I. et al. (2001). Pro-inflammatory and pro-oxidant properties of the HIV protein tat in a microglial cell line: attenuation by 17 beta-estradiol. *J. Neurochem.* 78: 1315–1324.

112 Bruce-Keller, A.J., Keeling, J.L., Keller, J.N. et al. (2000). Antiinflammatory effects of estrogen on microglial activation. *Endocrinology* 141: 3646–3656.

113 Vegeto, E., Pollio, G., Ciana, P., and Maggi, A. (2000). Estrogen blocks inducible nitric oxide synthase accumulation in LPS-activated microglia cells. *Exp. Gerontol.* 35: 1309–1316.

114 Hayashi, T., Yamada, K., Esaki, T. et al. (1998). Physiological concentrations of 17beta-estradiol inhibit the synthesis of nitric oxide synthase in macrophages via a receptor-mediated system. *J. Cardiovasc. Pharmacol.* 31: 292–298.

115 Barger, S.W., Chavis, J.A., and Drew, P.D. (2000). Dehydroepiandrosterone inhibits microglial nitric oxide production in a stimulus-specific manner. *J. Neurosci. Res.* 62: 503–509.

116 Vegeto, E., Bonincontro, C., Pollio, G. et al. (2001). Estrogen prevents the lipopolysaccharide-induced inflammatory response in microglia. *J. Neurosci.* 21: 1809–1818.

117 Chakrabarti, M., Haque, A., Banik, N.L. et al. (2014). Estrogen receptor agonists for attenuation of neuroinflammation and neurodegeneration. *Brain Res. Bull.* 109: 22–31.

118 McKhann, G.M., Knopman, D.S., Chertkow, H. et al. (2011). The diagnosis of dementia due to Alzheimer's disease: recommendations from the National Institute on Aging-Alzheimer's Association workgroups on diagnostic guidelines for Alzheimer's disease. *Alzheimers Dement.* 7: 263–269.

119 Lewis, D.K., Johnson, A.B., Stohlgren, S. et al. (2008). Effects of estrogen receptor agonists on regulation of the inflammatory response in astrocytes from young adult and middle-aged female rats. *J. Neuroimmunol.* 195: 47–59.

120 Kim, H., Bang, O.Y., Jung, M.W. et al. (2001). Neuroprotective effects of estrogen against beta-amyloid toxicity are mediated by estrogen receptors in cultured neuronal cells. *Neurosci. Lett.* 302: 58–62.

121 Zhao, L., Jin, C., Mao, Z. et al. (2007). Design, synthesis, and estrogenic activity of a novel estrogen receptor modulator – a hybrid structure of 17beta-estradiol and vitamin E in hippocampal neurons. *J. Med. Chem.* 50: 4471–4481.

122 Zhao, L. and Brinton, R.D. (2007). Estrogen receptor alpha and beta differentially regulate intracellular Ca(2+) dynamics leading to ERK phosphorylation and estrogen neuroprotection in hippocampal neurons. *Brain Res.* 1172: 48–59.

123 Grossmann, M., Thomas, M.C., Panagiotopoulos, S. et al. (2008). Low testosterone levels are common and associated with insulin resistance in men with diabetes. *J. Clin. Endocrinol. Metab.* 93: 1834–1840.

124 Lage, M.J., Barber, B.L., and Markus, R.A. (2007). Association between androgen-deprivation therapy and incidence of diabetes among males with prostate cancer. *Urology* 70: 1104–1108.

125 Bhasin, S., Parker, R.A., Sattler, F. et al. (2007). Effects of testosterone supplementation on whole body and regional fat mass and distribution in human immunodeficiency virus-infected men with abdominal obesity. *J. Clin. Endocrinol. Metab.* 92: 1049–1057.

126 Asih, P.R., Tegg, M.L., Sohrabi, H. et al. (2017). Multiple mechanisms linking type 2 diabetes and Alzheimer's disease: testosterone as a modifier. *J. Alzheimers Dis.* 59: 445–466.

127 Corbould, A. (2008). Effects of androgens on insulin action in women: is androgen excess a component of female metabolic syndrome? *Diabetes Metab. Res. Rev.* 24: 520–532.

128 Zang, H., Carlstrom, K., Arner, P., and Hirschberg, A.L. (2006). Effects of treatment with testosterone alone or in combination with estrogen on insulin sensitivity in postmenopausal women. *Fertil. Steril.* 86: 136–144.

129 Lv, W., Du, N., Liu, Y. et al. (2016). Low testosterone level and risk of Alzheimer's disease in the elderly men: a systematic review and meta-analysis. *Mol. Neurobiol.* 53: 2679–2684.

130 Xu, J., Xia, L.L., Song, N. et al. (2016). Testosterone, estradiol, and sex hormone-binding globulin in Alzheimer's disease: a meta-analysis. *Curr. Alzheimer Res.* 13: 215–222.

131 Bowen, R.L., Isley, J.P., and Atkinson, R.L. (2000). An association of elevated serum gonadotropin concentrations and Alzheimer disease. *J. Neuroendocrinol.* 12: 351–354.

132 Short, R.A., Bowen, R.L., O'Brien, P.C., and Graff-Radford, N.R. (2001). Elevated gonadotropin levels in patients with Alzheimer disease. *Mayo. Clin. Proc.* 76: 906–909.

133 Rodrigues, A., Queiroz, D.B., Honda, L. et al. (2008). Activation of toll-like receptor 4 (TLR4) by in vivo and in vitro exposure of rat epididymis to lipopolysaccharide from Escherichia Coli. *Biol. Reprod.* 79: 1135–1147.

134 Hyde, Z., Flicker, L., Almeida, O.P. et al. (2010). Higher luteinizing hormone is associated with poor memory recall: the health in men study. *J. Alzheimers Dis.* 19: 943–951.

135 Rodrigues, A., Queiróz, D.B.C., Honda, L. et al. (2008). Activation of toll-like receptor 4 (TLR4) by in vivo and in vitro exposure of rat epididymis to lipopolysaccharide from Escherichia Coli1. *Biol. Rep.* 79: 1135–1147.

136 Chu, C., Gao, G., and Huang, W. (2008). A study on co-localization of FSH and its receptor in rat hippocampus. *J. Mol. Histol.* 39: 49–55.

137 Lei, Z.M., Rao, C.V., Kornyei, J.L. et al. (1993). Novel expression of human chorionic gonadotropin/luteinizing hormone receptor gene in brain. *Endocrinology* 132: 2262–2270.

138 Bowen, R.L., Smith, M.A., Harris, P.L. et al. (2002). Elevated luteinizing hormone expression colocalizes with neurons vulnerable to Alzheimer's disease pathology. *J. Neurosci. Res.* 70: 514–518.

139 Bowen, R.L., Verdile, G., Liu, T. et al. (2004). Luteinizing hormone, a reproductive regulator that modulates the processing of amyloid-beta precursor protein and amyloid-beta deposition. *J. Biol. Chem.* 279: 20539–20545.

140 Casadesus, G., Webber, K.M., Atwood, C.S. et al. (2006). Luteinizing hormone modulates cognition and amyloid-beta deposition in Alzheimer APP transgenic mice. *Biochim. Biophys. Acta.* 1762: 447–452.

141 Wahjoepramono, E.J., Wijaya, L.K., Taddei, K. et al. (2011). Direct exposure of Guinea pig CNS to human luteinizing hormone increases cerebrospinal fluid and cerebral beta amyloid levels. *Neuroendocrinology* 94: 313–322.

142 Casadesus, G., Milliken, E.L., Webber, K.M. et al. (2007). Increases in luteinizing hormone are associated with declines in cognitive performance. *Mol. Cell Endocrinol.* 269: 107–111.

143 Berry, A., Tomidokoro, Y., Ghiso, J., and Thornton, J. (2008). Human chorionic gonadotropin (a luteinizing hormone homologue) decreases spatial memory and increases brain amyloid-beta levels in female rats. *Horm. Behav.* 54: 143–152.

144 Barron, A.M., Verdile, G., Taddei, K. et al. (2010). Effect of chronic hCG administration on Alzheimer's-related cognition and a beta accumulation in PS1KI mice. *Endocrinology* 151: 5380–5388.

145 Verdile, G., Yeap, B.B., Clarnette, R.M. et al. (2008). Luteinizing hormone levels are positively correlated with plasma amyloid-beta protein levels in elderly men. *J. Alzheimers Dis.* 14: 201–208.

146 Dubey, A.K., Herbert, J., Abbott, D.H., and Martensz, N.D. (1984). Serum and CSF concentrations of testosterone and LH related to negative feedback in male rhesus monkeys. *Neuroendocrinology* 39: 176–185.

147 Bagshawe, K.D., Orr, A.H., and Rushworth, A.G. (1968). Relationship between concentrations of human chorionic gonadotrophin in plasma and cerebrospinal fluid. *Nature* 217: 950–951.

148 Lukacs, H., Hiatt, E.S., Lei, Z.M., and Rao, C.V. (1995). Peripheral and intracerebroventricular administration of human chorionic gonadotropin alters several hippocampus-associated behaviors in cycling female rats. *Horm. Behav.* 29: 42–58.

149 Wilson, A.C., Salamat, M.S., Haasl, R.J. et al. (2006). Human neurons express type I GnRH receptor and respond to GnRH I by increasing luteinizing hormone expression. *J. Endocrinol.* 191: 651–663.

150 Palm, R., Chang, J., Blair, J. et al. (2014). Down-regulation of serum gonadotropins but not estrogen replacement improves cognition in aged-ovariectomized 3xTg AD female mice. *J. Neurochem.* 130: 115–125.

151 Lei, Z.M. and Rao, C.V. (2001). Neural actions of luteinizing hormone and human chorionic gonadotropin. *Semin. Reprod. Med.* 19: 103–109.

152 Lin, J., Li, X., Yuan, F. et al. (2010). Genetic ablation of luteinizing hormone receptor improves the amyloid pathology in a mouse model of Alzheimer disease. *J. Neuropathol. Exp. Neurol.* 69: 253–261.

153 Lee, C., Ji, I., Ryu, K. et al. (2002). Two defective heterozygous luteinizing hormone receptors can rescue hormone action. *J. Biol. Chem.* 277: 15795–15800.

154 Lee, C., Ji, I.J., and Ji, T.H. (2002). Use of defined-function mutants to access receptor-receptor interactions. *Methods* 27: 318–323.

155 Bowen, R.L., Perry, G., Xiong, C. et al. (2014). A clinical study of Lupron depot in the treatment of women with Alzheimer's disease: preservation of cognitive function in patients taking an Acetylcholinesterase inhibitor and treated with high dose Lupron over 48 weeks. *J. Alzheimers Dis.*

156 Rocca, W.A., Grossardt, B.R., and Shuster, L.T. (2014). Oophorectomy, estrogen, and dementia: a 2014 update. *Mol. Cell Endocrinol.* 389: 7–12.

157 Hogervorst, E., Williams, J., Budge, M. et al. (2000). The nature of the effect of female gonadal hormone replacement therapy on cognitive function in post-menopausal women: a meta-analysis. *Neuroscience* 101: 485–512.

158 Mulnard, R.A. (2000). Estrogen as a treatment for alzheimer disease. *JAMA* 284: 307–308.

159 Baldereschi, M., Di Carlo, A., Lepore, V. et al. (1998). Estrogen-replacement therapy and Alzheimer's disease in the Italian longitudinal study on aging. *Neurology* 50: 996–1002.

160 Kawas, C., Resnick, S., Morrison, A. et al. (1997). A prospective study of estrogen replacement therapy and the risk of developing Alzheimer's disease: the Baltimore longitudinal study of aging. *Neurology* 48: 1517–1521.

161 Tang, M.X., Jacobs, D., Stern, Y. et al. (1996). Effect of oestrogen during menopause on risk and age at onset of Alzheimer's disease. *Lancet.* 348: 429–432.

162 Brenner, D.E., Kukull, W.A., Stergachis, A. et al. (1994). Postmenopausal estrogen replacement therapy and the risk of Alzheimer's disease: a population-based case-control study. *Am. J. Epidemiol.* 140: 262–267.

163 Yaffe, K. (2001). Estrogens, selective estrogen receptor modulators, and dementia: what is the evidence? *Ann. N. Y. Acad. Sci.* 949: 215–222.

164 Espeland, M.A., Rapp, S.R., Shumaker, S.A. et al., Women's Health Initiative memory S (2004). Conjugated equine estrogens and global cognitive function in postmenopausal women: Women's Health Initiative memory study. *JAMA* 291: 2959–2968.

165 Shumaker, S.A., Legault, C., Rapp, S.R. et al. (2003). Estrogen plus progestin and the incidence of dementia and mild cognitive impairment in postmenopausal women: the Women's Health Initiative Memory Study: a randomized controlled trial. *JAMA* 289: 2651–2662.

166 Yaffe, K., Haan, M., Byers, A. et al. (2000). Estrogen use, APOE, and cognitive decline: evidence of gene-environment interaction. *Neurology* 54: 1949–1954.

167 Burkhardt, M.S., Foster, J.K., Laws, S.M. et al. (2004). Oestrogen replacement therapy may improve memory functioning in the absence of APOE epsilon4. *J. Alzheimers Dis.* 6: 221–228.

168 Henderson, V.W., Benke, K.S., Green, R.C. et al. (2005). Postmenopausal hormone therapy and Alzheimer's disease risk: interaction with age. *J. Neurol. Neurosurg. Psychiatry* 76: 103–105.

169 Shao, H., Breitner, J.C., Whitmer, R.A. et al. (2012). Hormone therapy and Alzheimer disease dementia: new findings from the Cache County study. *Neurology* 79: 1846–1852.

170 Marjoribanks, J., Farquhar, C., Roberts, H. et al. (2017). Long-term hormone therapy for perimenopausal and postmenopausal women. *Cochrane Database Syst. Rev.* 1: CD004143.

171 Imtiaz, B., Taipale, H., Tanskanen, A. et al. (2017). Risk of Alzheimer's disease among users of postmenopausal hormone therapy: a nationwide case-control study. *Maturitas* 98: 7–13.

172 Imtiaz, B., Tuppurainen, M., Rikkonen, T. et al. (2017). Postmenopausal hormone therapy and Alzheimer disease: a prospective cohort study. *Neurology* 88: 1062–1068.

173 Castelo-Branco, C., Fuste, P., Martinez de Osaba, M.J., and Gonzalez-Merlo, J. (1992). Hormone replacement therapy and changes on pituitary function. *Eur. J. Obstet. Gynecol. Reprod. Biol.* 43: 59–63.

174 Lambrinoudaki, I., Armeni, E., Rizos, D. et al. (2011). Sex hormones in postmenopausal women receiving low-dose hormone therapy: the effect of BMI. *Obesity (Silver Spring)* 19: 988–993.

175 Ushiroyama, T., Sakuma, K., Ikeda, A., and Ueki, M. (2004). Adequate reduction degree of pituitary gonadotropin levels in the clinical management of short-term hormone replacement therapy of women with menopausal symptoms. *J. Med.* 35: 281–294.

176 Ushiroyama, T., Sakai, M., Higashiyama, T. et al. (2001). Estrogen replacement therapy in postmenopausal women: a study of the efficacy of estriol and changes in plasma gonadotropin levels. *Gynecol. Endocrinol.* 15: 74–80.

177 Hogervorst, E. (2013). Effects of gonadal hormones on cognitive behaviour in elderly men and women. *J. Neuroendocrinol.* 25: 1182–1195.

178 Li, H.J., Zhou, B.L., Bai, L.L. et al. (2003). A tentative research of testosterone supplement therapy on male senile dementia. *Zhonghua Nan Ke Xue* 9: 193–196.

179 Cherrier, M.M., Matsumoto, A.M., Amory, J.K. et al. (2005). Testosterone improves spatial memory in men with Alzheimer disease and mild cognitive impairment. *Neurology* 64: 2063–2068.

180 Lu, P.H., Masterman, D.A., Mulnard, R. et al. (2006). Effects of testosterone on cognition and mood in male patients with mild Alzheimer disease and healthy elderly men. *Arch. Neurol.* 63: 177–185.

181 Kenny, A.M., Fabregas, G., Song, C. et al. (2004). Effects of testosterone on behavior, depression, and cognitive function in older men with mild cognitive loss. *J. Gerontol. A Biol. Sci. Med. Sci.* 59: 75–78.

182 Tan, R.S. and Pu, S.J. (2003). A pilot study on the effects of testosterone in hypogonadal aging male patients with Alzheimer's disease. *Aging Male* 6: 13–17.

183 Holland, J., Bandelow, S., and Hogervorst, E. (2011). Testosterone levels and cognition in elderly men: a review. *Maturitas* 69: 322–337.

184 Resnick, S.M., Matsumoto, A.M., Stephens-Shields, A.J. et al. (2017). Testosterone treatment and cognitive function in older men with low testosterone and age-associated memory impairment. *JAMA* 317: 717–727.

185 Jung, H.J. and Shin, H.S. (2016). Effect of testosterone replacement therapy on cognitive performance and depression in men with testosterone deficiency syndrome. *World J. Mens Health* 34: 194–199.

186 Huang, G., Wharton, W., Bhasin, S. et al. (2016). Effects of long-term testosterone administration on cognition in older men with low or low-to-normal testosterone concentrations: a prespecified secondary analysis of data from the randomised, double-blind, placebo-controlled TEAAM trial. *Lancet. Diabetes Endocrinol.* 4: 657–665.

187 Cherrier, M.M., Asthana, S., Plymate, S. et al. (2001). Testosterone supplementation improves spatial and verbal memory in healthy older men. *Neurology* 57: 80–88.

188 Cherrier, M.M., Plymate, S., Mohan, S. et al. (2004). Relationship between testosterone supplementation and insulin-like growth factor-I levels and cognition in healthy older men. *Psychoneuroendocrinology* 29: 65–82.

189 Cherrier, M.M., Matsumoto, A.M., Amory, J.K. et al. (2007). Characterization of verbal and spatial memory changes from moderate to supraphysiological increases in serum testosterone in healthy older men. *Psychoneuroendocrinology* 32: 72–79.

190 Haren, M.T., Wittert, G.A., Chapman, I.M. et al. (2005). Effect of oral testosterone undecanoate on visuospatial cognition, mood and quality of life in elderly men with low-normal gonadal status. *Maturitas* 50: 124–133.

191 Emmelot-Vonk, M.H., Verhaar, H.J., Nakhai Pour, H.R. et al. (2008). Effect of testosterone supplementation on functional mobility, cognition, and other parameters in older men: a randomized controlled trial. *JAMA* 299: 39–52.

192 Young, L.A., Neiss, M.B., Samuels, M.H. et al. (2010). Cognition is not modified by large but temporary changes in sex hormones in men. *J. Clin. Endocrinol. Metab.* 95: 280–288.

193 Matousek, R.H. and Sherwin, B.B. (2010). Sex steroid hormones and cognitive functioning in healthy, older men. *Horm. Behav.* 57: 352–359.

194 Muller, M., Aleman, A., Grobbee, D.E. et al. (2005). Endogenous sex hormone levels and cognitive function in aging men: is there an optimal level? *Neurology* 64: 866–871.

195 Barrett-Connor, E. (2005). Male testosterone: what is normal? *Clin. Endocrinol. (Oxf)* 62: 263–264.

196 Hogervorst, E., Matthews, F.E., and Brayne, C. (2010). Are optimal levels of testosterone associated with better cognitive function in healthy older women and men? *Biochim. Biophys. Acta* 1800: 1145–1152.

197 Raber, J., Bongers, G., LeFevour, A. et al. (2002). Androgens protect against apolipoprotein E4-induced cognitive deficits. *J. Neurosci.* 22: 5204–5209.

198 Wahjoepramono, E.J., Asih, P.R., Aniwiyanti, V. et al. (2016). The effects of testosterone supplementation on cognitive functioning in older men. *CNS Neurol. Disord. Drug Targets* 15: 337–343.

199 Asih, P.R., Wahjoepramono, E.J., Aniwiyanti, V. et al. (2015). Testosterone replacement therapy in older male subjective memory complainers: double-blind randomized crossover placebo-controlled clinical trial of physiological assessment and safety. *CNS Neurol. Disord. Drug Targets* 14: 576–586.

200 Asih, P.R., Chatterjee, P., Verdile, G. et al. (2014). Clearing the amyloid in Alzheimer's: progress towards earlier diagnosis and effective treatments – an update for clinicians. *Neurodegener. Dis. Manag.* 4: 363–378.

201 Rinnab, L., Gust, K., Hautmann, R.E., and Kufer, R. (2009). Testosterone replacement therapy and prostate cancer. The current position 67 years after the Huggins myth. *Urologe A* 48: 516–522.

202 Feneley, M.R. and Carruthers, M. (2012). Is testosterone treatment good for the prostate? Study of safety during long-term treatment. *J. Sex Med.* 9: 2138–2149.

203 Walsh, J.P. and Kitchens, A.C. (2015). Testosterone therapy and cardiovascular risk. *Trends Cardiovasc. Med.*, 25 (3): 250–257.

204 Yeap, B.B. (2015). Testosterone and cardiovascular disease risk. *Curr. Opin. Endocrinol. Diabetes Obes.* 22: 193–202.

205 Green, A.R., Parrott, E.L., Butterworth, M. et al. (2001). Comparisons of the effects of tamoxifen, toremifene and raloxifene on enzyme induction and gene expression in the ovariectomised rat uterus. *J. Endocrinol.* 170: 555–564.

206 Thomas, T., Bryant, M., Clark, L. et al. (2001). Estrogen and raloxifene activities on amyloid-beta-induced inflammatory reaction. *Microvasc. Res.* 61: 28–39.

207 Spampinato, S.F., Molinaro, G., Merlo, S. et al. (2012). Estrogen receptors and type 1 metabotropic glutamate receptors are interdependent in protecting cortical neurons against beta-amyloid toxicity. *Mol. Pharmacol.* 81: 12–20.

208 Benvenuti, S., Luciani, P., Vannelli, G.B. et al. (2005). Estrogen and selective estrogen receptor modulators exert neuroprotective effects and stimulate the expression of selective Alzheimer's disease indicator-1, a recently discovered antiapoptotic gene, in human neuroblast long-term cell cultures. *J. Clin. Endocrinol. Metab.* 90: 1775–1782.

209 Bagheri, M., Joghataei, M.T., Mohseni, S., and Roghani, M. (2011). Genistein ameliorates learning and memory deficits in amyloid beta(1-40) rat model of Alzheimer's disease. *Neurobiol. Learn Mem.* 95: 270–276.

210 Gray, N.E., Zweig, J.A., Kawamoto, C. et al. (2016). STX, a novel membrane estrogen receptor ligand, protects against amyloid-beta toxicity. *J. Alzheimers Dis.* 51: 391–403.

211 Simpkins, J.W. and Dykens, J.A. (2008). Mitochondrial mechanisms of estrogen neuroprotection. *Brain Res. Rev.* 57: 421–430.

212 Henderson, V.W., Ala, T., Sainani, K.L. et al. (2015). Raloxifene for women with Alzheimer disease: a randomized controlled pilot trial. *Neurology* 85: 1937–1944.

213 Pandey, D., Banerjee, S., Basu, M., and Mishra, N. (2016). Memory enhancement by Tamoxifen on amyloidosis mouse model. *Horm. Behav.* 79: 70–73.

214 Ohmichi, M., Tasaka, K., Kurachi, H., and Murata, Y. (2005). Molecular mechanism of action of selective estrogen receptor modulator in target tissues. *Endocr. J.* 52: 161–167.

215 Marin, R., Marrero-Alonso, J., Fernandez, C. et al. (2012). Estrogen receptors in lipid raft signalling complexes for neuroprotection. *Front Biosci. (Elite Ed)* (4): 1420–1433.

216 Adams, M.M., Fink, S.E., Shah, R.A. et al. (2002). Estrogen and aging affect the subcellular distribution of estrogen receptor-alpha in the hippocampus of female rats. *J. Neurosci.* 22: 3608–3614.

217 Milner, T.A., McEwen, B.S., Hayashi, S. et al. (2001). Ultrastructural evidence that hippocampal alpha estrogen receptors are located at extranuclear sites. *J. Comp. Neurol.* 429: 355–371.

218 Zhao, L., Mao, Z., Chen, S. et al. (2013). Early intervention with an estrogen receptor beta-selective phytoestrogenic formulation prolongs survival, improves spatial recognition memory, and slows progression of amyloid pathology in a female mouse model of Alzheimer's disease. *J. Alzheimers Dis.* 37: 403–419.

219 Zhao, L., Liu, S., Wang, Y. et al. (2015). Effects of Curculigoside on memory impairment and bone loss via anti-oxidative character in APP/PS1 mutated transgenic mice. *PLoS One* 10: e0133289.

220 Gao, W. and Dalton, J.T. (2007). Expanding the therapeutic use of androgens via selective androgen receptor modulators (SARMs). *Drug Discov. Today* 12: 241–248.

221 Venken, K., Boonen, S., Van Herck, E. et al. (2005). Bone and muscle protective potential of the prostate-sparing synthetic androgen 7alpha-methyl-19-nortestosterone: evidence from the aged orchidectomized male rat model. *Bone* 36: 663–670.

222 Shao, T.C., Li, H.L., Kasper, S. et al. (2006). Comparison of the growth-promoting effects of testosterone and 7-alpha-methyl-19-nor-testosterone (MENT) on the prostate and levator ani muscle of LPB-tag transgenic mice. *Prostate* 66: 369–376.

223 George, S., Petit, G.H., Gouras, G.K. et al. (2013). Nonsteroidal selective androgen receptor modulators and selective estrogen receptor beta agonists moderate cognitive deficits and amyloid-beta levels in a mouse model of Alzheimer's disease. *ACS Chem. Neurosci.* 4: 1537–1548.

224 Periti, P., Mazzei, T., and Mini, E. (2002). Clinical pharmacokinetics of depot leuprorelin. *Clin. Pharmacokinet.* 41: 485–504.

225 Bowen RL, Beaird H, Atwood CS, Smith MA, Rimm AA (2004) In 9th International Congress on AD., Philadelphia, USA.

226 D'Amico, A.V., Braccioforte, M.H., Moran, B.J., and Chen, M.H. (2010). Luteinizing-hormone releasing hormone therapy and the risk of death from Alzheimer disease. *Alzheimer Dis. Assoc. Disord.* 24: 85–89.

227 Bowen, R.L., Perry, G., Xiong, C. et al. (2015). A clinical study of lupron depot in the treatment of women with Alzheimer's disease: preservation of cognitive function in patients taking an acetylcholinesterase inhibitor and treated with high dose lupron over 48 weeks. *J. Alzheimers. Dis.* 44: 549–560.

228 Blair, J.A., Palm, R., Chang, J. et al. (2016). Luteinizing hormone downregulation but not estrogen replacement improves ovariectomy-associated cognition and spine density loss independently of treatment onset timing. *Horm. Behav.* 78: 60–66.

229 Gutierrez, H. and Davies, A.M. (2011). Regulation of neural process growth, elaboration and structural plasticity by NF-kappaB. *Trends Neurosci.* 34: 316–325.

13

The Link Between Exercise and Mediation of Alzheimer's Disease and Neurodegenerative Diseases

Belinda Brown[1,2] *and Tejal M. Shah*[3,4]

[1] *School of Psychology and Exercise Science, Murdoch University, Perth, WA, Australia*
[2] *Australian Alzheimer's Research Foundation, Ralph and Patricia Sarich Neuroscience Research Institute, Nedlands, WA, Australia*
[3] *Centre of Excellence for Alzheimer's Disease Research and Care, School of Medical and Health Sciences, Edith Cowan University, Joondalup, WA, Australia*
[4] *Department of Biomedical Sciences, Macquarie University, Sydney, NSW, Australia*

13.1 Introduction

Ageing is the greatest risk factor for neurodegenerative disorders. Although ageing is inevitable, the concept of successful physical and mental ageing [1] has led researchers to investigate the impact of lifestyle modifications on neuroprotection in older adults. Alzheimer's disease (AD) is the most common neurodegenerative disease. Currently, available AD therapeutic treatments mainly target the manifestations of clinical dementia, by which stage irreversible brain damage has already occurred. Yet these treatments have no effect on the course or inevitability of further neurodegeneration. In the last decade, newly developed sophisticated imaging methods, such as Pittsburgh compound B positron emission tomography (PiB-PET), have led to the understanding that the pathology of AD begins to develop decades before the onset of symptoms. Thus, attention in many research laboratories has shifted focus to identifying preventive treatments or lifestyle strategies that will preserve and/or enhance cognition, in middle-aged to older adults who are either disease-free or in early pre-clinical stages, with the hope of preventing or delaying the onset of AD and other neurodegenerative diseases. The term "lifestyle" encompasses numerous factors, including diet, exercise, employment, cognitive activities, and socialisation. Here we discuss the mounting evidence that physical activity/exercise[1] is neuroprotective due to its benefits to cognition and numerous other brain function parameters. Indeed, physical inactivity has been recognised as one of the seven greatest modifiable risk factors of AD [3] and 35% of all dementia cases are due to these lifestyle risk factors [4]. Pre-clinical and epidemiological studies now provide reasonable evidence to suggest that exercise may

---

1 It is important to note the distinction between physical activity and exercise used in this chapter: 'physical activity' refers to any physical movement resulting in increased heart rate and breathing (can include household activities, exercise, occupational activity, etc.); 'exercise' refers to any planned and structured physical activity that is conducted with the aim of improving or maintaining physical fitness. See [2].

Neurodegeneration and Alzheimer's Disease: The Role of Diabetes, Genetics, Hormones, and Lifestyle,
First Edition. Edited by Ralph N. Martins, Charles S. Brennan, W.M.A.D. Binosha Fernando,
Margaret A. Brennan and Stephanie J. Fuller.
© 2019 John Wiley & Sons Ltd. Published 2019 by John Wiley & Sons Ltd.

be a safe and effective strategy for delaying or even preventing cognitive impairment in later life.

Research indicates that brain plasticity is retained to some extent throughout adult life, and the promotion of repair and regeneration mechanisms can contribute to successful ageing. Cross-sectional and epidemiological studies have demonstrated that increases in physical activity and cardiovascular fitness in older adults are associated with improved cognition, as assessed by various neuropsychological tests [5, 6]. There is also robust literature indicating that the most significant form of exercise intervention for neuroprotection and brain health is aerobic exercise. Aerobic exercise, in particular, has been shown to reduce risk of cardiovascular diseases; it is also positively associated with biomarkers of brain health and enhanced cognitive performance [7, 8]. There is also some evidence that non-aerobic exercises, such as resistance and strength training, are also linked to enhanced cognition [9].

The current evidence supporting a link between exercise and cognition is reviewed in this chapter, and suggests that cognitive decline and dementia risk can be significantly reduced by undertaking regular physical activity [10, 11]. The purpose of this chapter is to summarise the existing evidence, with an emphasis on human cognitive performance. We discuss clinical implications and implementation of exercise interventions aimed at improving brain health. This chapter also includes discussion of potential mechanisms of action through which physical activity may mediate improved brain health and cognitive performance. This includes physiological changes occurring due to exercise-induced changes such as alterations in neurotransmitter levels, structural changes in the central nervous system, and other chemical, molecular, and cellular mechanisms.

13.2 Physical Activity Promotes Health and Well-being

It is well known that physical activity benefits major body organs and systems – the heart, skeletal muscles, bones, blood, the immune system, and the nervous system. Many studies have shown that increases in longevity can be achieved by undertaking 150–300 minutes of moderate intensity or 75–150 minutes of vigorous intensity aerobic activity per week, as recommended by major health organisations worldwide [12]. Importantly, non-communicable diseases such as hypertension, type 2 diabetes, and heart disease, all of which independently increase AD risk, are greatly reduced by physical activity. In fact, the well-documented numerous health benefits of physical activity in all age groups indicate that it should be encouraged throughout the human lifespan.

13.3 Neuroplasticity

Before evaluating the impact of exercise on cognition and brain health, it is necessary to understand the brain's capability to undergo change and repair. It was once believed that nerve cells could not be regenerated upon damage or injury, and that the corresponding brain functions would be permanently lost. However, there is now evidence that the brain continues to adjust and reorganise itself by forming new nerve cells [13] and neural connections throughout life. The term 'neuroplasticity' was coined to describe the concept of the brain's ability to compensate for injury or to respond to a stimulus [14]. Neuroplasticity is evident from the fact that rehabilitation techniques implemented at the correct time are known to aid significantly in recovering brain functions that have been damaged as a result of stroke, traumatic brain injury, or other cerebrovascular injuries. There is now considerable evidence that physical activity and exercise can enhance neuroplasticity and many aspects of cognition [15]. Moreover, there is much evidence that individuals with higher cardiovascular fitness have enhanced brain plasticity [16]. The molecular mechanisms through which physical activity mediates change at the cerebrovascular level, on specific neurodegenerative biomarkers and cognition are discussed further in this chapter.

13.4 The Link Between Physical Activity and Cognition Across the Human Lifespan

There is accumulating evidence that higher levels of physical activity are associated with better cognition throughout the lifespan [17–19]. Following a dose-response relationship, it has been shown that participating in lifelong physical activity provides significant benefits to memory and executive functioning (i.e. planning, organising, problem solving, and concentration) in middle-aged adults [20]. Physically active younger adults also have higher cognition than their sedentary counterparts, which is maintained over time. In studies of depression and mood disorders, which are known to increase the risk of cognitive impairment [21, 22], it has been shown that physical activity alleviates depression and improves mood, thereby promoting mental health in older adults [23, 24]. Figure 13.1 shows the neurocognitive benefits of physical activity/higher fitness levels across the lifespan.

13.4.1 Childhood

Observational and review studies indicate that physical activity, physical fitness, and physical education are positively associated with cognition and academic performance in school-aged children and preadolescents [25–27]. More specifically, enhanced processing speed and higher measures of neuroelectric responsiveness (brain-evoked potentials) and executive control processes have been associated with aerobic fitness in children [28, 29]. Furthermore, in children aged 10–13 years, a significant association between vigorous activity obtained outside school and academic achievement has been reported [30]. Intervention studies also report improved performance in academic and cognitive tasks following exercise programs [31, 32]; for example, improved executive function, and increased neuronal activity in the associated frontal brain region, have been observed in overweight children trained with aerobic exercise for 40 minutes per day, 5 days per week for 15 weeks, compared to a control group [32]. Combined, these studies provide evidence that physical activity can impact cognition as early as childhood. The positive benefits of exercise on cognition are again observed across adulthood and midlife, as discussed below.

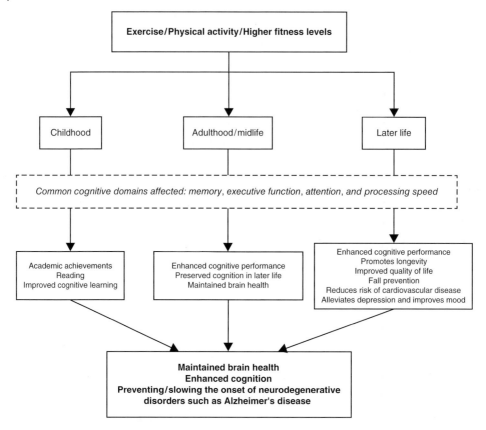

Figure 13.1 Influence of exercise and physical activity on brain health across the lifespan.

13.4.2 Adulthood and Midlife

Most studies exploring links between physical activity and cognition have been conducted in children or older adults, with little work completed on middle-aged cohorts. Nevertheless, a small number of studies with longitudinal follow-up have reported a positive relationship between staying physically active and maintaining cognition during midlife. For example, self-reported physical exercise at 36 years is associated with a slower rate of cognitive decline (verbal memory) between the ages of 43 and 53 years; and consistent regular exercise is required after 36 years of age to maintain brain health [33]. Moreover, low levels of physical activity in people between 35 and 55 years of age is a risk factor for poor cognitive function in middle age [34] and cardiovascular fitness at 18 years of age has been shown to be associated with cognition in later life [35]. Regular exercise, particularly in adulthood, has a lasting benefit on cognition in later life. Recommended activities include engagement in routine leisure activities, avoiding long hours of sitting, acute bouts of intense exercise, and engagement in workplace-based wellness programs [36].

Few studies have examined the role of exercise training on cognition in younger adults. One study of aerobic exercise training undertaken in individuals 21–45 years of age resulted in improved verbal memory in association with an increased cerebral blood volume in the hippocampus, as well as improved physical fitness levels [37]. Exercise-induced brain changes are discussed in more detail later in the chapter.

13.4.3 Older Adults

An array of evidence links higher levels of physical activity with enhanced cognition in later life and old age. The first studies to establish this link were primarily conducted in prospective cohort studies of healthy older adults. A pioneering study compared young and old racquet sportsmen, as well as runners and sedentary individuals, on simple, choice, and movement time tasks: Spirduso and colleagues observed that older athletes performed better than older sedentary adults, and produced similar results to the performance of young sedentary adults [38]. Studies mainly relying on self-reported questionnaires show that physical activity, mostly in the form of greater and more intense participation in leisure time physical activities, benefits cognition [39–43]. In another observational study, it was shown that women who reported walking the most showed decreased risk of cognitive decline over a five- to eight-year period [44]. Similarly, lower physical fitness was found to be associated with greater cognitive decline over a six-year period [45]. Table 13.1 includes a list of studies examining the relationship between physical activity, exercise, and measures of neurocognitive health in cognitively healthy older adults.

An important consideration when examining the link between physical activity and brain health is the type of physical activity (i.e. aerobic vs. resistance training) that may contribute to cognitive improvement. Many interventional studies have investigated whether aerobic exercise (i.e. contributes to increased cardiovascular fitness) is more likely to enhance cognition than other forms of exercise. For example, in a randomised

Table 13.1 Studies showing a relationship between physical activity, exercise, and neurocognitive measures in healthy older adults.

Type of research	Physical activity measurement/exercise type	Associated neuro-cognitive benefits	References
Observational	Higher cardiorespiratory fitness	Higher levels of cognition: including memory and executive functions	[5, 6, 46]
		Larger brain volume	[47–50]
		Protects against cognitive decline	[46]
	Higher levels of habitual physical activity	Higher levels of cognition: including memory and executive functions	[20, 39, 42, 43]
		Larger brain volume	[51–53]
		Protects against cognitive decline	[41, 44, 54]
		Reduced dementia risk	[55–59]
Interventional	Aerobic exercise	Improved cognition	[8, 60, 61]
		Increased brain volume	[7, 62]
	Resistance training	Improved cognition	[9, 63, 64]

controlled trial, a six-month walking intervention improved executive function, compared with a stretching and toning intervention [7, 65]. In another study, a reduction in reaction time (i.e. improved performance) was observed in the aerobic intervention group, when compared to an anaerobic intervention group [66]. However, a combination of two forms of exercise appears to provide even greater benefits, as a meta-analysis of 18 intervention studies revealed that a combination of aerobic and strength training provides greater benefit than aerobic exercise alone [67]. Some studies report that resistance training can also improve cognitive domains of executive functions, memory, and attention [9, 63]. However, aerobic and resistance training may enhance cognition differently depending on how they influence neurocognitive networks [68]. Overall, these studies indicate that aerobic exercise alone, or in combination with resistance anaerobic exercise, promotes an improvement in cognition among the elderly.

13.5 Physical Activity Reduces the Risk of Dementia and AD

Even though there is a plethora of evidence linking physical activity to cognition, this does not necessarily reflect an association between physical activity and dementia/AD risk. Thus, numerous studies have investigated the potential of physical activity to prevent, delay, or slow the progression of dementia, and have found that active older adults have a lower risk of incident dementia [55, 57, 59, 69, 70]. Indeed, it has been demonstrated that higher levels of physical activity at 65 years and above has been associated with a lower risk of developing dementia, compared with subjects exercising less than three times per week, at a six-year follow–up [56]. Furthermore, some well-cited longitudinal observational studies such as the Honolulu-Asia Aging Study and the Bronx Aging Study have demonstrated that walking and dancing (respectively) both contribute to a lowered risk of dementia [58, 69].

In regard to AD studies (as opposed to the above studies that investigated overall dementia risk only), there is evidence that regular and higher levels of physical activity lower the risk of developing AD [71–73]. Results from interventional studies also show that subjects at risk of AD can benefit from physical exercise [8, 74]. Individuals with mild cognitive impairment undertaking an aerobic and strength-training intervention (three times a week for 50 minutes over 6 months) showed improved cognition and an absence of cognitive decline [8]. Besides AD, physical activity also protects against the risk of developing Parkinson's disease, which is the second most common neurodegenerative disease after AD [75–77]. Although the interactions between the type, intensity, duration, and frequency of physical activity and its effects on cognitive domains remain to be determined, the following mechanisms may provide insight as to how exercise may enhance cognition.

13.6 Mechanisms Underlying the Relationship Between Exercise and Brain Health

As discussed in the previous sections of this chapter, there is compelling evidence that higher levels of physical activity can enhance cognitive function and reduce dementia/AD risk. Nevertheless, the mechanisms through which these associations may exist are still being determined. Research to date has highlighted a number of

Table 13.2 Mechanisms by which physical activity can protect the brain.

Mechanism	Method of assessment	Biological effects of physical activity (and a selection of references)
Modulation of Aβ levels (either via alterations to deposition and/or clearance)	Animal models	Decreased accumulation of Aβ in transgenic models following wheel running, increased Aβ clearance following wheel running in aged mice, and high-intensity exercise in transgenic mice increasing levels of neprilysin, insulin-degrading enzyme and other proteins which facilitate Aβ clearance [78, 79]
	Human studies: PET scanning	Decreased levels of brain Aβ in higher exercising individuals [80–82]
		No association found in MCI patients [83]
Enhancing BDNF production	Animals models	Increased BDNF mRNA in hippocampus in exercising animals [84]
	Human studies: blood sampling	Numerous studies have reported increased peripheral BDNF following acute bouts of exercise (for a comprehensive review see [85])
Enhancing IGF-1 production	Animal models	Wheel running induced uptake of blood IGF-1 by groups of neurons [86]
	Human studies: blood sampling	Six-month moderate- or high-intensity interventions were associated with increased levels of serum IGF-1 [63]
Increasing neurotransmitters	Animal models	Exercising was associated with increased levels of dopamine [87] and acetylcholine [88]
Increasing brain volume	Human studies: volumetric MRI	Increased grey-matter volume following a six-month intervention [7]
		Increased hippocampal volume following a one-year intervention [62]
Enhancing functional brain networks	Human studies: functional MRI	Enhanced brain connectivity in networks susceptible to age-related decline was observed in individuals following an exercise intervention [89]

potential mechanisms through which physical activity may modulate brain health, including influencing AD pathology (Aβ deposition and hyperphosphorylated tau levels), induction of growth factors (neurotrophins), alterations to hormone levels, and through reduction of cardiovascular and metabolic disease risk factors (Table 13.2 provides a brief overview of the mechanisms and studies discussed below).

13.6.1 Evidence from Molecular and Cellular Research

As described in other chapters, excessive production or reduced clearance/proteolysis of brain Aβ is a key part of AD pathogenesis. Animal studies have demonstrated that both soluble Aβ peptides and Aβ plaque levels are lowered by exercise in AD transgenic mice [78, 79, 90–93]. Furthermore, a recent study has indicated that the intensity of exercise may play an important role in lowering Aβ levels: high-intensity exercise was significantly more effective at lowering soluble Aβ, compared with low-intensity exercise and sedentary conditions [94]. Aβ is produced from the amyloid precursor protein (APP), which is cleaved via one of two competing pathways: the non-amyloidogenic pathway and amyloidogenic pathway [95]. Evidence from animal studies suggests that exercise may contribute to both the inhibition of APP processing, as well as enhancement of Aβ clearance in the brain. Indeed, decreased levels of APP cleavage fragments (αCTFs and βCTFs), have been observed in exercising transgenic mice, suggesting exercise contributes to decreasing Aβ processing by reducing APP processing [78, 90]. Furthermore, exercise-induced increases in activity of neprilysin and insulin-degrading enzyme (IDE), both known Aβ proteases, suggest a positive effect of exercise on Aβ degradation and clearance [94, 96]. Similarly, Maesako et al. [97] demonstrated the enzymatic activity of neprilysin was significantly higher in exercising transgenic mice compared with mice exposed to diet control, indicating that exercise may upregulate the enzymatic activity of neprilysin to a greater extent than caloric restriction. Nevertheless, Adlard and colleagues [78] reported reduced Aβ in the brains of mice following one month of exercise, independent of changes to IDE and neprilysin mRNA and protein levels, suggesting that only the enzymatic activity of these proteases is altered by exercise.

The accumulation of neurofibrillary tangles, comprising hyperphosphorylated tau, is associated with the development of clinical symptoms in AD [98]. Significant reductions in full-length and hyperphosphorylated tau have been observed in exercising tau-transgenic mice [99–101]. Furthermore, three [85] and five [90] months of forced wheel-running have been associated with a reversal of tau phosphorylation. Studying a human population, Liang and colleagues [80] reported lower exercise levels to be associated with higher cerebrospinal fluid (CSF) total tau and phosphorylated tau. With very recent advances in tau neuroimaging, the relationship between exercise and brain tau in human populations will likely be a highly studied topic in coming years.

13.6.2 Neurotrophins

A large quantity of research suggests that one of the most important ways exercise maintains brain health is through the induction of both neurotransmitters and neurotrophins. Low levels of many neurotransmitters are associated with AD; particularly acetylcholine which is the target for commonly used AD pharmaceutical treatments. Animal studies have shown that numerous neurotransmitters, including acetylcholine, serotonin, dopamine, epinephrine, and norepinephrine are all increased following exercise [87]. Thus, it is possible that the induction of neurotransmitters following exercise may contribute to enhanced cognitive function and/or prevention of cognitive decline. Nevertheless, to date, the most convincing evidence concerning the mechanisms underlying the association between physical activity and brain health indicates roles for growth factors, particularly for brain-derived neurotrophic factor (BDNF), insulin-like growth factor-1 (IGF-1), and vascular endothelial growth factor (VEGF).

Numerous studies have shown that BDNF levels are raised following exercise [102]: rat models demonstrated a positive dose-response in brain BDNF levels following wheel running, and in humans, BDNF has been measured in blood fractions, with higher levels of BDNF observed immediately following exercise [103–105]. BDNF is well-known to be associated with the growth, survival, and differentiation of neurons, and levels are reduced in the brains of people with AD [106]. Similarly, a reduction in IGF-1 expression and signalling has also been previously associated with more severe AD pathology, and it has been suggested that IGF-1 may have a protective role against AD [107, 108]. Similar to BDNF, IGF-1 plays a role in mediating physical activity-induced neuron growth and survival, and also has a positive effect on cerebral vasculature [109]. Physical activity has been shown to regulate levels of IGF-1 in the blood, and induce the uptake of circulating IGF-1 into the brain [110]. It is likely that a synergistic relationship between BDNF and IGF-1 exists. For example, the blocking of IGF-1 prevents the induction of BDNF in response to exercise. Furthermore, IGF-1 increases levels of the BDNF receptor, which in turn increases levels of BDNF signalling [111]. Lastly, VEGF likely plays an important role in angiogenic processes, but has also been identified as a neurotrophic factor [112]. Animal studies have observed an increased production of VEGF during exercise [113]. It is hypothesised that exercise-induced VEGF is an attempt to repair tissue damage to muscle and improve the vascular system, thus enabling the body to meet higher oxygen demands associated with exercise.

13.6.3 Hormonal Pathways

The modulation of gonadal hormones is another potential mechanism linking exercise to brain health. For example, levels of testosterone have been shown to be increased following various exercise regimens in both men and women throughout the lifespan [114–116]. There is evidence testosterone is neuroprotective, and it has been linked to the enhancement of neurogenesis and the reduction of Aβ levels [117, 118]. Age-related brain atrophy may be attenuated by maintenance of testosterone levels, and in the hippocampus, the neuroprotective actions of testosterone and dihydrotestosterone (a potent androgen) are mediated via binding to the androgen receptors [119]. This protective effect on neuronal health may have important implications on cognitive functioning, as higher levels of serum testosterone have been associated with cognitive performance in cognitively healthy older men [120]. As exercise enhances androgen synthesis, it is possible that neuroprotective effects of exercise are partially mediated by increases in testosterone. Indeed, one study has demonstrated that increased levels of hippocampal dihydrotestosterone mediated the induction of hippocampal neurogenesis in adult male mice undertaking low-intensity exercise [121]. Levels of testosterone in the brain have been shown to be lower post mortem, in those with neuropathological evidence of AD [122].

The literature regarding exercise and levels of oestrogens is more complicated. Pre-menopausal women experience decreased levels of oestrogen following exercise; however, after menopause, when oestrogen levels are naturally depleted, the literature remains equivocal as to the effect of exercise on oestrogen levels. Nevertheless, reports demonstrate that oestrogen plays a significant role in exercise-induced expression of *BDNF* mRNA [123]. Oestradiol has been shown to regulate both BDNF and APP levels, and it has positive influences on both cell proliferation and cell survival in the dentate gyrus. Indeed, early interest in this area arose from findings that female mice demonstrated higher levels of cell proliferation than males [124]. Nevertheless, it is important to recognise that the majority of this work has been performed on female rodents, and little is known about the effects of oestrogens on the hippocampus of humans (male or female). Similar to testosterone, oestrogen has been demonstrated to have a protective effect against AD and Aβ neurotoxicity - as the presence of oestrogen has been associated with neuronal resistance to AD-related toxicity [125].

13.6.4 Cardiovascular and Metabolic Mechanisms

Physical activity is a well-established protective factor against both cardiovascular disease and type 2 diabetes, and has been strongly associated with insulin sensitivity. For example, time spent watching television (i.e. sedentary time) has been found to correlate positively with serum insulin levels, whereas leisure-time physical activity has been found to be inversely associated with insulin levels [126]. This highlights another potential mechanism for the link between AD risk and physical activity, as insulin resistance, metabolic disease, and type 2 diabetes have been implicated in AD, and are associated with alterations in Aβ processing [127], oxidative stress, and chronic inflammation, all of which are thought to be pivotal in the development of AD pathology, as discussed in many other chapters of this book. There is already evidence that exercise can help reduce chronic inflammation, which is not only involved in insulin resistance and type 2 diabetes, but other age-associated chronic conditions such as cardiovascular disease and arthritis. Thus, increasing physical activity may reduce the risk of AD through the effect of reduced cardiovascular and metabolic disease risk combined with lower chronic inflammation.

13.6.5 Evidence from Neuroimaging Studies

Recent advances have provided researchers with the opportunity to visualise Aβ within the living human brain; thus, with studies of animal models already indicating a relationship between exercise and a lower accumulation rate of Aβ, the next step is to evaluate the relationship between physical activity levels and brain Aβ burden in large clinical studies. A number of epidemiological studies have already reported lower levels of brain Aβ in individuals reporting the highest levels of physical activity [80–82]. Importantly, in two of these studies, this finding was most salient in those at the greatest genetic risk of AD (i.e. carriers of the *APOE ε4* allele). We will discuss the important role genetics can play in the association between physical activity and AD risk later in this chapter. It is important to note that a recent study of memory complainers and individuals with mild cognitive impairment did not find an association between physical activity levels and brain Aβ [83]. Further research is required in this field to determine if physical activity is only linked to Aβ in those without clinical symptoms, or if physical activity can indeed play a role in delaying disease course once AD neuropathology has commenced.

Magnetic resonance imaging (MRI) can be used to measure the volume of the brain, and thus has been a useful tool in examining the relationship between physical activity and brain atrophy. For example, following a six-month aerobic exercise training intervention, a significant increase in grey and white matter volume of the prefrontal and temporal cortices has been observed [7]. Furthermore, a one-year aerobic exercise training program increased hippocampal volume by 2%, compared to the control subjects who experienced the expected age-related loss of volume of 1–2% [62]. It must be noted that studies in this field, similar to those of exercise and effects on Aβ, have primarily been conducted on cognitively healthy individuals. Thus, the effect of exercise on brain volume in those at the greatest risk of AD or dementia (i.e. those with a diagnosis of MCI) is not currently known. However, the mechanism whereby brain volume is protected by exercise may be via BDNF, as increases in BDNF levels are known to induce neurogenesis (generation of brain cells). It is hypothesised that exercise-induced increases in BDNF contribute to the conserving of brain volume, particularly in brain regions pertinent to memory and executive functions (i.e. frontal lobe and hippocampus).

Using functional magnetic resonance imaging (fMRI), functional connectivity analyses are used to characterise the way in which different brain regions may interact. In the first study of its kind, Voss et al. [89] reported that a one-year walking program enhanced the functional connectivity in network patterns that are susceptible to age-related disruptions. In addition to brain network connectivity, fMRI can also be used to evaluate activation in certain brain regions under particular conditions (i.e. carrying out specific cognitive tasks): this is known as task-evoked fMRI. One study utilising task-evoked fMRI investigated cardiovascular fitness, brain activation, and spatial learning in healthy middle-aged people. This study reported that fitness levels impact on brain regions involved in spatial learning: they found that cardiovascular fitness correlated positively with changes in brain activation in the medial frontal gyrus and the cuneus [128]. This intriguing area of research is still in its infancy, and future research will likely contribute to greater insights into the relationship between physical activity and brain health.

13.7 The Effect of Genetics on the Relationship Between Exercise and Brain Health

Both environmental and genetic factors contribute to AD risk; and in fact, environmental factors such as lifestyle most likely interact with genetic factors to influence AD risk (i.e. an individual's genetic make-up will most likely influence the level of benefits obtained from exercise). Similarly, genetic differences known to increase AD risk may be moderated by exercise. For example, the *APOE $\varepsilon 4$* allele is the strongest genetic risk factor for late-onset AD [129], and studies have shown that physical activity may play a role in moderating that increased risk. Various other *APOE* studies have shown that physical activity influences AD risk and brain amyloid deposition differently, depending on *APOE* genotype. For example, Podewils et al. [55] reported an association between physical activity and reduced AD risk: yet the association was only evident in carriers of the *APOE $\varepsilon 4$* allele. Furthermore, two studies of brain Aβ levels, reported that carriers of the *APOE $\varepsilon 4$* allele are more susceptible to increased amyloid deposition, yet only if they have a sedentary lifestyle. This relationship was reported by Head et al. [82] and Brown et al. [81], who found that brain Aβ burden (quantified by PiB-PET) was highest in sedentary *APOE $\varepsilon 4$* carriers, whereas in physically active individuals, *APOE* allele status did not appear to influence brain amyloid burden. These results suggest that *APOE $\varepsilon 4$* carriers gain the most benefit from exercise when considering amyloid pathology, and the results may reflect a greater clearance of brain Aβ due to exercise.

Differences in other genes that are relevant to brain health and function may also be modulated by physical activity to influence the risk of AD and cognitive decline. One such gene is the *BDNF* gene: individuals with the *BDNF* Val 66Met polymorphism have a reduced secretion of BDNF, which is associated with poorer memory, reduced hippocampal volumes, and lower memory-related activation in the hippocampus. Interestingly, physical activity has been associated with larger hippocampal volumes, with this finding only evident in non-carriers of the *BDNF* polymorphism [51]. This finding suggests that those with reduced secretion of BDNF (i.e. those with the *BDNF* polymorphism) may not receive the benefit from exercise in terms of enhanced brain volume. Of course, findings such as these do not indicate that individuals with particular genotypes do not get any other benefit from exercise: It is also clear that this field is still in the early stages of research, and over the coming years more will be known about this important topic.

13.8 Future Directions

Based on the literature presented in this chapter, physical activity plays a role in protecting the ageing brain and delaying the onset of neurodegenerative diseases such as AD. It is important to note that most of the studies discussed in this chapter evaluated the effect of physical activity/exercise in groups of cognitively healthy individuals (i.e. people without dementia), and that the effect of exercise on treating symptoms of neurodegenerative diseases are less understood. Nevertheless, numerous questions remain as to the use of exercise as a protective factor. Importantly, researchers are yet to identify the most effective exercise regimen (in terms of intensity, frequency, and duration) that will provide the greatest benefit to the brain. The type of exercise, i.e. aerobic or strength training or a combination of both, will likely be a focus of upcoming research studies. However, it is likely that the ideal exercise regimen to benefit the brain may differ from person to person. Using genetic studies, we may be able to provide individualised exercise prescriptions. For physical activity to be adopted as a preventative strategy for AD, we must have a comprehensive understanding of the biological mechanisms of this association. The use of emerging neuroimaging techniques in large exercise trials will help provide necessary evidence to establish physical activity as a well-recognised protective factor against neurodegeneration.

References

1. Rowe, J.W. and Kahn, R.L. (1997). Successful aging. *Gerontologist* 37: 433–440.
2. Caspersen, C.J., Powell, K.E., and Christenson, G.M. (1985). Physical activity, exercise, and physical fitness: definitions and distinctions for health-related research. *Public Health Rep.* 100: 126–131.
3. Barnes, D.E. and Yaffe, K. (2011). The projected effect of risk factor reduction on Alzheimer's disease prevalence. *Lancet Neurol.* 10: 819–828.
4. Livingston, G., Sommerlad, A., Orgeta, V. et al. (2017). Dementia prevention, intervention, and care. *Lancet* 390: 2673–2734.
5. Dupuy, O., Gauthier, C.J., Fraser, S.A. et al. (2015). Higher levels of cardiovascular fitness are associated with better executive function and prefrontal oxygenation in younger and older women. *Front. Hum. Neurosci.* 9: 66.

References

6 Hayes, S.M., Forman, D.E., and Verfaellie, M. (2014). Cardiorespiratory fitness is associated with cognitive performance in older but not younger adults. *J. Gerontol. B Psychol. Sci. Soc. Sci.*

7 Colcombe, S.J., Erickson, K.I., Scalf, P.E. et al. (2006). Aerobic exercise training increases brain volume in aging humans. *J. Gerontol. A Biol. Sci. Med. Sci.* 61: 1166–1170.

8 Lautenschlager, N.T., Cox, K.L., Flicker, L. et al. (2008). Effect of physical activity on cognitive function in older adults at risk for Alzheimer disease: a randomized trial. *JAMA* 300: 1027–1037.

9 Liu-Ambrose, T., Nagamatsu, L.S., Graf, P. et al. (2010). Resistance training and executive functions: a 12-month randomized controlled trial. *Arch. Intern. Med.* 170: 170–178.

10 Hamer, M. and Chida, Y. (2009). Physical activity and risk of neurodegenerative disease: a systematic review of prospective evidence. *Psychol. Med.* 39: 3–11.

11 Sofi, F., Valecchi, D., Bacci, D. et al. (2011). Physical activity and risk of cognitive decline: a meta-analysis of prospective studies. *J. Intern. Med.* 269: 107–117.

12 Reimers, C.D., Knapp, G., and Reimers, A.K. (2012). Does physical activity increase life expectancy? A review of the literature. *J. Aging Res.* 2012: 9.

13 Gage, F.H. and Temple, S. (2013). Neural stem cells: generating and regenerating the brain. *Neuron* 80: 588–601.

14 Bavelier, D. and Neville, H.J. (2002). Cross-modal plasticity: where and how? *Nat. Rev. Neurosci.* 3: 443–452.

15 Hötting, K. and Röder, B. (2013). Beneficial effects of physical exercise on neuroplasticity and cognition. *Neurosci. Biobehav. Rev.* 37: 2243–2257.

16 Hillman, C.H., Erickson, K.I., and Kramer, A.F. (2008). Be smart, exercise your heart: exercise effects on brain and cognition. *Nat. Rev. Neurosci.* 9: 58–65.

17 Kramer, A.F. and Erickson, K.I. (2007). Capitalizing on cortical plasticity: influence of physical activity on cognition and brain function. *Trends Cogn. Sci.* 11: 342–348.

18 Voss, M.W., Vivar, C., Kramer, A.F., and van Praag, H. (2013). Bridging animal and human models of exercise-induced brain plasticity. *Trends Cogn. Sci.* 17: 525–544.

19 Bielak, A.A., Cherbuin, N., Bunce, D., and Anstey, K.J. (2014). Preserved differentiation between physical activity and cognitive performance across young, middle, and older adulthood over 8 years. *J. Gerontol. Ser. B Psychol. Sci. Soc. Sci.* 69: 523–532.

20 Dregan, A. and Gulliford, M. (2013). Leisure-time physical activity over the life course and cognitive functioning in late mid-adult years: a cohort-based investigation. *Psychol. Med.* 43: 2447–2458.

21 Papazacharias, A. and Nardini, M. (2012). The relationship between depression and cognitive deficits. *Psychiatr. Danub.* 24: 179–182.

22 Marvel, C.L. and Paradiso, S. (2004). Cognitive and neurological impairment in mood disorders. *Psychiatr. Clin. North Am.* 27, 19-viii.

23 Strawbridge, W.J., Deleger, S., Roberts, R.E., and Kaplan, G.A. (2002). Physical activity reduces the risk of subsequent depression for older adults. *Am. J. Epidemiol.* 156: 328–334.

24 Lautenschlager, N.T., Almeida, O.P., Flicker, L., and Janca, A. (2004). Can physical activity improve the mental health of older adults? *Ann. Gen. Hosp. Psychiatry* 3: 12.

25 Sibley, B.A. and Etnier, J.L. (2003). The relationship between physical activity and cognition in children: a meta-analysis. *Pediatr. Exerc. Sci.* 15: 243–256.

26 Castelli, D.M., Hillman, C.H., Buck, S.M., and Erwin, H.E. (2007). Physical fitness and academic achievement in third- and fifth-grade students. *J. Sport Exerc. Psychol.* 29: 239.

27 Carlson, S.A., Fulton, J.E., Lee, S.M. et al. (2008). Physical education and academic achievement in elementary school: data from the early childhood longitudinal study. *Am. J. Public Health* 98: 721–727.

28 Buck, S.M., Hillman, C.H., and Castelli, D.M. (2008). The relation of aerobic fitness to stroop task performance in preadolescent children. *Med. Sci. Sports Exerc.* 40: 166–172.

29 Hillman, C.H., Castelli, D.M., and Buck, S.M. (2005). Aerobic fitness and neurocognitive function in healthy preadolescent children. *Med. Sci. Sports Exerc.* 37: 1967.

30 Coe, D.P., Pivarnik, J.M., Womack, C.J. et al. (2006). Effect of physical education and activity levels on academic achievement in children. *Med. Sci. Sports Exerc.* 38: 1515.

31 Donnelly, J.E., Greene, J.L., Gibson, C.A. et al. (2009). Physical Activity Across the Curriculum (PAAC): a randomized controlled trial to promote physical activity and diminish overweight and obesity in elementary school children. *Prev. Med.* 49: 336–341.

32 Davis, C.L., Tomporowski, P.D., Boyle, C.A. et al. (2007). Effects of aerobic exercise on overweight children's cognitive functioning: a randomized controlled trial. *Res. Q. Exerc. Sport* 78: 510–519.

33 Richards, M., Hardy, R., and Wadsworth, M.E. (2003). Does active leisure protect cognition? Evidence from a national birth cohort. *Soc. Sci. Med.* 56: 785–792.

34 Singh-Manoux, A., Hillsdon, M., Brunner, E., and Marmot, M. (2005). Effects of physical activity on cognitive functioning in middle age: evidence from the Whitehall II prospective cohort study. *Am. J. Public Health* 95: 2252.

35 Åberg, M.A., Pedersen, N.L., Torén, K. et al. (2009). Cardiovascular fitness is associated with cognition in young adulthood. *Proc. Natl. Acad. Sci. U.S.A.* 106: 20906–20911.

36 Ratey, J.J. and Loehr, J.E. (2011). The positive impact of physical activity on cognition during adulthood: a review of underlying mechanisms, evidence and recommendations. *Rev. Neurosci.* 22: 171–185.

37 Pereira, A.C., Huddleston, D.E., Brickman, A.M. et al. (2007). An *in vivo* correlate of exercise-induced neurogenesis in the adult dentate gyrus. *Proc. Natl. Acad. Sci. U.S.A.* 104: 5638–5643.

38 Spirduso, W.W. and Clifford, P. (1978). Replication of age and physical activity effects on reaction and movement time. *J Gerontol* 33 (1): 26–30.

39 Weuve, J., Kang, J.H., Manson, J.E. et al. (2004). Physical activity, including walking, and cognitive function in older women. *JAMA* 292: 1454–1461.

40 Angevaren, M., Vanhees, L., Wendel-Vos, W. et al. (2007). Intensity, but not duration, of physical activities is related to cognitive function. *Eur. J. Cardiovasc. Prev. Rehabil.* 14: 825–830.

41 Aichberger, M., Busch, M., Reischies, F. et al. (2010). Effect of physical inactivity on cognitive performance after 2.5 years of follow-up: longitudinal results from the Survey of Health, Ageing, and Retirement (SHARE). *GeroPsych* 23: 7.

42 Brown, B.M., Peiffer, J.J., Sohrabi, H.R. et al., and Group AR (2012). Intense physical activity is associated with cognitive performance in the elderly. *Transl. Psychiatry* 2: e191.

43 Hayes, S.M., Alosco, M.L., Hayes, J.P. et al. (2015). Physical activity is positively associated with episodic memory in aging. *J. Int. Neuropsychol. Soc.* 21: 780–790.

44 Yaffe, K., Barnes, D., Nevitt, M. et al. (2001). A prospective study of physical activity and cognitive decline in elderly women: women who walk. *Arch. Intern. Med.* 161: 1703–1708.

45 Barnes, D.E. et al. (2003). A longitudinal study of cardiorespiratory fitness and cognitive function in healthy older adults. *J Am Geriatr Soc* 51 (4): 459–465.

46 Barnes, D.E., Yaffe, K., Satariano, W.A., and Tager, I.B. (2003). A longitudinal study of cardiorespiratory fitness and cognitive function in healthy older adults. *J. Am. Geriatr. Soc.* 51: 459–465.

47 Dougherty, R.J., Schultz, S.A., Boots, E.A. et al. (2017). Relationships between cardiorespiratory fitness, hippocampal volume, and episodic memory in a population at risk for Alzheimer's disease. *Brain Behav.* 7: e00625.

48 Erickson, K.I., Prakash, R.S., Voss, M.W. et al. (2009). Aerobic fitness is associated with hippocampal volume in elderly humans. *Hippocampus* 19: 1030–1039.

49 Honea, R.A., Thomas, G.P., Harsha, A. et al. (2009). Cardiorespiratory fitness and preserved medial temporal lobe volume in Alzheimer disease. *Alzheimer Dis. Assoc. Disord.* 23: 188–197.

50 Tian, Q., Studenski, S.A., Resnick, S.M. et al. (2016). Midlife and late-life cardiorespiratory fitness and brain volume changes in late adulthood: results from the Baltimore longitudinal study of aging. *J. Gerontol. A Biol. Sci. Med. Sci.* 71: 124–130.

51 Brown, B.M., Bourgeat, P., Peiffer, J.J. et al., and Group AR (2014). Influence of BDNF Val66Met on the relationship between physical activity and brain volume. *Neurology* 83: 1345–1352.

52 Bugg, J.M. and Head, D. (2011). Exercise moderates age-related atrophy of the medial temporal lobe. *Neurobiol. Aging* 32: 506–514.

53 Smith, J.C., Nielson, K.A., Woodard, J.L. et al. (2014). Physical activity reduces hippocampal atrophy in elders at genetic risk for Alzheimer's disease. *Front. Aging Neurosci.* 6: 61.

54 Willey, J.Z., Gardener, H., Caunca, M.R. et al. (2016). Leisure-time physical activity associates with cognitive decline: the Northern Manhattan Study. *Neurology* 86: 1897–1903.

55 Podewils, L.J., Guallar, E., Kuller, L.H. et al. (2005). Physical activity, APOE genotype, and dementia risk: findings from the Cardiovascular Health Cognition Study. *Am. J. Epidemiol.* 161: 639–651.

56 Larson, E.B., Wang, L., Bowen, J.D. et al. (2006). Exercise is associated with reduced risk for incident dementia among persons 65 years of age and older. *Ann. Intern. Med.* 144: 73–81.

57 Rovio, S., Kareholt, I., Helkala, E.L. et al. (2005). Leisure-time physical activity at midlife and the risk of dementia and Alzheimer's disease. *Lancet Neurol.* 4: 705–711.

58 Verghese, J., Lipton, R.B., Katz, M.J. et al. (2003). Leisure activities and the risk of dementia in the elderly. *N. Engl. J. Med.* 348: 2508–2516.

59 Tan, Z.S., Spartano, N.L., Beiser, A.S. et al. (2017). Physical activity, brain volume, and dementia risk: The Framingham Study. *J. Gerontol. A Biol. Sci. Med. Sci.* 72: 789–795.

60 Vidoni, E.D., Johnson, D.K., Morris, J.K. et al. (2015). Dose-response of aerobic exercise on cognition: a community-based, pilot randomized controlled trial. *PLoS One* 10: e0131647.

61 Tamura, M., Nemoto, K., Kawaguchi, A. et al. (2015). Long-term mild-intensity exercise regimen preserves prefrontal cortical volume against aging. *Int. J. Geriatr. Psychiatry* 30: 686–694.

62 Erickson, K.I., Voss, M.W., Prakash, R.S. et al. (2011). Exercise training increases size of hippocampus and improves memory. *Proc. Natl. Acad. Sci. U.S.A.* 108: 3017–3022.

63 Cassilhas, R.C., Viana, V.A., Grassmann, V. et al. (2007). The impact of resistance exercise on the cognitive function of the elderly. *Med. Sci. Sports Exerc.* 39: 1401.

64 Tsai, C.L., Wang, C.H., Pan, C.Y., and Chen, F.C. (2015). The effects of long-term resistance exercise on the relationship between neurocognitive performance and GH, IGF-1, and homocysteine levels in the elderly. *Front. Behav. Neurosci.* 9: 23.

65 Kramer, A.F., Hahn, S., Cohen, N.J. et al. (1999). Ageing, fitness and neurocognitive function. *Nature* 400: 418–419.

66 Colcombe, S.J., Kramer, A.F., Erickson, K.I. et al. (2004). Cardiovascular fitness, cortical plasticity, and aging. *Proc. Natl. Acad. Sci. U.S.A.* 101: 3316–3321.

67 Colcombe, S. and Kramer, A.F. (2003). Fitness effects on the cognitive function of older adults a meta-analytic study. *Psychol. Sci.* 14: 125–130.

68 Cassilhas, R., Lee, K., Fernandes, J. et al. (2012). Spatial memory is improved by aerobic and resistance exercise through divergent molecular mechanisms. *Neuroscience* 202: 309–317.

69 Abbott, R.D., White, L.R., Ross, G.W. et al. (2004). Walking and dementia in physically capable elderly men. *JAMA* 292: 1447–1453.

70 Taaffe, D.R., Irie, F., Masaki, K.H. et al. (2008). Physical activity, physical function, and incident dementia in elderly men: the Honolulu–Asia Aging Study. *J. Gerontol. Ser. A Biol. Sci. Med. Sci.* 63: 529–535.

71 Lindsay, J., Laurin, D., Verreault, R. et al. (2002). Risk factors for Alzheimer's disease: a prospective analysis from the Canadian Study of Health and Aging. *Am. J. Epidemiol.* 156: 445–453.

72 Scarmeas, N., Luchsinger, J.A., Schupf, N. et al. (2009). Physical activity, diet, and risk of Alzheimer disease. *JAMA* 302: 627–637.

73 Jedrziewski, M.K., Lee, V.M.-Y., and Trojanowski, J.Q. (2005). Lowering the risk of Alzheimer's disease: evidence-based practices emerge from new research. *Alzheimer's Dement.* 1: 152–160.

74 Baker, L.D., Frank, L.L., Foster-Schubert, K. et al. (2010). Effects of aerobic exercise on mild cognitive impairment: a controlled trial. *Arch. Neurol.* 67: 71–79.

75 Xu, Q., Park, Y., Huang, X. et al. (2010). Physical activities and future risk of Parkinson disease. *Neurology* 75: 341–348.

76 Thacker, E.L., Chen, H., Patel, A.V. et al. (2008). Recreational physical activity and risk of Parkinson's disease. *Mov. Disord.* 23: 69–74.

77 Lesage, S. and Brice, A. (2009). Parkinson's disease: from monogenic forms to genetic susceptibility factors. *Hum. Mol. Genet.* 18: R48–R59.

78 Adlard, P.A., Perreau, V.M., Pop, V., and Cotman, C.W. (2005). Voluntary exercise decreases amyloid load in a transgenic model of Alzheimer's disease. *J. Neurosci.* 25: 4217–4221.

79 Um, H.S., Kang, E.B., Leem, Y.H. et al. (2008). Exercise training acts as a therapeutic strategy for reduction of the pathogenic phenotypes for Alzheimer's disease in an NSE/APPsw-transgenic model. *Int. J. Mol. Med.* 22: 529–539.

80 Liang, K.Y., Mintun, M.A., Fagan, A.M. et al. (2010). Exercise and Alzheimer's disease biomarkers in cognitively normal older adults. *Ann. Neurol.* 68: 311–318.

81 Brown, B.M., Peiffer, J.J., Taddei, K. et al. (2013). Physical activity and amyloid-beta plasma and brain levels: results from the Australian Imaging, Biomarkers and Lifestyle Study of Ageing. *Mol. Psychiatry* 18: 875–881.

82 Head, D., Bugg, J.M., Goate, A.M. et al. (2012). Exercise engagement as a moderator of the effects of APOE genotype on amyloid deposition. *Arch. Neurol.*

83 de Souto Barreto, P., Andrieu, S., Payoux, P. et al., and Multidomain Alzheimer Preventive Trial/Data Sharing Alzheimer Study G (2015). Physical activity and amyloid-beta brain levels in elderly adults with intact cognition and mild cognitive impairment. *J. Am. Geriatr. Soc.* 63: 1634–1639.

84 Neeper, S.A., Gomez-Pinilla, F., Choi, J., and Cotman, C.W. (1996). Physical activity increases mRNA for brain-derived neurotrophic factor and nerve growth factor in rat brain. *Brain Res.* 726: 49–56.

85 Um, H.S., Kang, E.B., Koo, J.H. et al. (2011). Treadmill exercise represses neuronal cell death in an aged transgenic mouse model of Alzheimer's disease. *Neurosci. Res.* 69: 161–173.

86 Carro, E., Nunez, A., Busiguina, S., and Torres-Aleman, I. (2000). Circulating insulin-like growth factor I mediates effects of exercise on the brain. *J. Neurosci.* 20: 2926–2933.

87 Sutoo, D. and Akiyama, K. (2003). Regulation of brain function by exercise. *Neurobiol. Dis.* 13: 1–14.

88 Fordyce, D.E. and Farrar, R.P. (1991). Enhancement of spatial learning in F344 rats by physical activity and related learning-associated alterations in hippocampal and cortical cholinergic functioning. *Behav. Brain Res.* 46: 123–133.

89 Voss, M.W., Prakash, R.S., Erickson, K.I. et al. (2010). Plasticity of brain networks in a randomized intervention trial of exercise training in older adults. *Front. Aging Neurosci.* 2.

90 Liu, H.L., Zhao, G., Zhang, H., and Shi, L.D. (2013). Long-term treadmill exercise inhibits the progression of Alzheimer's disease-like neuropathology in the hippocampus of APP/PS1 transgenic mice. *Behav. Brain Res.* 256: 261–272.

91 Yuede, C.M., Zimmerman, S.D., Dong, H. et al. (2009). Effects of voluntary and forced exercise on plaque deposition, hippocampal volume, and behavior in the Tg2576 mouse model of Alzheimer's disease. *Neurobiol. Dis.* 35: 426–432.

92 Nichol, K.E., Poon, W.W., Parachikova, A.I. et al. (2008). Exercise alters the immune profile in Tg2576 Alzheimer mice toward a response coincident with improved cognitive performance and decreased amyloid. *J. Neuroinflammation* 5: 13.

93 Zhao, G., Liu, H.L., Zhang, H., and Tong, X.J. (2015). Treadmill exercise enhances synaptic plasticity, but does not alter beta-amyloid deposition in hippocampi of aged APP/PS1 transgenic mice. *Neuroscience* 298: 357–366.

94 Tabuchi, M., Lone, S.R., Liu, S. et al. (2015). Sleep interacts with abeta to modulate intrinsic neuronal excitability. *Curr. Biol.* 25: 702–712.

95 Verdile, G., Fuller, S., Atwood, C.S. et al. (2004). The role of beta amyloid in Alzheimer's disease: still a cause of everything or the only one who got caught? *Pharmacol. Res.* 50: 397–409.

96 Lazarov, O., Robinson, J., Tang, Y.P. et al. (2005). Environmental enrichment reduces Abeta levels and amyloid deposition in transgenic mice. *Cell* 120: 701–713.

97 Maesako, M., Uemura, K., Kubota, M. et al. (2012). Exercise is more effective than diet control in preventing high fat diet-induced beta-amyloid deposition and memory deficit in amyloid precursor protein transgenic mice. *J. Biol. Chem.* 287: 23024–23033.

98 Giannakopoulos, P., Hof, P.R., Michel, J.P. et al. (1997). Cerebral cortex pathology in aging and Alzheimer's disease: a quantitative survey of large hospital-based geriatric and psychiatric cohorts. *Brain Res. Brain Res. Rev.* 25: 217–245.

99 Ohia-Nwoko, O., Montazari, S., Lau, Y.S., and Eriksen, J.L. (2014). Long-term treadmill exercise attenuates tau pathology in P301S tau transgenic mice. *Mol. Neurodegener.* 9: 54.

100 Belarbi, K., Burnouf, S., Fernandez-Gomez, F.J. et al. (2011). Beneficial effects of exercise in a transgenic mouse model of Alzheimer's disease-like Tau pathology. *Neurobiol. Dis.* 43: 486–494.

101 Fang, G., Zhao, J., Li, P. et al. (2017). Long-term treadmill exercise inhibits neuronal cell apoptosis and reduces tau phosphorylation in the cerebral cortex and hippocampus of aged rats. *Sci. Bull.* 62: 755–757.

102 Coelho, F.G., Gobbi, S., Andreatto, C.A. et al. (2013). Physical exercise modulates peripheral levels of brain-derived neurotrophic factor (BDNF): a systematic review of experimental studies in the elderly. *Arch. Gerontol. Geriatr.* 56: 10–15.

103 Marston, K.J., Newton, M.J., Brown, B.M. et al. (2017). Intense resistance exercise increases peripheral brain-derived neurotrophic factor. *J. Sci. Med. Sport* 20: 899–903.

104 Etnier, J.L., Wideman, L., Labban, J.D. et al. (2016). The effects of acute exercise on memory and brain-derived neurotrophic factor (BDNF). *J. Sport Exerc. Psychol.* 38: 331–340.

105 Szuhany, K.L., Bugatti, M., and Otto, M.W. (2015). A meta-analytic review of the effects of exercise on brain-derived neurotrophic factor. *J. Psychiatr. Res.* 60: 56–64.

106 Laske, C., Stransky, E., Leyhe, T. et al. (2007). BDNF serum and CSF concentrations in Alzheimer's disease, normal pressure hydrocephalus and healthy controls. *J. Psychiatr. Res.* 41: 387–394.

107 Steen, E., Terry, B.M., Rivera, E.J. et al. (2005). Impaired insulin and insulin-like growth factor expression and signaling mechanisms in Alzheimer's disease – is this type 3 diabetes? *J. Alzheimers Dis.* 7: 63–80.

108 Westwood, A.J., Beiser, A., Decarli, C. et al. (2014). Insulin-like growth factor-1 and risk of Alzheimer dementia and brain atrophy. *Neurology* 82: 1613–1619.

109 Aberg, M.A., Aberg, N.D., Hedbacker, H. et al. (2000). Peripheral infusion of IGF-I selectively induces neurogenesis in the adult rat hippocampus. *J. Neurosci.* 20: 2896–2903.

110 Trejo, J.L., Carro, E., and Torres-Aleman, I. (2001). Circulating insulin-like growth factor I mediates exercise-induced increases in the number of new neurons in the adult hippocampus. *J. Neurosci.* 21: 1628–1634.

111 McCusker, R.H., McCrea, K., Zunich, S. et al. (2006). Insulin-like growth factor-I enhances the biological activity of brain-derived neurotrophic factor on cerebrocortical neurons. *J. Neuroimmunol.* 179: 186–190.

112 Ogunshola, O.O., Antic, A., Donoghue, M.J. et al. (2002). Paracrine and autocrine functions of neuronal vascular endothelial growth factor (VEGF) in the central nervous system. *J. Biol. Chem.* 277: 11410–11415.

113 Ding, Y.H., Li, J., Zhou, Y. et al. (2006). Cerebral angiogenesis and expression of angiogenic factors in aging rats after exercise. *Curr. Neurovasc. Res.* 3: 15–23.

114 O'Leary, C.B., Lehman, C., Koltun, K. et al. (2013). Response of testosterone to prolonged aerobic exercise during different phases of the menstrual cycle. *Eur. J. Appl. Physiol.* 113: 2419–2424.

115 Hayes, L.D., Sculthorpe, N., Herbert, P. et al. (2015). Six weeks of conditioning exercise increases total, but not free testosterone in lifelong sedentary aging men. *Aging Male* 18: 195–200.

116 Geliebter, A., Ochner, C.N., Dambkowski, C.L., and Hashim, S.A. (2014). Obesity-related hormones and metabolic risk factors: a randomized trial of diet plus either strength or aerobic training versus diet alone in overweight participants. *J. Diabetes Obes.* 1: 1–7.

117 Leem, Y.H., Lim, H.J., Shim, S.B. et al. (2009). Repression of tau hyperphosphorylation by chronic endurance exercise in aged transgenic mouse model of tauopathies. *J. Neurosci. Res.* 87: 2561–2570.

118 Jessen, F., Amariglio, R.E., van Boxtel, M. et al., and Subjective Cognitive Decline Initiative Working G (2014). A conceptual framework for research on subjective cognitive decline in preclinical Alzheimer's disease. *Alzheimers Dement.* 10: 844–852.

119 Hammond, J., Le, Q., Goodyer, C. et al. (2001). Testosterone-mediated neuroprotection through the androgen receptor in human primary neurons. *J. Neurochem.* 77: 1319–1326.

120 Villain, N., Chetelat, G., Grassiot, B. et al., and Group AR (2012). Regional dynamics of amyloid-beta deposition in healthy elderly, mild cognitive impairment and Alzheimer's disease: a voxelwise PiB-PET longitudinal study. *Brain* 135: 2126–2139.

121 Okamoto, M., Hojo, Y., Inoue, K. et al. (2012). Mild exercise increases dihydrotestosterone in hippocampus providing evidence for androgenic mediation of neurogenesis. *Proc. Natl. Acad. Sci. U.S.A.* 109: 13100–13105.

122 Golden, E., Emiliano, A., Maudsley, S. et al. (2010). Circulating brain-derived neurotrophic factor and indices of metabolic and cardiovascular health: data from the Baltimore Longitudinal Study of Aging. *PLoS One* 5: e10099.

123 Berchtold, N.C., Kesslak, J.P., Pike, C.J. et al. (2001). Estrogen and exercise interact to regulate brain-derived neurotrophic factor mRNA and protein expression in the hippocampus. *Eur. J. Neurosci.* 14: 1992–2002.

124 Galea, L.A. and McEwen, B.S. (1999). Sex and seasonal differences in the rate of cell proliferation in the dentate gyrus of adult wild meadow voles. *Neuroscience* 89: 955–964.

125 Pike, C.J. (1999). Estrogen modulates neuronal Bcl-xL expression and beta-amyloid-induced apoptosis: relevance to Alzheimer's disease. *J. Neurochem.* 72: 1552–1563.

126 Ford, E.S., Li, C., Zhao, G. et al. (2010). Sedentary behavior, physical activity, and concentrations of insulin among US adults. *Metabolism* 59: 1268–1275.

127 Carro, E. and Torres-Aleman, I. (2004). The role of insulin and insulin-like growth factor I in the molecular and cellular mechanisms underlying the pathology of Alzheimer's disease. *Eur. J. Pharmacol.* 490: 127–133.

128 Holzschneider, K., Wolbers, T., Roder, B., and Hotting, K. (2012). Cardiovascular fitness modulates brain activation associated with spatial learning. *Neuroimage* 59: 3003–3014.

129 Corder, E.H., Saunders, A.M., Strittmatter, W.J. et al. (1993). Gene dose of apolipoprotein E type 4 allele and the risk of Alzheimer's disease in late onset families. *Science* 261: 921–923.

14

Current and Prospective Treatments for Alzheimer's Disease (and Other Neurodegenerative Diseases)
Steve Pedrini[1,5], *Mike Morici*[1] *and Ralph N. Martins*[1,2,3,4,5]

[1] *Centre of Excellence for Alzheimer's Disease Research and Care, School of Medical and Health Sciences, Edith Cowan University, Joondalup, WA, Australia*
[2] *Department of Biomedical Sciences, Macquarie University, Sydney, NSW, Australia*
[3] *School of Psychiatry and Clinical Neurosciences, University of Western Australia, Perth, WA, Australia*
[4] *KaRa Institute of Neurological Diseases, Sydney, NSW, Australia*
[5] *Australian Alzheimer's Research Foundation, Ralph and Patricia Sarich Neuroscience Research Institute, Nedlands, WA, Australia*

14.1 Introduction

Due to improved living conditions, more efficient health systems, and improvements in medical treatments, humans are likely to live longer than ever. However, with longer lifespans, the risk of conditions like age-related neurodegenerative diseases also increases. This underscores the importance of research into treatments and cures for such illnesses. It is also clear that the higher the number of individuals with dementia, the higher the cost to the community. By 2050, it is estimated that the number of people with Alzheimer's disease (AD) will be 130 million worldwide, with an overall cost to the community of around $1 trillion per annum (WHO Report 'Dementia a Public Health Priority', 2012). It is therefore desirable to find treatments that can delay disease onset, reduce symptoms, or even cure the disease, to increase the healthy lifespan of older individuals and to reduce the economic and social costs of providing care for affected individuals. For the moment however, most treatments only treat symptoms, including cognitive decline, depression, insomnia, aggression, and hallucinations. Here we mostly discuss treatments that influence cognitive function, as well as some potential treatments that may influence the development or course of the disease.

14.2 Current and Potential Medical Treatments

14.2.1 Treatments That Influence Neurotransmission

14.2.1.1 Cholinergic System
The majority of drugs currently approved for AD treatment affect the cholinergic system. Donepezil (Aricept™, chemical name: *2-[(1-benzylpiperidin-4-yl)methyl]-5, 6-dimethoxy-2,3-dihydroinden-1-one*) is an inhibitor of acetylcholinesterase [1–4].

Neurodegeneration and Alzheimer's Disease: The Role of Diabetes, Genetics, Hormones, and Lifestyle,
First Edition. Edited by Ralph N. Martins, Charles S. Brennan, W.M.A.D. Binosha Fernando,
Margaret A. Brennan and Stephanie J. Fuller.
© 2019 John Wiley & Sons Ltd. Published 2019 by John Wiley & Sons Ltd.

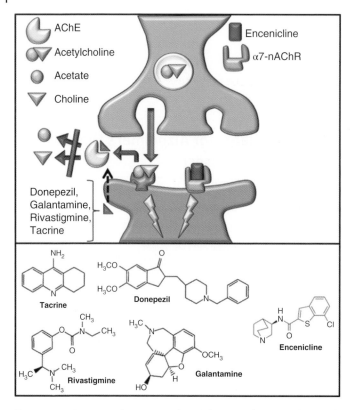

Figure 14.1 Diagram of synapse and site of action of commonly used AD drugs, and structure of commonly used AD drugs. (*See color plate section for the color representation of this figure.*)

In the cholinergic synapses, acetylcholinesterase degrades the neurotransmitter acetylcholine after its release from the presynapses into the synaptic space. By inhibiting its degradation, donepezil increases the availability of the neurotransmitter, enhancing cholinergic transmission (Figure 14.1). Although this drug does not affect the underlying causes of AD, it does delay cognitive impairment in patients affected by the disease. The most common side effects involve the gastrointestinal system including diarrhoea, nausea, and vomiting, in addition to dizziness, fatigue, and urinary incontinence. These relatively common effects usually occur at the beginning of treatment. Studies performed in a mouse model of AD have indicated that donepezil improves memory deficits and cognitive performances [5–7], increases synaptic density, and reduces Aβ and amyloid plaque levels [8]. There is also reduced microgliosis, astrocytosis, and Aβ-induced memory impairment and mitochondrial dysfunction [9, 10]. More than 200 clinical trials have involved donepezil and the majority of these have focused on AD. Results of an initial clinical trial were first reported in 1996, in which increasing doses from 1 to 5 mg/day for 12 weeks improved ADAS-cog (Alzheimer's Disease Assessment Scale-Cognitive Subscale test) scores without inducing hepatotoxicity [11]. Two later studies of mild to moderate AD found that 5 and 10 mg/day of donepezil improved cognition; these two clinical trials had a duration of six months. The same results were achieved using the same doses in a one-year clinical trial in which a small improvement in cognitive function was achieved [12, 13]. A study of hippocampal volume in 67 mild-to-moderate AD patients indicated that 5 and 10 mg/day of donepezil slowed the reduction of the hippocampal volume, paired with an improvement in the ADAS-cog score [14]. Subsequently, other clinical trials indicated improvements in cognition and memory in mild-to-moderate AD patients upon administration of donepezil [15–19]. One clinical trial for severe AD patients also found a modest improvement in cognition [20].

A study that evaluated non-responders after six months reported that continuing the treatment for an additional 12 weeks eventually resulted in benefits, indicating that the initial lack of efficacy does not necessarily mean treatment should be stopped [21]. Most recently, several studies have reported improved cognitive function in AD patients with high doses of donepezil (23 mg/day) versus the more commonly used dose (10 mg/day), although the most recent report showed no difference [22–25]. It has also been reported that donepezil increases blood flow in the frontal lobe, and in that prodromal AD, it reduces hippocampal atrophy [26, 27]. A one-year treatment with 10 mg/day of donepezil also reduced the atrophy progression in the basal forebrain area [28]. Due to the large number of clinical trials, it is not surprising that mixed results have been reported, but in general it is accepted that patients taking donepezil experience reduced cognitive decline and a reduced cost of care [29]. As donepezil is an approved drug for AD with reported beneficial effects, in recent years several studies have evaluated the option of co-treatments with the intent of further improving the cognitive performances of AD patients. Reportedly, donepezil treatments were tested in combination with ST101 (an acetylcholine release agent), cerebrolysin (a neurotrophic compound), idalopiridine (a 5-HT6 receptor antagonist), rosiglitazone (a type 2 diabetes treatment), ABT-126 (an α-7 nicotinic acetylcholine receptor agonist) and memantine (an N-Methyl-D-aspartate [NMDA] glutamate receptor antagonist), amongst others. Although the addition of the second drug to the donepezil treatment in some cases provided additional benefits compared to the donepezil treatment alone, further studies are needed to confirm such results [30–35]. Currently, a few clinical trials are recruiting patients to test donepezil alone (NCT02787746) or in combination with the ethanol extract of the seed of *Ziziphus jujuba* (DHP1401) (NCT03055741), DL-3-n-butylphtalide (a drug used for the treatment of ischemic stroke) (NCT02711683), and SUVN-502 (5-HT6 serotonin receptor antagonist) (NCT02580305). Other clinical trials are also recruiting healthy controls to evaluate the efficacy of transdermal patches of donepezil (NCT03438604, NCT03432195, NCT03259958, NCT02968719). Although donepezil has not been approved for the treatment of mild cognitive impairment (MCI), which is considered to be a common precursor to AD, it has been reported that donepezil delays the progression to AD by about one year [36] and improves cognitive scores [37]. Several clinical trials are currently evaluating, or have recently completed studying, the effect of donepezil in MCI patients (NCT01845636, NCT02769065, NCT00934375, NCT01658228). While being effective in AD, donepezil did not show any effect in attention deficit/hyperactivity disorder (ADHD) [38] and produced mixed results in vascular dementia studies [39]. Other clinical trials are currently evaluating donepezil for the treatment of Lewy body dementia and Parkinson's disease (PD) (NCT02415062, NCT02450786, NCT02345213).

Another approved medication that affects the cholinergic system is galantamine (Razadyne™, Reminyl™, Nivalin®, chemical name: *(4aS,6R, 8aS)-4a,5,9,10,11,12-Hexahydro-3-methoxy-11-methyl-6H-benzofuro[3a,3,2,ef][2]benzazepin-6-ol)*. Galantamine is an alkaloid isolated from the common snowdrop plant (*Galanthus woronowii*). It influences the cholinergic system in two ways: it is both a potent activator of the muscarinic and nicotinic receptors and a weak inhibitor of acetylcholinesterase [40]. Studies in AD animal models have reported that galantamine improves cognitive functions and reduces amyloid plaque levels in the brain [7, 41–43]. Just like donepezil, its major side effects are gastrointestinal, and include nausea, diarrhoea, vomiting, along with dizziness and agitation; however, these side effects tend to disappear with time. Almost 100 clinical trials have evaluated the effect of galantamine in AD and other conditions, and while there is consensus that the treatment improves the cognitive behaviour, the effects are rather modest. Several clinical trials spanning three to six month periods, testing doses ranging from 16 to 32 mg/day, showed improved cognition in comparison to placebo treatment [44–47]. Other clinical trials have shown positive effects of galantamine, improving daily activities, cognition, and attention in mild AD [48–52]. In patients with severe AD, the treatment has been found to have beneficial effects, as reported in several studies addressing the issue [53–55]. Long-term positive effects of galantamine treatment have been observed in AD patients, as the treatment stabilised cognition and improved regional cerebral blood flow [56], and other more recent studies have also indicated that galantamine treatment improves cognitive functions in AD patients [57–61]. Similar to donepezil, galantamine has also been tested in combination with other drugs, and the addition of a second drug improved cognitive functions over galantamine treatment alone in some, but not all cases [62–64]. In general, galantamine, like donepezil, delays the placing of patients in nursing homes [65] and pharmacokinetic studies have highlighted the cost-effectiveness of the galantamine treatment [66, 67]. For a brief period there were concerns about higher mortality upon galantamine treatment in two clinical trials in MCI patients [68]. Although the concerns about higher mortality were subsequently dismissed, the treatment failed to display positive effects in MCI patients [68]. Galantamine is currently being evaluated for diseases other than AD, such as vascular dementia and schizophrenia (NCT02098824, NCT01100775).

There is a third medicament approved for AD which affects the cholinergic system – rivastigmine (Exelon™, Rivastach Patch, chemical name: *(S)-3-[1-(dimethylamino) ethyl]phenyl N-ethyl-N-methylcarbamate)*. Rivastigmine is a reversible inhibitor of acetylcholinesterase and butyrylcholinesterase, and it is used for the treatment of mild to severe AD. While it was first developed in capsules, it is also currently available in transdermal patches which provide additional benefits and release the medicament over a 24-hour period. By being absorbed through the skin, rivastigmine bypasses the first-pass effect, thus results in fewer gastrointestinal side effects, allowing higher treatment doses. As with the other two approved drugs, side effects mostly affect the gastrointestinal system and include nausea, vomiting, diarrhoea, agitation, depression, and fatigue. Again, these side effects are more prominent at the beginning of the treatment and tend to disappear over time. As rivastigmine treatment improved cognition in AD animal models [7, 69, 70], more than 50 clinical trials have tested rivastigmine in AD. Early clinical trials evaluated the effect of rivastigmine capsules at doses of 1–4 and 6–12 mg/day and found a dose-dependent effect with improvements in cognition and daily living activities [71, 72]. In a 12-week study where donepezil and rivastigmine were tested in parallel, although both compounds resulted in improving the ADAS-cog score, donepezil was tolerated better [73]. However, rivastigmine is currently available in patches which display fewer gastrointestinal side effects [74, 75], and several more recent clinical trials using rivastigmine patches confirmed improvements in cognitive score [75–77]. While these clinical trials were relatively short, other clinical trials have evaluated the effect of longer treatment. One clinical trial evaluated rivastigmine over a five-year period and found that it slowed the cognitive decline, as measured by the Mini Mental State Examination (MMSE) [78] and one clinical trial will be evaluating the effects of the rivastigmine patch in the near future (NCT02703636). Other studies have also found rivastigmine patches to be beneficial to AD patients [79–81], and it has recently been found that co-treatment of rivastigmine with citicoline improves cognitive functions, but co-treatment with memantine does not show any additional benefits over rivastigmine treatment alone [82–84]. In addition, rivastigmine nasal spray (which results in higher bioavailability) and rivastigmine-hybrid drugs are also being investigated [85–87].

Rivastigmine has been tested for the treatment of Lewy body dementia and PD dementia. One study evaluated the effect of rivastigmine capsules in PD dementia, and found that after six months, rivastigmine treatment slightly improved cognition [88]. Rivastigmine has also been evaluated for the treatment of MCI (NCT01602198). In general, the three approved treatments for AD (donepezil, galantamine, and rivastigmine) have similar effects with similar side effects, although the rivastigmine patch treatment tends to have fewer side effects. In addition, rivastigmine seems to be more efficient as it also inhibits butyrylcholinesterase, another enzyme which can break down acetylcholine. For a subgroup of patients who have the specific butyrylcholinesterase K-genotype, who show a slower rate of cognitive decline compared to patients without the K-genotype, it has been found that the genotype influences the efficiency of the treatment. However, several studies show the dual inhibition of both cholinesterases maximises benefits, and that rivastigmine can also be of benefit in subcortical vascular dementia and PD dementia [89–92].

Ladostigil (TV-3326, chemical name: *[(N-propargyl-(3R) aminoindan-5-yl)-ethyl methyl carbamate]*) is a compound that combines the cholinesterase inhibitory activity (from rivastigmine) and monoamine oxidase inhibitory activity (from the anti-Parkinson drug rasagiline) [93] and has also been reported to be protective in AD by modulating the processing of amyloid precursor protein (APP) [94–96]. Two Phase II clinical trials in AD and MCI were recently terminated (NCT01354691, NCT01429623). However, although no further clinical trial is currently listed for ladostigil, rasagiline alone is currently being tested in a Phase II clinical trial (NCT02359552). GLN-1062 (memogain) is the inactive form of galantamine. It is more lipophilic than its precursor and is produced as a nasal spray. The main goals of the modification are to improve brain bioavailability and to reduce side effects. AD transgenic mice treated with intranasally-delivered memogain displayed improved scores in behavioural tests, and reduced numbers of amyloid plaques in the brain [42]. In initial clinical studies, GLN-1062 improved cognitive effects more efficiently than equivalent doses of galantamine, with fewer side effects [97]. In an initial trial using healthy young and old volunteers, memogain was found to be safe and well-tolerated (given at the same doses of galantamine and donepezil). Furthermore, GLN-1062 early side effects were not observable until given at a higher dose than galantamine [98].

In the past, the first acetylcholinesterase inhibitor approved for the treatment of AD was tacrine (Cognex™ chemical name: *1,2,3,4-tetrahydro-9-acridinamine monohydrochloride monohydrate*). However, due to liver toxicity [99] this treatment was discontinued once safer cholinesterase inhibitors reached the market. The efficacy of a non-toxic form of tacrine, named hupertacrine [100] as well as hybrids molecules of tacrine [101–106] are being investigated. Encenicline (EVP-6124, MT-4666 chemical name: *(R)-7-chloro-N-quinuclidin-3-yl benzo[b]thiophene-2-carboxamide*) is another molecule that affects the cholinergic system, specifically it is an agonist of the α-7-nicotinic acetylcholine receptor (α7-nAChR). So far, Phase I/II clinical trials have indicated that doses of up to 2 mg, in conjunction with either rivastigmine or donepezil, improve verbal and language fluency and attention without evident side effects [107]. However, in spite of promising results in Phase I/II, the development of the drug was halted during Phase III clinical trials, due to severe gastrointestinal side effects. Varenicline is an agonist of the α7-nicotinic acetylcholine receptor (α7-nAChR). Although early studies indicated that varenicline was able to reduce the toxic binding between Aβ and the acetylcholine receptor with consequent synaptic loss [108, 109], a Phase II clinical trial reported no benefits following varenicline treatment [110].

14.2.1.2 Other Neurotransmitters

Memantine (Exiba™, Namenda™, Axura®, Memary® chemical name: *3,5-Dimethyl-1-adamantanamine hydrochloride*) is the only approved drug for AD that does not affect the cholinergic system, and instead is an antagonist of the NMDA glutamate receptors in the brain. Its main action is to block the Ca^{2+} influx by binding to the NMDA receptors with a higher affinity than Mg^{2+} ions. This in turn reduces the release of glutamate in the synaptic regions, thus lowering the toxicity associated with high glutamate levels. Memantine is also a low-affinity antagonist of the α7-nAChR and a low-affinity antagonist of the 5-HT3 serotonin receptor. Several animal studies using AD models have reported that memantine is able to improve cognition, and reduce amyloid plaque numbers and AD-like pathology, either alone [43, 111–116] or in combination with acetylcholinesterase inhibitors [117, 118]. It has also been reported that memantine affects Aβ production and aggregation [119, 120]. Several clinical trials have reported that in general memantine improves cognitive behaviour, although results are mixed. Side effects include headache, confusion, sleepiness, dizziness, and high blood pressure. In mild-to-moderate AD, two six-month-long clinical trials evaluated the effect of memantine, and while one reported improved cognitive behaviour over placebo, the other failed to report statistically significant results. In general, memantine has not been found to be of significant benefit in the early stages of the disease [121, 122], though one report has indicated that memantine reduces agitation [123]. In mild-to-severe AD, several clinical trials have reported that memantine treatment improves cognitive behaviour, and reduces some other neurological symptoms associated with the disease, such as delusion, aggression, hallucinations, and irritability [124–126]. When given in combination with acetylcholinesterase inhibitors (donepezil, rivastigmine, galantamine), some studies have found that memantine increases the improvement in cognitive behaviour when compared to acetylcholinesterase inhibitor treatments on their own [64, 127–137], although some studies did not find such significant improvements [34, 83, 84, 138–140]. A Phase IV clinical trial is currently scheduled

(NCT03168997). Memantine has also been tested for other conditions such as Down Syndrome, vascular dementia, PD, Dementia with Lewy bodies and neuropathic pain, but in general, results of these studies have not reported significant improvements [141–143].

Treatments in Advanced Clinical Trials Prazosin (Vasoflex, Pressin, chemical name: *2-[4-(2-Furoyl)piperazin-1-yl]-6,7-dimethoxyquinazolin-4-amine*) is currently used for the treatment of hypertension, post-traumatic stress disorder, and panic disorder. Prazosin is a selective antagonist for the α1-adrenergic receptors located on vascular smooth muscle cells, where these receptors mediate the vasoconstrictive effects of norepinephrine and adrenaline. It is generally well-tolerated, and side effects include nausea, fatigue, and weakness. Since studies have linked α1-adrenergic receptors and AD [144] and that aggressive behaviour correlates with the number of α1-adrenoreceptors [145], it was thought that prazosin may be of value in the treatment of aggressive behaviour in AD patients. One study reported that prazosin at 6 mg/day for eight weeks improved the behavioural symptoms of AD patients who displayed agitation/aggression [146]. It has also been reported that prazosin reduces memory deterioration in a mouse model of AD [147], and advanced clinical trials were recently completed.

Also in Phase IV and III trials (NCT01832350, NCT02446132, NCT02442765, NCT02442778), are AVP-923 (Nuedexta, Zenvia chemical name: *dextromethorphan hydrobromide/quinidine sulfate*) and its second generation version, AVP-786, both of which involve the combination of two drugs, dextromethorphan (weak antagonist of NMDA receptors and agonist of sigma-1 receptors) and quinidine (used to treat irregular heartbeat and to increase the bioavailability of dextromethorphan). The main effect of these treatments is to reduce glutamate excitotoxicity, though studies have reported that the combination also reduces agitation in AD patients [148], and AVP-786 is currently being tested for treating agitation in AD [149]. However, AVP-923 is contraindicated in several groups of patients. These groups include people with heart problems, thrombocytopenia, lupus-like syndrome, and hepatitis. The dextromethorphan/quinidine combination has also been shown to be efficient for the treatment of pseudobulbar affect in dementia [150], and is being tested in diseases such as amyotrophic lateral sclerosis (ALS), multiple sclerosis (MS), and PD (NCT00573443, NCT00050232, NCT01767129).

ITI-007 is a 5-HT2A receptor antagonist (although it has also displayed affinity for dopamine receptors and serotonin transporter) [151–153] that is about to be evaluated in a Phase III clinical trial (NCT02817906) for the treatment of agitation in AD. It has also been tested for the treatment of schizophrenia.

Treatments in Early Research Phases There are many promising compounds going through earlier phases of testing.

BI 409306 (SUB 166499) is an inhibitor of phosphodiesterase 9A (PDE9A) which is involved in lowering the levels of cGMP. Synaptic transmission and plasticity of several brain areas affected in AD are modulated by cGMP through other messengers such as nitric oxide and glutamate. It has been reported that inhibition of PDE9A results in increased synaptic plasticity, enhanced memory, and improved behaviour in rodents [154, 155], although these results were achieved with PDE9A inhibitors other than BI 409306. In healthy males, the drug has been shown to be safe and well-tolerated [156], and a Phase I clinical trial in healthy volunteers indicated that the drug efficiently crosses the blood–brain barrier [157]. Two Phase II trials in AD patients have been completed, testing several doses of the drug, either alone, or in parallel with donepezil.

Neu-P11 (piromelatine) is a serotonin 5-HT1A/1D receptor agonist and a melatonin receptor agonist which has shown the capacity to improve object recognition in a rat model of AD (induced by intrahippocampal administration of Aβ42) and to reduce cellular loss [158]. A Phase II clinical trial in mild AD is recruiting participants (NCT02615002).

Riluzole (Rilutek®, chemical name: *6-trifluoromethoxy-2-benzothiazolamine*) is believed to alter glutamate excitotoxicity, by both modulating glutamate release and its post-synaptic effects. Riluzole has shown the capacity to provide neuroprotection against amyloid-induced damage in hippocampal neurons, and to improve cognitive and memory deficits in rodent models of AD [159–161]. Despite being an approved drug for ALS (for which more clinical trials are scheduled), following negative Phase II clinical trials results, it has been discontinued for the treatment of PD and Huntington disease [162, 163]. Currently, a Phase II clinical trial for mild AD is recruiting participants (NCT01703117).

Pimavanserin is a 5-HT2A receptor inverse agonist that has already been approved for the treatment of psychosis in PD [164]. A study in mouse models of AD indicated that this drug was able to reduce psychosis-like behaviours [165]. A one-year treatment Phase II clinical trial is currently ongoing (NCT03118947).

Allopregnanolone (clinical name: *3a,5a-tetrahydroprogesterone*) is a modulator of inhibitory γ-aminobutyric acid receptor (GABA-R) on several cell types in the brain, whose levels are reduced in the brains of AD patients [166–168]. Studies carried out in rodents indicate that allopregnanolone reduces amyloid deposition, increases learning and memory [169–171], and enhances the neurogenesis of dopaminergic neurons [172, 173], although some reports indicate that allopregnanolone treatment accelerates AD pathology [174, 175]. It is currently in Phase I clinical trials (NCT02221622) for the treatment of MCI and AD.

Discontinued (or not Currently Tested in Any Clinical Trials) Brexpiprazole (chemical name: *7-[4-[4-(1-benzothiophen-4-yl)piperazin-1-yl]butoxy]quinolin-2(1H)-one*) is an agonist of the dopamine receptor D2, and is currently approved for the treatment of schizophrenia, but it is being tested as adjuvant therapy in AD and in attention deficit hyperactivity disorders. Two Phase III clinical trials were recently completed and were evaluating doses ranging from 0.5 to 2 mg/day in AD patients for three months (NCT01862640, NCT01922258).

ORM-12741 is an α2c adrenergic receptor antagonist which has been tested in several Phase I trials that evaluated the safety and the dosage and, following a three-month Phase II trial, a small but significant memory improvement was reported [176]. Another Phase II clinical trial was recently completed (NCT02471196).

Dexpramipexole (R-Pramipexole, chemical name: *(R)-2-Amino-4,5,6,7-tetrahydro-6-(propylamino)benzothiazole*) is the optical enantiomer of a dopamine agonist (pramipexole), and it can be used at higher doses than pramipexole as it has a lower affinity for its receptor. However, it is believed that it also can protect neurons by acting as an antioxidant and free radical scavenger, beyond its main effect as dopamine agonist [177–179]. In addition, pramipexole has been shown to provide neuroprotection against Aβ-induced neurotoxicity [177, 180]. Several Phase I clinical trials tested single and repeated doses of the compound, and reported good tolerability and safety [181]; however, a small clinical trial in AD patients did not record any benefits of dexpramipexole [182].

Idalopirdine (chemical name: *2-(6-fluoro-1H-indol-3-yl)-ethyl-[3-(2,2,3,3-tetrafluoropropoxy)-benzyl]-amine*) is an antagonist of the serotonin 6H receptor, a receptor that is particularly expressed in the hippocampus and the cortex [183, 184], areas which are extremely affected in AD patients. It is an orally available drug, and has been tested in combination with cholinesterase inhibitors. A Phase II clinical trial measured the effect of 90 mg/day of idalopirdine in combination with 10 mg/day of donepezil for six months, and it was found that the combination of these two medicaments improved cognitive behaviour more than treatment with donepezil alone [35]. A Phase III clinical trial testing the effects of idalopirdine in conjunction with donepezil was recently completed. PF-5212377 (SAM760) is another serotonin 5-HT6 receptor antagonist, and this has been tested in Phase II trials in mild-to-moderate Alzheimer's patients (NCT01712074).

Intepirdine (RVT-101, SB-742457) is a serotonin 5-HT6 receptor antagonist which has been shown to improve learning in rodents [185, 186]. Some benefits from the drug were reported in clinical trials when it was tested at 35 mg/day (donepezil treatment alone was also included) [187]. A Phase III clinical trial tested RVT-101 in conjunction with donepezil in mild-to-moderate AD patients (NCT02585934), while another Phase III tested the compound alone (NCT02586909).

GSK239512 is a histamine H3 receptor antagonist which has been tested with the goal of increase cholinergic signalling. Clinical trials have tested doses of up to 80 mg/day and, while reportedly safe, it was only shown to improve episodic memory [188, 189]. No further clinical trials are currently listed.

14.2.2 Cholesterol-Lowering Medications

As discussed in other chapters of this book, hypercholesterolemia is considered a risk factor for AD, therefore medications aimed at reducing cholesterol levels have been tested for effectiveness in treating AD.

Simvastatin (Zocor®, Lipex®) and atorvastatin (Lipitor®, Zarator®) are HMG-CoA reductase inhibitors widely approved and prescribed for hypercholesterolemia, as they inhibit the synthesis of cholesterol. In previous years, there was growing evidence which indicated that the use of statins seemed to be protective in AD; this was detailed in several scientific reports [190–192]. Statins have also been tested in non-demented individuals. In the first study, pravastatin was given for up to six months at 10 mg/day doses and did not decrease plasma levels of Aβ40 and Aβ42 [193]. Following these results, a second study was performed in hypercholesterolemic patients. Simvastatin at 40 mg/day for 6 weeks then 80 mg/day for 30 weeks did not alter plasma levels of Aβ40 and Aβ42, and neither did atorvastatin at doses of 20 mg/day for 6 weeks, then 40 mg/day for 6 weeks, and finally 80 mg/day for 24 weeks [194]. However, these statins need to be evaluated differently, as plasma Aβ40 and Aβ42 levels are not established biomarkers of AD or AD risk [195]. More encouragingly, when the analysis was performed on the cerebrospinal fluid (CSF) of hypercholesterolemic dementia-free subjects, reduced levels of phospho-tau were observed following the administration of simvastatin at 40 mg/day but not pravastatin at 80 mg/day for 14 weeks. However, no differences in CSF Aβ40, Aβ42, total tau, or soluble APPα levels were observed [196]. In one trial, simvastatin at doses up to 80 mg/day for 26 weeks had no significant effect on CSF Aβ40 or Aβ42 levels in AD patients. However, in post-hoc analysis, it was found to decrease CSF Aβ40 levels along with 24S-hydroxycholesterol levels in patients with mild AD (but not severe AD), though had no significant effect on the more aggregable Aβ42 [197]. In another trial, 19 patients with AD received simvastatin at a dose of 20 mg/day for 12 weeks. The drug significantly reduced the levels of CSF sAPPα and sAPPβ, but did not affect the levels of CSF tau, phospho-tau, Aβ42, or plasma Aβ42 [198]. In accordance with these articles, simvastatin at doses of 20 mg/day in AD patients for 12 months in another study did not decrease CSF Aβ42 levels. However, based on the APP isoform analysis, the treatment may favour non-amyloidogenic APP processing, as more sAPPα was observed at the endpoint [199]. A later study found that simvastatin at up to 80 mg/day for 12 weeks decreased brain cholesterol levels but did not affect AD biomarkers such as plasma Aβ40 (as mentioned earlier, not necessarily a good AD biomarker), CSF Aβ40 and Aβ42, tau or phospho-tau. In addition, 24S-hydroxycholesterol, 27-hydroxycholesterol, and 7-hydroxycholesterol levels were unchanged in CSF [200]. Many other studies have been carried out, yet Cochrane database systematic reviews have indicated that there is no convincing evidence that statins provide any benefit on the primary outcome measures of ADAS-Cog or MMSE, and no clear benefit in preventing dementia [201, 202]. It is now thought that statins may provide some protective effect long before the potential onset of the disease, by reducing vascular risk factors [203], yet once the disease has started, the protective effect disappears. Atorvastatin and simvastatin are currently not being tested in clinical trials for AD, although simvastatin is currently in a Phase IV clinical trial for MCI (NCT00842920).

Although deferiprone is mostly known as an iron chelator, it has been shown to have the ability to reduce the levels of Aβ40, Aβ42 and BACE1 in cholesterol-fed rabbits, in addition to reducing the cholesterol-induced tau-phosphorylation. These results suggest that the protective effects of deferiprone may be achieved through reduction of cholesterol and iron in the plasma rather than chelation of iron in the brain (which was unaffected in this study). A Phase II clinical trial is currently recruiting MCI, prodromal AD, and mild AD patients (NCT03234686).

14.2.3 Immunotherapy

Immunotherapy for AD is currently being tested with the aim of removing Aβ plaques from the brain. Immunotherapy can be divided into two types: active immunotherapy and passive immunotherapy. Active immunotherapy involves the stimulation of the immune system by injecting substances (such as antigens) which can trigger an immune response. Passive immunotherapy on the other hand, rather than activating the immune system, involves the injection of agents such as antibodies, that directly attack their targets (i.e. senile plaques for Aβ immunotherapy) (Figure 14.2).

Active immunotherapy involves the host producing antibodies following injection of a specific antigen, whereas passive immunotherapy involves direct injection of purified specific antibodies.

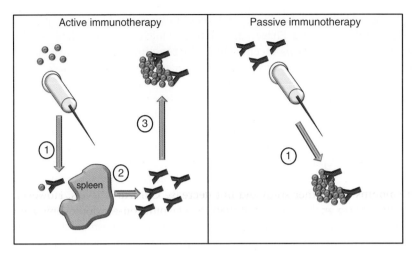

Figure 14.2 Active and passive immunotherapy. (*See color plate section for the color representation of this figure.*)

14.2.3.1 Active Immunotherapy (Aβ)

AN-1792 was the first immunotherapy compound tested and the peptide consisted of the full-length Aβ peptide. Although vaccination with Aβ in murine models of AD showed promising results [204, 205], in a Phase II clinical trial, four patients developed meningoencephalitis [206] and in 2002 the development of this vaccine was terminated. Post-mortem evaluation of patients who received the vaccine continued after vaccine production was stopped, and it was reported that the vaccine was efficient in removing plaques from the brain, although it also resulted in T-cell infiltration and overall inflammation [207].

CAD106 immunisation involved the use of Aβ 1–6 fragments as antigens. In murine models, this immunisation reduced the accumulation of amyloid in the brain [208]. A Phase I clinical trial in people with mild-to-moderate AD indicated that the vaccine elicited an immune response without causing encephalitis [209]. Subsequently, Phase II clinical trials with intramuscular and subcutaneous injections tested the tolerability of different doses and antibody response following injection for longer periods. Results indicated that responders had prolonged antibody titres and administration of the antigen was tolerated [210, 211]. It is currently being tested in further Phase II/III clinical trials (NCT02565511).

ABvac40 is an active vaccine which targets the C-terminal end of Aβ40. A recently terminated Phase I clinical trial reported the vaccine was safe and well tolerated [212] and a Phase II clinical trial is currently recruiting MCI/AD patients (NCT03461276).

UB-311 vaccine was generated using two copies of Aβ1–14 fragments linked to different helper T-cell epitopes in a Th2-biased delivery system. Safety and tolerability were tested in primates. Studies in mice reported that the vaccine was able to reduce Aβ oligomers and plaques, while an initial clinical trial indicated that the vaccine was effective, although cognitive improvements were more prominent in the mild AD group rather than in patients in a more advanced stage of the disease [213]. Currently a Phase II clinical trial is ongoing in mild AD patients (NCT02551809).

Another vaccine Lu AF20513 is based on three repetitions of the Aβ 1–12 sequence, and is currently being tested in a Phase I trial (NCT02388152). Preliminary results in animal models indicated that this vaccine elicits a strong immune response paired with a reduction in AD-like pathology, without inducing microglial or astrocytic activation [214].

ACC-001 is a discontinued active immunotherapeutic compound whose peptide spanned the first seven amino acids of the Aβ sequence, again developed with the intention of avoiding the inflammatory response elicited by longer Aβ fragments (see AN-1792). Tested in several Phase II clinical trials, it was generally found to be safe, but some adverse events were reported [215–218].

AD02 is a peptide that resembles the six amino acids at the N-terminus of Aβ. A Phase I clinical trial indicated that AD02 immunisation is safe and well-tolerated, and no meningoencephalitis cases were reported [219]. AD02-induced antibodies are characterised by selectivity for aggregated Aβ forms, thus theoretically have an absence of reactivity with related molecules such as APP and secreted APPα [220], which should therefore reduce unwanted immune reactions. Further clinical trials are not being carried out on this peptide.

ACI-24 is a liposome vaccine based on the tetrapalmitoylated Aβ 1–15 fragment, again based on a sequence of Aβ that is not expected to generate an unwanted inflammatory response. In murine models, the vaccine induces a non-inflammatory antibody response and reduces the level of insoluble Aβ40 and Aβ42 [221].

14.2.3.2 Active Immunotherapy (tau)

AADvac1 is an active immunotherapy peptide consisting of amino acids 294–305 of the tau sequence. In animal models, initial studies reported beneficial effects, while also displaying safety properties [222]. An initial Phase I clinical trial also reported that the vaccine was generally safe, and that the vaccine provoked a strong immune response [223]. A Phase II clinical trial is currently ongoing (NCT02579252).

ACI-35 is a liposomal vaccine which consists of 16 copies of tau fragments including phosphorylation at positions S396 and S404. In mouse models of AD, ACI-35 injection induces antibodies directed against phosphorylated tau, and it extends lifespan, without inducing inflammation or T-cell activation [224].

14.2.3.3 Passive Immunotherapy (Aβ)

In contrast to active immunotherapy, passive immunotherapy has more ongoing clinical trials, and more compounds have been tested.

Aducanumab (BIIB037) is a human IgG1 monoclonal antibody against a conformational epitope of Aβ. Recent results have highlighted that in human and mouse models of AD, aducanumab reduces amyloid plaque load and restores calcium homeostasis [225–227]. However, in one study, some adverse effects were reported in more than one-half of patients given a higher dose [228, 229]. Aducanumab is currently recruiting patients in two Phase III clinical trials (NCT02484547, NCT02477800), while a Phase I clinical trial is ongoing (NCT01677572).

Solanezumab is a monoclonal IgG1 antibody raised against the central sequence of Aβ and targets soluble, not fibrillar, Aβ. An initial study using different doses of solanezumab reported increased levels of Aβ in plasma and CSF, although no changes in cognitive scores were recorded [230]. Increased levels of plasma Aβ were subsequently confirmed in a Japanese study which also reported that the vaccine was safe and well-tolerated [231]. In two Phase III clinical trials in mild to moderate AD, solanezumab at first failed to produce significant improvements, although the assessment of secondary outcome measures indicated that it can be beneficial in mild AD [232, 233]. An additional double-blind Phase III clinical trial failed to associate solanezumab treatment with improved cognitive performances [234]. However, in spite of these latest results, a Phase II/III clinical trial is enrolling patients (NCT01760005) while a Phase III clinical trial is currently ongoing (NCT02008357).

Gantenerumab (RG1450) is another IgG1 antibody that binds to fibrillar Aβ (1–11 domain), and by recruiting microglia, generates a cell-mediated clearance of amyloid plaques which does not alter plasma Aβ levels [235]. In another mouse model study, gantenerumab, in combination with a beta-site amyloid precursor protein-cleaving enzyme (BACE) inhibitor (see later 'Targeting the Aβ-producing Pathway'), was able to reduce the amyloid plaque number [236]. The Phase I clinical trial reported that the compound is generally safe, although it may induce inflammation when injected at the highest dose [237]. A Phase III clinical trial, which was stopped early for futility, indicated that higher doses of gantenerumab may be necessary [238]. It is currently in two Phase III clinical trials for patients with mild AD or prodromal AD (NCT02051608, NCT01224106) and two more Phase III clinical trials are planned, but not yet recruiting (NCT03443973, NCT03444870).

Crenezumab is an IgG4 immunoglobulin that recognises oligomeric and fibrillar Aβ species better than monomeric ones. By using the IgG4 subclass, there is a reduced risk of Fcγ-receptor activation with consequent reduction of pro-inflammatory cytokines, such as TNFα. Plaque reduction was observed following crenezumab treatment in a mouse model of AD, in which microglia were responsible for the uptake of Aβ [239]. However, data reported at the 2014 AAIC Conference indicated that crenezumab failed to meet expectations in two Phase II clinical trials (http://www.alzforum.org/news/conference-coverage/crenezumab-disappoints-phase-2-researchers-remain-hopeful). Nevertheless, a Phase III clinical trial is currently recruiting patients (NCT03114657) while another Phase II is ongoing (NCT02670083).

In addition to these compounds which are at a more advanced stage, other compounds are being tested in earlier phases in clinical trials.

BAN2401 is a human IgG1 that binds to large Aβ protofibrils with the intent of enhancing their clearance, which was observed while using the murine version (mAb158) that reduces the levels of amyloid in the brain in a mouse model of AD [240]. A Phase I clinical trial in mild-to-moderate AD patients reported that BAN2401 was tolerated at doses up to 10 mg kg^{-1} [241] and a Phase II clinical trial is ongoing (NCT01767311).

LY3002813 is an IgG2 antibody which targets a pyroglutamate form of Aβ, present in amyloid plaques, with the goal of dissolving existing senile plaques present in the brain. In mice, mE8 antibody (the murine version) was able to reduce plaques without causing microhaemorrhages [242]. Co-treatment with BACE inhibitors LY2811376 (see later inhibitors of Aβ productions) reduced plaques in a mouse transgenic model of AD by around 80%, far better than either compound tested alone (http://www.alzforum.org/news/conference-coverage/anti-amyloid-therapies-combine-forces-knock-out-plaques). A Phase I clinical trial testing intravenous and subcutaneous injection is currently ongoing in patients with AD (NCT02624778) while a Phase II clinical trial is testing LY3002813 in combination with another BACE inhibitor LY3202626 (NCT03367403).

Gamunex, is an IntraVenous Immunoglobulin (IVIg) mix purified from human plasma. It has been tested in AD as the immunoglobulins include natural antibodies against Aβ, as well as anti-inflammatory antibodies. Several studies performed in mice indicated beneficial effects of IVIg injections [243–246]. However, while the first studies in humans also reported beneficial effects of IVIg [247, 248], subsequent Phase II and Phase III clinical trials have failed to confirm early results [249, 250]. The use of such a product is also questionable, as meeting the huge demand for it would be almost impossible.

AAB-003 is a modified version of the former AAB-001 (bapineuzumab, see below), with the intent of reducing microglial activation and imaging abnormalities, which were a complication of AAB-001 treatment [251, 252] (see later discontinued compounds). Recently published data in humans reported a dose-dependent increase in plasma Aβ with increasing doses of AAB-003 (0.5–8 mg kg^{-1}) [253]. Although imaging abnormalities were still present in some patients, they appeared at a higher dose in comparison with bapineuzumab, indicating that AAB-003 is less prone to causing microglial activation [253]. Two Phase I clinical trials (NCT01193608, NCT01369225) were recently completed.

Bapineuzumab (see above AAB-001) is an IgG1 antibody that binds to soluble and fibrillar Aβ and the murine version 3D6 had shown the capacity to clear plaques and improve behaviour in mouse models, although it also induced micro-haemorrhages and increased the levels of pro-inflammatory cytokines [254–258]. Several clinical trials were performed and, in addition to some side effects at the highest dose, no major differences were observed between placebo and treated groups [259–264].

Another discontinued immunoglobulin is ponezumab, an IgG2A mapped against amino acids 33–40 of the Aβ1–40 sequence [265]. In aged transgenic mice, the murine analogue was able to increase Aβ levels in plasma without causing micro-haemorrhages [266] and to reduce the rate of cerebral vascular amyloid [267]. When tested in humans, ponezumab injections did not display any safety concerns and increased the plasma levels of Aβ; unfortunately cognitive function tests indicated no improvements [268–271].

SAR228810 and MED1814 are two additional antibodies that have been tested intravenously or subcutaneously in Phase I clinical trials to assess their safety features (NCT02036645, NCT01485302), but no additional clinical trials are scheduled.

14.2.3.4 Passive Immunotherapy (tau)

RO7105705 is an antibody directed against tau for which a recently terminated Phase I clinical trial in mild-to-moderate AD was followed by a Phase II clinical trial in prodromal-to-mild AD which is recruiting participants (NCT03289143).

In a Phase I clinical trial in patients with progressive supranuclear palsy (PSP) ABBV-8E12 has shown a safety profile at different doses [272]. Based on the safety information obtained in this initial study, Phase II clinical trials have been listed in early AD patients (NCT02880956) and in PSP patients (NCT03391765, NCT02985879).

BIIB076 is a human anti-tau monoclonal antibody which has been reported to cross the BBB in monkeys, and it is currently being tested in a Phase I clinical trial (NCT03056729).

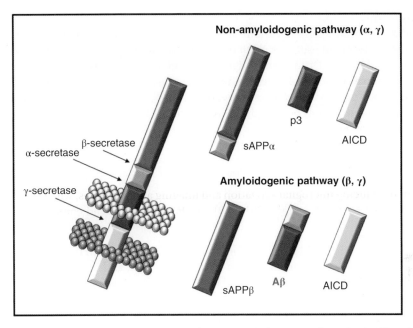

Figure 14.3 APP cleavage pathways. In the non-amyloidogenic pathway (top), APP is cleaved by α-secretase then γ-secretase, which leads to the generation of sAPPα, the non-amyloidogenic p3 fragment, and AICD. In the amyloidogenic pathway (bottom), APP is cleaved by β-secretase then γ-secretase, which leads to the generation of sAPPβ, Aβ, and AICD. (*See color plate section for the color representation of this figure.*)

RG7345 (RO6926496) is a monoclonal antibody that is directed against the phosphorylated epitope S422 of tau, generated by immunising rabbits with the sequence 416–430 of tau. This site, when phosphorylated, has been shown to be important in relocating tau [273]. In a mouse model of AD, injection of the antibody was found to reduce the accumulation of tau pathology [274]. However, no clinical trials are planned.

14.2.4 Targeting the Aβ-Producing Pathway

Aβ is a proteolytic fragment generated from a longer transmembrane protein – the amyloid precursor protein – APP. Aβ is usually 40–42 amino acids long, and is the main component of the amyloid plaques in the AD brain. It is considered, especially in small oligomer form, to be the main toxic agent responsible for the synaptic loss and neuronal death that is associated with the disease. APP is cleaved via two major pathways. In the non-amyloidogenic pathway, APP is cleaved by α-secretase, at a site in the middle of the Aβ sequence; this is followed by the γ-secretase cleavage. This pathway does not generate Aβ, instead produces secreted/soluble APP cleaved at the α-cleavage site (sAPPα), the small proteolytic fragment p3, and a C-terminal fragment (often referred to as the amyloid precursor protein intracellular domain or AICD). In the alternative amyloidogenic pathway, APP is first cleaved by β-secretase (known as BACE-1), and the subsequent cleavage by γ-secretase generates the Aβ peptide and sAPPβ (as well as the C-terminal fragment) and this is considered the pathological amyloidogenic pathway (see Figure 14.3). In general, therapies aimed at these three secretases are aiming to increase α-secretase activity and/or inhibit the β or γ-secretase activities.

14.2.4.1 α-Secretase

Acitretin (soriatane) is an agonist of the retinoic acid receptor which has long been approved for the treatment of psoriasis. With regards to AD, acitretin has been shown to increase the expression of A Disintegrin and Metalloproteinase 10 (ADAM-10), which is considered to be an α-secretase. In the murine model of AD it has been reported that it can cross the blood–brain barrier and reduce Aβ levels [275, 276]. In a Phase II clinical trial, the drug reduced the levels of sAPPβ and increased the levels of sAPPα, although levels of Aβ were unchanged [277].

14.2.4.2 β-Secretase

Verubecestat (MK-8931) is a BACE1/2 inhibitor currently in Phase III clinical trials. Studies in animals and humans have indicated that this BACE inhibitor lowers the levels of brain Aβ and CSF Aβ without causing unwanted events [278–280]. A Phase III clinical trial was recently terminated (NCT01739348) while another Phase III clinical trial is ongoing (NCT01953601).

Lanabecestat (AZD3293, LY3314814) is an orally active BACE1 inhibitor that has been shown to reduce the levels of Aβ and sAPPβ in mice, guinea pigs, and dogs, in plasma, CSF, and brain tissue [281]. In a Phase I clinical trial, several doses were evaluated and it was reported that the compound was generally safe and induced a marked reduction in levels of Aβ in CSF and plasma [282, 283]. Currently in Phase II/III, these trials will evaluate the effect of the drug when given for 78 and 104 weeks to AD patients (NCT02245737, NCT02783573).

Elenbecestat (E2609) is a BACE inhibitor which has been widely tested in Phase I clinical trials, and it has been reported that the drug is well tolerated and reduces the levels of plasma Aβ up to 90% and CSF Aβ up to 80% [284]. A large Phase II trial is currently recruiting and will involve MCI and mild-to-moderate AD (NCT02322021); two other Phase III clinical trials are also recruiting patients (NCT03036280, NCT02956486).

Another BACE inhibitor, JNJ54861911, has been tested in several clinical trials, involving both healthy controls and AD patients. In a recent report, the company indicated that the drug is well tolerated and can decrease CSF Aβ levels by 90% at daily doses of 90 mg, paralleled by a decrease in sAPPβ and an increase in sAPPα [284]. Three Phase II/III clinical trials are recruiting participants (NCT02406027, NCT02569398, NCT01760005).

CNP520 is another BACE inhibitor, and two Phase II/III clinical trials (NCT02565511, NCT03131453) are currently recruiting AD patients to test it [285]. Many other BACE inhibitors have previously been tested in clinical trials and their development has been discontinued.

LY3202626, a BACE inhibitor that can be administered orally, will be evaluated in two Phase II clinical trials involving AD patients, either taken alone (NCT02791191) or in combination with LY3002813 (see above 'Immunotheraphy') (NCT03367403).

Thalidomide (Thalidomid®) is a compound which is currently prescribed for inflammatory conditions and several types of cancer, although it was formerly withdrawn from the market following numerous cases of severe birth defects (due to administration to mothers for the treatment of morning sickness). However, several early studies using mouse models of AD indicated that thalidomide was beneficial as it inhibited BACE1 [286–289]. Nevertheless, a more recent study failed to confirm the beneficial effects of the drug, due to poor tolerability and frequent adverse events [290].

14.2.4.3 γ-Secretase

γ-Secretase is the last enzyme involved in Aβ generation. As mentioned, after β-secretase cleavage (which generates sAPPβ and C99 – the C-terminal fragment that still includes Aβ), the C99 is cleaved by γ-secretase to generate Aβ and the AICD. Unfortunately, inhibition of γ-secretase, while inhibiting Aβ generation, also inhibits many other proteases and protein processing steps (for example Notch), and these additional events have been reported to cause adverse events. To avoid this problem, compound design has shifted from making γ-secretase inhibitors (which inhibit indiscriminately all protein processing) to γ-secretase modulators (which preferentially inhibit Aβ cleavage at position 42, while not affecting cleavages which generate shorter Aβ peptides and/or Notch). Readers should be reminded here that the longer Aβ42 peptides are more prone to aggregation, and are more amyloidogenic and more toxic than the shorter forms of Aβ, thus shifting γ-secretase cleavage towards producing a greater proportion of Aβ40 peptides is theoretically desirable.

Inhibitors With respect to γ-secretase inhibitors, two inhibitory compounds reached advanced testing stages, yet both are now discontinued.

Semagacestat (LY450139) was the first γ-secretase inhibitor to reach a Phase III clinical trial. In Phase II, despite consistently lowering Aβ plasma levels [291, 292], adverse side effects, mostly involving skin, were reported [292]. A Phase III clinical trial was terminated before the supposed final date because of major side effects such as skin cancer and infections [293].

Avagacestat (BMS-708163) is a selective inhibitor of γ-secretase (while not affecting Notch processing) which has been shown to reduce CSF Aβ levels in rats. In spite of being ruled safe in initial studies [294], the drug testing was halted after two Phase II clinical trials reported benefits were modest, yet were paired with numerous side effects, mostly gastrointestinal-related, but also including other unwanted effects such as non-melanoma skin cancer [295]. In a prodromal AD cohort, avagacestat was found to be inefficient, and the frequency of adverse side effects was found to correlate with dose size [296].

Modulators Ibuprofen (Advil™, Nuprin™, Motrin™) is a non-specific anti-inflammatory drug (NSAID) which gained attention when reports indicated that chronic administration of the drug reduced AD risk [297]. Its effect was attributed to its capacity to modulate γ-secretase and its ability to scavenge nitric oxide radicals. In addition, it was reported that it was able to reduce cytokine-induced Aβ release [298, 299]. In transgenic mice, ibuprofen treatment was found to reduce Aβ levels, plaques, and improve cognitive performances [300–304]. Further studies have highlighted the possibility that ibuprofen effects in mice were due to a direct effect on pro-inflammatory molecules such as interleukin-1β and α1-anti-chymotrypsin, rather than on cyclooxygenase-1 or -2 (COX-1/2) [305, 306]. However, a clinical trial indicated that no overall differences between placebo and treated groups were observable, except for a subset of AD patients that consisted of *APOE* ε4-carriers [307]. A combination of ibuprofen and cromolyn sodium (ALZT-OP1) [308] is currently being tested in a Phase III clinical trial (NCT02547818).

Flurizan™ (R-flurbiprofen, MCP7869, Tarenflurbil) is a NSAID related to ibuprofen, and is the optical enantiomer of S-flurbiprofen. It causes fewer side effects because it is not active on COX enzymes. Studies suggested that the drug has a direct effect on γ-secretase, that it lowers Aβ42 production, and reduces learning impairment in animals [309–313]. However, although encouraging results were obtained in a Phase II clinical trial involving mild AD patients [314], the drug did not show any beneficial effects in a Phase III clinical trial [315]. Nevertheless, a more recent study indicated that tarenflurbil can be effectively delivered to the brain through intranasal delivery [316], and further studies may be carried out, although no clinical trials are scheduled.

EVP-0962 (EVP-0015962) is a γ-secretase modulator that has been reported to reduce Aβ42 with a consequent increase in levels of the shorter Aβ38 in cells, while decreasing plaques, and neuroinflammation in a mouse model of AD [317]. A Phase II clinical trial with doses from 10 to 200 mg/day of EVP-0962 was recently terminated.

CHF5074 was believed to be a γ-secretase modulator, but studies in transgenic models of AD have indicated that the drug has a wider range of action which includes lowering tau and modulating synaptic plasticity and microglia [318]. Studies in AD animal models have indicated that CHF5074 treatment is able to reduce Aβ levels and amyloid plaques in the brain and to restore visual memory [319–322]. In clinical trials, administration of the drug did not induce any unwanted side effects [323] however, there were no significant differences between drug and placebo following neuropsychological tests, except in *APOE ε4* carriers [324]. No clinical trials are currently ongoing or recruiting patients.

14.2.5 Other Compounds Affecting Aβ

Azeliragon (PF-04494700) is an inhibitor of the receptor for advanced glycation end-products (RAGE) which (despite the name) functions as a receptor for the immunoglobulin superfamily. As RAGE is overexpressed in the hippocampus of AD patients and in transgenic mouse models of AD, and toxic changes occur upon RAGE binding to Aβ, current strategies are aimed at inhibiting its downstream effects [325–330]. A small initial trial indicated that azeraligon is safe and well-tolerated [331] and a larger 18-month Phase III clinical trial in mild AD patients is ongoing (NCT02080364). However, it is likely to be important to treat with RAGE inhibitors in early AD stages, preferably at asymptomatic stages, to gain most benefit.

Diabetes and related conditions such as insulin resistance, metabolic syndrome, obesity, and hyperinsulinaemia have all been reported to be risk factors for AD. It has been reported that the insulin receptor is downregulated in AD [332], and that reduced insulin signalling is linked to AD [333]. In fact, increasing signalling has been proven to be beneficial in the disease by preventing Aβ aggregation [334], by regulating tau phosphorylation [335], and by reducing inflammation, glucose toxicity, and production of advanced glycation end products. Previous clinical trials have reported beneficial effects following insulin treatment [336–339], and nasal insulin – insulin administered in the form of a nasal spray – is now being tested in AD: Phase I and II/III clinical trials are currently ongoing or recruiting AD patients (NCT01595646, NCT01767909, NCT02462161).

Nilotinib is an approved anti-cancer medication that acts as tyrosine kinase Abelson inhibitor. Recent reports have shown that nilotinib enhances amyloid clearance in mouse models of AD [340–342], and a Phase II clinical trial in mild-to-moderate AD (NCT02947893) is currently recruiting patients. Additionally, nilotinib has also produced encouraging results in Parkinson's mouse models [343–345].

Thiethylperazine is an activator of the ABCC1 transporter, which has been shown to play a prominent role in amyloid clearance from the brain [346, 347]. Accordingly, treatment with thiethylperazine has been shown to reduce the amyloid load in the brain of AD-model transgenic mice [348], and a Phase II clinical trial is currently scheduled in early to mild AD (NCT03417986).

Bryostatin is a protein kinase C (PKC) activator which has demonstrated the capacity to improve memory functions and to prevent synaptic loss in mouse models of AD, through a mechanism that shifts the APP processing towards the non-amyloidogenic sAPPα pathway [349–352]. An initial clinical trial provided positive results, and a subsequent Phase II clinical trial in moderately severe to severe AD patients is ongoing (NCT02431468).

NPT088 is a laboratory-engineered protein consisting of a fragment of human IgG and a fragment of a bacteriophage M13 protein, which had previously been shown to interact with amyloid [353]. Administration of NTP088 in mouse models of AD resulted in a broad range of positive effects such as improved cognitive performance, reduced brain atrophy, and reduced amyloid plaque and phospho-tau pathology [354]. A Phase I clinical trial in mild to moderate AD is recruiting participants (NCT03008161).

Vorinostat is an anti-cancer drug that acts as a histone deacetylation (HDAC) inhibitor, mostly inhibiting class I HDAC but not class II HDAC. Several studies have reported vorinostat may have beneficial effects as it can reduce Aβ25–35-induced toxicity in neuronal cells, it can also improve memory performance in mice, which may be a consequence of its anti-inflammatory effects, its capacity to increase apoJ, and to maintain H3 acetylation [355–359]. A Phase I clinical trial in mild AD (NCT03056495) is currently enrolling participants.

Oxaloacetate is a compound that removes excess glutamate in the nervous system by enhancing the activity of glutamate oxaloacetate transaminase (GOT), an enzyme responsible for its clearance. Indeed, *in vivo* administration of recombinant GOT reversed the toxic effects of Aβ, suggesting that targeting this pathway could reduce glutamate-related toxicity [360, 361]. After an initial study reported that oxaloacetate was generally safe [362] a Phase I clinical trial is enrolling participants (NCT02593318).

Bexarotene is an agonist of the retinoid X receptor (RXR) which has been linked to AD in the past, as its activation induces the expression of α-secretase (therefore shifting APP processing towards the non-amyloidogenic pathway, as discussed above), and also enhances Aβ uptake [276, 363]. Early studies indicated positive results as bexarotene reversed the deficit in an AD mouse model; however, in later animal studies, results were contradictory [190, 364–368]. Results from a clinical trial indicated that while the primary outcome was negative, bexarotene did reduce brain amyloid levels in *APOE ε4* non-carriers [369].

PQ912 is an inhibitor of the metalloenzyme glutaminyl cyclase. This enzyme is overexpressed in the brain and the blood of AD patients and generates a modified form of Aβ that tends to produce aggregates [370–373]. Furthermore, a recent report indicated that glutaminyl cyclase activity correlates with Aβ CSF levels in AD patients [374]. The use of PQ912 in mouse models has proven to be beneficial [375] supporting results from earlier reports which evaluated other glutaminyl cyclase inhibitors in animal studies [376–378]. A Phase II clinical trial was recently terminated (NCT02389413) and for the moment, no other trials are recruiting or ongoing.

ELND005 (scyllo-inositol; cyclohexane-1,2,3,4,5,6-hexol, a stereoisomer of inositol) has the capacity to prevent Aβ aggregation and to stabilise small Aβ42 aggregates [379].

Scyllo-inositol has been shown to be protective in *in vitro* and in mouse models of AD [380–386]. A Phase II clinical trial reported that doses of 250 mg/day reduces Aβ in the CSF [387], however no further clinical trials are currently planned.

PBT2 is a Cu/Zn ionophore related to 8-hydroxyquinoline. It attenuates the toxicity caused by metal ions and has been shown to reduce metal-induced Aβ aggregation. Reports have indicated that PBT2 promotes Aβ degradation, inhibits glutamate-mediated excitotoxicity, and restores synaptic spine density in a murine model of AD [388–390]. Clinical trials have also reported beneficial effects of PBT2 treatment in AD [391, 392], such as the lowering of CSF Aβ42. However, the results of a 12-month small double-blind trial of PBT2 at 250 mg/day showed no significant differences between PBT2 and controls in fluorodeoxyglucose-PET, MRI volumetrics, blood Aβ biomarkers, or cognition/function over the course of the double-blind phase [393], and the conclusion was that the individual variation in this small trial prevented a good evaluation of PBT2, and larger trials are necessary. The first generation Cu/Zn ionophore compound PBT1 (also known as clioquinol) had shown promising *in vitro* and *in vivo* results, as well as beneficial effects in a Phase II clinical trial, but displayed toxicity at high doses [394–398].

14.2.6 Other Compounds Affecting Tau

TRx0237 is an inhibitor of tau aggregation and is a replacement formulation for an initial product, Rember (TRx0014). The drug is based on methylene blue, and it modulates tau aggregation by inhibiting the formation of new aggregates in addition to dissolving existing ones. Methylene blue has been reported to be beneficial in AD in improving clearance of Aβ and in modulating β-secretase and mitochondrial antioxidant activity [399–404]. A Phase III clinical trial for AD and frontotemporal dementia was recently terminated, while a Phase II/III clinical trial is currently enrolling (NCT03446001).

Liraglutide (Glucagon-Like Peptide-1 [GLP1]) is an anti-diabetic drug which has repeatedly been linked to cognitive and memory improvements in mouse models of AD. In addition to enhancing synaptic plasticity and reducing amyloid load in the brain, its main effect appears to be the modulation of tau phosphorylation through a mechanism that involves GSK-3β [405–414]. A Phase II clinical trial is enrolling patients (NCT01843075).

LM11A-31 is a small compound which acts as a p75 neurotrophic receptor (p75NTR) ligand that reduces tau phosphorylation and misfolding. As p75NTR has previously been linked to AD [415, 416], several reports have subsequently targeted it and indicated that AD mouse models treated with LM11A-31 displayed reduced cognitive defects, neurite degeneration, and inflammatory changes by limiting microglial activation [417–420]. A Phase I/II clinical trial in mild-to-moderate AD is recruiting participants (NCT03069014).

TPI287 is a microtubule-stabilising drug that has been tested in several types of cancer [421–424]. It is currently being tested in a Phase I clinical trial in AD patients (NCT01966666) for its capacity to stabilise tau.

Tideglusib is a GSK3β inhibitor being tested in AD and PSP. In animal models, it has so far displayed beneficial effects such as reducing neuronal loss and promoting neurogenesis [425, 426]. A small trial indicated that tideglusib can improve cognitive functions compared to placebo [427]; however, a subsequent larger Phase II clinical trial did not report any clinical benefits following treatment with tideglusib [428].

14.2.7 Inflammatory Targets

The last part of this chapter discusses molecules that affect inflammatory pathways. Although some of these compounds, such as ibuprofen, were discussed earlier in this chapter due to their ability to affect other pathways as well as inflammation, in this section we will discuss compounds that only affect inflammation.

Pioglitazone is a Peroxisome Proliferator-Activated Receptor-γ (PPAR-γ) agonist which has been tested in several mouse models of AD. It has been found to lead to improved cognition and memory performances, reduced Aβ pathology, and reduced synaptic defects [429–436]. Improved cognition and memory performances have also been observed in clinical trials [437, 438]. One Phase III clinical trial is ongoing in MCI patients (NCT01931566) while another Phase III trial is enrolling MCI patients (NCT02284906).

Sargramostim (Leukine®) is a synthetic glycoprotein that resembles granulocyte-macrophage colony-stimulating factor (GM-CSF), and has the goal of stimulating the innate immune system. In animal models, it has been shown to reverse cognitive impairment and amyloidosis [439]. Its tolerability is currently being tested in Phase II clinical trials in AD patients (NCT01409915).

Neflamapimod (VX-745) is another compound that has been tested in two recently terminated Phase II clinical trials (NCT02423122, NCT02423200), and acts as a p38 mitogen-activated protein kinase (MAPK) inhibitor. It has been reported that p38 MAPK stimulates the release of pro-inflammatory cytokines in response to several stimuli, including Aβ42 [440] and its inhibition has been proven to be beneficial in AD animal models [441–444]. In rats, VX-745 reduced neuroinflammation while in parallel improved performances in the water maze [445]. As the results from the initial clinical trials were positive (significant improvement in episodic memory) [446], one Phase II clinical trial is enrolling participants (NCT03402659).

COR388 is a bacterial protease inhibitor which targets pathogens in the brain and CSF of AD patients (https://www.businesswire.com/news/home/20180104005431/en/Cortexyme-Initiates-Phase-1-Clinical-Development-COR388). A Phase I clinical trial is recruiting participants (NCT03418688).

Minocycline is an anti-inflammatory compound that inhibits microglial activation and has been shown to be protective in several studies involving animal models of AD [447–452]. A Phase II clinical trial was recently terminated.

GC021109 is a small compound that binds the microglial P2Y6 receptor, and in pre-clinical studies was found to lower inflammation and Aβ levels (https://gliacure.com/gliacure-enters-first-in-human-clinical-trial-in-alzheimers-disease). A Phase I clinical trial has just been completed.

Naproxen is a non-selective COX inhibitor, while celecoxib and rofecoxib are both COX-2 inhibitors. Interest in these drugs for the treatment of AD arose when it appeared that anti-inflammatory drugs may reduce the pathology of the disease [453–455], but subsequent clinical trials failed to confirm such results [456–461]. No clinical trials are listed for any of the aforementioned drugs.

Prednisone is a corticosteroid that is already used to treat several other conditions such as arthritis, autoimmune diseases, and MS. It has been trialled for the treatment of AD; however, as clinical trials failed to demonstrate improvements [462, 463], the drug testing was halted.

14.3 Conclusions

Current treatments for AD provide some symptomatic relief, yet only provide benefit for around 12 months due to the neurodegeneration progressing further. The list of treatments in this review is not comprehensive, yet shows that a wide range of potential targets are being investigated, and demonstrates that many clinical trials are underway. However, drug treatments need to be developed for the earliest possible stages of AD, to have the best possible chance of halting or slowing the pathogenesis, and to preserve cognitive function. The availability of brain amyloid imaging and MRI scans, as well as developing biomarker tests, will help determine whether treatments are slowing the pathological advances of the disease (in pre-symptomatic stages). This will therefore facilitate drug testing at earlier stages, and speed up the discovery of potentially disease-altering drugs to help reduce the burden of this debilitating disease.

References

1 Jann, M.W. (1998). Pharmacology and clinical efficacy of cholinesterase inhibitors. *Am. J. Health Syst. Pharm.* 55 (Suppl 2): S22–S25.
2 Jann, M.W., Shirley, K.L., and Small, G.W. (2002). Clinical pharmacokinetics and pharmacodynamics of cholinesterase inhibitors. *Clin. Pharmacokinet.* 41: 719–739.
3 Bryson, H.M. and Benfield, P. (1997). Donepezil. *Drugs Aging* 10: 234, 240–239; discussion , 231.
4 Doody, R.S. (1999). Clinical profile of donepezil in the treatment of Alzheimer's disease. *Gerontology* 45 (Suppl 1): 23–32.
5 Dong, H., Csernansky, C.A., Martin, M.V. et al. (2005). Acetylcholinesterase inhibitors ameliorate behavioral deficits in the Tg2576 mouse model of Alzheimer's disease. *Psychopharmacology* 181: 145–152.
6 Romberg, C., Mattson, M.P., Mughal, M.R. et al. (2011). Impaired attention in the 3xTgAD mouse model of Alzheimer's disease: rescue by donepezil (Aricept). *J. Neurosci.* 31: 3500–3507.
7 Van Dam, D., Abramowski, D., Staufenbiel, M., and De Deyn, P.P. (2005). Symptomatic effect of donepezil, rivastigmine, galantamine and memantine on cognitive deficits in the APP23 model. *Psychopharmacology* 180: 177–190.
8 Dong, H., Yuede, C.M., Coughlan, C.A. et al. (2009). Effects of donepezil on amyloid-beta and synapse density in the Tg2576 mouse model of Alzheimer's disease. *Brain Res.* 1303: 169–178.
9 Kim, H.G., Moon, M., Choi, J.G. et al. (2014). Donepezil inhibits the amyloid-beta oligomer-induced microglial activation in vitro and in vivo. *Neurotoxicology* 40: 23–32.

10 Ye, C.Y., Lei, Y., Tang, X.C., and Zhang, H.Y. (2015). Donepezil attenuates Abeta-associated mitochondrial dysfunction and reduces mitochondrial Abeta accumulation in vivo and in vitro. *Neuropharmacology* 95: 29–36.

11 Rogers, S.L. and Friedhoff, L.T. (1996). The efficacy and safety of donepezil in patients with Alzheimer's disease: results of a US Multicentre, Randomized, Double-Blind, Placebo-Controlled Trial. The Donepezil Study Group. *Dementia* 7: 293–303.

12 Burns, A., Rossor, M., Hecker, J. et al. (1999). The effects of donepezil in Alzheimer's disease – results from a multinational trial. *Dement. Geriatr. Cogn. Disord.* 10: 237–244.

13 Rogers, S.L., Farlow, M.R., Doody, R.S. et al. (1998). A 24-week, double-blind, placebo-controlled trial of donepezil in patients with Alzheimer's disease: Donepezil Study Group. *Neurology* 50: 136–145.

14 Krishnan, K.R., Charles, H.C., Doraiswamy, P.M. et al. (2003). Randomized, placebo-controlled trial of the effects of donepezil on neuronal markers and hippocampal volumes in Alzheimer's disease. *Am. J. Psychiatry* 160: 2003–2011.

15 Cummings, J.L., McRae, T., and Zhang, R. (2006). Effects of donepezil on neuropsychiatric symptoms in patients with dementia and severe behavioral disorders. *Am. J. Geriatr. Psychiatry* 14: 605–612.

16 Gauthier, S., Feldman, H., Hecker, J. et al. (2002). Efficacy of donepezil on behavioral symptoms in patients with moderate to severe Alzheimer's disease. *Int. Psychogeriatr.* 14: 389–404.

17 Homma, A., Takeda, M., Imai, Y. et al. (2000). Clinical efficacy and safety of donepezil on cognitive and global function in patients with Alzheimer's disease: a 24-week, multicenter, double-blind, placebo-controlled study in Japan. E2020 Study Group. *Dement. Geriatr. Cogn. Disord.* 11: 299–313.

18 Matthews, H.P., Korbey, J., Wilkinson, D.G., and Rowden, J. (2000). Donepezil in Alzheimer's disease: eighteen month results from Southampton Memory Clinic. *Int. J. Geriatr. Psychiatry* 15: 713–720.

19 Seltzer, B., Zolnouni, P., Nunez, M. et al. (2004). Efficacy of donepezil in early-stage Alzheimer disease: a randomized placebo-controlled trial. *Arch. Neurol.* 61: 1852–1856.

20 Winblad, B., Black, S.E., Homma, A. et al. (2009). Donepezil treatment in severe Alzheimer's disease: a pooled analysis of three clinical trials. *Curr. Med. Res. Opin.* 25: 2577–2587.

21 Johannsen, P., Salmon, E., Hampel, H. et al. (2006). Assessing therapeutic efficacy in a progressive disease: a study of donepezil in Alzheimer's disease. *CNS Drugs* 20: 311–325.

22 Cummings, J.L., Geldmacher, D., Farlow, M. et al. (2013). High-dose donepezil (23 mg/day) for the treatment of moderate and severe Alzheimer's disease: drug profile and clinical guidelines. *CNS Neurosci. Ther.* 19: 294–301.

23 Farlow, M.R., Salloway, S., Tariot, P.N. et al. (2010). Effectiveness and tolerability of high-dose (23 mg/d) versus standard-dose (10 mg/d) donepezil in moderate to severe Alzheimer's disease: a 24-week, randomized, double-blind study. *Clin. Ther.* 32: 1234–1251.

24 Ferris, S.H., Schmitt, F.A., Saxton, J. et al. (2011). Analyzing the impact of 23 mg/day donepezil on language dysfunction in moderate to severe Alzheimer's disease. *Alzheimers Res. Ther.* 3: 22.

25 Homma, A., Atarashi, H., Kubota, N. et al. (2016). Efficacy and safety of sustained release Donepezil high dose versus immediate release Donepezil standard dose in Japanese patients with severe Alzheimer's disease: a randomized, double-blind trial. *J. Alzheimers Dis.* 52: 345–357.

26 Dubois, B., Chupin, M., Hampel, H. et al. (2015). Donepezil decreases annual rate of hippocampal atrophy in suspected prodromal Alzheimer's disease. *Alzheimers Dement.* 11: 1041–1049.

27 Shimizu, S., Kanetaka, H., Hirose, D. et al. (2015). Differential effects of acetylcholinesterase inhibitors on clinical responses and cerebral blood flow changes in patients with Alzheimer's disease: a 12-month, randomized, and open-label trial. *Dement. Geriatr. Cogn. Dis. Extra* 5: 135–146.

28 Cavedo, E., Grothe, M.J., Colliot, O. et al. (2017). Reduced basal forebrain atrophy progression in a randomized Donepezil trial in prodromal Alzheimer's disease. *Sci. Rep.* 7.

29 Lopez-Bastida, J., Hart, W., Garcia-Perez, L., and Linertova, R. (2009). Cost-effectiveness of donepezil in the treatment of mild or moderate Alzheimer's disease. *J. Alzheimers Dis.* 16: 399–407.

30 Alvarez, X.A., Cacabelos, R., Sampedro, C. et al. (2011). Combination treatment in Alzheimer's disease: results of a randomized, controlled trial with cerebrolysin and donepezil. *Curr. Alzheimer Res.* 8: 583–591.

31 Florian, H., Meier, A., Gauthier, S. et al. (2016). Efficacy and safety of ABT-126 in subjects with mild-to-moderate Alzheimer's disease on stable doses of acetylcholinesterase inhibitors: a randomized, double-blind, placebo-controlled study. *J. Alzheimers Dis.* 51: 1237–1247.

32 Gauthier, S., Rountree, S., Finn, B. et al. (2015). Effects of the acetylcholine release agent ST101 with Donepezil in Alzheimer's disease: a randomized phase 2 study. *J. Alzheimers Dis.* 48: 473–481.

33 Harrington, C., Sawchak, S., Chiang, C. et al. (2011). Rosiglitazone does not improve cognition or global function when used as adjunctive therapy to AChE inhibitors in mild-to-moderate Alzheimer's disease: two phase 3 studies. *Curr. Alzheimer Res.* 8: 592–606.

34 Howard, R., McShane, R., Lindesay, J. et al. (2012). Donepezil and memantine for moderate-to-severe Alzheimer's disease. *N. Engl. J. Med.* 366: 893–903.

35 Wilkinson, D., Windfeld, K., and Colding-Jorgensen, E. (2014). Safety and efficacy of idalopirdine, a 5-HT6 receptor antagonist, in patients with moderate Alzheimer's disease (LADDER): a randomised, double-blind, placebo-controlled phase 2 trial. *Lancet Neurol.* 13: 1092–1099.

36 Petersen, R.C., Thomas, R.G., Grundman, M. et al. (2005). Vitamin E and donepezil for the treatment of mild cognitive impairment. *N. Engl. J. Med.* 352: 2379–2388.

37 Salloway, S., Ferris, S., Kluger, A. et al. (2004). Efficacy of donepezil in mild cognitive impairment: a randomized placebo-controlled trial. *Neurology* 63: 651–657.

38 Wilens, T.E., Waxmonsky, J., Scott, M. et al. (2005). An open trial of adjunctive donepezil in attention-deficit/hyperactivity disorder. *J. Child Adolesc. Psychopharmacol.* 15: 947–955.

39 Roman, G.C., Salloway, S., Black, S.E. et al. (2010). Randomized, placebo-controlled, clinical trial of donepezil in vascular dementia: differential effects by hippocampal size. *Stroke* 41: 1213–1221.

40 Maelicke, A., Samochocki, M., Jostock, R. et al. (2001). Allosteric sensitization of nicotinic receptors by galantamine, a new treatment strategy for Alzheimer's disease. *Biol. Psychiatry* 49: 279–288.

41 Bhattacharya, S., Haertel, C., Maelicke, A., and Montag, D. (2014). Galantamine slows down plaque formation and behavioral decline in the 5XFAD mouse model of Alzheimer's disease. *PLoS One* 9: e89454.

42 Bhattacharya, S., Maelicke, A., and Montag, D. (2015). Nasal application of the galantamine pro-drug memogain slows down plaque deposition and ameliorates behavior in 5X familial Alzheimer's disease mice. *J. Alzheimers Dis.* 46: 123–136.

43 Van Dam, D. and De Deyn, P.P. (2006). Cognitive evaluation of disease-modifying efficacy of galantamine and memantine in the APP23 model. *Eur. Neuropsychopharmacol.* 16: 59–69.

44 Tariot, P.N., Solomon, P.R., Morris, J.C. et al. (2000). A 5-month, randomized, placebo-controlled trial of galantamine in AD. The Galantamine USA-10 Study Group. *Neurology* 54: 2269–2276.

45 Wilcock, G.K., Lilienfeld, S., and Gaens, E. (2000). Efficacy and safety of galantamine in patients with mild to moderate Alzheimer's disease: multicentre randomised controlled trial. Galantamine International-1 Study Group. *BMJ* 321: 1445–1449.

46 Raskind, M.A., Peskind, E.R., Wessel, T., and Yuan, W. (2000). Galantamine in AD: a 6-month randomized, placebo-controlled trial with a 6-month extension. The Galantamine USA-1 Study Group. *Neurology* 54: 2261–2268.

47 Rockwood, K., Mintzer, J., Truyen, L. et al. (2001). Effects of a flexible galantamine dose in Alzheimer's disease: a randomised, controlled trial. *J. Neurol. Neurosurg. Psychiatry* 71: 589–595.

48 Herrmann, N., Rabheru, K., Wang, J., and Binder, C. (2005). Galantamine treatment of problematic behavior in Alzheimer disease: post-hoc analysis of pooled data from three large trials. *Am. J. Geriatr. Psychiatry* 13: 527–534.

49 Kavanagh, S., Gaudig, M., Van Baelen, B. et al. (2011). Galantamine and behavior in Alzheimer disease: analysis of four trials. *Acta Neurol. Scand.* 124: 302–308.

50 Orgogozo, J.M., Small, G.W., Hammond, G. et al. (2004). Effects of galantamine in patients with mild Alzheimer's disease. *Curr. Med. Res. Opin.* 20: 1815–1820.

51 Vellas, B., Cunha, L., Gertz, H.J. et al. (2005). Early onset effects of galantamine treatment on attention in patients with Alzheimer's disease. *Curr. Med. Res. Opin.* 21: 1423–1429.

52 Brodaty, H., Corey-Bloom, J., Potocnik, F.C. et al. (2005). Galantamine prolonged-release formulation in the treatment of mild to moderate Alzheimer's disease. *Dement. Geriatr. Cogn. Disord.* 20: 120–132.

53 Burns, A., Bernabei, R., Bullock, R. et al. (2009). Safety and efficacy of galantamine (Reminyl) in severe Alzheimer's disease (the SERAD study): a randomised, placebo-controlled, double-blind trial. *Lancet Neurol.* 8: 39–47.

54 Marcusson, J., Bullock, R., Gauthier, S. et al. (2003). Galantamine demonstrates efficacy and safety in elderly patients with Alzheimer disease. *Alzheimer Dis. Assoc. Disord.* 17 (Suppl 3): S86–S91.

55 Wilkinson, D.G., Hock, C., Farlow, M. et al. (2002). Galantamine provides broad benefits in patients with 'advanced moderate' Alzheimer's disease (MMSE < or = 12) for up to six months. *Int. J. Clin. Pract.* 56: 509–514.

56 Keller, C., Kadir, A., Forsberg, A. et al. (2011). Long-term effects of galantamine treatment on brain functional activities as measured by PET in Alzheimer's disease patients. *J. Alzheimers Dis.* 24: 109–123.

57 Kavanagh, S., Van Baelen, B., and Schauble, B. (2011). Long-term effects of galantamine on cognitive function in Alzheimer's disease: a large-scale international retrospective study. *J. Alzheimers Dis.* 27: 521–530.

58 Nakagawa, R., Ohnishi, T., Kobayashi, H. et al. (2017). Long-term effect of galantamine on cognitive function in patients with Alzheimer's disease versus a simulated disease trajectory: an observational study in the clinical setting. *Neuropsychiatr. Dis. Treat.* 13: 1115–1124.

59 Nakano, Y., Matsuzono, K., Yamashita, T. et al. (2015). Long-term efficacy of galantamine in Alzheimer's disease: the Okayama Galantamine Study (OGS). *J. Alzheimers Dis.* 47: 609–617.

60 Nakayama, S., Suda, A., Nakanishi, A. et al. (2017). Galantamine response associates with agitation and the prefrontal cortex in patients with Alzheimer's disease. *J. Alzheimers Dis.* 57: 267–273.

61 Park, J.J., Choi, S.H., Kim, S. et al. (2016). Effect of galantamine on attention in patients with Alzheimer's disease combined with cerebrovascular disease. *Geriatr. Gerontol. Int.* 10: 1661–1666.

62 Caramelli, P., Laks, J., Palmini, A.L. et al. (2014). Effects of galantamine and galantamine combined with nimodipine on cognitive speed and quality of life in mixed dementia: a 24-week, randomized, placebo-controlled exploratory trial (the REMIX study). *Arq. Neuropsiquiatr.* 72: 411–417.

63 Hishikawa, N., Fukui, Y., Sato, K. et al. (2016). Comprehensive effects of galantamine and cilostazol combination therapy on patients with Alzheimer's disease with asymptomatic lacunar infarction. *Geriatr. Gerontol. Int.* 10: 1384–1391.

64 Matsuzono, K., Hishikawa, N., Ohta, Y. et al. (2015). Combination therapy of cholinesterase inhibitor (Donepezil or Galantamine) plus Memantine in the Okayama Memantine Study. *J. Alzheimers Dis.* 45: 771–780.

65 Feldman, H.H., Pirttila, T., Dartigues, J.F. et al. (2009). Treatment with galantamine and time to nursing home placement in Alzheimer's disease patients with and without cerebrovascular disease. *Int. J. Geriatr. Psychiatry* 24: 479–488.

66 Hyde, C., Peters, J., Bond, M. et al. (2013). Evolution of the evidence on the effectiveness and cost-effectiveness of acetylcholinesterase inhibitors and memantine for Alzheimer's disease: systematic review and economic model. *Age Ageing* 42: 14–20.

67 Suh, G.H., Jung, H.Y., Lee, C.U., and Choi, S. (2008). Economic and clinical benefits of galantamine in the treatment of mild to moderate Alzheimer's disease in a Korean population: a 52-week prospective study. *J. Korean Med. Sci.* 23: 10–17.

68 Loy, C. and Schneider, L. (2006). Galantamine for Alzheimer's disease and mild cognitive impairment. *Cochrane Database Syst. Rev.* (1): CD001747.

69 Francis, B.M., Yang, J., Hajderi, E. et al. (2012). Reduced tissue levels of noradrenaline are associated with behavioral phenotypes of the TgCRND8 mouse model of Alzheimer's disease. *Neuropsychopharmacology* 37: 1934–1944.

70 Mohamed, L.A., Keller, J.N., and Kaddoumi, A. (2016). Role of P-glycoprotein in mediating rivastigmine effect on amyloid-beta brain load and related pathology in Alzheimer's disease mouse model. *Biochim. Biophys. Acta* 1862: 778–787.

71 Rosler, M., Anand, R., Cicin-Sain, A. et al. (1999). Efficacy and safety of rivastigmine in patients with Alzheimer's disease: international randomised controlled trial. *BMJ* 318: 633–638.

72 Farlow, M., Anand, R., Messina, J. Jr. et al. (2000). A 52-week study of the efficacy of rivastigmine in patients with mild to moderately severe Alzheimer's disease. *Eur. Neurol.* 44: 236–241.

73 Wilkinson, D.G., Passmore, A.P., Bullock, R. et al. (2002). A multinational, randomised, 12-week, comparative study of donepezil and rivastigmine in patients with mild to moderate Alzheimer's disease. *Int. J. Clin. Pract.* 56: 441–446.

74 Grossberg, G.T., Olin, J.T., Somogyi, M., and Meng, X. (2011). Dose effects associated with rivastigmine transdermal patch in patients with mild-to-moderate Alzheimer's disease. *Int. J. Clin. Pract.* 65: 465–471.

75 Winblad, B., Cummings, J., Andreasen, N. et al. (2007). A six-month double-blind, randomized, placebo-controlled study of a transdermal patch in Alzheimer's disease – rivastigmine patch versus capsule. *Int. J. Geriatr. Psychiatry* 22: 456–467.

76 Farlow, M.R., Grossberg, G.T., Sadowsky, C.H. et al. (2013). A 24-week, randomized, controlled trial of rivastigmine patch 13.3 mg/24 h versus 4.6 mg/24 h in severe Alzheimer's dementia. *CNS Neurosci. Ther.* 19: 745–752.

77 Nakamura, Y., Imai, Y., Shigeta, M. et al. (2011). A 24-week, randomized, double-blind, placebo-controlled study to evaluate the efficacy, safety and tolerability of the rivastigmine patch in Japanese patients with Alzheimer's disease. *Dement. Geriatr. Cogn. Dis. Extra* 1: 163–179.

78 Small, G.W., Kaufer, D., Mendiondo, M.S. et al. (2005). Cognitive performance in Alzheimer's disease patients receiving rivastigmine for up to 5 years. *Int. J. Clin. Pract.* 59: 473–477.

79 Kim, Y.K., Lim, K.B., Lee, S.C. et al. (2014). Effects of a rivastigmine patch on self-care activities in patients with Alzheimer's disease plus cerebrovascular disease. *Dement. Geriatr. Cogn. Dis. Extra* 4: 395–401.

80 Nakamura, Y., Strohmaier, C., Tamura, K. et al. (2015). A 24-week, randomized, controlled study to evaluate the tolerability, safety and efficacy of 2 different titration schemes of the rivastigmine patch in Japanese patients with mild to moderate Alzheimer's disease. *Dement. Geriatr. Cogn. Dis. Extra* 5: 361–374.

81 Zhang, Z.X., Hong, Z., Wang, Y.P. et al. (2016). Rivastigmine patch in Chinese patients with probable Alzheimer's disease: a 24-week, Randomized, Double-Blind Parallel-Group Study comparing rivastigmine patch (9.5 mg/24 h) with capsule (6 mg twice daily). *CNS Neurosci. Ther.* 22: 488–496.

82 Castagna, A., Cotroneo, A.M., Ruotolo, G., and Gareri, P. (2016). The CITIRIVAD Study: CITIcoline plus RIVAstigmine in elderly patients affected with Dementia Study. *Clin. Drug Investig.* 36: 1059–1065.

83 Grossberg, G.T., Farlow, M.R., Meng, X., and Velting, D.M. (2015). Evaluating high-dose rivastigmine patch in severe Alzheimer's disease: analyses with concomitant memantine usage as a factor. *Curr. Alzheimer Res.* 12: 53–60.

84 Yoon, S.J., Choi, S.H., Na, H.R. et al. (2017). Effects on agitation with rivastigmine patch monotherapy and combination therapy with memantine in mild to moderate Alzheimer's disease: a multicenter 24-week prospective randomized open-label study (the Korean EXelon Patch and combination with mEmantine Comparative Trial study). *Geriatr. Gerontol. Int.* 17: 494–499.

85 Chen, Z., Digiacomo, M., Tu, Y. et al. (2017). Discovery of novel rivastigmine-hydroxycinnamic acid hybrids as multi-targeted agents for Alzheimer's disease. *Eur. J. Med. Chem.* 125: 784–792.

86 Morgan, T.M. and Soh, B. (2017). Absolute bioavailability and safety of a novel rivastigmine nasal spray in healthy elderly individuals. *Br. J. Clin. Pharmacol.* 83: 510–516.

87 Xiao, G., Li, Y., Qiang, X. et al. (2017). Design, synthesis and biological evaluation of 4′-aminochalcone-rivastigmine hybrids as multifunctional agents for the treatment of Alzheimer's disease. *Bioorg. Med. Chem.* 25: 1030–1041.

88 Poewe, W., Wolters, E., Emre, M. et al. (2006). Long-term benefits of rivastigmine in dementia associated with Parkinson's disease: an active treatment extension study. *Mov. Disord.* 21: 456–461.

89 Bullock, R., Touchon, J., Bergman, H. et al. (2005). Rivastigmine and donepezil treatment in moderate to moderately-severe Alzheimer's disease over a 2-year period. *Curr. Med. Res. Opin.* 21: 1317–1327.

90 Blesa, R., Bullock, R., He, Y. et al. (2006). Effect of butyrylcholinesterase genotype on the response to rivastigmine or donepezil in younger patients with Alzheimer's disease. *Pharmacogenet. Genomics* 16: 771–774.

91 Ferris, S., Nordberg, A., Soininen, H. et al. (2009). Progression from mild cognitive impairment to Alzheimer's disease: effects of sex, butyrylcholinesterase genotype, and rivastigmine treatment. *Pharmacogenet. Genomics* 19: 635–646.

92 Kandiah, N., Pai, M.C., Senanarong, V. et al. (2017). Rivastigmine: the advantages of dual inhibition of acetylcholinesterase and butyrylcholinesterase and its role in subcortical vascular dementia and Parkinson's disease dementia. *Clin. Interv. Aging* 12: 697–707.

93 Weinstock, M., Kirschbaum-Slager, N., Lazarovici, P. et al. (2001). Neuroprotective effects of novel cholinesterase inhibitors derived from rasagiline as potential anti-Alzheimer drugs. *Ann. N.Y. Acad. Sci.* 939: 148–161.

94 Yogev-Falach, M., Bar-Am, O., Amit, T. et al. (2006). A multifunctional, neuroprotective drug, ladostigil (TV3326), regulates holo-APP translation and processing. *FASEB J.* 20: 2177–2179.

95 Youdim, M.B., Amit, T., Bar-Am, O. et al. (2006). Implications of co-morbidity for etiology and treatment of neurodegenerative diseases with multifunctional neuroprotective-neurorescue drugs; ladostigil. *Neurotox. Res.* 10: 181–192.

96 Youdim, M.B., Amit, T., Bar-Am, O. et al. (2003). Amyloid processing and signal transduction properties of antiparkinson-antialzheimer neuroprotective drugs rasagiline and TV3326. *Ann. N.Y. Acad. Sci.* 993: 378, 387–386; discussion , 393.

97 Maelicke, A., Hoeffle-Maas, A., Ludwig, J. et al. (2010). Memogain is a galantamine pro-drug having dramatically reduced adverse effects and enhanced efficacy. *J. Mol. Neurosci.* 40: 135–137.

98 Baakman, A.C., t Hart, E., Kay, D.G. et al. (2016). First in human study with a prodrug of galantamine: improved benefit-risk ratio? *Alzheimers Dement. (N.Y.)* 2: 13–22.

99 Watkins, P.B., Zimmerman, H.J., Knapp, M.J. et al. (1994). Hepatotoxic effects of tacrine administration in patients with Alzheimer's disease. *JAMA* 271: 992–998.

100 Chioua, M., Perez, M., Bautista-Aguilera, O.M. et al. (2015). Development of HuperTacrines as non-toxic, cholinesterase inhibitors for the potential treatment of Alzheimer's disease. *Mini Rev. Med. Chem.* 15: 648–658.

101 Cen, J., Guo, H., Hong, C. et al. (2018). Development of tacrine-bifendate conjugates with improved cholinesterase inhibitory and pro-cognitive efficacy and reduced hepatotoxicity. *Eur. J. Med. Chem.* 144: 128–136.

102 Chen, Y., Zhu, J., Mo, J. et al. (2018). Synthesis and bioevaluation of new tacrine-cinnamic acid hybrids as cholinesterase inhibitors against Alzheimer's disease. *J. Enzyme Inhib. Med. Chem.* 33: 290–302.

103 Hepnarova, V., Korabecny, J., Matouskova, L. et al. (2018). The concept of hybrid molecules of tacrine and benzyl quinolone carboxylic acid (BQCA) as multifunctional agents for Alzheimer's disease. *Eur. J. Med. Chem.* 150: 292–306.

104 Hiremathad, A., Keri, R.S., Esteves, A.R. et al. (2018). Novel Tacrine-Hydroxyphenylbenzimidazole hybrids as potential multitarget drug candidates for Alzheimer's disease. *Eur. J. Med. Chem.* 148: 255–267.

105 Li, X., Wang, H., Xu, Y. et al. (2017). Novel Vilazodone-Tacrine hybrids as potential multitarget-directed ligands for the treatment of Alzheimer's disease accompanied with depression: design, synthesis, and biological evaluation. *ACS Chem. Neurosci.* 8: 2708–2721.

106 Spilovska, K., Korabecny, J., Sepsova, V. et al. (2017). Novel Tacrine-Scutellarin hybrids as multipotent anti-Alzheimer's agents: design, synthesis and biological evaluation. *ACS Chem. Neurosci.* 22: https://doi.org/10.3390/molecules22061006.

107 Deardorff, W.J., Shobassy, A., and Grossberg, G.T. (2015). Safety and clinical effects of EVP-6124 in subjects with Alzheimer's disease currently or previously receiving an acetylcholinesterase inhibitor medication. *Expert Rev. Neurother.* 15: 7–17.

108 Lilja, A.M., Porras, O., Storelli, E. et al. (2011). Functional interactions of fibrillar and oligomeric amyloid-beta with alpha7 nicotinic receptors in Alzheimer's disease. *J. Alzheimers Dis.* 23: 335–347.

109 Ni, R., Marutle, A., and Nordberg, A. (2013). Modulation of alpha7 nicotinic acetylcholine receptor and fibrillar amyloid-beta interactions in Alzheimer's disease brain. *J. Alzheimers Dis.* 33: 841–851.

110 Kim, S.Y., Choi, S.H., Rollema, H. et al. (2014). Phase II crossover trial of varenicline in mild-to-moderate Alzheimer's disease. *Dement. Geriatr. Cogn. Disord.* 37: 232–245.

111 Dong, H., Yuede, C.M., Coughlan, C. et al. (2008). Effects of memantine on neuronal structure and conditioned fear in the Tg2576 mouse model of Alzheimer's disease. *Neuropsychopharmacology* 33: 3226–3236.

112 Filali, M., Lalonde, R., and Rivest, S. (2011). Subchronic memantine administration on spatial learning, exploratory activity, and nest-building in an APP/PS1 mouse model of Alzheimer's disease. *Neuropharmacology* 60: 930–936.

113 Tan, Y., Liu, T.R., Hu, S.W. et al. (2014). Acute coronary syndrome remodels the protein cargo and functions of high-density lipoprotein subfractions. *PLoS One* 9: e94264.

114 Minkeviciene, R., Banerjee, P., and Tanila, H. (2004). Memantine improves spatial learning in a transgenic mouse model of Alzheimer's disease. *J. Pharmacol. Exp. Ther.* 311: 677–682.

115 Scholtzova, H., Wadghiri, Y.Z., Douadi, M. et al. (2008). Memantine leads to behavioral improvement and amyloid reduction in Alzheimer's-disease-model transgenic mice shown as by micromagnetic resonance imaging. *J. Neurosci. Res.* 86: 2784–2791.

116 Martinez-Coria, H., Green, K.N., Billings, L.M. et al. (2010). Memantine improves cognition and reduces Alzheimer's-like neuropathology in transgenic mice. *Am. J. Pathol.* 176: 870–880.

117 Nagakura, A., Shitaka, Y., Yarimizu, J., and Matsuoka, N. (2013). Characterization of cognitive deficits in a transgenic mouse model of Alzheimer's disease and effects of donepezil and memantine. *Eur. J. Pharmacol.* 703: 53–61.

118 Neumeister, K.L. and Riepe, M.W. (2012). Synergistic effects of antidementia drugs on spatial learning and recall in the APP23 transgenic mouse model of Alzheimer's disease. *J. Alzheimers Dis.* 30: 245–251.

119 Ito, K., Tatebe, T., Suzuki, K. et al. (2017). Memantine reduces the production of amyloid-beta peptides through modulation of amyloid precursor protein trafficking. *PLoS One* 798: 16–25.

120 Takahashi-Ito, K., Makino, M., Okado, K., and Tomita, T. (2017). Memantine inhibits beta-amyloid aggregation and disassembles preformed beta-amyloid aggregates. *Biochem. Biophys. Res. Commun.* 493: 158–163.

121 Doody, R.S., Tariot, P.N., Pfeiffer, E. et al. (2007). Meta-analysis of six-month memantine trials in Alzheimer's disease. *Alzheimers Dement.* 3: 7–17.

122 Schneider, L.S., Dagerman, K.S., Higgins, J.P., and McShane, R. (2011). Lack of evidence for the efficacy of memantine in mild Alzheimer disease. *Arch. Neurol.* 68: 991–998.

123 Zhang, N., Wei, C., Du, H. et al. (2015). The effect of Memantine on cognitive function and behavioral and psychological symptoms in mild-to-moderate Alzheimer's disease patients. *Dement. Geriatr. Cogn. Disord.* 40: 85–93.

124 Gauthier, S., Loft, H., and Cummings, J. (2008). Improvement in behavioural symptoms in patients with moderate to severe Alzheimer's disease by memantine: a pooled data analysis. *Int. J. Geriatr. Psychiatry* 23: 537–545.

125 Reisberg, B., Doody, R., Stöffler, A. et al. (2003). Memantine in moderate-to-severe Alzheimer's disease. *N. Engl. J. Med.* 348: 1333–1341.

126 Winblad, B., Jones, R.W., Wirth, Y. et al. (2007). Memantine in moderate to severe Alzheimer's disease: a meta-analysis of randomised clinical trials. *Dement. Geriatr. Cogn. Disord.* 24: 20–27.

127 Tariot, P.N., Farlow, M.R., Grossberg, G.T. et al. (2004). Memantine treatment in patients with moderate to severe Alzheimer disease already receiving donepezil: a randomized controlled trial. *JAMA* 291: 317–324.

128 Cummings, J.L., Schneider, E., Tariot, P.N., and Graham, S.M. (2006). Behavioral effects of memantine in Alzheimer disease patients receiving donepezil treatment. *Neurology* 67: 57–63.

129 Feldman, H.H., Schmitt, F.A., and Olin, J.T. (2006). Activities of daily living in moderate-to-severe Alzheimer disease: an analysis of the treatment effects of memantine in patients receiving stable donepezil treatment. *Alzheimer Dis. Assoc. Disord.* 20: 263–268.

130 Riordan, K.C., Hoffman Snyder, C.R., Wellik, K.E. et al. (2011). Effectiveness of adding memantine to an Alzheimer dementia treatment regimen which already includes stable donepezil therapy: a critically appraised topic. *Neurologist* 17: 121–123.

131 Schmitt, F.A., van Dyck, C.H., Wichems, C.H., and Olin, J.T. (2006). Cognitive response to memantine in moderate to severe Alzheimer disease patients already receiving donepezil: an exploratory reanalysis. *Alzheimer Dis. Assoc. Disord.* 20: 255–262.

132 van Dyck, C.H., Schmitt, F.A., and Olin, J.T. (2006). A responder analysis of memantine treatment in patients with Alzheimer disease maintained on donepezil. *Am. J. Geriatr. Psychiatry* 14: 428–437.

133 Riepe, M.W., Adler, G., Ibach, B. et al. (2007). Domain-specific improvement of cognition on memantine in patients with Alzheimer's disease treated with rivastigmine. *Dement. Geriatr. Cogn. Disord.* 23: 301–306.

134 Gareri, P., Putignano, D., Castagna, A. et al. (2014). Retrospective study on the benefits of combined Memantine and cholinEsterase inhibitor treatMent in AGEd Patients affected with Alzheimer's Disease: the MEMAGE study. *J. Alzheimers Dis.* 41: 633–640.

135 Gauthier, S. and Molinuevo, J.L. (2013). Benefits of combined cholinesterase inhibitor and memantine treatment in moderate-severe Alzheimer's disease. *Alzheimers Dement.* 9: 326–331.

136 Grossberg, G.T., Manes, F., Allegri, R.F. et al. (2013). The safety, tolerability, and efficacy of once-daily memantine (28 mg): a multinational, randomized, double-blind, placebo-controlled trial in patients with moderate-to-severe Alzheimer's disease taking cholinesterase inhibitors. *CNS Drugs* 27: 469–478.

137 Chen, R., Chan, P.T., Chu, H. et al. (2017). Treatment effects between monotherapy of donepezil versus combination with memantine for Alzheimer disease: a meta-analysis. *PLoS One* 12: e0183586.

138 Porsteinsson, A.P., Grossberg, G.T., Mintzer, J., and Olin, J.T. (2008). Memantine treatment in patients with mild to moderate Alzheimer's disease already receiving a cholinesterase inhibitor: a randomized, double-blind, placebo-controlled trial. *Curr. Alzheimer Res.* 5: 83–89.

139 Choi, S.H., Park, K.W., Na, D.L. et al. (2011). Tolerability and efficacy of memantine add-on therapy to rivastigmine transdermal patches in mild to moderate Alzheimer's disease: a multicenter, randomized, open-label, parallel-group study. *Curr. Med. Res. Opin.* 27: 1375–1383.

140 Farlow, M.R., Alva, G., Meng, X., and Olin, J.T. (2010). A 25-week, open-label trial investigating rivastigmine transdermal patches with concomitant memantine in mild-to-moderate Alzheimer's disease: a post hoc analysis. *Curr. Med. Res. Opin.* 26: 263–269.

141 Hanney, M., Prasher, V., Williams, N. et al. (2012). Memantine for dementia in adults older than 40 years with Down's syndrome (MEADOWS): a randomised, double-blind, placebo-controlled trial. *Lancet* 379: 528–536.

142 Rogers, M., Rasheed, A., Moradimehr, A., and Baumrucker, S.J. (2009). Memantine (Namenda) for neuropathic pain. *Am. J. Hosp. Palliat. Care* 26: 57–59.

143 Wilcock, G., Mobius, H.J., and Stoffler, A. (2002). A double-blind, placebo-controlled multicentre study of memantine in mild to moderate vascular dementia (MMM500). *Int. Clin. Psychopharmacol.* 17: 297–305.

144 Haase, N., Herse, F., Spallek, B. et al. (2013). Amyloid-beta peptides activate alpha1-adrenergic cardiovascular receptors. *Hypertension* 62: 966–972.

145 Sharp, S.I., Ballard, C.G., Chen, C.P., and Francis, P.T. (2007). Aggressive behavior and neuroleptic medication are associated with increased number of alpha1-adrenoceptors in patients with Alzheimer disease. *Am. J. Geriatr. Psychiatry* 15: 435–437.

146 Wang, L.Y., Shofer, J.B., Rohde, K. et al. (2009). Prazosin for the treatment of behavioral symptoms in patients with Alzheimer disease with agitation and aggression. *Am. J. Geriatr. Psychiatry* 17: 744–751.

147 Katsouri, L., Vizcaychipi, M.P., McArthur, S. et al. (2013). Prazosin, an alpha(1)-adrenoceptor antagonist, prevents memory deterioration in the APP23 transgenic mouse model of Alzheimer's disease. *Neurobiol. Aging* 34: 1105–1115.

148 Cummings, J.L., Lyketsos, C.G., Peskind, E.R. et al. (2015). Effect of dextromethorphan-quinidine on agitation in patients with Alzheimer disease dementia: a randomized clinical trial. *JAMA* 314: 1242–1254.

149 Garay, R.P. and Grossberg, G.T. (2017). AVP-786 for the treatment of agitation in dementia of the Alzheimer's type. *Expert Opin. Investig. Drugs* 26: 121–132.

150 Doody, R.S., D'Amico, S., Cutler, A.J. et al. (2016). An open-label study to assess safety, tolerability, and effectiveness of dextromethorphan/quinidine for pseudobulbar affect in dementia: PRISM II results. *CNS Spectr.* 21: 450–459.

151 Davis, R.E., Vanover, K.E., Zhou, Y. et al. (2015). ITI-007 demonstrates brain occupancy at serotonin 5-HT(2)A and dopamine D(2) receptors and serotonin transporters using positron emission tomography in healthy volunteers. *Psychopharmacology* 232: 2863–2872.

152 Snyder, G.L., Vanover, K.E., Zhu, H. et al. (2015). Functional profile of a novel modulator of serotonin, dopamine, and glutamate neurotransmission. *Psychopharmacology* 232: 605–621.

153 Li, P., Zhang, Q., Robichaud, A.J. et al. (2014). Discovery of a tetracyclic quinoxaline derivative as a potent and orally active multifunctional drug candidate for the treatment of neuropsychiatric and neurological disorders. *J. Med. Chem.* 57: 2670–2682.

154 Hutson, P.H., Finger, E.N., Magliaro, B.C. et al. (2011). The selective phosphodiesterase 9 (PDE9) inhibitor PF-04447943 (6-[(3S,4S)-4-methyl-1-(pyrimidin-2-ylmethyl)pyrrolidin-3-yl]-1-(tetrahydro-2H-pyran-4-yl)-1,5-dihydro-4H-pyrazolo[3,4-d]pyrimidin-4-one) enhances synaptic plasticity and cognitive function in rodents. *Neuropharmacology* 61: 665–676.

155 van der Staay, F.J., Rutten, K., Barfacker, L. et al. (2008). The novel selective PDE9 inhibitor BAY 73-6691 improves learning and memory in rodents. *Neuropharmacology* 55: 908–918.

156 Moschetti, V., Boland, K., Feifel, U. et al. (2016). First-in-human study assessing safety, tolerability and pharmacokinetics of BI 409306, a selective phosphodiesterase 9A inhibitor, in healthy males. *Br. J. Clin. Pharmacol.*

157 Boland, K., Moschetti, V., Dansirikul, C. et al. (2017). A phase I, randomized, proof-of-clinical-mechanism study assessing the pharmacokinetics and pharmacodynamics of the oral PDE9A inhibitor BI 409306 in healthy male volunteers. *Hum. Psychopharmacol.* 32.

158 He, P., Ouyang, X., Zhou, S. et al. (2013). A novel melatonin agonist Neu-P11 facilitates memory performance and improves cognitive impairment in a rat model of Alzheimer' disease. *Horm. Behav.* 64: 1–7.

159 Ren, S.C., Shao, H., Ji, W.G. et al. (2015). Riluzole prevents soluble Abeta1-42 oligomers-induced perturbation of spontaneous discharge in the hippocampal CA1 region of rats. *Amyloid* 22: 36–44.

160 Hunsberger, H.C., Weitzner, D.S., Rudy, C.C. et al. (2015). Riluzole rescues glutamate alterations, cognitive deficits, and tau pathology associated with P301L tau expression. *J. Neurochem.* 135: 381–394.

161 Mokhtari, Z., Baluchnejadmojarad, T., Nikbakht, F. et al. (2017). Riluzole ameliorates learning and memory deficits in Abeta25-35-induced rat model of Alzheimer's disease and is independent of cholinoceptor activation. *Biomed. Pharmacother.* 87: 135–144.

162 Bensimon, G., Ludolph, A., Agid, Y. et al. (2009). Riluzole treatment, survival and diagnostic criteria in Parkinson plus disorders: the NNIPPS study. *Brain* 132: 156–171.

163 Landwehrmeyer, G.B., Dubois, B., de Yebenes, J.G. et al. (2007). Riluzole in Huntington's disease: a 3-year, randomized controlled study. *Ann. Neurol.* 62: 262–272.

164 Kitten, A.K., Hallowell, S.A., Saklad, S.R., and Evoy, K.E. (2018). Pimavanserin: a novel drug approved to treat Parkinson's disease psychosis. *Innov. Clin. Neurosci.* 15: 16–22.

165 Price, D.L., Bonhaus, D.W., and McFarland, K. (2012). Pimavanserin, a 5-HT2A receptor inverse agonist, reverses psychosis-like behaviors in a rodent model of Alzheimer's disease. *Behav. Pharmacol.* 23: 426–433.

166 Luchetti, S., Huitinga, I., and Swaab, D.F. (2011). Neurosteroid and GABA-A receptor alterations in Alzheimer's disease, Parkinson's disease and multiple sclerosis. *Neuroscience* 191: 6–21.

167 Naylor, J.C., Kilts, J.D., Hulette, C.M. et al. (2010). Allopregnanolone levels are reduced in temporal cortex in patients with Alzheimer's disease compared to cognitively intact control subjects. *Biochim. Biophys. Acta* 1801: 951–959.

168 Marx, C.E., Trost, W.T., Shampine, L.J. et al. (2006). The neurosteroid allopregnanolone is reduced in prefrontal cortex in Alzheimer's disease. *Biol. Psychiatry* 60: 1287–1294.

169 Chen, S., Wang, J.M., Irwin, R.W. et al. (2011). Allopregnanolone promotes regeneration and reduces beta-amyloid burden in a preclinical model of Alzheimer's disease. *PLoS One* 6: e24293.

170 Wang, J.M., Singh, C., Liu, L. et al. (2010). Allopregnanolone reverses neurogenic and cognitive deficits in mouse model of Alzheimer's disease. *Proc. Natl. Acad. Sci. U.S.A.* 107: 6498–6503.

171 Singh, C., Liu, L., Wang, J.M. et al. (2012). Allopregnanolone restores hippocampal-dependent learning and memory and neural progenitor survival in aging 3xTgAD and nonTg mice. *Neurobiol. Aging* 33: 1493–1506.

172 Zhang, P., Xie, M.Q., Ding, Y.Q. et al. (2015). Allopregnanolone enhances the neurogenesis of midbrain dopaminergic neurons in APPswe/PSEN1 mice. *Neuroscience* 290: 214–226.

173 Sun, C., Ou, X., Farley, J.M. et al. (2012). Allopregnanolone increases the number of dopaminergic neurons in substantia nigra of a triple transgenic mouse model of Alzheimer's disease. *Curr. Alzheimer Res.* 9: 473–480.

174 Bengtsson, S.K., Johansson, M., Backstrom, T. et al. (2013). Brief but chronic increase in allopregnanolone cause accelerated AD pathology differently in two mouse models. *Curr. Alzheimer Res.* 10: 38–47.

175 Bengtsson, S.K., Johansson, M., Backstrom, T., and Wang, M. (2012). Chronic allopregnanolone treatment accelerates Alzheimer's disease development in AbetaPP(Swe)PSEN1(DeltaE9) mice. *J. Alzheimers Dis.* 31: 71–84.

176 Rinne, J.O., Wesnes, K., Cummings, J.L. et al. (2017). Tolerability of ORM-12741 and effects on episodic memory in patients with Alzheimer's disease. *Alzheimers Dement. (N.Y.)* 3: 1–9.

177 Abramova, N.A., Cassarino, D.S., Khan, S.M. et al. (2002). Inhibition by R(+) or S(−) pramipexole of caspase activation and cell death induced by methylpyridinium ion or beta amyloid peptide in SH-SY5Y neuroblastoma. *J. Neurosci. Res.* 67: 494–500.

178 Boscolo, A., Starr, J.A., Sanchez, V. et al. (2012). The abolishment of anesthesia-induced cognitive impairment by timely protection of mitochondria in the developing rat brain: the importance of free oxygen radicals and mitochondrial integrity. *Neurobiol. Dis.* 45: 1031–1041.

179 Fujita, Y., Izawa, Y., Ali, N. et al. (2006). Pramipexole protects against H2O2-induced PC12 cell death. *Naunyn-Schmiedeberg's Arch. Pharmacol.* 372: 257–266.

180 Uberti, D., Bianchi, I., Olivari, L. et al. (2007). Pramipexole prevents neurotoxicity induced by oligomers of beta-amyloid. *Eur. J. Pharmacol.* 569: 194–196.

181 Bozik, M.E., Mather, J.L., Kramer, W.G. et al. (2011). Safety, tolerability, and pharmacokinetics of KNS-760704 (dexpramipexole) in healthy adult subjects. *J. Clin. Pharmacol.* 51: 1177–1185.

182 Bennett, J., Burns, J., Welch, P., and Bothwell, R. (2016). Safety and tolerability of R(+) pramipexole in mild-to-moderate Alzheimer's disease. *J. Alzheimers Dis.* 49: 1179–1187.

183 Gerard, C., Martres, M.P., Lefevre, K. et al. (1997). Immuno-localization of serotonin 5-HT6 receptor-like material in the rat central nervous system. *Brain Res.* 746: 207–219.

184 Marazziti, D., Baroni, S., Pirone, A. et al. (2013). Serotonin receptor of type 6 (5-HT6) in human prefrontal cortex and hippocampus post-mortem: an immunohistochemical and immunofluorescence study. *Neurochem. Int.* 62: 182–188.

185 Callaghan, C.K., Hok, V., Della-Chiesa, A. et al. (2012). Age-related declines in delayed non-match-to-sample performance (DNMS) are reversed by the novel 5HT6 receptor antagonist SB742457. *Neuropharmacology* 63: 890–897.

186 de Bruin, N.M., van Drimmelen, M., Kops, M. et al. (2013). Effects of risperidone, clozapine and the 5-HT6 antagonist GSK-742457 on PCP-induced deficits in reversal learning in the two-lever operant task in male Sprague Dawley rats. *Behav. Brain Res.* 244: 15–28.

187 Maher-Edwards, G., Dixon, R., Hunter, J. et al. (2011). SB-742457 and donepezil in Alzheimer disease: a randomized, placebo-controlled study. *Int. J. Geriatr. Psychiatry* 26: 536–544.

188 Grove, R.A., Harrington, C.M., Mahler, A. et al. (2014). A randomized, double-blind, placebo-controlled, 16-week study of the H3 receptor antagonist, GSK239512 as a monotherapy in subjects with mild-to-moderate Alzheimer's disease. *Curr. Alzheimer Res.* 11: 47–58.

189 Nathan, P.J., Boardley, R., Scott, N. et al. (2013). The safety, tolerability, pharmacokinetics and cognitive effects of GSK239512, a selective histamine H(3) receptor antagonist in patients with mild to moderate Alzheimer's disease: a preliminary investigation. *Curr. Alzheimer Res.* 10: 240–251.

190 Cramer, P.E., Cirrito, J.R., Wesson, D.W. et al. (2012). ApoE-directed therapeutics rapidly clear beta-amyloid and reverse deficits in AD mouse models. *Science* 335: 1503–1506.

191 Wolozin, B., Wang, S.W., Li, N.C. et al. (2007). Simvastatin is associated with a reduced incidence of dementia and Parkinson's disease. *BMC Med.* 5: 20.

192 Yaffe, K., Barrett-Connor, E., Lin, F., and Grady, D. (2002). Serum lipoprotein levels, statin use, and cognitive function in older women. *Arch. Neurol.* 59: 378–384.

193 Ishii, K., Tokuda, T., Matsushima, T. et al. (2003). Pravastatin at 10 mg/day does not decrease plasma levels of either amyloid-beta (Abeta) 40 or Abeta 42 in humans. *Neurosci. Lett.* 350: 161–164.

194 Hoglund, K., Wiklund, O., Vanderstichele, H. et al. (2004). Plasma levels of beta-amyloid(1-40), beta-amyloid(1-42), and total beta-amyloid remain unaffected in adult patients with hypercholesterolemia after treatment with statins. *Arch. Neurol.* 61: 333–337.

195 Lue, L.F., Guerra, A., and Walker, D.G. (2017). Amyloid Beta and tau as Alzheimer's disease blood biomarkers: promise from new technologies. *Neurol. Ther.* 6: 25–36.

196 Riekse, R.G., Li, G., Petrie, E.C. et al. (2006). Effect of statins on Alzheimer's disease biomarkers in cerebrospinal fluid. *J. Alzheimers Dis.* 10: 399–406.

197 Simons, M., Schwarzler, F., Lutjohann, D. et al. (2002). Treatment with simvastatin in normocholesterolemic patients with Alzheimer's disease: A 26-week randomized, placebo-controlled, double-blind trial. *Ann. Neurol.* 52: 346–350.

198 Sjogren, M., Gustafsson, K., Syversen, S. et al. (2003). Treatment with simvastatin in patients with Alzheimer's disease lowers both alpha- and beta-cleaved amyloid precursor protein. *Dement. Geriatr. Cogn. Disord.* 16: 25–30.

199 Hoglund, K., Thelen, K.M., Syversen, S. et al. (2005). The effect of simvastatin treatment on the amyloid precursor protein and brain cholesterol metabolism in patients with Alzheimer's disease. *Dement. Geriatr. Cogn. Disord.* 19: 256–265.

200 Serrano-Pozo, A., Vega, G.L., Lutjohann, D. et al. (2010). Effects of simvastatin on cholesterol metabolism and Alzheimer disease biomarkers. *Alzheimer Dis. Assoc. Disord.* 24: 220–226.

201 McGuinness, B., Craig, D., Bullock, R. et al. (2014). Statins for the treatment of dementia. *Cochrane Database Syst. Rev.* CD007514. https://doi.org/10.1002/14651858.CD007514.pub2.

202 McGuinness, B., Craig, D., Bullock, R., and Passmore, P. (2016). Statins for the prevention of dementia. *Cochrane Database Syst. Rev.* CD003160. https://doi.org/10.1002/14651858.CD003160.pub3.

203 Rakesh, G., Szabo, S.T., Alexopoulos, G.S., and Zannas, A.S. (2017). Strategies for dementia prevention: latest evidence and implications. *Ther. Adv. Chronic Dis.* 8: 121–136.

204 Schenk, D., Barbour, R., Dunn, W. et al. (1999). Immunization with amyloid-beta attenuates Alzheimer-disease-like pathology in the PDAPP mouse. *Nature* 400: 173–177.

205 Janus, C., Pearson, J., McLaurin, J. et al. (2000). A beta peptide immunization reduces behavioural impairment and plaques in a model of Alzheimer's disease. *Nature* 408: 979–982.

206 Orgogozo, J.M., Gilman, S., Dartigues, J.F. et al. (2003). Subacute meningoencephalitis in a subset of patients with AD after Abeta42 immunization. *Neurology* 61: 46–54.

207 Nicoll, J.A., Wilkinson, D., Holmes, C. et al. (2003). Neuropathology of human Alzheimer disease after immunization with amyloid-beta peptide: a case report. *Nat. Med.* 9: 448–452.

208 Wiessner, C., Wiederhold, K.H., Tissot, A.C. et al. (2011). The second-generation active Abeta immunotherapy CAD106 reduces amyloid accumulation in APP transgenic mice while minimizing potential side effects. *J. Neurosci.* 31: 9323–9331.

209 Winblad, B., Andreasen, N., Minthon, L. et al. (2012). Safety, tolerability, and antibody response of active Abeta immunotherapy with CAD106 in patients with Alzheimer's disease: randomised, double-blind, placebo-controlled, first-in-human study. *Lancet Neurol.* 11: 597–604.

210 Farlow, M.R., Andreasen, N., Riviere, M.E. et al. (2015). Long-term treatment with active Abeta immunotherapy with CAD106 in mild Alzheimer's disease. *Alzheimers Res. Ther.* 7: 23.

211 Vandenberghe, R., Riviere, M.E., Caputo, A. et al. (2017). Active Abeta immunotherapy CAD106 in Alzheimer's disease: a phase 2b study. *Alzheimers Dement. (N.Y.)* 3: 10–22.

212 Lacosta, A.M., Pascual-Lucas, M., Pesini, P. et al. (2018). Safety, tolerability and immunogenicity of an active anti-Abeta40 vaccine (ABvac40) in patients with Alzheimer's disease: a randomised, double-blind, placebo-controlled, phase I trial. *Alzheimers Res. Ther.* 10: 12.

213 Wang, C.Y., Wang, P.N., Chiu, M.J. et al. (2017). UB-311, a novel UBITh((R)) amyloid beta peptide vaccine for mild Alzheimer's disease. *Alzheimers Dement. (N.Y.)* 3: 262–272.

214 Davtyan, H., Ghochikyan, A., Petrushina, I. et al. (2013). Immunogenicity, efficacy, safety, and mechanism of action of epitope vaccine (Lu AF20513) for Alzheimer's disease: prelude to a clinical trial. *J. Neurosci.* 33: 4923–4934.

215 Arai, H., Suzuki, H., and Yoshiyama, T. (2015). Vanutide cridificar and the QS-21 adjuvant in Japanese subjects with mild to moderate Alzheimer's disease: results from two phase 2 studies. *Curr. Alzheimer Res.* 12: 242–254.

216 Pasquier, F., Sadowsky, C., Holstein, A. et al. (2016). Two phase 2 multiple ascending-dose studies of Vanutide Cridificar (ACC-001) and QS-21 adjuvant in mild-to-moderate Alzheimer's Disease. *J. Alzheimers Dis.* 51: 1131–1143.

217 Hull, M., Sadowsky, C., Arai, H. et al. (2017). Long-term extensions of randomized vaccination trials of ACC-001 and QS-21 in mild to moderate Alzheimer's disease. *Curr. Alzheimer Res.* 14: 696–708.

218 Ketter, N., Liu, E., Di, J. et al. (2016). A randomized, double-blind, phase 2 study of the effects of the vaccine Vanutide Cridificar with QS-21 adjuvant on immunogenicity, safety and amyloid imaging in patients with mild to moderate Alzheimer's disease. *J. Prev. Alzheimers Dis.* 3: 192–201.

219 Schneeberger, A., Hendrix, S., Mandler, M. et al. (2015). Results from a Phase II Study to assess the clinical and immunological activity of AFFITOPE(R) AD02 in patients with early Alzheimer's disease. *J. Prev. Alzheimers Dis.* 2: 103–114.

220 Mandler, M., Santic, R., Gruber, P. et al. (2015). Tailoring the antibody response to aggregated Ass using novel Alzheimer-vaccines. *PLoS One* 10: e0115237.

221 Muhs, A., Hickman, D.T., Pihlgren, M. et al. (2007). Liposomal vaccines with conformation-specific amyloid peptide antigens define immune response and efficacy in APP transgenic mice. *Proc. Natl. Acad. Sci. U.S.A.* 104: 9810–9815.

222 Kontsekova, E., Zilka, N., Kovacech, B. et al. (2014). First-in-man tau vaccine targeting structural determinants essential for pathological tau-tau interaction reduces tau oligomerisation and neurofibrillary degeneration in an Alzheimer's disease model. *Alzheimers Res. Ther.* 6: 44.

223 Novak, P., Schmidt, R., Kontsekova, E. et al. (2017). Safety and immunogenicity of the tau vaccine AADvac1 in patients with Alzheimer's disease: a randomised, double-blind, placebo-controlled, phase 1 trial. *Lancet Neurol.* 16: 123–134.

224 Theunis, C., Crespo-Biel, N., Gafner, V. et al. (2013). Efficacy and safety of a liposome-based vaccine against protein tau, assessed in tau.P301L mice that model tauopathy. *PLoS One* 8: e72301.

225 Gamage, K.K. and Kumar, S. (2017). Aducanumab therapy ameliorates calcium overload in a mouse model of Alzheimer's disease. *J. Neurosci.* 37: 4430–4432.

226 Kastanenka, K.V., Bussiere, T., Shakerdge, N. et al. (2016). Immunotherapy with Aducanumab restores calcium homeostasis in Tg2576 Mice. *J. Neurosci.* 36: 12549–12558.

227 Sevigny, J., Chiao, P., Bussiere, T. et al. (2016). The antibody aducanumab reduces Abeta plaques in Alzheimer's disease. *Nature* 537: 50–56.

228 Piazza, F. and Winblad, B. (2016). Amyloid-Related Imaging Abnormalities (ARIA) in immunotherapy trials for Alzheimer's disease: need for prognostic biomarkers? *J. Alzheimers Dis.* 52: 417–420.

229 Ferrero, J., Williams, L., Stella, H. et al. (2016). First-in-human, double-blind, placebo-controlled, single-dose escalation study of aducanumab (BIIB037) in mild-to-moderate Alzheimer's disease. *Alzheimers Dement. (N.Y.)* 2: 169–176.

230 Siemers, E.R., Friedrich, S., Dean, R.A. et al. (2010). Safety and changes in plasma and cerebrospinal fluid amyloid beta after a single administration of an amyloid beta monoclonal antibody in subjects with Alzheimer disease. *Clin. Neuropharmacol.* 33: 67–73.

231 Uenaka, K., Nakano, M., Willis, B.A. et al. (2012). Comparison of pharmacokinetics, pharmacodynamics, safety, and tolerability of the amyloid beta monoclonal antibody solanezumab in Japanese and white patients with mild to moderate alzheimer disease. *Clin. Neuropharmacol.* 35: 25–29.

232 Doody, R.S., Thomas, R.G., Farlow, M. et al. (2014). Phase 3 trials of solanezumab for mild-to-moderate Alzheimer's disease. *N. Engl. J. Med.* 370: 311–321.

233 Siemers, E.R., Sundell, K.L., Carlson, C. et al. (2016). Phase 3 solanezumab trials: Secondary outcomes in mild Alzheimer's disease patients. *Alzheimers Dement.* 12: 110–120.

234 Honig, L.S., Vellas, B., Woodward, M. et al. (2018). Trial of Solanezumab for mild dementia due to Alzheimer's disease. *N. Engl. J. Med.* 378: 321–330.

235 Bohrmann, B., Baumann, K., Benz, J. et al. (2012). Gantenerumab: a novel human anti-Abeta antibody demonstrates sustained cerebral amyloid-beta binding and elicits cell-mediated removal of human amyloid-beta. *J. Alzheimers Dis.* 28: 49–69.

236 Jacobsen, H., Ozmen, L., Caruso, A. et al. (2014). Combined treatment with a BACE inhibitor and anti-Abeta antibody gantenerumab enhances amyloid reduction in APPLondon mice. *J. Neurosci.* 34: 11621–11630.

237 Ostrowitzki, S., Deptula, D., Thurfjell, L. et al. (2012). Mechanism of amyloid removal in patients with Alzheimer disease treated with gantenerumab. *Arch. Neurol.* 69: 198–207.

238 Ostrowitzki, S., Lasser, R.A., Dorflinger, E. et al. (2017). A phase III randomized trial of gantenerumab in prodromal Alzheimer's disease. *Alzheimers Res. Ther.* 9: 95.

239 Adolfsson, O., Pihlgren, M., Toni, N. et al. (2012). An effector-reduced anti-beta-amyloid (Abeta) antibody with unique abeta binding properties promotes neuroprotection and glial engulfment of Abeta. *J. Neurosci.* 32: 9677–9689.

240 Tucker, S., Moller, C., Tegerstedt, K. et al. (2015). The murine version of BAN2401 (mAb158) selectively reduces amyloid-beta protofibrils in brain and cerebrospinal fluid of tg-ArcSwe mice. *J. Alzheimers Dis.* 43: 575–588.

241 Logovinsky, V., Satlin, A., Lai, R. et al. (2016). Safety and tolerability of BAN2401 – a clinical study in Alzheimer's disease with a protofibril selective Abeta antibody. *Alzheimers Res. Ther.* 8: 14.

242 Demattos, R.B., Lu, J., Tang, Y. et al. (2012). A plaque-specific antibody clears existing beta-amyloid plaques in Alzheimer's disease mice. *Neuron* 76: 908–920.

243 Lahiri, D.K. and Ray, B. (2014). Intravenous immunoglobulin treatment preserves and protects primary rat hippocampal neurons and primary human brain cultures against oxidative insults. *Curr. Alzheimer Res.* 11: 645–654.

244 Magga, J., Puli, L., Pihlaja, R. et al. (2010). Human intravenous immunoglobulin provides protection against Abeta toxicity by multiple mechanisms in a mouse model of Alzheimer's disease. *J. Neuroinflam.* 7: 90.

245 Puli, L., Pomeshchik, Y., Olas, K. et al. (2012). Effects of human intravenous immunoglobulin on amyloid pathology and neuroinflammation in a mouse model of Alzheimer's disease. *J. Neuroinflammation* 9: 105.

246 St-Amour, I., Pare, I., Tremblay, C. et al. (2014). IVIg protects the 3xTg-AD mouse model of Alzheimer's disease from memory deficit and Abeta pathology. *J. Neuroinflammation* 11: 54.

247 Dodel, R.C., Du, Y., Depboylu, C. et al. (2004). Intravenous immunoglobulins containing antibodies against beta-amyloid for the treatment of Alzheimer's disease. *J. Neurol. Neurosurg. Psychiatry* 75: 1472–1474.

248 Relkin, N.R., Szabo, P., Adamiak, B. et al. (2009). 18-month study of intravenous immunoglobulin for treatment of mild Alzheimer disease. *Neurobiol. Aging* 30: 1728–1736.

249 Dodel, R., Rominger, A., Bartenstein, P. et al. (2013). Intravenous immunoglobulin for treatment of mild-to-moderate Alzheimer's disease: a phase 2, randomised, double-blind, placebo-controlled, dose-finding trial. *Lancet Neurol.* 12: 233–243.

250 Relkin, N.R., Thomas, R.G., Rissman, R.A. et al. (2017). A phase 3 trial of IV immunoglobulin for Alzheimer disease. *Neurology* 88: 1768–1775.

251 Crespi, G.A., Ascher, D.B., Parker, M.W., and Miles, L.A. (2014). Crystallization and preliminary X-ray diffraction analysis of the Fab portion of the Alzheimer's disease immunotherapy candidate bapineuzumab complexed with amyloid-beta. *Acta Crystallogr. F Struct. Biol. Commun.* 70: 374–377.

252 Moreth, J., Mavoungou, C., and Schindowski, K. (2013). Passive anti-amyloid immunotherapy in Alzheimer's disease: what are the most promising targets? *Immun. Ageing* 10: 18.

253 Delnomdedieu, M., Duvvuri, S., Li, D.J. et al. (2016). First-In-Human safety and long-term exposure data for AAB-003 (PF-05236812) and biomarkers after intravenous infusions of escalating doses in patients with mild to moderate Alzheimer's disease. *Alzheimers Res. Ther.* 8: 12.

254 Bouter, Y., Lopez Noguerola, J.S., Tucholla, P. et al. (2015). Abeta targets of the biosimilar antibodies of Bapineuzumab, Crenezumab, Solanezumab in comparison to an antibody against Ntruncated Abeta in sporadic Alzheimer disease cases and mouse models. *Acta Neuropathol.* 130: 713–729.

255 Zago, W., Buttini, M., Comery, T.A. et al. (2012). Neutralization of soluble, synaptotoxic amyloid beta species by antibodies is epitope specific. *J. Neurosci.* 32: 2696–2702.

256 Zago, W., Schroeter, S., Guido, T. et al. (2013). Vascular alterations in PDAPP mice after anti-Abeta immunotherapy: Implications for amyloid-related imaging abnormalities. *Alzheimers Dement.* 9: S105–S115.

257 Abushouk, A.I., Elmaraezy, A., Aglan, A. et al. (2017). Bapineuzumab for mild to moderate Alzheimer's disease: a meta-analysis of randomized controlled trials. *BMC Neurol.* 17: 66.

258 Ketter, N., Brashear, H.R., Bogert, J. et al. (2017). Central review of amyloid-related imaging abnormalities in two phase III clinical trials of Bapineuzumab in mild-to-moderate Alzheimer's disease patients. *J. Alzheimers Dis.* 57: 557–573.

259 Arrighi, H.M., Barakos, J., Barkhof, F. et al. (2016). Amyloid-related imaging abnormalities-haemosiderin (ARIA-H) in patients with Alzheimer's disease treated with bapineuzumab: a historical, prospective secondary analysis. *J. Neurol. Neurosurg. Psychiatry* 87: 106–112.

260 Blennow, K., Zetterberg, H., Rinne, J.O. et al. (2012). Effect of immunotherapy with bapineuzumab on cerebrospinal fluid biomarker levels in patients with mild to moderate Alzheimer disease. *Arch. Neurol.* 69: 1002–1010.

261 Melancon, D., Morris, K., Ketter, N. et al. (2016). Bapineuzumab for mild to moderate Alzheimer's disease in two global, randomized, phase 3 trials. *J. Neurol. Neurosurg. Psychiatry* 8: 18.

262 Salloway, S., Sperling, R., Fox, N.C. et al. (2014). Two phase 3 trials of bapineuzumab in mild-to-moderate Alzheimer's disease. *N. Engl. J. Med.* 370: 322–333.

263 Salloway, S., Sperling, R., Gilman, S. et al. (2009). A phase 2 multiple ascending dose trial of bapineuzumab in mild to moderate Alzheimer disease. *Neurology* 73: 2061–2070.

264 Vandenberghe, R., Rinne, J.O., Boada, M. et al. (2016). Bapineuzumab for mild to moderate Alzheimer's disease in two global, randomized, phase 3 trials. *Alzheimers Res. Ther.* 8: 18.

265 La Porte, S.L., Bollini, S.S., Lanz, T.A. et al. (2012). Structural basis of C-terminal beta-amyloid peptide binding by the antibody ponezumab for the treatment of Alzheimer's disease. *J. Mol. Biol.* 421: 525–536.

266 Freeman, G.B., Brown, T.P., Wallace, K., and Bales, K.R. (2012). Chronic administration of an aglycosylated murine antibody of ponezumab does not worsen microhemorrhages in aged Tg2576 mice. *Curr. Alzheimer Res.* 9: 1059–1068.

267 Bales, K.R., O'Neill, S.M., Pozdnyakov, N. et al. (2016). Passive immunotherapy targeting amyloid-beta reduces cerebral amyloid angiopathy and improves vascular reactivity. *Brain* 139: 563–577.

268 Burstein, A.H., Zhao, Q., Ross, J. et al. (2013). Safety and pharmacology of ponezumab (PF-04360365) after a single 10-minute intravenous infusion in subjects with mild to moderate Alzheimer disease. *Clin. Neuropharmacol.* 36: 8–13.

269 Landen, J.W., Zhao, Q., Cohen, S. et al. (2013). Safety and pharmacology of a single intravenous dose of ponezumab in subjects with mild-to-moderate Alzheimer disease: a phase I, randomized, placebo-controlled, double-blind, dose-escalation study. *Clin. Neuropharmacol.* 36: 14–23.

270 Miyoshi, I., Fujimoto, Y., Yamada, M. et al. (2013). Safety and pharmacokinetics of PF-04360365 following a single-dose intravenous infusion in Japanese subjects with mild-to-moderate Alzheimer's disease: a multicenter, randomized, double-blind, placebo-controlled, dose-escalation study. *Int. J. Clin. Pharmacol. Ther.* 51: 911–923.

271 Landen, J.W., Andreasen, N., Cronenberger, C.L. et al. (2017). Ponezumab in mild-to-moderate Alzheimer's disease: Randomized phase II PET-PIB study. *Alzheimers Dement. (N.Y.)* 3: 393–401.

272 West, T., Hu, Y., Verghese, P.B. et al. (2017). Preclinical and clinical development of ABBV-8E12, a humanized anti-tau antibody, for treatment of Alzheimer's disease and other tauopathies. *J. Prev. Alzheimers Dis.* 4: 236–241.

273 Buee, L., Bussiere, T., Buee-Scherrer, V. et al. (2000). Tau protein isoforms, phosphorylation and role in neurodegenerative disorders. *Brain Res. Brain Res. Rev.* 33: 95–130.

274 Collin, L., Bohrmann, B., Gopfert, U. et al. (2014). Neuronal uptake of tau/pS422 antibody and reduced progression of tau pathology in a mouse model of Alzheimer's disease. *Brain* 137: 2834–2846.

275 Holthoewer, D., Endres, K., Schuck, F. et al. (2012). Acitretin, an enhancer of alpha-secretase expression, crosses the blood-brain barrier and is not eliminated by P-glycoprotein. *Neurodegener. Dis.* 10: 224–228.

276 Tippmann, F., Hundt, J., Schneider, A. et al. (2009). Up-regulation of the alpha-secretase ADAM10 by retinoic acid receptors and acitretin. *FASEB J.* 23: 1643–1654.

277 Endres, K., Fahrenholz, F., Lotz, J. et al. (2014). Increased CSF APPs-alpha levels in patients with Alzheimer disease treated with acitretin. *Neurology* 83: 1930–1935.

278 Kennedy, M.E., Stamford, A.W., Chen, X. et al. (2016). The BACE1 inhibitor verubecestat (MK-8931) reduces CNS beta-amyloid in animal models and in Alzheimer's disease patients. *Sci. Transl. Med.* 8: 363ra150.

279 Scott, J.D., Li, S.W., Brunskill, A.P. et al. (2016). Discovery of the 3-imino-1,2,4-thiadiazinane 1,1-dioxide derivative Verubecestat (MK-8931)-a beta-site amyloid precursor protein cleaving enzyme 1 inhibitor for the treatment of Alzheimer's disease. *J. Med. Chem.* 59: 10435–10450.

280 Villarreal, S., Zhao, F., Hyde, L.A. et al. (2017). Chronic Verubecestat treatment suppresses amyloid accumulation in advanced aged Tg2576-AbetaPPswe mice without inducing microhemorrhage. *J. Alzheimers Dis.* 59: 1393–1413.

281 Eketjall, S., Janson, J., Kaspersson, K. et al. (2016). AZD3293: a novel, orally active BACE1 inhibitor with high potency and permeability and markedly slow off-rate kinetics. *J. Alzheimers Dis.* 50: 1109–1123.

282 Cebers, G., Alexander, R.C., Haeberlein, S.B. et al. (2017). AZD3293: pharmacokinetic and pharmacodynamic effects in healthy subjects and patients with Alzheimer's disease. *J. Alzheimers Dis.* 55: 1039–1053.

283 Sakamoto, K., Matsuki, S., Matsuguma, K. et al. (2017). BACE1 inhibitor Lanabecestat (AZD3293) in a Phase 1 Study of Healthy Japanese subjects: pharmacokinetics and effects on plasma and cerebrospinal fluid Abeta peptides. *J. Clin. Pharmacol.* https://doi.org/10.1002/jcph.950.

284 Yan, R. (2016). Stepping closer to treating Alzheimer's disease patients with BACE1 inhibitor drugs. *Transl. Neurodegener.* 5: 13.

285 Lopez Lopez, C., Caputo, A., Liu, F. et al. (2017). The Alzheimer's prevention initiative generation program: evaluating CNP520 efficacy in the prevention of Alzheimer's disease. *J. Prev. Alzheimers Dis.* 4: 242–246.

286 Alkam, T., Nitta, A., Mizoguchi, H. et al. (2008). Restraining tumor necrosis factor-alpha by thalidomide prevents the amyloid beta-induced impairment of recognition memory in mice. *Behav. Brain Res.* 189: 100–106.

287 Greig, N.H., Giordano, T., Zhu, X. et al. (2004). Thalidomide-based TNF-alpha inhibitors for neurodegenerative diseases. *Acta Neurobiol. Exp. (Wars)* 64: 1–9.

288 He, P., Cheng, X., Staufenbiel, M. et al. (2013). Long-term treatment of thalidomide ameliorates amyloid-like pathology through inhibition of beta-secretase in a mouse model of Alzheimer's disease. *PLoS One* 8: e55091.

289 Tweedie, D., Ferguson, R.A., Fishman, K. et al. (2012). Tumor necrosis factor-alpha synthesis inhibitor 3,6'-dithiothalidomide attenuates markers of inflammation, Alzheimer pathology and behavioral deficits in animal models of neuroinflammation and Alzheimer's disease. *J. Neuroinflammation* 9: 106.

290 Decourt, B., Drumm-Gurnee, D., Wilson, J. et al. (2017). Poor safety and tolerability hamper reaching a potentially therapeutic dose in the use of thalidomide for Alzheimer's disease: results from a double-blind, placebo-controlled trial. *Curr. Alzheimer Res.* 14: 403–411.

291 Siemers, E.R., Quinn, J.F., Kaye, J. et al. (2006). Effects of a gamma-secretase inhibitor in a randomized study of patients with Alzheimer disease. *Neurology* 66: 602–604.

292 Fleisher, A.S., Raman, R., Siemers, E.R. et al. (2008). Phase 2 safety trial targeting amyloid beta production with a gamma-secretase inhibitor in Alzheimer disease. *Arch. Neurol.* 65: 1031–1038.

293 Doody, R.S., Raman, R., Farlow, M. et al. (2013). A phase 3 trial of semagacestat for treatment of Alzheimer's disease. *N. Engl. J. Med.* 369: 341–350.

294 Tong, G., Wang, J.S., Sverdlov, O. et al. (2012). Multicenter, randomized, double-blind, placebo-controlled, single-ascending dose study of the oral gamma-secretase inhibitor BMS-708163 (Avagacestat): tolerability profile, pharmacokinetic parameters, and pharmacodynamic markers. *Clin. Ther.* 34: 654–667.

295 Coric, V., van Dyck, C.H., Salloway, S. et al. (2012). Safety and tolerability of the gamma-secretase inhibitor avagacestat in a phase 2 study of mild to moderate Alzheimer disease. *Arch. Neurol.* 69: 1430–1440.

296 Coric, V., Salloway, S., van Dyck, C.H. et al. (2015). Targeting prodromal Alzheimer disease with avagacestat: a randomized clinical trial. *JAMA Neurol.* 72: 1324–1333.

297 in 't Veld, B.A., Launer, L.J., Hoes, A.W. et al. (1998). NSAIDs and incident Alzheimer's disease: the Rotterdam Study. *Neurobiol. Aging* 19: 607–611.

298 Asanuma, M., Nishibayashi-Asanuma, S., Miyazaki, I. et al. (2001). Neuroprotective effects of non-steroidal anti-inflammatory drugs by direct scavenging of nitric oxide radicals. *J. Neurochem.* 76: 1895–1904.

299 Blasko, I., Apochal, A., Boeck, G. et al. (2001). Ibuprofen decreases cytokine-induced amyloid beta production in neuronal cells. *Neurobiol. Dis.* 8: 1094–1101.

300 Lim, G.P., Yang, F., Chu, T. et al. (2000). Ibuprofen suppresses plaque pathology and inflammation in a mouse model for Alzheimer's disease. *J. Neurosci.* 20: 5709–5714.

301 Lim, G.P., Yang, F., Chu, T. et al. (2001). Ibuprofen effects on Alzheimer pathology and open field activity in APPsw transgenic mice. *Neurobiol. Aging* 22: 983–991.

302 McKee, A.C., Carreras, I., Hossain, L. et al. (2008). Ibuprofen reduces Abeta, hyperphosphorylated tau and memory deficits in Alzheimer mice. *Brain Res.* 1207: 225–236.

303 Van Dam, D., Coen, K., and De Deyn, P.P. (2010). Ibuprofen modifies cognitive disease progression in an Alzheimer's mouse model. *J. Psychopharmacol.* 24: 383–388.

304 Yan, Q., Zhang, J., Liu, H. et al. (2003). Anti-inflammatory drug therapy alters beta-amyloid processing and deposition in an animal model of Alzheimer's disease. *J. Neurosci.* 23: 7504–7509.

305 Morihara, T., Teter, B., Yang, F. et al. (2005). Ibuprofen suppresses interleukin-1beta induction of pro-amyloidogenic alpha1-antichymotrypsin to ameliorate beta-amyloid (Abeta) pathology in Alzheimer's models. *Neuropsychopharmacology* 30: 1111–1120.

306 Park, S.A., Chevallier, N., Tejwani, K. et al. (2016). Deficiency in either COX-1 or COX-2 genes does not affect amyloid beta protein burden in amyloid precursor protein transgenic mice. *Biochem. Biophys. Res. Commun.* 478: 286–292.

307 Pasqualetti, P., Bonomini, C., Dal Forno, G. et al. (2009). A randomized controlled study on effects of ibuprofen on cognitive progression of Alzheimer's disease. *Aging Clin. Exp. Res.* 21: 102–110.

308 Panza, F., Seripa, D., Solfrizzi, V. et al. (2016). Emerging drugs to reduce abnormal beta-amyloid protein in Alzheimer's disease patients. *Expert Opin. Emerg. Drugs* 21: 377–391.

309 Eriksen, J.L., Sagi, S.A., Smith, T.E. et al. (2003). NSAIDs and enantiomers of flurbiprofen target gamma-secretase and lower Abeta 42 in vivo. *J. Clin. Invest.* 112: 440–449.

310 Kukar, T., Prescott, S., Eriksen, J.L. et al. (2007). Chronic administration of R-flurbiprofen attenuates learning impairments in transgenic amyloid precursor protein mice. *BMC Neurosci.* 8: 54.

311 Weggen, S., Eriksen, J.L., Das, P. et al. (2001). A subset of NSAIDs lower amyloidogenic Abeta42 independently of cyclooxygenase activity. *Nature* 414: 212–216.

312 Weggen, S., Eriksen, J.L., Sagi, S.A. et al. (2003). Evidence that nonsteroidal anti-inflammatory drugs decrease amyloid beta 42 production by direct modulation of gamma-secretase activity. *J. Biol. Chem.* 278: 31831–31837.

313 Ettcheto, M., Sanchez-Lopez, E., Pons, L. et al. (2017). Dexibuprofen prevents neurodegeneration and cognitive decline in APPswe/PS1dE9 through multiple signaling pathways. *Redox Biol.* 13: 345–352.

314 Wilcock, G.K., Black, S.E., Hendrix, S.B. et al. (2008). Efficacy and safety of tarenflurbil in mild to moderate Alzheimer's disease: a randomised phase II trial. *Lancet Neurol.* 7: 483–493.

315 Green, R.C., Schneider, L.S., Amato, D.A. et al. (2009). Effect of tarenflurbil on cognitive decline and activities of daily living in patients with mild Alzheimer disease: a randomized controlled trial. *JAMA* 302: 2557–2564.

316 Muntimadugu, E., Dhommati, R., Jain, A. et al. (2016). Intranasal delivery of nanoparticle encapsulated tarenflurbil: a potential brain targeting strategy for Alzheimer's disease. *Eur. J. Pharm. Sci.* 92: 224–234.

317 Rogers, K., Felsenstein, K.M., Hrdlicka, L. et al. (2012). Modulation of gamma-secretase by EVP-0015962 reduces amyloid deposition and behavioral deficits in Tg2576 mice. *Mol. Neurodegener.* 7: 61.

318 Sivilia, S., Lorenzini, L., Giuliani, A. et al. (2013). Multi-target action of the novel anti-Alzheimer compound CHF5074: in vivo study of long term treatment in Tg2576 mice. *BMC Neurosci.* 14: 44.

319 Imbimbo, B.P., Del Giudice, E., Colavito, D. et al. (2007). 1-(3′,4′-Dichloro-2-fluoro[1,1′-biphenyl]-4-yl)-cyclopropanecarboxylic acid (CHF5074), a novel gamma-secretase modulator, reduces brain beta-amyloid pathology in a transgenic mouse model of Alzheimer's disease without causing peripheral toxicity. *J. Pharmacol. Exp. Ther.* 323: 822–830.

320 Imbimbo, B.P., Giardino, L., Sivilia, S. et al. (2010). CHF5074, a novel gamma-secretase modulator, restores hippocampal neurogenesis potential and reverses contextual memory deficit in a transgenic mouse model of Alzheimer's disease. *J. Alzheimers Dis.* 20: 159–173.

321 Imbimbo, B.P., Hutter-Paier, B., Villetti, G. et al. (2009). CHF5074, a novel gamma-secretase modulator, attenuates brain beta-amyloid pathology and learning deficit in a mouse model of Alzheimer's disease. *Br. J. Pharmacol.* 156: 982–993.

322 Giuliani, A., Beggiato, S., Baldassarro, V.A. et al. (2013). CHF5074 restores visual memory ability and pre-synaptic cortical acetylcholine release in pre-plaque Tg2576 mice. *J. Neurochem.* 124: 613–620.

323 Imbimbo, B.P., Frigerio, E., Breda, M. et al. (2013). Pharmacokinetics and pharmacodynamics of CHF5074 after short-term administration in healthy subjects. *Alzheimer Dis. Assoc. Disord.* 27: 278–286.

324 Ross, J., Sharma, S., Winston, J. et al. (2013). CHF5074 reduces biomarkers of neuroinflammation in patients with mild cognitive impairment: a 12-week, double-blind, placebo-controlled study. *Curr. Alzheimer Res.* 10: 742–753.

325 Lue, L.F., Yan, S.D., Stern, D.M., and Walker, D.G. (2005). Preventing activation of receptor for advanced glycation endproducts in Alzheimer's disease. *Curr. Drug Targets CNS Neurol. Disord.* 4: 249–266.

326 Yan, S.D., Chen, X., Fu, J. et al. (1996). RAGE and amyloid-beta peptide neurotoxicity in Alzheimer's disease. *Nature* 382: 685–691.

327 Choi, B.R., Cho, W.H., Kim, J. et al. (2014). Increased expression of the receptor for advanced glycation end products in neurons and astrocytes in a triple transgenic mouse model of Alzheimer's disease. *Exp. Mol. Med.* 46: e75.

328 Deane, R., Singh, I., Sagare, A.P. et al. (2012). A multimodal RAGE-specific inhibitor reduces amyloid beta-mediated brain disorder in a mouse model of Alzheimer disease. *J. Clin. Invest.* 122: 1377–1392.

329 Kook, S.Y., Hong, H.S., Moon, M. et al. (2012). Abeta(1)(−)(4)(2)-RAGE interaction disrupts tight junctions of the blood-brain barrier via Ca(2)(+)-calcineurin signaling. *J. Neurosci.* 32: 8845–8854.

330 Lubitz, I., Ricny, J., Atrakchi-Baranes, D. et al. (2016). High dietary advanced glycation end products are associated with poorer spatial learning and accelerated Abeta deposition in an Alzheimer mouse model. *Exp. Mol. Med.* 15: 309–316.

331 Sabbagh, M.N., Agro, A., Bell, J. et al. (2011). PF-04494700, an oral inhibitor of receptor for advanced glycation end products (RAGE), in Alzheimer disease. *Alzheimer Dis. Assoc. Disord.* 25: 206–212.

332 Steen, E., Terry, B.M., Rivera, E.J. et al. (2005). Impaired insulin and insulin-like growth factor expression and signaling mechanisms in Alzheimer's disease – is this type 3 diabetes? *J. Alzheimers Dis.* 7: 63–80.

333 Schioth, H.B., Craft, S., Brooks, S.J. et al. (2012). Brain insulin signaling and Alzheimer's disease: current evidence and future directions. *Mol. Neurobiol.* 46: 4–10.

334 De Felice, F.G., Vieira, M.N., Bomfim, T.R. et al. (2009). Protection of synapses against Alzheimer's-linked toxins: insulin signaling prevents the pathogenic binding of Abeta oligomers. *Proc. Natl. Acad. Sci. U.S.A.* 106: 1971–1976.

335 Hong, M. and Lee, V.M. (1997). Insulin and insulin-like growth factor-1 regulate tau phosphorylation in cultured human neurons. *J. Biol. Chem.* 272: 19547–19553.

336 Claxton, A., Baker, L.D., Wilkinson, C.W. et al. (2013). Sex and ApoE genotype differences in treatment response to two doses of intranasal insulin in adults with mild cognitive impairment or Alzheimer's disease. *J. Alzheimers Dis.* 35: 789–797.

337 Claxton, A., Baker, L.D., Hanson, A. et al. (2015). Long-acting intranasal insulin detemir improves cognition for adults with mild cognitive impairment or early-stage Alzheimer's disease dementia. *J. Alzheimers Dis.* 44: 897–906.

338 Craft, S., Baker, L.D., Montine, T.J. et al. (2012). Intranasal insulin therapy for Alzheimer disease and amnestic mild cognitive impairment: a pilot clinical trial. *Arch. Neurol.* 69: 29–38.

339 Craft, S., Claxton, A., Baker, L.D. et al. (2017). Effects of regular and long-acting insulin on cognition and Alzheimer's disease biomarkers: a pilot clinical trial. *J. Alzheimers Dis.* 57: 1325–1334.

340 Lonskaya, I., Hebron, M., Chen, W. et al. (2014). Tau deletion impairs intracellular beta-amyloid-42 clearance and leads to more extracellular plaque deposition in gene transfer models. *Mol. Neurodegener.* 9: 46.

341 Lonskaya, I., Hebron, M.L., Desforges, N.M. et al. (2013). Tyrosine kinase inhibition increases functional parkin-Beclin-1 interaction and enhances amyloid clearance and cognitive performance. *EMBO Mol. Med.* 5: 1247–1262.

342 Lonskaya, I., Hebron, M.L., Desforges, N.M. et al. (2014). Nilotinib-induced autophagic changes increase endogenous parkin level and ubiquitination, leading to amyloid clearance. *J. Mol. Med. (Berl.)* 92: 373–386.

343 Hebron, M.L., Lonskaya, I., and Moussa, C.E. (2013). Nilotinib reverses loss of dopamine neurons and improves motor behavior via autophagic degradation of alpha-synuclein in Parkinson's disease models. *Hum. Mol. Genet.* 22: 3315–3328.

344 Karuppagounder, S.S., Brahmachari, S., Lee, Y. et al. (2014). The c-Abl inhibitor, nilotinib, protects dopaminergic neurons in a preclinical animal model of Parkinson's disease. *Sci. Rep.* 4: 4874.

345 Tanabe, A., Yamamura, Y., Kasahara, J. et al. (2014). A novel tyrosine kinase inhibitor AMN107 (nilotinib) normalizes striatal motor behaviors in a mouse model of Parkinson's disease. *Front. Cell Neurosci.* 8: 50.

346 Hofrichter, J., Krohn, M., Schumacher, T. et al. (2013). Reduced Alzheimer's disease pathology by St. John's Wort treatment is independent of hyperforin and facilitated by ABCC1 and microglia activation in mice. *Curr. Alzheimer Res.* 10: 1057–1069.

347 Krohn, M., Bracke, A., Avchalumov, Y. et al. (2015). Accumulation of murine amyloid-beta mimics early Alzheimer's disease. *Brain* 138: 2370–2382.

348 Krohn, M., Lange, C., Hofrichter, J. et al. (2011). Cerebral amyloid-beta proteostasis is regulated by the membrane transport protein ABCC1 in mice. *J. Clin. Invest.* 121: 3924–3931.

349 Etcheberrigaray, R., Tan, M., Dewachter, I. et al. (2004). Therapeutic effects of PKC activators in Alzheimer's disease transgenic mice. *Proc. Natl. Acad. Sci. U.S.A.* 101: 11141–11146.

350 Hongpaisan, J., Sun, M.K., and Alkon, D.L. (2011). PKC epsilon activation prevents synaptic loss, Abeta elevation, and cognitive deficits in Alzheimer's disease transgenic mice. *J. Neurosci.* 31: 630–643.

351 Khan, T.K., Nelson, T.J., Verma, V.A. et al. (2009). A cellular model of Alzheimer's disease therapeutic efficacy: PKC activation reverses Abeta-induced biomarker abnormality on cultured fibroblasts. *Neurobiol. Dis.* 34: 332–339.

352 Schrott, L.M., Jackson, K., Yi, P. et al. (2015). Acute oral Bryostatin-1 administration improves learning deficits in the APP/PS1 transgenic mouse model of Alzheimer's disease. *Curr. Alzheimer Res.* 12: 22–31.

353 Krishnan, R., Tsubery, H., Proschitsky, M.Y. et al. (2014). A bacteriophage capsid protein provides a general amyloid interaction motif (GAIM) that binds and remodels misfolded protein assemblies. *J. Mol. Biol.* 426: 2500–2519.

354 Levenson, J.M., Schroeter, S., Carroll, J.C. et al. (2016). NPT088 reduces both amyloid-beta and tau pathologies in transgenic mice. *Alzheimers Dement. (N.Y.)* 2: 141–155.

355 Benito, E., Urbanke, H., Ramachandran, B. et al. (2015). HDAC inhibitor-dependent transcriptome and memory reinstatement in cognitive decline models. *J. Clin. Invest.* 125: 3572–3584.

356 Kilgore, M., Miller, C.A., Fass, D.M. et al. (2010). Inhibitors of class 1 histone deacetylases reverse contextual memory deficits in a mouse model of Alzheimer's disease. *Neuropsychopharmacology* 35: 870–880.

357 Nuutinen, T., Suuronen, T., Kauppinen, A., and Salminen, A. (2010). Valproic acid stimulates clusterin expression in human astrocytes: implications for Alzheimer's disease. *Neurosci. Lett.* 475: 64–68.

358 Sharma, S. and Taliyan, R. (2016). Epigenetic modifications by inhibiting histone deacetylases reverse memory impairment in insulin resistance induced cognitive deficit in mice. *Neuropharmacology* 105: 285–297.

359 Meng, J., Li, Y., Camarillo, C. et al. (2014). The anti-tumor histone deacetylase inhibitor SAHA and the natural flavonoid curcumin exhibit synergistic neuroprotection against amyloid-beta toxicity. *PLoS One* 9: e85570.

360 Zhang, D., Mably, A.J., Walsh, D.M., and Rowan, M.J. (2017). Peripheral interventions enhancing brain glutamate homeostasis relieve amyloid beta- and

TNFalpha-mediated synaptic plasticity disruption in the rat hippocampus. *Cereb. Cortex.* 27: 3724–3735.

361 Zhang, D., Qi, Y., Klyubin, I. et al. (2017). Targeting glutamatergic and cellular prion protein mechanisms of amyloid beta-mediated persistent synaptic plasticity disruption: longitudinal studies. *Neuropharmacology* 121: 231–246.

362 Swerdlow, R.H., Bothwell, R., Hutfles, L. et al. (2016). Tolerability and pharmacokinetics of oxaloacetate 100 mg capsules in Alzheimer's subjects. *BBA Clin.* 5: 120–123.

363 Yamanaka, M., Ishikawa, T., Griep, A. et al. (2012). PPARgamma/RXRalpha-induced and CD36-mediated microglial amyloid-beta phagocytosis results in cognitive improvement in amyloid precursor protein/presenilin 1 mice. *J. Neurosci.* 32: 17321–17331.

364 Balducci, C., Paladini, A., Micotti, E. et al. (2015). The continuing failure of bexarotene in Alzheimer's disease mice. *J. Alzheimers Dis.* 46: 471–482.

365 LaClair, K.D., Manaye, K.F., Lee, D.L. et al. (2013). Treatment with bexarotene, a compound that increases apolipoprotein-E, provides no cognitive benefit in mutant APP/PS1 mice. *Mol. Neurodegener.* 8: 18.

366 O'Hare, E., Jeggo, R., Kim, E.M. et al. (2016). Lack of support for bexarotene as a treatment for Alzheimer's disease. *Neuropharmacology* 100: 124–130.

367 Corona, A.W., Kodoma, N., Casali, B.T., and Landreth, G.E. (2016). ABCA1 is necessary for bexarotene-mediated clearance of soluble amyloid beta from the hippocampus of APP/PS1 mice. *J. Neuroimmune Pharmacol.* 11: 61–72.

368 Mariani, M.M., Malm, T., Lamb, R. et al. (2017). Neuronally-directed effects of RXR activation in a mouse model of Alzheimer's disease. *Sci. Rep.* 7: 42270.

369 Cummings, J.L., Zhong, K., Kinney, J.W. et al. (2016). Double-blind, placebo-controlled, proof-of-concept trial of bexarotene Xin moderate Alzheimer's disease. *Alzheimers Res. Ther.* 8: 4.

370 Frost, J.L., Le, K.X., Cynis, H. et al. (2013). Pyroglutamate-3 amyloid-beta deposition in the brains of humans, non-human primates, canines, and Alzheimer disease-like transgenic mouse models. *Am. J. Pathol.* 183: 369–381.

371 Morawski, M., Schilling, S., Kreuzberger, M. et al. (2014). Glutaminyl cyclase in human cortex: correlation with (pGlu)-amyloid-beta load and cognitive decline in Alzheimer's disease. *J. Alzheimers Dis.* 39: 385–400.

372 Hartlage-Rubsamen, M., Morawski, M., Waniek, A. et al. (2011). Glutaminyl cyclase contributes to the formation of focal and diffuse pyroglutamate (pGlu)-Abeta deposits in hippocampus via distinct cellular mechanisms. *Acta Neuropathol.* 121: 705–719.

373 Valenti, M.T., Bolognin, S., Zanatta, C. et al. (2013). Increased glutaminyl cyclase expression in peripheral blood of Alzheimer's disease patients. *J. Alzheimers Dis.* 34: 263–271.

374 Bridel, C., Hoffmann, T., Meyer, A. et al. (2017). Glutaminyl cyclase activity correlates with levels of Abeta peptides and mediators of angiogenesis in cerebrospinal fluid of Alzheimer's disease patients. *Alzheimers Res. Ther.* 9: 38.

375 Hoffmann, T., Meyer, A., Heiser, U. et al. (2017). Glutaminyl cyclase inhibitor PQ912 improves cognition in mouse models of Alzheimer's disease-studies on relation to effective target occupancy. *J. Pharmacol. Exp. Ther.* 362: 119–130.

376 Schilling, S., Zeitschel, U., Hoffmann, T. et al. (2008). Glutaminyl cyclase inhibition attenuates pyroglutamate Abeta and Alzheimer's disease-like pathology. *Nat. Med.* 14: 1106–1111.

377 Jawhar, S., Wirths, O., Schilling, S. et al. (2011). Overexpression of glutaminyl cyclase, the enzyme responsible for pyroglutamate A{beta} formation, induces behavioral deficits, and glutaminyl cyclase knock-out rescues the behavioral phenotype in 5XFAD mice. *J. Biol. Chem.* 286: 4454–4460.

378 Song, H., Chang, Y.J., Moon, M. et al. (2015). Inhibition of glutaminyl cyclase ameliorates amyloid pathology in an animal model of Alzheimer's disease via the modulation of gamma-secretase activity. *J. Alzheimers Dis.* 43: 797–807.

379 McLaurin, J., Golomb, R., Jurewicz, A. et al. (2000). Inositol stereoisomers stabilize an oligomeric aggregate of Alzheimer amyloid beta peptide and inhibit abeta-induced toxicity. *J Biol Chem* 275: 18495–18502.

380 Hawkes, C.A., Deng, L.H., Shaw, J.E. et al. (2010). Small molecule beta-amyloid inhibitors that stabilize protofibrillar structures in vitro improve cognition and pathology in a mouse model of Alzheimer's disease. *Eur. J. Neurosci.* 31: 203–213.

381 Dorr, A., Sahota, B., Chinta, L.V. et al. (2012). Amyloid-beta-dependent compromise of microvascular structure and function in a model of Alzheimer's disease. *Brain* 135: 3039–3050.

382 Fenili, D., Brown, M., Rappaport, R., and McLaurin, J. (2007). Properties of scyllo-inositol as a therapeutic treatment of AD-like pathology. *J. Mol. Med. (Berl.)* 85: 603–611.

383 Jin, M. and Selkoe, D.J. (2015). Systematic analysis of time-dependent neural effects of soluble amyloid beta oligomers in culture and in vivo: prevention by scyllo-inositol. *Neurobiol. Dis.* 82: 152–163.

384 Lai, A.Y. and McLaurin, J. (2012). Inhibition of amyloid-beta peptide aggregation rescues the autophagic deficits in the TgCRND8 mouse model of Alzheimer disease. *Biochim. Biophys. Acta* 1822: 1629–1637.

385 Townsend, M., Cleary, J.P., Mehta, T. et al. (2006). Orally available compound prevents deficits in memory caused by the Alzheimer amyloid-beta oligomers. *Ann. Neurol.* 60: 668–676.

386 Liu, M., Jevtic, S., Markham-Coultes, K. et al. (2018). Investigating the efficacy of a combination Abeta-targeted treatment in a mouse model of Alzheimer's disease. *Brain Res.* 1678: 138–145.

387 Salloway, S., Sperling, R., Keren, R. et al. (2011). A phase 2 randomized trial of ELND005, scyllo-inositol, in mild to moderate Alzheimer disease. *Neurology* 77: 1253–1262.

388 Adlard, P.A., Bica, L., White, A.R. et al. (2011). Metal ionophore treatment restores dendritic spine density and synaptic protein levels in a mouse model of Alzheimer's disease. *PLoS One* 6: e17669.

389 Crouch, P.J., Savva, M.S., Hung, L.W. et al. (2011). The Alzheimer's therapeutic PBT2 promotes amyloid-beta degradation and GSK3 phosphorylation via a metal chaperone activity. *J. Neurochem.* 119: 220–230.

390 Johanssen, T., Suphantarida, N., Donnelly, P.S. et al. (2015). PBT2 inhibits glutamate-induced excitotoxicity in neurons through metal-mediated preconditioning. *Neurobiol. Dis.* 81: 176–185.

391 Faux, N.G., Ritchie, C.W., Gunn, A. et al. (2010). PBT2 rapidly improves cognition in Alzheimer's disease: additional phase II analyses. *J. Alzheimers Dis.* 20: 509–516.

392 Lannfelt, L., Blennow, K., Zetterberg, H. et al. (2008). Safety, efficacy, and biomarker findings of PBT2 in targeting Abeta as a modifying therapy for Alzheimer's disease: a phase IIa, double-blind, randomised, placebo-controlled trial. *Lancet Neurol.* 7: 779–786.

393 Villemagne, V.L., Rowe, C.C., Barnham, K.J. et al. (2017). A randomized, exploratory molecular imaging study targeting amyloid beta with a novel 8-OH quinoline in Alzheimer's disease: the PBT2-204 IMAGINE study. *Alzheimers Dement. (N.Y.)* 3: 622–635.

394 Ritchie, C.W., Bush, A.I., Mackinnon, A. et al. (2003). Metal-protein attenuation with iodochlorhydroxyquin (clioquinol) targeting Abeta amyloid deposition and toxicity in Alzheimer disease: a pilot phase 2 clinical trial. *Arch. Neurol.* 60: 1685–1691.

395 Abramov, A.Y., Canevari, L., and Duchen, M.R. (2003). Changes in intracellular calcium and glutathione in astrocytes as the primary mechanism of amyloid neurotoxicity. *J. Neurosci.* 23: 5088–5095.

396 Cherny, R.A., Atwood, C.S., Xilinas, M.E. et al. (2001). Treatment with a copper-zinc chelator markedly and rapidly inhibits beta-amyloid accumulation in Alzheimer's disease transgenic mice. *Neuron* 30: 665–676.

397 Matlack, K.E., Tardiff, D.F., Narayan, P. et al. (2014). Clioquinol promotes the degradation of metal-dependent amyloid-beta (Abeta) oligomers to restore endocytosis and ameliorate Abeta toxicity. *Proc. Natl. Acad. Sci. U.S.A.* 111: 4013–4018.

398 Zhang, Y.H., Raymick, J., Sarkar, S. et al. (2013). Efficacy and toxicity of clioquinol treatment and A-beta42 inoculation in the APP/PSI mouse model of Alzheimer's disease. *Curr. Alzheimer Res.* 10: 494–506.

399 Deiana, S., Harrington, C.R., Wischik, C.M., and Riedel, G. (2009). Methylthioninium chloride reverses cognitive deficits induced by scopolamine: comparison with rivastigmine. *Psychopharmacology* 202: 53–65.

400 Medina, D.X., Caccamo, A., and Oddo, S. (2011). Methylene blue reduces abeta levels and rescues early cognitive deficit by increasing proteasome activity. *Brain Pathol.* 21: 140–149.

401 Riha, P.D., Rojas, J.C., and Gonzalez-Lima, F. (2011). Beneficial network effects of methylene blue in an amnestic model. *Neuroimage* 54: 2623–2634.

402 Wen, Y., Li, W., Poteet, E.C. et al. (2011). Alternative mitochondrial electron transfer as a novel strategy for neuroprotection. *J. Biol. Chem.* 286: 16504–16515.

403 Atamna, H. and Kumar, R. (2010). Protective role of methylene blue in Alzheimer's disease via mitochondria and cytochrome c oxidase. *J. Alzheimers Dis.* 20 (Suppl 2): S439–S452.

404 Mori, T., Koyama, N., Segawa, T. et al. (2014). Methylene blue modulates beta-secretase, reverses cerebral amyloidosis, and improves cognition in transgenic mice. *J. Biol. Chem.* 289: 30303–30317.

405 Batista, A.F., Forny-Germano, L., Clarke, J.R. et al. (2018). The diabetes drug liraglutide reverses cognitive impairment in mice and attenuates insulin receptor and synaptic pathology in a non-human primate model of Alzheimer's disease. *J. Pathol.* 245 (1): 85–100.

406 Chen, S., Sun, J., Zhao, G. et al. (2017). Liraglutide improves water maze learning and memory performance while reduces hyperphosphorylation of tau and neurofilaments in APP/PS1/tau triple transgenic mice. *J. Pathol.* 42: 2326–2335.

407 Hansen, H.H., Fabricius, K., Barkholt, P. et al. (2015). The GLP-1 receptor agonist liraglutide improves memory function and increases hippocampal CA1 neuronal numbers in a senescence-accelerated mouse model of Alzheimer's disease. *J. Alzheimers Dis.* 46: 877–888.

408 Long-Smith, C.M., Manning, S., McClean, P.L. et al. (2013). The diabetes drug liraglutide ameliorates aberrant insulin receptor localisation and signalling in parallel with decreasing both amyloid-beta plaque and glial pathology in a mouse model of Alzheimer's disease. *Neuromolecular Med.* 15: 102–114.

409 McClean, P.L., Gault, V.A., Harriott, P., and Holscher, C. (2010). Glucagon-like peptide-1 analogues enhance synaptic plasticity in the brain: a link between diabetes and Alzheimer's disease. *Eur. J. Pharmacol.* 630: 158–162.

410 McClean, P.L. and Holscher, C. (2014). Liraglutide can reverse memory impairment, synaptic loss and reduce plaque load in aged APP/PS1 mice, a model of Alzheimer's disease. *Neuropharmacology* 76 (Pt A): 57–67.

411 McClean, P.L., Jalewa, J., and Holscher, C. (2015). Prophylactic liraglutide treatment prevents amyloid plaque deposition, chronic inflammation and memory impairment in APP/PS1 mice. *Behav. Brain Res.* 293: 96–106.

412 Qi, L., Chen, Z., Wang, Y. et al. (2017). Subcutaneous liraglutide ameliorates methylglyoxal-induced Alzheimer-like tau pathology and cognitive impairment by modulating tau hyperphosphorylation and glycogen synthase kinase-3beta. *Am. J. Transl. Res.* 9: 247–260.

413 Qi, L., Ke, L., Liu, X. et al. (2016). Subcutaneous administration of liraglutide ameliorates learning and memory impairment by modulating tau hyperphosphorylation via the glycogen synthase kinase-3beta pathway in an amyloid beta protein induced alzheimer disease mouse model. *Eur. J. Pharmacol.* 783: 23–32.

414 Yang, Y., Zhang, J., Ma, D. et al. (2013). Subcutaneous administration of liraglutide ameliorates Alzheimer-associated tau hyperphosphorylation in rats with type 2 diabetes. *J. Alzheimers Dis.* 37: 637–648.

415 Zeng, F., Lu, J.J., Zhou, X.F., and Wang, Y.J. (2011). Roles of p75NTR in the pathogenesis of Alzheimer's disease: a novel therapeutic target. *Biochem. Pharmacol.* 82: 1500–1509.

416 Zhou, X.F. and Wang, Y.J. (2011). The p75NTR extracellular domain: a potential molecule regulating the solubility and removal of amyloid-beta. *Prion* 5: 161–163.

417 James, M.L., Belichenko, N.P., Shuhendler, A.J. et al. (2017). [(18)F]GE-180 PET detects reduced microglia activation after LM11A-31 therapy in a mouse model of Alzheimer's disease. *Theranostics* 7: 1422–1436.

418 Knowles, J.K., Simmons, D.A., Nguyen, T.V. et al. (2013). Small molecule p75NTR ligand prevents cognitive deficits and neurite degeneration in an Alzheimer's mouse model. *Neurobiol. Aging* 34: 2052–2063.

419 Nguyen, T.V., Shen, L., Vander Griend, L. et al. (2014). Small molecule p75NTR ligands reduce pathological phosphorylation and misfolding of tau, inflammatory changes, cholinergic degeneration, and cognitive deficits in AbetaPP(L/S) transgenic mice. *J. Alzheimers Dis.* 42: 459–483.

420 Simmons, D.A., Knowles, J.K., Belichenko, N.P. et al. (2014). A small molecule p75NTR ligand, LM11A-31, reverses cholinergic neurite dystrophy in Alzheimer's disease mouse models with mid- to late-stage disease progression. *PLoS One* 9: e102136.

421 Mitchell, D., Bergendahl, G., Ferguson, W. et al. (2016). A Phase 1 trial of TPI 287 as a single agent and in combination with temozolomide in patients with refractory or recurrent neuroblastoma or medulloblastoma. *Pediatr. Blood Cancer* 63: 39–46.

422 McQuade, J.L., Posada, L.P., Lecagoonporn, S. et al. (2016). A phase I study of TPI 287 in combination with temozolomide for patients with metastatic melanoma. *Melanoma Res.* 26 (6): 604–608.

423 Fitzgerald, D.P., Emerson, D.L., Qian, Y. et al. (2012). TPI-287, a new taxane family member, reduces the brain metastatic colonization of breast cancer cells. *Mol. Cancer Ther.* 11: 1959–1967.

424 Zumbar, C.T., Usubalieva, A., King, P.D. et al. (2018). The CNS penetrating taxane TPI 287 and the AURKA inhibitor alisertib induce synergistic apoptosis in glioblastoma cells. *J Neurooncol.* 137 (3): 481–492.

425 Morales-Garcia, J.A., Luna-Medina, R., Alonso-Gil, S. et al. (2012). Glycogen synthase kinase 3 inhibition promotes adult hippocampal neurogenesis in vitro and in vivo. *ACS Chem. Neurosci.* 3: 963–971.

426 Sereno, L., Coma, M., Rodriguez, M. et al. (2009). A novel GSK-3beta inhibitor reduces Alzheimer's pathology and rescues neuronal loss in vivo. *Neurobiol. Dis.* 35: 359–367.

427 del Ser, T., Steinwachs, K.C., Gertz, H.J. et al. (2013). Treatment of Alzheimer's disease with the GSK-3 inhibitor tideglusib: a pilot study. *J. Alzheimers Dis.* 33: 205–215.

428 Lovestone, S., Boada, M., Dubois, B. et al. (2015). A phase II trial of tideglusib in Alzheimer's disease. *J. Alzheimers Dis.* 45: 75–88.

429 Chen, J., Li, S., Sun, W., and Li, J. (2015). Anti-diabetes drug pioglitazone ameliorates synaptic defects in AD transgenic mice by inhibiting cyclin-dependent kinase5 activity. *PLoS One* 10: e0123864.

430 Gupta, R. and Gupta, L.K. (2012). Improvement in long term and visuo-spatial memory following chronic pioglitazone in mouse model of Alzheimer's disease. *Pharmacol. Biochem. Behav.* 102: 184–190.

431 Heneka, M.T., Sastre, M., Dumitrescu-Ozimek, L. et al. (2005). Acute treatment with the PPARgamma agonist pioglitazone and ibuprofen reduces glial inflammation and Abeta1-42 levels in APPV717I transgenic mice. *Brain* 128: 1442–1453.

432 Papadopoulos, P., Rosa-Neto, P., Rochford, J., and Hamel, E. (2013). Pioglitazone improves reversal learning and exerts mixed cerebrovascular effects in a mouse model of Alzheimer's disease with combined amyloid-beta and cerebrovascular pathology. *PLoS One* 8: e68612.

433 Searcy, J.L., Phelps, J.T., Pancani, T. et al. (2012). Long-term pioglitazone treatment improves learning and attenuates pathological markers in a mouse model of Alzheimer's disease. *J. Alzheimers Dis.* 30: 943–961.

434 Skerrett, R., Pellegrino, M.P., Casali, B.T. et al. (2015). Combined liver X receptor/peroxisome proliferator-activated receptor gamma agonist treatment reduces amyloid beta levels and improves behavior in amyloid precursor protein/presenilin 1 mice. *J. Biol. Chem.* 290: 21591–21602.

435 Toba, J., Nikkuni, M., Ishizeki, M. et al. (2016). PPARgamma agonist pioglitazone improves cerebellar dysfunction at pre-Abeta deposition stage in APPswe/PS1dE9 Alzheimer's disease model mice. *Biochem. Biophys. Res. Commun.* 473: 1039–1044.

436 Yang, S., Chen, Z., Cao, M. et al. (2017). Pioglitazone ameliorates Abeta42 deposition in rats with diet-induced insulin resistance associated with AKT/GSK3beta activation. *Mol. Med. Rep.* 15: 2588–2594.

437 Hanyu, H., Sato, T., Kiuchi, A. et al. (2009). Pioglitazone improved cognition in a pilot study on patients with Alzheimer's disease and mild cognitive impairment with diabetes mellitus. *J. Am. Geriatr. Soc.* 57: 177–179.

438 Sato, T., Hanyu, H., Hirao, K. et al. (2011). Efficacy of PPAR-gamma agonist pioglitazone in mild Alzheimer disease. *Neurobiol. Aging* 32: 1626–1633.

439 Boyd, T.D., Bennett, S.P., Mori, T. et al. (2010). GM-CSF upregulated in rheumatoid arthritis reverses cognitive impairment and amyloidosis in Alzheimer mice. *J. Alzheimers Dis.* 21: 507–518.

440 Bachstetter, A.D., Xing, B., de Almeida, L. et al. (2011). Microglial p38alpha MAPK is a key regulator of proinflammatory cytokine up-regulation induced by toll-like receptor (TLR) ligands or beta-amyloid (Abeta). *J. Neuroinflammation* 8: 79.

441 Giraldo, E., Lloret, A., Fuchsberger, T., and Vina, J. (2014). Abeta and tau toxicities in Alzheimer's are linked via oxidative stress-induced p38 activation: protective role of vitamin E. *Redox Biol.* 2: 873–877.

442 Schnoder, L., Hao, W., Qin, Y. et al. (2016). Deficiency of neuronal p38alpha MAPK attenuates amyloid pathology in Alzheimer disease mouse and cell models through facilitating lysosomal degradation of BACE1. *J. Biol. Chem.* 291: 2067–2079.

443 Zou, L., Qin, H., He, Y. et al. (2012). Inhibiting p38 mitogen-activated protein kinase attenuates cerebral ischemic injury in Swedish mutant amyloid precursor protein transgenic mice. *Neural Regen. Res.* 7: 1088–1094.

444 Roy, S.M., Grum-Tokars, V.L., Schavocky, J.P. et al. (2015). Targeting human central nervous system protein kinases: an isoform selective p38alphaMAPK inhibitor that attenuates disease progression in Alzheimer's disease mouse models. *ACS Chem. Neurosci.* 6: 666–680.

445 Alam, J.J. (2015). Selective brain-targeted antagonism of p38 MAPKalpha reduces hippocampal IL-1beta levels and improves Morris Water Maze performance in aged rats. *J. Alzheimers Dis.* 48: 219–227.

446 Alam, J., Blackburn, K., and Patrick, D. (2017). Neflamapimod: clinical phase 2b-ready oral small molecule inhibitor of p38alpha to reverse synaptic dysfunction in early Alzheimer's disease. *J. Prev. Alzheimers Dis.* 4: 273–278.

447 Biscaro, B., Lindvall, O., Tesco, G. et al. (2012). Inhibition of microglial activation protects hippocampal neurogenesis and improves cognitive deficits in a transgenic mouse model for Alzheimer's disease. *Neurodegener. Dis.* 9: 187–198.

448 Cai, Z., Yan, Y., and Wang, Y. (2013). Minocycline alleviates beta-amyloid protein and tau pathology via restraining neuroinflammation induced by diabetic metabolic disorder. *Clin. Interv. Aging* 8: 1089–1095.

449 Choi, Y., Kim, H.S., Shin, K.Y. et al. (2007). Minocycline attenuates neuronal cell death and improves cognitive impairment in Alzheimer's disease models. *Neuropsychopharmacology* 32: 2393–2404.

450 El-Shimy, I.A., Heikal, O.A., and Hamdi, N. (2015). Minocycline attenuates Abeta oligomers-induced pro-inflammatory phenotype in primary microglia while enhancing Abeta fibrils phagocytosis. *Neurosci. Lett.* 609: 36–41.

451 Ferretti, M.T., Allard, S., Partridge, V. et al. (2012). Minocycline corrects early, pre-plaque neuroinflammation and inhibits BACE-1 in a transgenic model of Alzheimer's disease-like amyloid pathology. *J. Neuroinflammation* 9: 62.

452 Garcez, M.L., Mina, F., Bellettini-Santos, T. et al. (2017). Minocycline reduces inflammatory parameters in the brain structures and serum and reverses memory impairment caused by the administration of amyloid beta (1-42) in mice. *Prog. Neuropsychopharmacol. Biol. Psychiatry* 77: 23–31.

453 Kim, S., Chang, W.E., Kumar, R., and Klimov, D.K. (2011). Naproxen interferes with the assembly of Abeta oligomers implicated in Alzheimer's disease. *Biophys. J.* 100: 2024–2032.

454 Hirohata, M., Ono, K., Naiki, H., and Yamada, M. (2005). Non-steroidal anti-inflammatory drugs have anti-amyloidogenic effects for Alzheimer's beta-amyloid fibrils in vitro. *Neuropharmacology* 49: 1088–1099.

455 Scali, C., Giovannini, M.G., Prosperi, C. et al. (2003). The selective cyclooxygenase-2 inhibitor rofecoxib suppresses brain inflammation and protects cholinergic neurons from excitotoxic degeneration in vivo. *Neuroscience* 117: 909–919.

456 Martin, B.K., Szekely, C., Brandt, J. et al. (2008). Cognitive function over time in the Alzheimer's Disease Anti-inflammatory Prevention Trial (ADAPT): results of a randomized, controlled trial of naproxen and celecoxib. *Arch. Neurol.* 65: 896–905.

457 Aisen, P.S., Schafer, K.A., Grundman, M. et al. (2003). Effects of rofecoxib or naproxen vs placebo on Alzheimer disease progression: a randomized controlled trial. *JAMA* 289: 2819–2826.

458 Lyketsos, C.G., Breitner, J.C., Green, R.C. et al. (2007). Naproxen and celecoxib do not prevent AD in early results from a randomized controlled trial. *Neurology* 68: 1800–1808.

459 Reines, S.A., Block, G.A., Morris, J.C. et al. (2004). Rofecoxib: no effect on Alzheimer's disease in a 1-year, randomized, blinded, controlled study. *Neurology* 62: 66–71.

460 Alzheimer's Disease Anti-inflammatory Prevention Trial Research Group (2013). Results of a follow-up study to the randomized Alzheimer's Disease Anti-inflammatory Prevention Trial (ADAPT). *Alzheimers Dement.* 9: 714–723.

461 Fields, C., Drye, L., Vaidya, V., and Lyketsos, C. (2012). Celecoxib or naproxen treatment does not benefit depressive symptoms in persons age 70 and older: findings from a randomized controlled trial. *Am. J. Geriatr. Psychiatry* 20: 505–513.

462 Aisen, P.S., Marin, D., Altstiel, L. et al. (1996). A pilot study of prednisone in Alzheimer's disease. *Dementia* 7: 201–206.

463 Aisen, P.S., Davis, K.L., Berg, J.D. et al. (2000). A randomized controlled trial of prednisone in Alzheimer's disease. Alzheimer's Disease Cooperative Study. *Neurology* 54: 588–593.

15

The Role of Genetics in Alzheimer's Disease and Parkinson's Disease

Tenielle Porter[1,2], Aleksandra K. Gozt[1], Francis L. Mastaglia[3] and Simon M. Laws[1,2,4]

[1] *Collaborative Genomic Group, School of Medical and Health Sciences, Centre of Excellence for Alzheimer's Disease Research and Care, Edith Cowan University, Joondalup, WA, Australia*
[2] *Cooperative Research Centre for Mental Health, Carlton, VIC, Australia*
[3] *Institute for Immunology and Infectious Diseases, Murdoch University, Murdoch, WA, Australia*
[4] *Faculty of Health Sciences, School of Pharmacy and Biomedical Sciences, Curtin Health Innovation Research Institute, Curtin University, Bentley, WA, Australia*

15.1 Introduction

The term 'Neurodegenerative brain diseases' is an umbrella term that covers a spectrum of disorders which are generally adult-onset diseases, and which share several overlapping clinical, pathologic, and molecular characteristics. Pathologically they are characterised by a progressive and insidious loss of function or structure of neuronal populations of the central nervous system (CNS), with the particular neuronal populations first affected usually being specific to a disease, for example hippocampal neurons in Alzheimer's disease (AD) and dopaminergic neurons in Parkinson's disease (PD). As diseases progress, the neuronal loss spreads to other brain regions leading to a common morphological characteristic of neurodegeneration – significant macroscopic atrophy. Further, most neurodegenerative diseases are proteinopathies, and are associated with the toxic accumulation of aggregates of misfolded proteins [1], the deposition of which may be pathognomonic, e.g. the accumulation of Aβ-amyloid (Aβ) in AD. Alternatively the particular deposits may be seen in several diseases, e.g. the hyperphosphorylated tau protein seen in AD as well as in frontotemporal lobar degeneration (FTD). Clinically they also share several characteristics, for example dementia is a clinical characteristic of not only AD and FTD but also PD.

As with many conditions, genetics play a major role in neurodegenerative diseases. In general, a highly complex interaction between multiple genetic risk factors and environmental and lifestyle factors together modify the risk of developing a given disease at a particular stage of life. However, some neurodegenerative diseases are also genetically characterised by a small monogenic component, which invariably leads to disease through the Mendelian inheritance of dominant or recessive mutations. In this chapter, we discuss the current understanding of research into the genetics that underpins the two major neurodegenerative disease – Alzheimer's disease and Parkinson's disease.

15.2 Genetics of Alzheimer's Disease

AD is the most prevalent form of dementia, accounting for 50–75% of all dementia cases and affecting 23–35 million people worldwide [2]. In Australia over 350 000 people live with AD or another form of dementia, which since 2013 is the second leading cause of death [3]. Advancing age is the greatest risk factor for developing AD [4]. A family history of AD is also a strong risk factor, making genetic factors arguably the next greatest single contributor to an individual's risk of developing AD. It has been estimated from twin and family studies that up to 80% of AD cases have a genetic contribution [5, 6]. In addition to this, epidemiological and animal studies suggest that the likelihood with which an individual may develop AD can also be influenced by numerous environmental and lifestyle factors. As such, AD risk can be seen to be influenced by a highly complex interaction between genetic and environmental/lifestyle factors.

AD can be classified into two broad categories (Figure 15.1). The first category is early-onset Alzheimer's disease (EOAD) which accounts for <10% of patients with AD and presents with an age of onset <65 years. Approximately 35–60% of EOAD patients have a strong familial AD history (EOFAD) and, of these, 10–15% present with a Mendelian pattern of inheritance of highly penetrant gene variants (Figure 15.2) [8]; this form is termed Autosomal Dominant Alzheimer's Disease (ADAD). As such approximately up to 90% of EOAD cases are of an unknown genetic aetiology, potentially explained by epigenetic dysregulation or other genetic mechanisms [8]. The second category covers the more common late-onset Alzheimer's disease (LOAD), and includes those with an age of onset >65 years. LOAD accounts for >90% of patients, and is attributed to genetic risk factors with reduced penetrance (Figure 15.2).

The history of gene discovery in LOAD is as complex and heterogeneous as the disease itself. Commencing over 30 years ago, our knowledge of the genetics underpinning the aetiology of the disease has greatly improved with advances in gene variant discovery. Whilst the advent of genome-wide association studies (GWAS) has been fundamental to the rapid expansion of the genetic understanding of AD, with over 30 AD genetic risk loci identified with varying effect sizes (Figure 15.2) [9–22], these risk loci account for

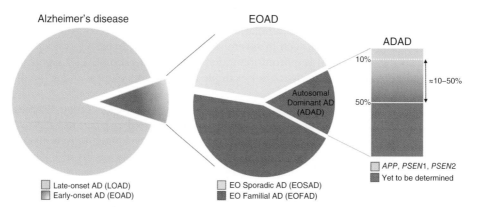

Figure 15.1 Diagrammatic representation of the relationship between the different forms of Alzheimer's disease (AD). EOAD, Early-onset AD; LOAD, Late-onset AD; ADAD, Autosomal Dominant AD; EOFAD, Early-onset Familial AD; LOFAD, Late-onset Familial AD; *APP*, Amyloid Precursor Protein; *PSEN1*, Presenilin 1; *PSEN2*, Presenilin 2.

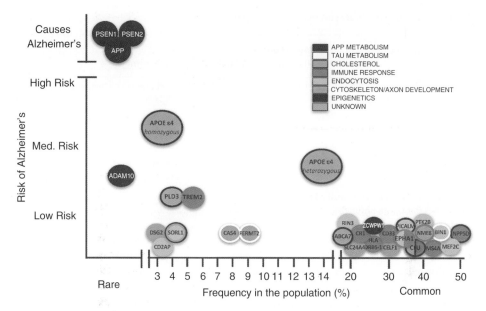

Figure 15.2 Rare and common genetic variants which contribute to Alzheimer's disease risk. Distributed by frequency in population and AD risk-effect size. Genes are colour-coded by probable pathway through which they are involved in AD pathogenesis. Source: Modified from Karch and Goate, 2015 [7]. (*See color plate section for the color representation of this figure.*)

under 50% of heritability that has been seen in AD [23]. Studies that have implemented next-generation sequencing (NGS) strategies [24–29] suggest the potential for identifying more risk loci responsible for disease heritability. In the first component of this chapter we review the established genetic loci for EOFAD, focusing on ADAD, as well as genetic loci implicated as genetic risk factors for LOAD through large-scale GWAS, with a particular emphasis on classifying the latter by biological pathways.

15.3 Autosomal Dominant AD (ADAD)

ADAD is defined as a dominantly inherited form of AD with pathological confirmation and generally presenting with an age of onset between 30 and 50 years of age [30]. Currently it is estimated that anywhere between approximately 10% [8] to approximately 50% [31] of ADAD cases are caused by over 280 mutations in three genes (Table 15.1) that were identified in large pedigrees with AD through linkage analyses. These three genes are the amyloid precursor protein (*APP*) gene located on chromosome 21, the presenilin 1 (*PSEN1*) gene located on chromosome 14, and the presenilin 2 (*PSEN2*) gene located on chromosome 1 [33–37].

15.3.1 Understanding the Importance of APP and the Presenilins in AD

The deposition of aggregated Aβ in senile plaques in the brain is a hallmark of AD pathology. This peptide is a normal cleavage product of the APP protein mentioned above, a transmembrane protein found in most tissues of the body. In AD, it is believed

Table 15.1 Identified loci and causative genes in ADAD.

Gene	Genomic location	Mutations	Age at onset (range, yrs.)	Freq. [31][a]	Mechanism
APP	21q21.3	51[b]	45–60	15–20%	↑β-secretase cleavage (↑Aβ40, ↑Aβ42) ↑γ-secretase cleavage (↑Aβ42)
PSEN1	14q24.3	219[b]	24–65	75–80%	Alters γ-secretase conformation (↑Aβ42)
PSEN2	1q31-q42	16[b]	39–75	<5%	Alters γ-secretase conformation (↑Aβ42)

a) Within the 50% of EOFAD with a known genetic aetiology.
b) Excludes those with no/unclear pathogenic effect (www.molgen.ua.ac.be/ADMutations) [32], retrieved 15 August 2016.

that an imbalance in Aβ production occurs, and/or reduced clearance of the peptide from the brain, leading to an excess of Aβ peptides in the brain; these aggregate into toxic small fibrils, disrupting synaptic function and cell membrane integrity and causing oxidative stress. Aβ is produced mostly in one of two isoforms; Aβ40 (terminates at Val40), the most common form, and Aβ42 (terminates at Ala42), the less common, yet more toxic form of the peptide. Cleavage of APP can occur either via the amyloidogenic pathway, or the non-amyloidogenic pathway, the latter precluding production of full-length Aβ40 or Aβ42. The cleavage of APP with α-secretase (followed by γ-secretase) produces non-amyloidogenic fragments, while cleavage of APP with BACE-1 (β-site APP-cleaving enzyme, also known as β-secretase) and γ-secretase results in Aβ40 or Aβ42 peptide production. Aβ peptides, particularly Aβ42, aggregate readily, resulting in the formation of small oligomers, eventually insoluble fibrils, which over time aggregate in the brain as plaques. Aβ42 is neurotoxic, especially in small oligomer form: it induces free-radical production and increasing oxidative stress, as mentioned above. The overproduction (or reduced clearance) of Aβ42 together with oxidative stress leads to inflammatory and further oxidative changes including mitochondrial malfunction, eventually resulting in neuronal loss and associated cognitive decline. This is widely accepted as the course of development of AD neuropathology, and is known as the 'amyloid cascade hypothesis' [38–40].

These discoveries of ADAD-causing genes were central to the development of our current understanding of AD pathological changes and pivotal in providing strong supporting evidence to the amyloid cascade hypothesis [38–40]. Briefly, all the mutations in these three genes increase the production of the Aβ peptide (either or both of Aβ40 and Aβ42) [41] as the mutations either cluster around the Aβ sequence within APP, near the β- and γ-secretase cleavage sites, or are within genes (*PSEN1/PSEN2*) for proteins that are integral components (catalytic subunit) of the γ-secretase complex [32]. These known mutations in the currently identified ADAD genes account for a significant proportion of ADAD cases, yet it is believed that further as yet unidentified mutations in ADAD-causing genes may exist. Whilst mutations or copy-number variations in other genes have been suggested to cause AD, including two previously linked with frontotemporal dementia (microtubule associated protein tau [*MAPT*; 17q21.31] and charged multivesicular body protein 2B [*CHMP2B*; 3p11.2]) [42], their causal nature for AD cannot be validated until autopsy-confirmation of AD is made. As such we focus in this next section on the three aforementioned established ADAD genes; *APP*, *PSEN1*, and *PSEN2*.

15.4 Amyloid Precursor Protein (*APP*)

The *APP* gene is approximately 300 kb in length and located on the minus strand of chromosome 21 (21q21.3) [43]. Comprising 18 exons, the gene encodes for the APP protein, a ubiquitously expressed type 1 transmembrane protein. Proteolytic cleavage of APP protein can be either via the non-amyloidogenic pathway (involving the α-secretase and γ-secretase enzymes, which cleaves APP within the Aβ sequence), or via the amyloidogenic pathway using the β-secretase (BACE-1) and γ-secretase enzymes, which generates the Aβ peptides that can aggregate into toxic fibrils, then eventually into the amyloid plaques seen in both ADAD and sporadic AD. To date, 51 different pathogenic mutations in the *APP* gene have been observed across 121 different families that express the ADAD phenotype (www.molgen.ua.ac.be/ADMutations) [32]. Of these, 25 are missense mutations which occur mostly around the β- and γ-secretase cleavage sites that are located on exons 16 and 17 [43]. The other 26 mutations are duplications that overlap with the *APP* genetic locus and up to five other neighbouring genes.

As discussed earlier, the mutations result in the generation of atypical levels of Aβ peptides [41], thus encouraging the aggregation into the toxic fibrils that are central to the pathogenesis of the disease, ADAD in particular. However, the specific pathological consequences of *APP* mutations largely depend on the position that they occur relative to the β- and γ-secretase coding sites. For example, there are 12 *APP* gene mutations that occur between residues 714 and 717 of the γ-secretase cleavage site (www.molgen.ua.ac.be/ADMutations) [32], which are all believed to instigate ADAD by altering the ratio of Aβ40 : Aβ42 peptides through the modification of γ-secretase activity that preferentially results in greater production of Aβ42 [44–47]. Conversely, mutations in the vicinity of the β-secretase cleavage site, such as the 'Swedish mutation' (KM670/671NL), increase β-secretase cleavage, producing increased amounts of both Aβ40 and Aβ42 [48], thus providing more substrate for fibrilisation and aggregation [49, 50], and similarly, the duplication of *APP* again causes AD through an overall increase in the production of Aβ peptides. Whilst these *APP* mutations are pathogenic, a rare variant (A673T) conferring resilience to dementia has also been reported, though it is likely limited to members of the original Icelandic and Finnish discovery kindreds [51–55].

15.5 Presenilin 1 (*PSEN1*)

The presenilin 1 gene (*PSEN1*), located on chromosome 14 (14q24.3), consists of 10 coding and 2 noncoding exons and spans approximately 87 kb [43]. It encodes for the PS1 protein, an integral membrane protein comprising 9 transmembrane domains and a cytoplasmic hydrophilic loop domain [30]. The PS1 protein, along with nicastrin, anterior pharynx-defective-1, and presenilin enhancer 2, constitutes the γ-secretase complex [56, 57]. Currently over 200 different *PSEN1* mutations have been identified amongst some 480 families with ADAD pedigrees (www.molgen.ua.ac.be/ADMutations) [32]. Most of these are missense mutations, but include in-frame deletions or insertion [58–60]. Unlike *APP* mutations, *PSEN1* has a wide distribution of mutations across the entirety of the gene (with the exception of the first three exons), although with an increased density in exons 5–8 [43]. Due to the integral role of PS1 as the catalytic subunit of the γ-secretase complex [32] mutations in the gene primarily alter the configuration of the γ-secretase complex resulting in altered enzymatic activity and ability to cleave transmembrane regions of various membrane-bound proteins, including APP [43]. As such, the physiological outcomes of *PSEN1* mutations include an increased production of Aβ42 [61], altering the Aβ42:Aβ40 ratio and increasing formation of toxic oligomeric species [62].

PSEN1 mutations are unique relative to those occurring in other ADAD associated genes, in that they have been associated with a distinct, atypical ADAD presentation. Firstly, *PSEN1* mutation carriers generally develop symptoms earlier than *APP* or *PSEN2* mutation carriers, at around 30–50 years of age [30]. Secondly, there is also considerable phenotypic heterogeneity, with individuals often exhibiting what is referred to as 'variant Alzheimer's disease' (vAD), in which the typical features of ADAD are accompanied by additional physical symptoms such as myoclonus, seizures, extrapyramidal signs, and spastic paraparesis [31]. Lastly, the neuropathological features caused by the *PSEN1* mutations, particularly those in exons 8 and 9, also tend to differ from typical AD features, with the presence of large, diffuse, Aβ-amyloid positive structures known as 'cotton-wool plaques': these lack the typical AD features of mature Aβ-amyloid plaques, such as the congophillic plaque cores, neuritic pathological changes and accompanying signs of inflammation [63, 64].

15.6 Presenilin 2 (*PSEN2*)

Of the three genes known to be implicated in ADAD, the presenilin 2 gene (*PSEN2*), located on chromosome 1 (1q31-q42) [30] and 26 kb in length [43], was discovered most recently. This gene encodes for the PS2 protein, which is a homologue of PS1, and is a constituent of the γ-secretase complex. Currently, 16 pathogenic *PSEN2* mutations, affecting exons 4–7 and 12, have been identified in 34 families (http://www.molgen.ua.ac.be/ADMutations) [32]. As PS2 also serves as a main catalytic subunit of the γ-secretase complex, independent of PS1 [57], mutations also alter γ-secretase activity resulting in an increased production of Aβ42 and altered Aβ42:Aβ40 ratio [61, 62]. PS2-dependent γ-secretase activity is predominant in microglia, and is responsible for functions which include intracellular signalling, gene expression, and modulating the release of pro-inflammatory cytokines [65].

PSEN2 mutation carriers appear to exhibit considerable phenotypic heterogeneity. Firstly, they typically display milder symptoms [43], likely due to the lower brain being more severely affected in contrast to the upper-cortical regions in *PSEN1* mutation carriers [37]. Secondly, the age of disease onset is highly variable compared to other ADAD mutations (Table 15.1) ranging from 39 to 75 years of age [31]. The possession of *PSEN2* mutations in sporadic AD cases (e.g. Val148Ile) suggests that age of disease onset may be influenced by interactions with other AD risk factors. A GWAS of nine families carrying the *PSEN2* Asn141Ile mutation identified several candidate-modifier loci (including apolipoprotein E [*APOE*]) which may influence the age of AD onset [66]. Finally, *PSEN2* mutations carriers tend to also suffer from additional physiological abnormalities, for example, dilated cardiomyopathy [67] and the presence of Lewy bodies [68] which have been reported in Ser130Leu and the Ala85Val mutations, respectively.

15.7 Genetic Contributions to Sporadic Late-Onset AD (LOAD)

With the likely involvement of multiple genes and environmental factors, and a myriad of possible interactions between them, LOAD (heritability 70–80%) [6] is a far more genetically complex disease than EOFAD, and ADAD in particular, which are almost completely determined through genetic components (heritability between 90% and 100%) [69]. Prior to the technological advances that led to the development of large-scale GWAS, only one genetic risk factor for LOAD was well-established, being the *APOE* ε4 allele (described in detail below). Since then, researchers have identified a number of different genes that are thought to alter an individual's susceptibility to developing the disease. Such discoveries have been made either through the application of GWAS, on ever-increasing datasets, or through the application of NGS techniques to uncover rare variants (Table 15.2) [9–22, 24–26, 29, 70].

The identification of these LOAD-associated gene loci has been highly beneficial in increasing our understanding of the underlying causes or contributors to AD pathogenesis. Whilst the direct causal variants or indeed the actual genes are generally not necessarily obvious from GWAS, due to the number of genes in close proximity to the associated marker, these studies have provided an ever-broadening evidence base that implicates several biological pathways in AD pathogenesis. AD-associated genes arising from GWAS likely affect the Aβ-amyloid cascade or tau pathology through one or more distinct biological pathways (Table 15.2). This growing body of literature provides strong evidence for the involvement of lipid/cholesterol metabolism, the immune response, and endocytosis in the development of AD. The following is a brief summary of genes that have been found to be associated with AD using GWAS, classified according to these commonly implicated biological pathways: cholesterol metabolism, immune response, and endocytosis. Where possible, the mechanisms by which the gene products are thought to be implicated in AD are also described.

15.8 Cholesterol Metabolism

There is substantial evidence that pathways involved in cholesterol metabolism are significantly implicated in AD pathogenesis, particularly due to the fact that *APOE*, shown to be a major genetic risk factor for LOAD more than two decades ago, plays a key role in this pathway [71]. More recent evidence at the genetic level has been provided in GWAS, where variants in other genes also involved in cholesterol metabolism have been identified, chief amongst these are *CLU*, *ABCA7*, and *SORL1* [14, 15, 18, 19, 22].

15.8.1 Apolipoprotein E (*APOE*)

The *APOE* gene is located on the long arm of chromosome 19 (19q13.2) and consists of 4 exons that encode a 299 AA, ~34 kDa pleiotropic glycoprotein (apoE) [72] that

Table 15.2 AD risk loci, grouped by biological pathway, and their proposed mechanisms of association.

	Gene	Genomic location	Proposed mechanisms of AD association[a]
Biological pathway/mechanism of AD association	**Cholesterol metabolism**		
	APOE	19q13.2	APP metabolism/Aβ clearance
	CLU	8p21.1	APP metabolism/Aβ clearance, immune response
	ABCA7	19p13.3	APP metabolism, Immune response
	Immune response		
	CR1	1q32	APP metabolism/Aβ clearance
	CD33	19q13.3	APP metabolism/Aβ clearance
	MS4A4A/6A	11q12.2	unknown[b]
	TREM2	6q21.1	Aβ clearance
	HLA-DRB1/DRB5	6p21.32	unknown[b]
	INPP5D	2q37.1	unknown[b]
	MEF2C	5q14.3	Synaptic function
	Endocytosis		
	BIN1	2q14.3	Immune response, synaptic activity, tau toxicity
	PICALM	11q14	APP metabolism
	CD2AP	6q12	Cytoskeletal function, synaptic function, Aβ clearance
	EPHA1	7q34	Cytoskeletal function, synaptic function, immune response
	SORL1	11q23.2	APP metabolism, lipid metabolism
	RIN3-SLC24A4	14q32.12	APP metabolism?
	Other pathways		
	ADAM10	15g21.3	APP metabolism
	PLD3	19q13.2	APP metabolism
	PTK2B	8p21.2	Synaptic function
	CELF1	11p11.2	Cytoskeletal/axonal function, tau toxicity
	NME8	7p14.1	Cytoskeletal/axonal function, immune response
	CASS4	20q13.31	Cytoskeletal/axonal function, tau metabolism
	FERMT2	14q22.1	Cytoskeletal/axonal function, tau metabolism
	ZCWPW1	7q22.1	Epigenetic regulation

APOE, Apolipoprotein E; CLU, Clusterin; ABCA7, ATP-binding cassette transporter A7; CR1, Complement receptor 1; CD33, myeloid cell surface antigen CD33; MS4A, membrane spanning 4 domains, subfamily A; TREM2, triggering receptor expressed on myeloid cells 2; HLA-DRB1/DRB5, major histocompatibility complex class II, DRβ1 and DRβ5; INPP5D, inositol polyphosphate-5-phosphatase; MEF2C, myocyte enhancer factor 2C; BIN1, bridging integrator 1; PICALM, phosphatidylinositol binding clathrin assembly lymphoid myeloid protein; CD2AP, CD2-associated protein; EPHA1, EPH receptor A1; SORL1, sortilin-related receptor, LDLR class A repeats containing; RIN3-SLC24A4, rab interactor 3-solute carrier family 24 sodium/potassium/calcium exchanger, member 4 locus; ADAM10, A Disintegrin And Metalloprotease 10; PLD3, phospholipase D3; PTK2B, protein tyrosine kinase 2β; CELF1, CUGBP, elav-like family member 1; NME8, NME/NM23 family member 8; CASS4, cas scaffolding protein family member 4; FERMT2, fermitin family member 2; ZCWPW1, zinc finger, CW type with PWWP domain 1.
a) In addition to classified biological pathway;
b) Unknown, designates that proposed mechanism of involvement in AD pathogenesis is yet to be determined.

is synthesised in the liver, brain, and macrophages. In the periphery it mediates cholesterol transport and metabolism [73]. In the CNS, where apoE is chiefly synthesised by microglia and astrocytes, in addition to cholesterol transport to neurons via apoE receptors [73], it also plays an important role in neuroplasticity and inflammatory processes [7]. The *APOE* gene is polymorphic, with three major alleles denoted *APOE* ε2, *APOE* ε3, and *APOE* ε4. These are the result of cysteine/arginine substitutions at residues 112 and 158 (ε2, Cys112/Cys158; ε3, Cys112/Arg158; ε4, Arg112/Arg158) [73]. In the general population, these alleles have estimated frequencies of 8.4%, 77.9%, and 13.7%, respectively [74].

AD genetic linkage studies have revealed that carriage of the *APOE* ε4 allele is associated with an elevated risk of developing AD [75, 76]. This risk for AD appears to increase with *APOE* ε4 dosage in the order of ε4/ε4> ε4/ε3> ε4/ε2> ε3/ε3> ε3/ε2> ε2/ε2 [76–78]. However, unlike the ADAD genes discussed above, carriage of the *APOE* ε4 allele is neither necessary nor sufficient for development of AD. Rather the implication is that the combination of *APOE* alleles that an individual possesses determines whether their risk of developing AD is higher or lower than average. It is estimated that ≈40% individuals with LOAD carry an *APOE* ε4 allele [74], with the risk of developing LOAD increasing 4- and 15-fold with the carriage of one and two *APOE* ε4 alleles, respectively [75, 76]. Conversely, carriage of the *APOE* ε2 allele is associated with a reduced risk and a delayed age of onset of AD [78]. The subsequent and consistent replication of these findings across multiple populations and ethnicities has led to the consensus that *APOE* ε4 is the strongest genetic risk factor for LOAD.

The two amino acid changes alter the physical structure of apoE to some extent, such that the three protein isoforms apoE2, apoE3, and apoE4 which are produced from the three alleles have different affinities for binding to Aβ peptides, apoE receptors, and certain lipids [79–81]. It is these differences in the three isoforms that are believed to be responsible for the respective associations with the risk and progression of AD. Human and animal studies have also indicated that the manner in which Aβ peptides aggregate and are cleared is influenced by the apoE isoforms present [82]. Furthermore, ApoE is known to regulate Aβ metabolism indirectly through interactions with the receptor: low-density lipoprotein receptor-related protein-1 (LRP1) [83], and cholesterol levels are also known to influence Aβ production [82]. The aspects of cholesterol and Aβ metabolism linked to apoE4 are thought to be less effective (compared to apoE2 and apoE3), and may confer AD risk through both a reduction in the clearance of Aβ peptides and an increase in Aβ-amyloid aggregation [84]. ApoE4 has been shown *in vitro* and in animal studies to promote a far greater level of Aβ fibril formation and amyloid deposition relative to apoE3 [85, 86], findings which have been confirmed by clinical neuropathological and neuroimaging studies [87–90]. It has also been suggested that *APOE* risk may be mediated through a more simplistic signalling pathway that imparts an isoform-dependent impact on the transcription of APP, in a manner that reflects the AD risk each isoform confers [91]. Finally, apoE4 also influences a person's likelihood of developing cardiovascular problems, as it increases LDL and VLDL levels: it has a greater binding affinity than the other two apoE forms for triglyceride-rich VLVL, leading to downregulation of LDL receptors (interestingly apoE2 also increases cardiovascular disease risk, though for a different reason – apoE2 has an impaired LDL receptor binding) [92]. This is relevant to AD, since cardiovascular disease and associated health problems such as midlife obesity, hypertension, diabetes, and metabolic syndrome are all known to increase the risk of AD, as discussed in much greater detail in other chapters. Collectively, these studies indicate that apoE plays a central role in AD and that genetic variation, particularly *APOE* ε4, significantly underpins not only the risk of developing AD through altered Aβ metabolism and clearance, but also increases the risk of other conditions known to be AD risk factors.

15.8.2 Clusterin (*CLU*)

The human *clusterin* (*CLU*) gene is a 16-kb single-copy gene which comprises nine exons and is located on chromosome 8 (8p21-p12) [93]. The gene encodes for the clusterin (CLU) protein, also known as apolipoprotein J (apoJ), a highly conserved stress-activated chaperone glycoprotein that plays a role in apoptosis, complement regulation, lipid transports, membrane protection, and cell–cell interactions [94]. *CLU* mRNA has been detected in nearly all mammalian tissue types. However, it is expressed in particularly high amounts within several types of neuronal cells (e.g. cortical and hippocampal astrocytes, as well as pyramidal neurons of the hippocampus) [95–98], and it is also found in cerebrospinal fluid (CSF) and blood plasma [98]. GWAS have identified several *CLU* single nucleotide polymorphisms (SNPs – when a single DNA nucleotide in a particular sequence varies between members of the same species), all of which have been consistently found to confer protection against LOAD (rs11136000, rs9331888, rs2279590, rs7982, and rs7012010) [14, 15, 18, 22], whilst a further SNP, rs9331896, was reported in the mega-meta GWAS [19]. Whilst the functional impacts of these SNPs remain to be elucidated, expression of an alternative splice variant has been linked to rs9331888 [99]; and plasma clusterin levels, previously linked with brain atrophy, disease severity, and disease progression [100–103], are reported to be associated with both rs9331888 and rs11136000 [99, 104–109].

Prior to the identification of risk alleles, clusterin had already been implicated in AD pathogenesis many years earlier. For example, clusterin had already been detected in Aβ-amyloid plaques, and elevated levels of *CLU* mRNA had been detected in the hippocampus [110, 111]. Recent studies have confirmed *CLU* mRNA is expressed in elevated levels in the brains of AD patients [112, 113].

CLU is believed to play a protective role in AD pathogenesis through its interactions with Aβ-amyloid, and the neuroinflammatory, oxidative stress and cell apoptotic processes that are associated with AD [114]. Purified CLU interacts at high affinity with Aβ, forming 1:1 stoichiometric complexes [111, 115], and it influences fibril formation *in vitro* [116–118]. CLU-deficient *APP*-transgenic mice have reduced fibril formation, fewer dystrophic neurites, and altered soluble Aβ-amyloid levels [119]. CLU likely influences Aβ clearance, deposition, and neuritic toxicity. ApoE-deficient and CLU-deficient *APP*-transgenic mice exhibit earlier and more extensive Aβ-amyloid deposition compared with control mice [120]. This has led to the hypothesis that CLU plays a protective role in AD through influencing the way in which Aβ-amyloid aggregates, deposits, and is cleared in the AD brain. CLU is implicated in the neuroinflammatory process associated with AD, through modulating the membrane attack complex and inhibiting the inflammatory responses that occur as a result of complement activation [94]. As neuroinflammation is a hallmark symptom of AD, it is possible that those SNPs which alter *CLU* gene expression or impact its function as an Aβ-amyloid response agent may affect AD pathogenesis. Lastly, the protective properties of CLU in AD have also been attributed to its role in oxidative stress and cell apoptosis. It is hypothesised that CLU interacts with other proteins directly (e.g. Bax) [121] and mediates the DNA repair pathways (e.g. the non-homologous end-joining and double-strand break pathways) [114] that are implicated in oxidative stress in a way that minimises the negative effects that are associated with these events.

AD risk is increased in people with cardiovascular disease, as mentioned earlier. As CLU plays a major role in lipid transport – a process highly relevant in cardiovascular health – it is important to note that plasma CLU levels were found in a study of Sardinian aged people to be significantly related to the most atherogenic components of lipid profiles (total cholesterol and LDL), especially in women [122]. This suggests CLU protein levels can modulate cardiovascular metabolic risk factors, and indicates that, like apoE, CLU may influence AD risk via multiple pathways. This suggestion is supported by the finding that plasma fatty-acid distribution and/or body mass index (investigated in a population of Alaskan eskimos) is influenced by SNPs in the *CLU* gene, including one linked to AD above (rs11136000) [123]. This further supports the role of genetic variation in not only significantly underpinning AD risk, but also the risk for developing other conditions that are themselves risk factors for AD, such as cardiovascular disease and diabetes.

15.8.3 ATP-Binding Cassette Transporter A7 (*ABCA7*)

The *ATP-binding cassette transporter A7* (*ABCA7*) gene is located on chromosome 19 (19p13.3). The gene encodes for the ABCA7 protein, a large 220 kDa [124] protein that is a member of the ABC transporter superfamily. ABCA7 protein facilitates the transport of a wide range of phospholipids (and to a lesser extent, cholesterol, as well) across cell membranes [125]. *ABCA7* is predominantly expressed in peripheral myolymphatic tissues, however two transcripts generated through alternate splicing are expressed in the brain [126]. In particular, *ABCA7* expression has been reported in hippocampal CA1 neurons and is notably present (at levels 10-fold higher) within microglia [127].

To date, GWAS have identified several SNPs within the *ABCA7* gene which are associated with an increased chance of developing LOAD; these include rs3764650 [14, 15, 22] and rs4147929, the latter identified in the mega-meta GWAS [19]. For example, the rs3764650T allele has been found to decrease AD risk, and is associated with increased *ABCA7* expression [128]. However, the pathological mechanisms by which these polymorphisms affect the function of the ABCA7 protein and are associated with AD is unclear. *ABCA7* expression is increased in AD individuals, yet the protective SNP just mentioned (rs3764650T) increases *ABCA7* expression. It may be that increased *ABCA7* expression would normally decrease AD risk, yet, once AD pathogenesis has started, higher ABCA7 levels are an inadequate compensatory change [129]. In support of this, *ABCA7* expression has been associated with neuritic plaque burden and advanced cognitive decline [112, 129], and increased expression of the gene has been found to correlate positively with microglial phagocytosis, via the C1q complement pathway, of apoptotic cells, synthetic substrates, and Aβ [125, 130, 131]. Moreover, ABCA7 has been found to promote cholesterol efflux and inhibit Aβ secretion *in vitro* [132], and a loss of ABCA7, as in an ABCA7-deficient transgenic mouse model causes an increase in brain Aβ-amyloid deposition [125]. In recent genetic studies, an *ABCA7* frameshift deletion has been found to be associated with an increased risk of AD in African Americans, for whom the deletion is relatively common (15%) [133], and within a large EOAD cohort, premature termination codon (PTC) mutations were 5 times more common than in a control population, 10 novel PTC mutations were only observed in patients, and PTC mutation carriers in general had an increased familial AD load [134]. In other recent studies, *ABCA7* loss of function variants (also believed to be due to PTC mutations) have been linked with other neuropathologies, such as Parkinson's disease, diffuse Lewy body disease, and vascular dementia [135].

Whilst not fully elucidated, ABCA7's normal biological function is largely believed to involve maintenance of lipid homeostasis within immunogenic cells, albeit that knocking out *ABCA7* has been shown to have only a modest phenotypic impact in mice [125, 136]. However, this may be considered consistent with a chronic functional impairment that would manifest in AD with a later age of onset [137]. Overall, ABCA7 influences the pathogenesis of AD and other neuropathologies, and it is likely that ABCA7 influences Aβ-amyloid related pathways, interacts with ApoE and lipid metabolism, and plays a role in the immune system, though further studies are required to help elucidate the importance of each of these roles in the various neuropathologies.

15.9 Immune Response

Although common to many neurodegenerative disorders, neuroinflammation and thus dysregulation of the immune response has long been recognised as one of the pathological characteristics of AD, where activated glial cells are observed to surround Aβ-amyloid plaques. Further evidence is provided through the association of several genes with AD that play central roles in this pathway, principal among these being complement receptor 1 (*CR1*), myeloid cell surface antigen CD33 (*CD33*), and membrane spanning 4 domains, subfamily A (*MS4A*) [15, 18, 19, 22]. Other AD-associated genes linked with roles in immune response, such as *CLU* and *ABCA7* [14, 18], already mentioned in the section above, add further weight to the involvement of this pathway, as does the association of rare variants in *TREM2* (triggering receptor expressed on myeloid cells 2) [24, 25].

15.9.1 Complement Receptor 1 (*CR1*)

The *CR1* gene is located on chromosome 1 (1q32.2) within a genetic cluster of complement-related proteins [138]. The gene encodes the CR1 protein: a large, type 1 transmembrane glycoprotein [139] that plays a major role in immune system function as a receptor for the activated form of the C3 and C4 complement proteins (C3b and C4b, respectively) [140]. CR1 presents as four isoforms which differ in terms of size (CR1-C (190 kDa), CR1-A (220 kDa), CR1-B (250 kDa), and CR1-D (280 kDa)), and variation due to genetic duplications and deletions [141], and differ considerably in relative frequency (CR1-A: 83%, CR1-B: 15%, CR1-C: 1%, and CR1-D: <1%) [141]. The main structural difference is due to the two larger isoforms possessing an additional binding site for C3b and C4b [138]. CR1 is expressed on phagocytic cells, where it plays a role in the ingestion and removal of complement-activated particles [142].

To date, GWAS have shown consistent replication of association of *CR1* SNPs with AD [14, 15, 18, 19, 22], the two most common of which are rs6656401, which tags several other AD-associated SNPs in *CR1*, and rs3818361, which is associated with an elevated risk of LOAD in *APOE* ε4 carriers [19]. Further evidence to support a link between *CR1* SNPs comes from studies investigating the impact upon AD-related phenotypes. These studies report: the association of rs6656401 with elevated levels of Aβ42 in CSF [139, 143], correlation of *CR1* SNPs with MRI characteristics of the disease [144] and neuritic plaque burden [145] in brains with AD, and decreased episodic memory in combination with the *APOE* ε4 allele [146]. Whilst the functional significance of these SNPs remains unknown and further investigation is required, several lines of evidence that emerged prior to the association of *CR1* SNPs with AD pointed towards a role for compliment in AD pathogenesis. Specifically, several types of brain cells (e.g. neurons, glia) are sources of complement in the brain [147–149], and an increase in complement factors has been reported in cortical regions affected by AD [150]. Moreover, the complement system is also known to be activated by material sourced from neuritic plaques and neurofibrillary tangles (NFT) [151, 152]. Therefore, it has been suggested that the manifestation of plaques and tangles may be responsible for activating the complement pathways [153], which could exacerbate AD pathologic change. On the other hand, it is also speculated that CR1 functions as a vehicle that helps facilitate the removal of Aβ from the brain and that genetic variability in the *CR1* gene alters the underlying structure of the protein that affects the rate of this clearance [138]. The relationship with AD is further complicated by the encoding of high-expression and low-expression alleles [140], which have different effects on the complement cascade and thus most likely Aβ clearance and thus AD pathogenesis. Further research is thus warranted to fully elucidate the role of CR1 in AD pathogenesis.

15.9.2 *CD33* (Myeloid Cell Surface Antigen *CD33*; Sialic Acid-Binding Immunoglobulin-Like Lectin 3)

The *CD33* gene is located on chromosome 19 (19q13.3) and encodes for CD33, which is a member of the sialic acid-binding immunoglobulin (Ig)-like lectins (Siglecs) family of receptors [156, 157]. *CD33* has been found to be expressed on the surface of myeloid progenitor cells, mature monocytes, and macrophages as well as microglia [156–160]. CD33 is reported to play a role in regulating innate immunity, since it has been observed to be implicated in several processes which include adhesion processes in immune and malignant cells, the inhibition of monocytic cytokine release, and immune cell growth [161]. CD33 is also reported to be involved in clathrin-independent receptor-mediated endocytosis [162].

The rs3826656 SNP, proximal to *CD33* was found to be associated with increased AD risk in an initial family-based GWAS [11] and subsequently an additional proximal SNP in the *CD33* promotor region, rs3865444, has been linked with reduced AD risk in larger GWAS [15, 19, 22]. The functional implications are that the mildly protective allele rs3865444 increases expression of *CD33*, lacking exon 2 (the sialic-acid binding domain), on the surface membrane of monocytes [156]. In fact, this SNP is a proxy for the co-inherited exon 2 SNP, rs12459419, which regulates the ability of CD33 to inhibit microglial activation (and thus phagocytosis) by modulating exon 2 splicing efficiency [156].

The *CD33* risk allele rs3865444 is associated with a greater number of activated human microglia, the diminished internalisation of Aβ, and the accumulation of amyloid plaques and NFT, as indicated by *in vivo* imaging [158]. Furthermore, microglial expression of *CD33* mRNA is increased in AD autopsy brain tissue, and higher *CD33* expression levels have also been reported to be associated with more advanced cognitive decline [157]. *In vitro* studies in immortalised microglial cells show that whilst *CD33* expression inhibits Aβ phagocytosis, this effect is ameliorated when the *CD33* being expressed lacks exon 2 [157], as is the case with the minor T allele of rs3865444. It is generally thought that CD33 may be implicated in AD by playing a role in the uptake and clearance of Aβ (and thus potentiating its toxicity) by microglia via interactions with sialic acids [163] and impacting other microglial-mediated neuroinflammatory pathways [164].

15.9.3 Membrane Spanning 4 Domains, Subfamily A (*MS4A*)

The *membrane-spanning 4-domains, subfamily A* (*MS4A*) is a cluster of genetic loci located on chromosome 11 (11q12.2) that encode for several proteins (i.e. MS4A4A, MS4A4E, MS4A6A, and MS4A6E) known to play a role in the inflammatory response [7]. Whilst the gene family is yet to be comprehensively characterised, MS4A proteins are known to have a similar structure to B-lymphocyte antigen CD20 [165, 166] which is responsible for the regulation of calcium influx following its activation [167]. SNPs within this cluster of genes have been reported to be associated with AD in several GWAS [14, 15, 19, 22, 168, 169], with the two most implicated genes being *MS4A4A* and *MS4A6A*. However, due to the complex structure of this region other genes in this region may also contain AD-associated variants. Despite many reports of AD association with this family of genes in several GWAS, the actual impact these genes have on AD pathogenesis is yet to be determined.

MS4A genes are highly expressed in haematopoietic cells such as monocytes and myeloid cells [170], whilst *in vitro* studies of primary adult microglial cell cultures report the expression of *MS4A4A* and *MS4A6A*, both of which were downregulated in response to the induction of neuroinflammation [171]. This suggests that *MS4A* genetic variants, at least within *MS4A4A* and *MS4A6A*, may impact AD pathology through modifying the function of microglia. Furthermore, correlation analysis of gene expression with AD pathological hallmarks shows that these markers are associated with more advanced Braak tangle and plaque stages [112, 113]. The paucity of knowledge regarding the role of these genes in AD pathogenesis, combined with constant replication of association signals, strongly suggests that further functional analysis is warranted.

15.9.4 Triggering Receptor Expressed on Myeloid Cells 2 (*TREM2*)

The *TREM2* gene located on chromosome 6 (6q21.1) encodes for a type 1 transmembrane receptor protein that is expressed on myeloid cells. Genetic variation, specifically homozygous mutations, within *TREM2* have previously been associated with Nasu-Hakola disease [172, 173]. This autosomal recessive disease, also known as polycystic lipomembranous osteodysplasia with sclerosing leukoencephalopathy (PLOSL) is a form of dementia that presents with multiple bone cysts and progressive neurodegeneration leading to dementia [174–177]. Studies of LOAD suggest that multiple rare, coding variants in *TREM2* increase the risk of AD. Of these variants, R47H (rs75932628), initially reported in an Icelandic population [25] and a European population [24], is the most frequent, and its association with LOAD has been substantiated in several subsequent studies [178–180]. This missense mutation confers an approximately 2-fold increased risk for LOAD [24, 25, 181–183], though reports have varied from 1.7- to 3.4-fold increased risk [180, 184]. Phenotypically, LOAD *TREM2* mutation carriers present with more extensive brain atrophy than LOAD *TREM2* mutation non-carriers [185]. In addition, an endophenotype-based GWAS approach identified variants within *TREM2* that are associated with CSF tau levels [186]. The *TREM2* R47H variant has also been reported to be associated with other neurodegenerative disorders, as it has been linked with an increased risk for Parkinson's disease, frontotemporal dementia, and amyotrophic lateral sclerosis [183, 187–189].

In the CNS, TREM2 is primarily expressed on microglia where it stimulates phagocytosis and suppresses inflammation [190]. Whilst the exact pathogenic mechanism by which *TREM2* variants increase risk for LOAD is yet to be fully understood, some studies suggested a role in AD by increasing neurodegeneration through neuroinflammation and dysregulation of the immune response [191, 192]. Since the inhibition of TREM2 activity reduces the phagocytic potential of microglial cells, it has also been suggested that genetic variation may also inhibit clearance of apoptotic neurons [193]. Recent studies however have shed more light on TREM2 normal function, as it was found that TREM2 promotes microglial survival by activating the Wnt/β-catenin signalling pathway: TREM2 was found to stabilise β-catenin by inhibiting its degradation via the Akt/GSK3β signalling pathway [194]. Since APOE has been identified as a ligand for the TREM2 microglial receptor, it is possible that ApoE polymorphisms may also influence TREM2-mediated microglial phagocytosis [195], further complicating studies of this protein's influence in AD, and indicating more studies are required to understand how all these AD-associated proteins and pathways influence each other.

15.9.5 Further Genetic Associations Implicating the Immune Response

There are several other gene candidates identified in the AD mega-meta GWAS [19] that can be added to the growing list of immune-system-related genes that have been associated with AD. A prime example of this is the major histocompatibility complex class II, DRβ1 and DRβ5 (*HLA-DRB1/DRB5*) gene locus, which is a member of the major histocompatibility complex (MHC, specifically MHC class II), a highly polymorphic region located on chromosome 6 (6p21.32) that is responsible for numerous immune responses [196] and has been the focus of significant study with respect to neurodegenerative disease. The HLA-locus has been reported in GWAS to be associated with multiple sclerosis [197–199], FTLD [200], and PD [201–205], the latter of which is discussed in the second component of this chapter. *HLA-DRB1* variants are also well known to be associated with rheumatoid arthritis and systemic lupus erythematosus (SLE) [206], whereas *HLA-DRB5* (as well as *HLA-DRB3* and -*DRB4*) have been associated with type 1 diabetes [207].

With respect to AD, genetic variation at the HLA-locus was first reported nearly 40 years ago [208]; however, the much more recent mega-meta GWAS [19] has provided the most comprehensive study of these genes. The associated locus also included *HLA-DRB6*, *HLA-DQA1*, and *HLA-DQB1*, with the strongest AD-associated marker being rs9271192 [19], findings that have been replicated [209] and consolidated due to the finding of an association of *HLA-DRB1* with total brain volume [210] and brain DNA methylation [211]. The association of *HLA-DRB1/HLA-DRB5* with both AD and PD suggests that this locus may play a similar role in the inflammatory responses that underpin the pathogenesis of both diseases. Since the locus is also associated with autoimmune conditions, comparisons of the inflammatory responses in all these conditions and differences caused by the allelic variations will help reveal more information on how these immune responses are related to disease pathogenesis.

Further significant evidence to support the role of the immune response in AD is provided by the association with AD of an intronic SNP (rs35349669) in the inositol polyphosphate-5-phosphatase (*INPP5D*) gene, located on chromosome 2 (2q37.1). This association was reported in the same large GWAS meta-analyses [19] and subsequently replicated [212]. The role that *INPP5D* plays in several inflammatory responses and regulation of cytokine signalling has been extensively studied [213, 214], particularly with respect to its negative regulation of inflammatory cytokine release, B-cell proliferation, chemotaxis, and activation [215–219]. How *INPP5D* functions with respect to immune response and inflammation in the brain remains unclear, however it is likely through its role in negative regulation that it may play a role in the suppression of inflammatory cytokine release from CNS myeloid cells such as microglia. Further, INPP5D binds CD2AP, encoded by an AD-linked gene involved in endocytosis (discussed below), to form a complex that controls the degradation of the IgE receptor FcεRIγ [220].

Finally, the myocyte enhancer factor 2C (*MEF2C*) gene located on the chromosome 5 (5q14.3), which is a member of the MEF2 family of transcription factors that have an essential role in myogenesis, is also reported to play a role in the regulation of B-cell proliferation, which is an integral part of the adaptive immune system [221]. Further, *MEF2C* modulates transcription factors with anti-inflammatory roles in endothelial cells [222]. The mega-meta-analysis GWAS reported a SNP (rs190982) within *MEF2C* that was associated with a reduced risk for AD [19, 212]. However, the association may be ethnicity-dependent, as in a study of a Han Chinese cohort, the rs190982 SNP was not found to be associated with LOAD [223]. Whilst the exact mechanism of association for *MEF2C* in AD in some populations is not understood, it is reported that *MEF2C* is integral to neuronal development [224] and is suggested to be important in hippocampal-dependent learning and memory [225]. In the case of the latter, this is mediated through the protein-limiting excessive synapse formation during activity-dependent refinement of synaptic connectivity [226]. Further evidence to support a role for MEF2C in cognitive performance comes from a large GWAS [55], which showed an association between AD-linked variants in *MEF2C* and cognitive ability.

15.10 Endocytosis

Endocytosis dysfunction has been linked to the development of AD, as endocytic pathways play critical roles in several mechanisms that are central to AD pathogenesis, including normal APP metabolism, synaptic activity, and neurotransmitter release, all of which are disrupted in AD. Several genes that have been identified in LOAD GWAS play important roles in endocytosis and synaptic function (including *BIN1*, *PICALM*, *CD2AP*, *EPHA1*, and *SORL1*) [14, 15, 18, 19, 22], thus providing further evidence at the genetic level for the importance of this pathway in AD pathogenesis.

15.10.1 Bridging Integrator 1 (*BIN1*)

The *bridging integrator 1* (*BIN1*) gene, previously known as *amphiphysin 2*, is located on the long arm of chromosome 2 (2q14.3) and is differentially spliced into at least 10 major isoforms: 2 which are expressed ubiquitously, 7 of which are expressed in the brain, and 1 that is expressed exclusively in muscular tissue [227, 228]. BIN1 is believed to be significantly involved in regulating endocytosis and trafficking, particularly in clathrin-mediated endocytosis in neurons, as it is able to bind to the GTPase dynamin [229, 230] and interact with clathrin and AP2/a-adaptin [231, 232]. A recent study has also shown that *BIN1* is expressed in high levels in mature oligodendrocytes, that it is upregulated during post-natal myelination, and that a loss of BIN1 significantly correlates with the extent of demyelination in multiple sclerosis lesions [233].

The initial association between the *BIN1* gene locus and AD risk was reported by the GERARD1 (Genetic and Environmental Risk in AD Consortium 1) GWAS [14] and replicated in subsequent GWAS and independent candidate gene analyses, which have identified several associated SNPs (rs6733839, rs744373, rs7561528, rs12989701) [228, 234–236]. Amongst these, the rs7561528 SNP has been found to correlate with magnetic resonance imaging measures of entorhinal and temporal-pole cortical thicknesses in AD brains [144]. Other studies have reported that BIN1 protein levels are altered in aged mice, AD mouse models, and human AD brains [237, 238], whilst higher BIN1 mRNA expression levels have been found to be associated with a delayed age of onset of AD [112].

Early research into the likely role *BIN1* plays in neurodegeneration and AD pathogenesis indicated mechanisms could involve modulation of tau pathology, endocytosis/trafficking, inflammation, calcium homeostasis, cell senescence, and apoptosis [228]. Of these, the first two pathways have received the greatest amount of attention from the AD research community. Later studies provided several lines of evidence supporting a role for BIN1 in modulating tau processing. BIN1 (i) forms tubular membrane structures that link the microtubule cytoskeleton to the cellular membrane, (ii) interacts with cytoplasmic linker protein 170 (CLP-170: a microtubule-associated protein), which is thought to increase the intrinsic tubulating capacity of BIN1 [239], (iii) interacts with tau proteins in human neuroblastoma cells and in mouse brain homogenates [237], and (iv) when knocked down in *Drosophila* AD models suppresses tau-induced toxicity [237]. Furthermore, rs59335482, which is in linkage disequilibrium with the AD-associated SNP rs744373, has been shown to be associated with tau-load (but not Aβ-amyloid-load) in AD brains [237]. However, more recent studies in AD brain failed to co-localise Bin1 with tau tangles, suggesting that other pathways may play a significant role in mediating risk for AD [240].

As indicated above, BIN1 plays a significant role in the endocytic pathway, and amphiphysin 1 and *BIN1* knockout mice exhibit deficiencies in endocytic protein scaffolding and synaptic vesicle recycling [241]. Furthermore, recent data suggest that BIN1 is essential in facilitating the endocytic recycling of endosomes [242]. Thus it may be that BIN1 plays a role in modulating the intracellular trafficking of large molecules (like APP, Aβ-amyloid, and/or ApoE) that are internalised through endo-lysosomal trafficking [243]. Recent studies have provided further explanations of BIN1's potential role in AD, as it was shown that a depletion of BIN1 increases cellular BACE1 levels through impaired endosomal trafficking, lowering BACE1 degradation in lysosomes, and thus causing an increase in Aβ production [244]. Similarly, other recent studies of

BIN1 and CD2AP (discussed below) show they control Aβ generation in axonal and dendritic early endosomes (respectively), and when BIN1 levels are reduced, BACE1 is trapped in the tubules of early endosomes and is not sorted for degradation in dendrites. The resulting convergence of APP and BACE 1 in early endosomes increases the generation of Aβ [245]. Tau processing may also be affected however, as it has been shown recently that reduced levels of BIN1 also promote tau pathology, by increasing aggregate internalisation by endocytosis and endosomal trafficking [246].

15.10.2 Phosphatidylinositol Binding Clathrin Assembly Lymphoid Myeloid Protein (PICALM)

The *phosphatidylinositol binding clathrin assembly lymphoid myeloid protein* (*PICALM*) gene is located on the long arm of chromosome 11 (11q14) and encodes for the PICALM protein. Currently, 23 alternative transcripts of the *PICALM* gene have been identified, many of which are expressed in the human brain [247]. PICALM isoforms have been found to be particularly abundant in neurons, astrocytes, and the endothelial cells of brain blood vessels [247]. The PICALM protein is thought to play a critical function in the mediation of clathrin-coated pit endocytosis, where it is involved in clathrin assembly, recruiting clathrin and adaptor protein complex 2 (AP2) to the cell membrane, and determining the amount of cell membrane that can be recycled by regulating the size of the clathrin cage [247]. PICALM also plays a role in the fusion of synaptic vesicles to the presynaptic cleft via the VAMP2 pathway [248]. Evidence supporting the role of PICALM in clathrin-mediated endocytic processes has been well documented in laboratory models, such as *Drosophila* [249] and yeast [250], where in both the deletion of the *PICALM* homologue results in impaired clathrin-mediated endocytosis. Whilst this phenotype was not observed in a transgenic mouse model, the mice did exhibit abnormal iron metabolism, which is noteworthy since iron metabolism is also known to be implicated in APP processing [251].

AD GWAS have identified two genetic variants (rs3851179 and rs541458) located upstream from the *PICALM* gene that are associated with a reduced risk of LOAD [14, 18, 19]. The exact functional effect of these variants remain to be determined, however *PICALM* has been implicated in AD pathogenesis through an impact on one or all of APP metabolism, Aβ clearance, or Aβ toxicity. The most prominent of these is the role in APP metabolism via endocytosis. PICALM co-localises with APP under both *in vitro* and *in vivo* circumstances [252], and varying degrees of *PICALM* expression have been observed to modulate APP metabolism *in vivo* [252]. More specifically, decreased *PICALM* expression leads to increased concentrations of APP at the cell surface, whilst increased *PICALM* expression facilitates greater internalisation of APP [253]. As such, PICALM may impact APP metabolism through its effects on APP localisation, and lead to altered Aβ levels through favouring of alternate cleavage pathways. Similarly, other studies have shown that reducing *PICALM* expression leads to altered APP trafficking *in vitro*, whilst the overexpression of *PICALM in vivo* is associated with an increased deposition of Aβ-amyloid plaques in AD transgenic mice [252].

There is also significant evidence to support a role for PICALM in Aβ clearance. PICALM isoforms have been found to be robustly expressed in the microvessels of the brain, suggesting that PICALM protein may facilitate the clearance of Aβ across the blood–brain barrier (BBB) [253]. This is supported through the *PICALM* risk-allele rs541458 being associated with reduced levels of Aβ in the CSF of AD patients and controls [143]. Further, PICALM is able to bind to autophagosomes suggesting that PICALM may play a role in autophagy-mediated clearance of Aβ [254]. This is supported by the findings of more recent studies which showed that PICALM also affects the internalisation, cellular localisation, and trafficking of SNAREs (receptors required for combining phagophores – autophagosome precursors), thus modulating macroautophagy [255]. This was found to influence the clearance of tau.

Other potential links between PICALM's role in endocytosis and AD have also been found recently. For example, PICALM is involved in cholesterol homeostasis, as a loss of PICALM was found to increase cellular cholesterol pool size: it was found that PICALM-deficient cells had enhanced internalisation of LDL receptors, due to higher LDLR (low density lipoprotein receptor) expression [256], and many studies have shown cholesterol and lipid dysregulation are involved in AD pathogenesis. Another study has found that depletion of PICALM can reduce the expression of BACE1, suggesting this effect may be employed to slow the development of AD [257].

It has also been hypothesised that PICALM may reduce the risk of AD by way of reducing cellular damage that is associated with excitotoxicity. This suggestion is based on the finding that PICALM is able to modulate Aβ-induced toxicity in yeast [258]. From the brain function point of view, recent quantitative electroencephalography (EEG) investigations of a cohort of people divided into groups according to the *PICALM* rs3851179 A and G alleles found that there was an increase in 'beta relative power' in the carriers of the AD-risk *PICALM* GG genotype. This means there were changes in the cortical excitatory-inhibitory balance, and these changes were found to be greater in the older (over 50 years of age) subjects of the cohort [259]. Other recent investigations in a Chinese cohort aged 50–82 years found the *PICALM* rs541458 polymorphism influenced executive function and processing speed, brain structure and functional connectivity [260].

15.10.3 CD2-Associated Protein (*CD2AP*)

The *CD2-associated protein* (*CD2AP*) gene is located on chromosome 6 (6q12) and encodes for the CD2AP protein, which is a scaffolding protein involved in actin-based cytoskeletal reorganisation [261], receptor-mediated endocytosis [15], and vesicular trafficking [262]. In humans, the CD2AP protein has been found to be highly expressed in plasmacytoid dendritic cells (innate immune cells that accumulate in peripheral lymphoid organs and circulate throughout the blood stream), whilst western blot analysis has also confirmed the expression of *CD2AP* in brain tissue, although the extent to which this occurs appears to be dependent on gene dosage [262]. GWAS have identified three *CD2AP* SNPs, rs9296559, rs9349407, and rs10948363, which are associated with an increased risk of AD [15, 19, 22, 263]. Furthermore, the *CD2AP* rs9349407 has been associated with an increased neuritic plaque burden [264].

The suppression of *CD2AP* expression in a cell-culture model results in decreased APP expression on the cell membrane, a decreased release of Aβ peptides, and a lower Aβ42/Aβ40 ratio [262]. Furthermore, complete loss of *CD2AP* expression in the brains of PS1APP mice also caused a decrease in the Aβ42/Aβ40 ratio, whereas there was no effect on Aβ-amyloid deposition or accumulation in PS1APP mice in which only a single copy of the *CD2AP* gene was expressed [262]. Cells of *CD2AP*-deficient mice exhibit abnormal lysosomal functioning, suggesting that *CD2AP* is a likely regulator of vesicular trafficking to the lysosome [265]. Although the effect of the SNPs have not been properly characterised as yet, the limited literature seems to suggest that CD2AP plays a role in AD pathogenesis by impacting APP metabolism/clearance via an endocytic pathway. In support of this, a recent study already mentioned above by Ubelmann et al. [245] concerning BIN1 and CD2AP, showed that loss of function of either BIN1 or CD2AP causes an increased generation of Aβ (through different mechanisms), with loss of CD2AP causing APP to become trapped at the limiting membrane of early endosomes, preventing it from being sorted for degradation in dendrites [245].

15.10.4 Further Genetic Associations Implicating Endocytosis

Several other genetic associations provide further evidence that disruptions to endocytosis are critical in the pathogenesis of AD. One such example is the *sortilin-related receptor, LDLR class A repeats containing (SORL1)* gene on chromosome 11 (11q24.1). Initially associated with AD through candidate gene-based approaches [266, 267], variants in *SORL1* have been subsequently linked with modifying AD risk in several GWAS [268–272] including the largest to date, where the SNP rs11218343 was associated with a reduced AD risk [19]. SORL1 is a member of the Vsp10p domain-receptor family; it is expressed throughout the brain [273], and it plays a role in vesicle trafficking from the cell surface to the Golgi-endoplasmic reticulum [274]. SORL1 has been shown to play a role in directing APP to endocytic pathways for recycling [267] and more recent studies have shown SORL1 interacts with cytosolic adaptors involved in anterograde and retrograde movement of APP between the trans-Golgi network and early endosomes, thereby influencing the delivery of APP to endocytic compartments that favour amyloidogenic breakdown [275, 276]. SORL1 is also involved in the uptake of lipoproteins, including apoE-containing particles via endocytotic pathways [267]. *In vivo* studies report elevated Aβ-amyloid levels in *SORL1*-deficient mice [277] and reduced mRNA expression in AD brain samples [278]. Recent genetic studies of German and Dutch subjects investigated 19 *SORL1* SNP variants, and linked *SORL1* genetic variants with tau metabolism, for example *SORL1* rs2070045-G allele has been linked with increased CSF-tau and more hippocampal atrophy [279]. The different SNPs appear to cause distinct neuropathological features, including changes in tau metabolism as just mentioned, deposition of senile plaques (rs668387), and loss of grey-matter volume (rs3824968); one interestingly has a gender bias, with females showing a greater cognitive decline (rs2070045) [280].

Also reported in the largest GWAS to date [19] is rs10498633 in the vicinity of the *rab interactor 3 (RIN3)* on chromosome14 (14q32.12), though other genes, including *solute carrier family 24 sodium/potassium/calcium exchanger, member 4 (SLC24A4)* are also located in the vicinity of this variant. However, *RIN3* is suggested to be a strong functional candidate for this locus, as it may modify disease risk by impacting APP trafficking (and therefore Aβ generation) through the early endocytic pathway where it activates GTPase Rab5 and is critical to membrane budding and trafficking [281–283]. Further evidence to support a role for RIN3 in AD pathogenesis through the endocytic pathway is provided through its interaction with two other AD-linked genes involved in this pathway, namely the aforementioned *BIN1* and *CD2AP* [284]. Interestingly, this is another association that may depend on ethnicity, as a recent study has found that the rs10498633 polymorphism doesn't appear to be linked to AD risk in a Han Chinese population, similar to the lack of link to AD risk found with the SNP rs190982 in *MEF2C* that we mentioned earlier [285].

Modification of LOAD risk by the SNP rs11767557, upstream of the *EPH receptor A1* (*EPHA1*) gene on chromosome 7 (7q34) [286], was first reported in 2010 [168] and subsequently replicated in several larger studies [12, 15, 19, 22, 287]. As a member of the ephrin family of tyrosine kinase receptors, *EPHA1* binds to membrane-bound ephrin-A ligands on adjacent cells resulting in contact-dependent, bidirectional signalling to adjacent cells [288]. This family of genes are crucial for nervous system development [289, 290] whilst also being critical to synaptic plasticity and axonal guidance [291, 292]. *EPHA1* may also modify AD risk through a role in the immune system as it is expressed by CD4-positive T lymphocytes and monocytes [293] and plays a role in the regulation of T-cell interactions through the integrin pathway [294]. EPHA1 has also been reported to be a substrate for ADAM10 [295, 296], suggesting that a further mechanism of association for *EPHA1* is potentially via the α-secretase pathway. As mentioned, rs11767557 is not located directly within the *EPHA1* gene and, whilst located close to the gene, there are several other genes that may be implicated, through being located within the region of linkage disequilibrium defined by this SNP.

15.10.5 Variants in *APP* and Genes for APP-Metabolising Proteins

In addition to their established role in ADAD, there is a growing body of literature to indicate the existence of further genetic variants in *APP* and genes for APP-metabolising proteins (e.g. *PSEN1*, *PSEN2*) in modifying risk for LOAD. Novel, rare variants have been discovered in *APP* that are suggestive of both increasing (N660Y) [27] and, as mentioned earlier, decreasing (A673T) [51] AD risk. There is further evidence that polymorphisms may significantly modify risk of LOAD risk, a particular example being a polymorphism in *PSEN1* (E318G) that significantly modifies risk in *APOE* ε4 carriers [28]. As discussed previously, PS1 and PS2 are integral constituents of the γ-secretase complex, where mutations within the respective genes significantly increase the amyloidogenic processing of APP. A further major secretase important in metabolising APP is α-secretase, encoded by the *ADAM10* (*a disintegrin and metalloprotease 10*) gene (Chr15q21.3), which is involved in the 'non-amyloidogenic' pathway [297]. Rare coding variants in *ADAM10*, Q170H, and R181G, have been identified in several LOAD pedigrees [29, 298]. These variants have been shown to increase Aβ levels in *in vitro* cell-based studies [29], and *in vivo* to significantly reduce α-secretase cleavage of APP and thus resulting in elevated Aβ deposition, likely due to a resultant favouring of the amyloidogenic processing of APP [298]. Finally, a polymorphism, rs638405, in the beta-site APP cleaving enzyme 1 (*BACE1*) gene (Chr11q23.3) has been discovered; however, associations with AD risk have been controversial, with some studies finding an increased risk with some genotypes, often depending on *APOE* ε4 status, whereas other studies suggest the polymorphism has no effect on AD risk [299, 300]. Overall, these reports demonstrate clearly that genetic variation in *APP* and genes for APP-metabolising proteins can alter risk for LOAD and not only provide further evidence to support the amyloid hypothesis, but also for the targets for which therapeutic interventions can be identified.

15.10.6 Further Mechanisms Implicated Through Genetic Associations

Whilst the majority of genetic associations uncovered through GWAS and NGS approaches can be grouped within the aforementioned biological pathways, several other recent genetic associations suggest the involvement of other biological pathways that drive their putative mechanisms of association with AD. A 'Next-Generation Sequencing' approach that employed whole exome sequencing of LOAD families with subsequent genotyping validation identified a genetic variant (V232M) in the *phospholipase D3* (*PLD3*) gene [26], located on chromosome 19 (19q13.2). The enzyme PLD3 is a member of the phospholipase D (PLD) family, members of which are involved in catalysing the hydrolysis of membrane phospholipids [301]. Whilst its role in AD is poorly understood, *in vitro* studies suggest that it may influence APP processing, albeit by an unknown mechanism [26]. The association of *PLD3* with AD is controversial due to a current lack of replication in several subsequent studies [16, 302–304], though the most recent study, which analysed data from a large sample set of approximately 40 000 subjects, suggests a modest increase in AD genetic risk for this V232M variant [305]; however, the exact effect of the variant on AD pathogenesis is still unknown.

Several other loci, where the putative roles in AD pathogenesis are still ambiguous, were identified in a large LOAD GWAS meta-analysis [19]. Zinc finger, CW type with *PWWP domain 1* (*ZCWPW1*) gene located on chromosome 7 (7q22.1) harbours a genetic variant (rs1476679) associated with modifying risk for AD [19] that has subsequently been replicated [212] and reported to be associated with regulatory functions [306] and AD neuropathological features [307]. Whilst these findings support the genetic association of *ZCWPW1* with AD the only insight into the functional mechanisms of association is that of a role in epigenetics through its reported role as a histone-modification reader [308]. More recent studies have shown that this polymorphism influences grey-matter density in specific brain areas, at the mild cognitive impairment (MCI) stage [309], that it is associated with cognitive linear rate of change [310], and that it influences NFT accumulation [311].

The rs28834970 SNP in the *protein tyrosine kinase 2β* (*PTK2B*) gene on chromosome 8 (8p21.2) has been associated with increased AD risk [19]. The *PTK2B* gene encodes a cytoplasmic protein tyrosine kinase which is activated by neurotrophic factors that are important in neuronal differentiation and survival, and which is involved in activation of the map kinase signalling pathway, actin reorganisation in association with focal adhesions, calcium-induced regulation of ion channels, and regulation of neuronal activity through acting as a signalling intermediate to neuropeptide activated receptors or neurotransmitters [312, 313]. It was suggested that PTK2B's involvement in AD pathogenesis involves the bringing together of Aβ-amyloid and tau pathologies, through its activation of GSK3 [314], which has been reported to play an important role in Aβ-amyloid-induced NFT formation [315], and a very recent study has shown that PTD2B interacts with tau *in vitro*, and that it co-localises with hyperphosphorylated and oligomeric tau in AD brains [316]. A further gene whose mechanism of association with AD may also involve tau metabolism [317, 318] is *fermitin family member 2* (*FERMT2*), located on chromosome 14 (14q22.1), and in which the rs17125944 SNP reportedly increases AD risk by about 15% [19]. *FERMT2* is part of a class of focal adhesion proteins that connect cells to the extracellular matrix (ECM) and actin cytoskeleton [319]. FERMT2's links with AD neuropathology appear to be via modulating Aβ peptide production, as recent studies have found that low levels of FERMT2 result in an increase in Aβ peptide production by raising levels of mature APP at the cell surface and increasing APP recycling [320], whereas recent genomic association studies have indicated that *FERMT2* appears to influence CSF Aβ42 levels [321].

The *cas scaffolding protein family member 4* (*CASS4*) gene located on chromosome 20 (20q13.31; associated variant rs7274581 [19]) has been implicated in tau metabolism as well as APP metabolism [322]. *CASS4* is a comparatively understudied gene for which the protein has a putative normal function in focal adhesion integrity, and cell spreading [323]. In keeping with the theory that CASS4 is involved in tau metabolism, a recent study has suggested CASS4 is likely to be a tau toxicity modulator [316]. In addition to involvement with tau metabolism, the potential involvement in cytoskeletal function and axonal transport may also be the mechanism of association that links the next two genes with AD. The first of these, the *CUGBP, elav-like family member 1* (*CELF1*) gene, located on chromosome 11 (11p11.2), has predominantly been linked to regulation of gene expression [324], however preliminary functional analyses with respect to AD suggests a possible link to both cytoskeletal function/transport and tau metabolism [318]. Another GWAS study found that the rs10838725 at the *CELF1* locus appears to be relevant to both AD and obesity (which happens to be a risk factor for AD) [325], and a recent study has found that, as with *ZCWPW1*, the *CELF1* polymorphism has been linked to cognitive linear rate of change in AD [310], It is plausible that *CELF1* may not be the actual gene responsible for the discovered AD locus [19] but rather a proxy for other genes in this gene-rich region of chromosome 11.

Little if anything is understood about the role in AD of the *NME/NM23 family member 8* (*NME8*) gene, located on chromosome 7 (7p14.1) and why the rs2718058 SNP is reportedly associated with modifying AD risk [19]. However, the NM23 family, which encodes nucleoside diphosphate kinase (NDPK), is suggested to play a role in neuronal cell proliferation, differentiation, and neurite outgrowth [326–328], and *NME8* mutations are known to result in primary ciliary dyskinesia type 6 [329], suggesting a potential role in innate immunity and inflammation. Furthermore, the association with AD has been confirmed in subsequent studies, which showed associations of the polymorphism with occipital gyrus atrophy, cerebral glucose usage, and cognitive decline [330].

15.11 Genetics of Parkinson's Disease

Parkinson's disease (PD) is a chronic neurodegenerative disease, second only to Alzheimer's disease in its global prevalence. Although most cases are sporadic, it has long been known that on rare occasions the condition may be familial, and it has been suspected that there may be a genetic susceptibility even in sporadic cases. The current understanding of the genetic contribution dates from the ground-breaking discovery in 1997 of a mutation in the α-synuclein (*SNCA*) gene as the cause of the disease in a large Italian American family (the Contursi kindred) with autosomal dominant inheritance [331]. This proved to be of critical importance not only as it was the first gene associated with familial PD, but more importantly because it was subsequently shown that α-synuclein is the major protein component of the Lewy bodies which are the neuropathological hallmark of PD [332], and this finding has since led to major advances in our understanding of the pathogenesis of the disease. Over the next

18 years a series of additional monogenic forms of PD have been identified and there has also been increasing recognition of the importance of common genetic variants in some of these genes, and in a number of other genes, in determining an individual's risk of developing PD. It is now generally accepted that the genetic contribution to PD is complex and that genetic factors probably contribute to some degree to most, if not all forms of the disease [333]. In this second component of the chapter we review genetic loci associated with both monogenic and late-onset sporadic forms of PD.

15.12 Monogenic forms of PD

Mutations in a number of genes encoding a variety of proteins with diverse cellular functions have now been implicated in causing familial PD [334, 335] and are estimated to account for ~5–10% of all cases of PD. As shown in Table 15.3, these are associated with different patterns of inheritance and a spectrum of clinical phenotypes which ranges from early-onset to classical late-onset PD, and in some families may include additional features such as dementia, dystonia (involuntary muscle contractions), pyramidal tract, and autonomic involvement (symptoms include spasticity, weakness, difficulty swallowing, urinary leakage, and dizziness).

15.12.1 Autosomal Dominant Forms

A number of genetic loci and mutations have been associated with autosomal dominant Parkinson's disease (ADPD): PARK 1 and 4 (*SNCA*), PARK 8 (*LRRK2*), PARK 11 (*GIGYF2*), PARK 17 (*VPS35*), and PARK 18 (*EIF4G1*). In addition, mutations in a number of the spinocerebellar ataxia (SCA) genes (*ATXN2*, *ATXN3*, *TBP*) have been associated with the development of PD in some families [336, 337].

15.12.1.1 PARK 1 (*SNCA*)
Although *SNCA* mutations represent the prototypic form of ADPD, it is now recognised that they are in fact a rare cause of PD and have been reported in only a relatively small number of families, mainly of European ancestry. Point mutations, including the original A53T mutation, the A30P, E46K mutations [338], and the more recently identified G51D, H50Q, and A53E mutations [339–341], have been reported only rarely, whereas gene duplications have been found in ~1–2% of autosomal dominant families [333].

Triplications of the *SNCA* gene have also been identified in rare families, such as the large Iowa kindred which had previously been assigned the PARK 4 locus [342]. Such gene multiplications lead to increased expression of wild-type α-synuclein and a gene-dose effect which is reflected in a more severe clinical phenotype. The clinical phenotype is similar to that of idiopathic PD, but most *SNCA* mutations and multiplications are associated with an earlier age at onset than sporadic PD (<50 years), and non-motor features such as dementia, depression, and psychotic features are common. Other atypical features such as myoclonus, pyramidal, and autonomic involvement and central hypoventilation are also present in some families [339, 343]. The motor manifestations are usually levodopa-responsive, however the rate of decline tends to be faster than in idiopathic cases [344].

Table 15.3 Identified loci and causative genes in familial Parkinson's disease.

PARK locus	Genomic location	Gene	Phenotype	Suggested biological pathways
Autosomal dominant				
PARK 1 & 4	4q21	SNCA	EOPD	Synaptic vesicle formation, UPS dysfunction, dopamine release, microtubule function
PARK 5	4p13	UCHL1[a]	Classical PD	UPS dysfunction
PARK 8	12q12	LRRK2	Classical PD	Autophagy, mitochondrial dysfunction, immune response
PARK 11	2q37	GIGYF2[a]	LOPD	IGF signalling
PARK 13	2p12	HTRA2	LOPD	Apoptosis (caspase-dependent), mitochondrial dysfunction
PARK 17	16q11.2	VPS35	Classical PD	Endocytosis, endosome-lysosome transport
PARK 18	3q27.1	EIF4G1[a]	Classical PD	Eukaryote translation, mRNA degradation via UPS
Autosomal recessive				
PARK 2	6q25.2-q27	PRKN	EOPD	Ubiquitin mediated proteolysis, mitochondrial dysfunction, mitophagy
PARK 6	1p35-p36	PINK 1	EOPD	Mitochondrial dysfunction, mitophagy
PARK 7	1p36	DJ-1	EOPD	Oxidative stress, mitochondrial dysfunction
PARK 9	1p36	ATP13A2	Kufor-Rakeb Syndrome; JPD	Metal transport (divalent transition metal cations)
PARK 14	22q12-q13	PLA2G6	EOPD-dystonia	Phospholipid metabolism, remodelling
PARK 15	22q12-q13	FBXO7	JPD-pyramidal signs	UPS dysfunction, mitophagy

EOPD, early-onset Parkinson's disease; LOPD, late-onset Parkinson's disease; JPD, juvenile Parkinson's disease; SNCA, alpha-synuclein; UCHL1, ubiquitin carboxy-terminal hydrolase L1; LRRK2, leucine-rich repeat kinase 2; GIGYF2, PERQ amino acid-rich with GYF domain-containing protein 2; HTRA2, HtrA serine peptidase 2; VPS35, vacuolar protein sorting 35; EIF4G1, eukaryotic translation initiation factor 4 gamma 1; PRKN, parkin; PINK 1, PTEN-induced putative kinase 1; DJ-1, protein deglycase DJ-1; ATP13A2, probable cation-transporting ATPase 13A2; PLA2G6, phospholipase A2 group 6; FBXO7, F-box protein 7; UPS, ubiquitin-proteasome system; IGF, insulin-like growth factor.
a) Requires confirmation.

15.12.1.2 PARK 8 (LRRK2)

It is now recognised that mutations in the *leucine-rich repeat kinase 2* gene (*LRRK2*) [345, 346] are the most common cause of ADPD, accounting for ~5% of familial PD in Northern European and North American populations, and bridge the gap between hereditary and sporadic PD [337, 347]. The frequency of *LRRK2* mutations has been found to vary considerably in different populations, ranging from ~10% in Italian and Portuguese families, ~20% in Ashkenazy Jewish PD cases, and ~40% in North African Berber cases [337]. Penetrance is incomplete and age-related, and has varied from ~30–70% in different families, accounting for the lack of a family history in some cases with late-onset PD [348]. The age at onset is typically in the 60s, and the clinical phenotype is usually indistinguishable from late-onset idiopathic PD, although atypical features are present in some families. A number of pathogenic mutations have been identified in the GTPase (Ras of complex protein, ROC) domain of the gene (R1441C/G/H, A1442P) [349], but the most prevalent is the G2019S mutation in the kinase domain, which is common in Southern European and North African populations and Ashkenazy Jews [350, 351], but is rare in Asian populations [352]. Two common *LRRK2* variants (G2385A and R1628P) have however been shown to be risk factors for the sporadic form of PD in Chinese and Japanese people [352, 353]. The kinase domain *LRRK2* mutations have been shown to result in an increased kinase activity and a presumed toxic gain of function [354], whereas mutations in the ROC domain of the gene cause increased intracellular degradation of *LRRK2* [349]. LRRK2 has been shown to have kinase-like and GTPase domains, and recent studies have shown that it enhances IL-1β signalling, through phosphorylation of RCAN1 (an inhibitor of phosphatase 3B) which positively regulates inflammatory signals, providing evidence that LRRK2 is normally involved in immune response signalling [355].

15.12.1.3 PARK 11 (*GIGYF2*)

Linkage to chromosome 2q was first established in sibling pairs and 150 PD families in 2002 [356]. Heterozygous mutations in the *GIGYF2* gene at 2q37, which encodes the Grb10-interacting GYF protein-2, were later identified in Italian and French families with ADPD, with incomplete penetrance and a clinical phenotype resembling that of idiopathic PD [357]. However, a number of subsequent studies in other populations have cast doubt on this association [358, 359]. A recent meta-analysis of suggested PD-causing mutations found N56S and N457T to be risk factors for PD in Caucasians, though not in Asians, and several other variants were found to be not related to PD [360].

15.12.1.4 PARK 17 (*VPS35*)

Mutations in the *VPS35* gene which encodes a core component of the retromer cargo-recognition complex were first identified in Swiss, Austrian, and American families with late-onset ADPD using NGS, and this has since been confirmed in other cohorts [361, 362]. The most common mutation is the heterozygous missense Asp620Asn mutation which has been found in 1% of French families with ADPD, a frequency similar to that of *SNCA* multiplications and *SCA2* CAG expansions in familial PD [363]. Several other *VPS35* mutations and variants have since also been identified in other populations [364]. The clinical phenotype of *PARK17* closely resembles that of idiopathic PD, with onset between 45 and 59 years of age and a good response to treatment with levodopa [364], whereas pathologically, the Asp620Asn variant causes defects in endosomal trafficking and retromer formation [365].

15.12.1.5 PARK 18 (*EIF4G1*)

A heterozygous missense mutation (R1205H) in the *eukaryotic translation initiation factor 4-gamma* (*EIF4G1*) gene on 3q27 was first identified in a large French family with ADPD and a classical late-onset PD phenotype, then four additional mutations were found in other families with ADPD and Lewy body disease [366]. Functional studies showed that the R1205H and A502V variants impair formation of the larger EIF4 complex and were compatible with a dominant-negative loss-of-function mechanism of neurodegeneration. However, subsequent studies have so far failed to confirm the association with *EIF4G1* variants in other large PD cohorts [367–369].

15.12.2 Autosomal Recessive Forms

Six genetic loci and genes have been associated with recessively-inherited forms of PD (meaning both genes passed on from parents must be abnormal to cause disease): PARK 2 (*PRKN*), PARK 6 (*PINK 1*), PARK 7 (*DJ-1*), PARK 9 (*ATP13A2*), PARK 14 (*PLA2G6*), and PARK 15 (*FBXO7*) as listed in Table 15.3.

15.12.2.1 PARK 2 (*PRKN*)

Mutations in the *PRKN* gene, which encodes the E3 ubiquitin ligase parkin, are the most common cause of recessively-inherited early-onset Parkinson's disease (EOPD, onset <45 years of age), and may also occur in individuals with late-onset PD (>60 years of age) who have a family history of PD [370, 371]. The frequency of pathogenic *PRKN* mutations is age-related, and the likelihood of carrying a mutation is greater, the earlier the age of onset of the disease. In one study, *PRKN* mutations were found in 49% of EOPD families, and the age at symptom onset ranged from 7 to 58 years [370]. *PRKN* mutations also occur in ~18% of cases of isolated PD with onset under 40 years of age [372], and in 77% of cases with onset before the age of 20 years [370]. The clinical phenotype is usually that of levodopa-responsive parkinsonism, yet with certain features such as symmetry of motor disturbances, slower progression, and a more benign clinical course with infrequent cognitive and vegetative changes. Other atypical features may include hyperreflexia, dystonia, gait abnormalities, and diurnal fluctuation [373].

A wide variety of gene mutations have been reported, including exon deletions and multiplications as well as point mutations, and homozygous, heterozygous (mutation in only one copy of the gene), or compound heterozygous (mutations in both gene copies, mutations being different) mutations may occur in different individuals [370]. In patients with a single heterozygous mutation, it may be difficult to be certain that the mutation is pathogenic, as opposed to being an incidental finding. However, heterozygous mutations may act as susceptibility alleles for late-onset PD [374]. Genotype–phenotype correlations have shown that individuals with heterozygous or compound heterozygous mutations tend to have an earlier age of onset of PD [375].

15.12.2.2 PARK 6 (*PINK 1*)

Mutations in the PTEN (phosphatase and tensin homolog)-induced putative kinase 1 (*PINK 1*) gene, which encodes the mitochondrial serine/threonine kinase PINK 1, combine to form the second most common cause of early-onset autosomal recessive PD. Homozygous missense and nonsense mutations have been identified in various racial and ethnic populations and may account for ~1% of cases of sporadic EOPD [376]. The pathogenic significance of single heterozygous mutations in individual patients is less certain, but may nevertheless be associated with a subclinical dopaminergic deficit and, as in the case of *PRKN*, may act as a risk allele for the development of late-onset PD [337]. Heterozygous offspring of patients with homozygous mutations may also have mild clinical signs [377]. The clinical phenotype is similar to that of *PARK 2*, but onset is usually between 40 and 50 years of age, and may include dystonia, pyramidal signs, and sleep benefit (better motor function just after waking) in some families [337]. Functional studies have shown that parkin and PINK 1 are part of a common pathway and that mutations in *PINK 1* interfere with the E3 ubiquitin-protein ligase function of parkin and the autophagic removal of damaged mitochondria (mitophagy) from cells [378]. Such studies are showing that deficiencies in either of these two enzymes increases oxidative stress due to the accumulation of dysfunctional mitochondria, and that this may also lead to degeneration due to inflammation, dendritic changes, and apoptosis [379, 380].

15.12.2.3 PARK 7 (*DJ-1*)

Homozygous or heterozygous missense mutations in *DJ-1*, as well as exon deletions, have been identified in a small number of consanguineous families as the cause of EOPD levodopa-responsive PD with onset at 20–30 years of age, slow progression, and associated dystonia and psychiatric features in some cases [381]. In some families, there are also features of amyotrophic lateral sclerosis. Subsequent studies have shown that *DJ-1* mutations are a rare cause of EOPD, being found in only ~0.2–1% of cases and are not found in late-onset sporadic PD [382, 383]. Although the cellular function of DJ-1 is not fully understood, it is known to protect against oxidative stress and to have a role in maintaining endoplasmic reticulum-mitochondrial coupling [384]. Experimental studies have shown that DJ-1, PINK 1, and parkin are part of a common molecular pathway and interact to form a ubiquitin E3 ligase complex which promotes degradation of unfolded or misfolded proteins in cells [385].

15.12.2.4 PARK 9 (*ATP13A2*)

Mutations in the *ATP13A2* gene which encodes a lysosomal P-type ATPase (ATP13A2) have been identified as the cause of the Kufor-Rabek syndrome, which is a rare form of levodopa-responsive juvenile-onset parkinsonism, with onset between 10 and 30 years of age, and which is associated with spasticity, dystonia, dementia, and supranuclear ophthalmoplegia (eye movement difficulty, especially looking up) [386, 387]. Multiple homozygous or compound heterozygous mutations comprising missense mutations or small gene rearrangements were found in the 11 families that have been reported in the literature [388]. Single heterozygous *ATP13A2* mutations also occur in some cases of EOPD [389] and may also confer susceptibility for the development of sporadic late-onset PD. The role played by ATP13A2 in the development of PD has been clarified by recent studies which have shown that it is involved in zinc homeostasis, and that a reduced expression of the protein results in impaired lysosomal and mitochondrial function as well as the accumulation of α-synuclein [380, 388].

15.12.2.5 PARK 14 (*PLA2G6*)

One early-onset form of PD is caused by homozygous or compound heterozygous mutations in the *PLA2G6* gene that encodes phospholipase A2. Only a few families of Indian, Pakistani, Japanese, and Chinese origin have been reported, some being consanguineous, with onset in the early 30s. This form of PD is levodopa-responsive PD; symptoms can include dystonia (involuntary muscle contractions), pyramidal features (such as plantar extension and overactive reflexes), and cognitive and personality changes. Pathological changes include frontotemporal lobar atrophy on brain MRI and in some cases iron accumulation in the basal ganglia [390–392]. Recent studies have also shown that PLA2G6 protein accumulates in the Lewy bodies of both PARK 14 and idiopathic PD cases, in the brain stem [393], that the PLA2G6 protein plays a role in calcium signalling, specifically the store-operated calcium signalling pathway, and that dysfunction of PLA2G6 results in disruptions to autophagy, dopaminergic neurons, and levodopa-sensitive motor functions [394]. This latter finding in idiopathic PD was suggested to reveal one of the pathogenic mechanisms contributing to PD.

15.12.2.6 PARK 15 (*FBXO7*)

Mutations in the gene which encodes the *F-box protein 7* (*FBXO7*) lead to an early-onset parkinsonian-pyramidal syndrome which has been reported in consanguineous families of various racial backgrounds [395]. The onset is usually in the first two decades of life, with gait abnormalities and slowly progressive spasticity and extrapyramidal manifestations, which may be responsive to treatment with levodopa. Homozygous and compound heterozygous mutations have been reported in different families [395]. Recent studies have shown that the FBXO7 protein is part of a complex involved in ubiquitination and proteasome function [396].

15.12.3 Genetic Contributions to Late-Onset Sporadic PD (LOPD)

A number of susceptibility alleles for late-onset Parkinson's disease (LOPD) were first identified in case-control association studies in relatively small patient populations. These studies showed that, in addition to their involvement in causing monogenic disease, common variants in some of the familial PD genes such as *SNCA*, *LRRK2*, and *UCHL1* are also risk alleles for LOPD. In addition, genes associated with other neurodegenerative diseases (e.g. *MAPT* and *glucocerebroside*, *GCA*), or genes that have immune-inflammatory functions, may also have modifying effects. Over the past 15 years, GWAS in increasingly larger populations of affected and unaffected individuals have allowed confirmation of previously identified major gene associations (e.g. *SNCA* and *MAPT*) and have also identified an increasing number of previously unrecognised genetic loci associated with disease risk (including *PARK 16*, *BST1*, *GAK-DGKQ*, *HLA-DRB5*, *RIT2*, and others) [204, 397–400]. The individual contributions of these variants is quite small; however their frequency in the population means that their cumulative effects can be quite substantial [401]. Recent studies have also shown that variations in genes with detoxifying functions may influence susceptibility to environmental toxins such as pesticides and solvents, and may be important in determining the risk of developing PD [402, 403].

15.12.4 Common Variants in PD Genes

The NACP-Rep1 polymorphic dinucleotide repeat in the vicinity of the *SNCA* gene has been associated with PD risk, but this has varied in different populations [404, 405]. Polymorphisms in other non-coding regions of the *SNCA* gene have also been linked to disease risk, both in Caucasian and non-Caucasian populations [398, 406–408], as well as interactions with *MAPT* alleles [409]. Linkage to several *LRRK2* polymorphisms has been found in large case-control studies and in GWAS [398, 410]. The low-penetrance *LRRK2* mutation G2019S is frequently associated with both familial and sporadic PD in South European, Middle Eastern, and North African populations, while the G2385A and R1628P variants have been shown to be associated with an increased risk of developing sporadic LOPD in Asia [352, 353]. Heterozygous mutations in *PRKN*, *ATP13A2* and common variants in *EIF4G1*, *VPS3* may also contribute to the risk of developing sporadic PD, but this has yet to be proven.

15.12.5 Glucocerebrosidase (*GBA*)

Following the observation that some patients with Gaucher's disease may develop atypical parkinsonism later in life, it has been recognised that homozygous or heterozygous mutations in the *glucocerebrosidase GBA* gene, that encodes the lysosomal enzyme β-glucocerebrosidase, can increase the risk of PD. The association has been confirmed in various racial groups, with a carrier frequency ranging from 3% to 4% in British, European, and American patient cohorts [411–413] and 2–9% in Asian populations [414–416], to 15–18% in Ashkenazi Jews [417, 418]. Patients with *GBA* mutations are more likely to have other affected relatives as well as an earlier age of onset of PD, and atypical features including cognitive symptoms and dementia [413, 418, 419]. It has also been found that *GBA* mutations are a significant risk factor for diffuse Lewy body dementia, with an odds ratio of 8.28 in *GBA1* mutation carriers in a large multicentre study [420]. Mutant forms of GBA have been shown to exert a toxic gain of function and promote the accumulation of α-synuclein, both in non-neural cells and in brain tissue [421].

15.12.6 Immune-Inflammatory Genes

Immune-inflammatory mechanisms are thought to play a critical role in the initiation of the neurodegenerative process in PD and there is increasing evidence that genetic variants in PD genes and genes encoding inflammatory mediators may enhance the severity of the inflammatory process [422, 423]. Variations in a number of the familial PD genes including *SNCA*, *LRRK2*, *PRKN*, *PINK 1*, and *GBA1* have been shown to activate microglia, which are the innate immune cells of the CNS and may modulate the release of inflammatory mediators such as TNFα and IL-1β and enhance the production of reactive oxygen species and nitric oxide [424]. In addition, polymorphisms in *IL-1B*, *IL-6*, *IL-8*, *IL-10*, *IL-18*, and *TNFα* have been associated with an increased risk of developing PD [423]. Independent confirmation of the importance of the immune-inflammatory process has been provided by studies of HLA associations. A GWAS of a large American PD cohort initially showed an association with a noncoding variant of *HLA-DRA* (HLA class II histocompatibility antigen, DR alpha chain) [201]. Subsequent studies in other cohorts showed that multiple loci within the *HLA* region appear to be involved, including *HLA-DR5*, *HLA-DRB1*, and *HLA-DQB1* [202–204]. A recent analysis of GWAS data found that autoimmune diseases such as rheumatoid arthritis, ulcerative colitis, and Crohn's disease share genetic loci with PD, including loci linked to *GAK* (cyclin G-associated kinase), *HLA-DRB5*, *LRRK2*, and *MAPT*. Replication then confirmed the involvement of *MAPT*, *HLA*, *LRRK2*, *TRIM10*, and *SETD1A* in PD [425]. Such studies are again adding to our understanding of mechanisms behind the pathogenic changes in PD.

15.12.7 Mitochondrial DNA Variants

Mitochondrial DNA (mtDNA) codes for 13 respiratory-chain proteins that are essential for the synthesis of the intracellular energy source ATP; and a defect in respiratory chain complex 1 has been documented in the substantia nigra of PD brains. Mitochondrial DNA polymorphisms and haplogroups have been found to have modifying effects on the risk of developing PD. In a study of 949 individuals of European ancestry, the risk of PD was significantly lower in individuals who carried the J or K mtDNA haplogroups and the associated 10398G SNP within the NADH dehydrogenase 3 (ND3) gene, which is a subunit of complex I of the respiratory enzyme chain [426]. A subsequent larger UK study of 9214 PD cases confirmed the reduced risk associated with carriage of the J and K haplogroups and the JT super-haplogroup, whereas carriage of the H super-haplogroup increased the risk of PD [427]. Studies of mitochondrial DNA variants that lead to PD have helped to reveal the complex homeostasis of mitochondrial production and autophagy, involving their dynamic fission/fusion cycle, and showing the requirement for mitochondrial DNA maintenance as well as the requirement of other genes already mentioned above such as *PINK 1* and *PRKN* [428].

15.13 Conclusion

As has been discussed, genetics plays a significant role in underpinning susceptibility to both AD and PD. In the case of the autosomal dominant forms of these diseases, highly penetrant causal mutations have been discovered that result in the development of either ADAD or ADPD through the Mendelian inheritance of dominant or recessive mutations, whilst, on the other hand, sporadic forms of each disease are generally characterised by a highly complex interaction between multiple genetic risk factors and environmental and lifestyle factors, which together modify the risk of developing either disease. In the case of AD, increasing age is still the dominant factor leading to an increased risk of the late-onset form of the disease. However, genetic factors are arguably the next greatest single contributor to an individual's risk, through modifying susceptibility to other diseases (e.g. diabetes, cardiovascular disease), themselves considered risk factors for AD, or being moderated by, or moderating the impact of, lifestyle factors.

Genetic studies of neurodegenerative disease such as AD and PD have provided the research field with a more comprehensive understanding of the genetic basis of each disease and concurrently a greater understanding of biological pathways involved in disease pathogenesis. The latter holds the key to the eventual development of treatments for both diseases. In addition to genetics, it will be important to understand the role of lifestyle factors that modify disease risk in conjunction with these genetic factors, as understanding the interaction or moderating effects will be crucial in developing early disease-modifying interventions. For example, in AD, the potential success of developing early preventative strategies focusing on modifying key lifestyle factors such as diet, exercise, and sleep will be highly dependent on targeting the right intervention, to the right person (based on their genetics), at the right time.

References

1 Soto, C. and Estrada, L.D. (2008). Protein misfolding and neurodegeneration. *Arch. Neurol.* 65: 184–189.
2 ADI (2015) Alzheimer's Disease International (ADI), London.
3 ABS, Causes of Death, Australia 2014. ABS cat. no.3303.0.,ABS, www.abs.gov.au/ausstats/abs@.nsf/0/47E19CA15036B04BCA2577570014668B?Opendocument.
4 Flicker, L. (2010). Modifiable lifestyle risk factors for Alzheimer's disease. *J. Alzheimers Dis.* 20: 803–811.
5 Ashford, J.W. and Mortimer, J.A. (2002). Non-familial Alzheimer's disease is mainly due to genetic factors. *J. Alzheimers Dis.* 4: 169–177.
6 Gatz, M., Reynolds, C.A., Fratiglioni, L. et al. (2006). Role of genes and environments for explaining Alzheimer disease. *Arch. Gen. Psychiatry* 63: 168–174.
7 Karch, C.M. and Goate, A.M. (2015). Alzheimer's disease risk genes and mechanisms of disease pathogenesis. *Biol. Psychiatry* 77: 43–51.
8 Cacace, R., Sleegers, K., and Van Broeckhoven, C. (2016). Molecular genetics of early-onset Alzheimer's disease revisited. *Alzheimers Dement* 12: 733–748.
9 Abraham, R., Moskvina, V., Sims, R. et al. (2008). A genome-wide association study for late-onset Alzheimer's disease using DNA pooling. *BMC Med. Genet.* 1: 44.
10 Beecham, G.W., Martin, E.R., Li, Y.J. et al. (2009). Genome-wide association study implicates a chromosome 12 risk locus for late-onset Alzheimer disease. *Am. J. Hum. Genet.* 84: 35–43.
11 Bertram, L., Lange, C., Mullin, K. et al. (2008). Genome-wide association analysis reveals putative Alzheimer's disease susceptibility loci in addition to APOE. *Am. J. Hum. Genet.* 83: 623–632.
12 Carrasquillo, M.M., Zou, F., Pankratz, V.S. et al. (2009). Genetic variation in PCDH11X is associated with susceptibility to late-onset Alzheimer's disease. *Nat. Genet.* 41: 192–198.
13 Grupe, A., Abraham, R., Li, Y. et al. (2007). Evidence for novel susceptibility genes for late-onset Alzheimer's disease from a genome-wide association study of putative functional variants. *Hum. Mol. Genet.* 16: 865–873.
14 Harold, D., Abraham, R., Hollingworth, P. et al. (2009). Genome-wide association study identifies variants at CLU and PICALM associated with Alzheimer's disease. *Nat. Genet.* 41: 1088–1093.
15 Hollingworth, P., Harold, D., Sims, R. et al. (2011). Common variants at ABCA7, MS4A6A/MS4A4E, EPHA1, CD33 and CD2AP are associated with Alzheimer's disease. *Nat. Genet.* 43: 429–435.
16 Hooli, B.V., Lill, C.M., Mullin, K. et al. (2015). PLD3 gene variants and Alzheimer's disease. *Nature* 520: E7–E8.
17 Jun, G., Ibrahim-Verbaas, C.A., Vronskaya, M. et al. (2016). A novel Alzheimer disease locus located near the gene encoding tau protein. *Mol. Psychiatry* 21: 108–117.
18 Lambert, J.C., Heath, S., Even, G. et al. (2009). Genome-wide association study identifies variants at CLU and CR1 associated with Alzheimer's disease. *Nat. Genet.* 41: 1094–1099.
19 Lambert, J.C., Ibrahim-Verbaas, C.A., Harold, D. et al., European Alzheimer's Disease I, Genetic, Environmental Risk in Alzheimer's D, Alzheimer's Disease Genetic

C, Cohorts for H, Aging Research in Genomic E (2013). Meta-analysis of 74,046 individuals identifies 11 new susceptibility loci for Alzheimer's disease. *Nat. Genet.* 45: 1452–1458.
20 Li, H., Wetten, S., Li, L. et al. (2008). Candidate single-nucleotide polymorphisms from a genomewide association study of Alzheimer disease. *Arch. Neurol.* 65: 45–53.
21 Naj, A.C., Beecham, G.W., Martin, E.R. et al. (2010). Dementia revealed: novel chromosome 6 locus for late-onset Alzheimer disease provides genetic evidence for folate-pathway abnormalities. *PLos Genet.* 6: e1001130.
22 Naj, A.C., Jun, G., Beecham, G.W. et al. (2011). Common variants at MS4A4/MS4A6E, CD2AP, CD33 and EPHA1 are associated with late-onset Alzheimer's disease. *Nat. Genet.*
23 Bertram, L. and Tanzi, R.E. (2012). The genetics of Alzheimer's disease. *Prog. Mol. Biol. Transl. Sci.* 107: 79–100.
24 Guerreiro, R., Wojtas, A., Bras, J. et al., Alzheimer Genetic Analysis G (2013). TREM2 variants in Alzheimer's disease. *N. Engl. J. Med.* 368: 117–127.
25 Jonsson, T., Stefansson, H., Steinberg, S. et al. (2013). Variant of TREM2 associated with the risk of Alzheimer's disease. *N. Engl. J. Med.* 368: 107–116.
26 Cruchaga, C., Karch, C.M., Jin, S.C. et al. (2014). Rare coding variants in the phospholipase D3 gene confer risk for Alzheimer's disease. *Nature* 505: 550–554.
27 Cruchaga, C., Haller, G., Chakraverty, S. et al., Consortium N-LNFS (2012). Rare variants in APP, PSEN1 and PSEN2 increase risk for AD in late-onset Alzheimer's disease families. *PLoS One* 7: e31039.
28 Benitez, B.A., Karch, C.M., Cai, Y. et al., Alzheimer's Disease Neuroimaging I, Genetic, Environmental Risk for Alzheimer's Disease Consortium G. (2013). The PSEN1, p.E318G variant increases the risk of Alzheimer's disease in APOE-epsilon4 carriers. *PLos Genet.* 9: e1003685.
29 Kim, M., Suh, J., Romano, D. et al. (2009). Potential late-onset Alzheimer's disease-associated mutations in the ADAM10 gene attenuate {alpha}-secretase activity. *Hum. Mol. Genet.* 18: 3987–3996.
30 Bateman, R.J., Aisen, P.S., De Strooper, B. et al. (2011). Autosomal-dominant Alzheimer's disease: a review and proposal for the prevention of Alzheimer's disease. *Alzheimers Res. Ther.* 3: 1.
31 Wu, L., Rosa-Neto, P., Hsiung, G.Y. et al. (2012). Early-onset familial Alzheimer's disease (EOFAD). *Can. J. Neurol. Sci.* 39: 436–445.
32 Cruts, M., Theuns, J., and Van Broeckhoven, C. (2012). Locus-specific mutation databases for neurodegenerative brain diseases. *Hum. Mutat.* 33: 1340–1344.
33 Sherrington, R., Rogaev, E.I., Liang, Y. et al. (1995). Cloning of a gene bearing missense mutations in early-onset familial Alzheimer's disease. *Nature* 375: 754–760.
34 Goate, A., Chartier-Harlin, M.C., Mullan, M. et al. (1991). Segregation of a missense mutation in the amyloid precursor protein gene with familial Alzheimer's disease. *Nature* 349: 704–706.
35 Levy-Lahad, E., Wasco, W., Poorkaj, P. et al. (1995). Candidate gene for the chromosome 1 familial Alzheimer's disease locus. *Science* 269: 973–977.
36 Levy-Lahad, E., Wijsman, E.M., Nemens, E. et al. (1995). A familial Alzheimer's disease locus on chromosome 1. *Science* 269: 970–973.

37 Rogaev, E.I., Sherrington, R., Rogaeva, E.A. et al. (1995). Familial Alzheimer's disease in kindreds with missense mutations in a gene on chromosome 1 related to the Alzheimer's disease type 3 gene. *Nature* 376: 775–778.
38 Hardy, J.A. and Higgins, G.A. (1992). Alzheimer's disease: the amyloid cascade hypothesis. *Science* 256: 184–185.
39 Hardy, J. and Selkoe, D.J. (2002). The amyloid hypothesis of Alzheimer's disease: progress and problems on the road to therapeutics. *Science* 297: 353–356.
40 Selkoe, D.J. and Hardy, J. (2016). The amyloid hypothesis of Alzheimer's disease at 25 years. *EMBO Mol. Med.* 8: 595–608.
41 Borchelt, D.R., Thinakaran, G., Eckman, C.B. et al. (1996). Familial Alzheimer's disease-linked presenilin 1 variants elevate Abeta1-42/1-40 ratio in vitro and in vivo. *Neuron* 17: 1005–1013.
42 Hooli, B.V., Kovacs-Vajna, Z.M., Mullin, K. et al. (2014). Rare autosomal copy number variations in early-onset familial Alzheimer's disease. *Mol. Psychiatry* 19: 676–681.
43 Ghani, M. and Rogaeva, E. (2014). Autosomal dominant Alzheimer's disease: underlying causes. In: *Neurodegenerative Diseases: Clinical Aspects, Molecular Genetics and Biomarkers* (ed. E. Scarpini), 27–47. London, UK: Springer London.
44 Haass, C., Hung, A.Y., Selkoe, D.J., and Teplow, D.B. (1994). Mutations associated with a locus for familial Alzheimer's disease result in alternative processing of amyloid beta-protein precursor. *J. Biol. Chem.* 269: 17741–17748.
45 Kumar-Singh, S., De Jonghe, C., Cruts, M. et al. (2000). Nonfibrillar diffuse amyloid deposition due to a gamma(42)-secretase site mutation points to an essential role for N-truncated A beta(42) in Alzheimer's disease. *Hum. Mol. Genet.* 9: 2589–2598.
46 Herl, L., Thomas, A.V., Lill, C.M. et al. (2009). Mutations in amyloid precursor protein affect its interactions with presenilin/gamma-secretase. *Mol. Cell Neurosci.* 41: 166–174.
47 Stenh, C., Nilsberth, C., Hammarback, J. et al. (2002). The Arctic mutation interferes with processing of the amyloid precursor protein. *Neuroreport* 13: 1857–1860.
48 Citron, M., Oltersdorf, T., Haass, C. et al. (1992). Mutation of the beta-amyloid precursor protein in familial Alzheimer's disease increases beta-protein production. *Nature* 360: 672–674.
49 Kirkitadze, M.D., Condron, M.M., and Teplow, D.B. (2001). Identification and characterization of key kinetic intermediates in amyloid beta-protein fibrillogenesis. *J. Mol. Biol.* 312: 1103–1119.
50 Citron, M., Vigo-Pelfrey, C., Teplow, D.B. et al. (1994). Excessive production of amyloid beta-protein by peripheral cells of symptomatic and presymptomatic patients carrying the Swedish familial Alzheimer disease mutation. *Proc. Natl. Acad. Sci. U.S.A.* 91: 11993–11997.
51 Jonsson, T., Atwal, J.K., Steinberg, S. et al. (2012). A mutation in APP protects against Alzheimer's disease and age-related cognitive decline. *Nature* 488: 96–99.
52 Kero, M., Paetau, A., Polvikoski, T. et al. (2013). Amyloid precursor protein (APP) A673T mutation in the elderly Finnish population. *Neurobiol. Aging* 34 (1518): e1511–e1513.
53 Maloney, J.A., Bainbridge, T., Gustafson, A. et al. (2014). Molecular mechanisms of Alzheimer disease protection by the A673T allele of amyloid precursor protein. *J. Biol. Chem.* 289: 30990–31000.

54 Bamne, M.N., Demirci, F.Y., Berman, S. et al. (2014). Investigation of an amyloid precursor protein protective mutation (A673T) in a North American case-control sample of late-onset Alzheimer's disease. *Neurobiol. Aging* 35 (1779): e1715–e1776.

55 Davies, G., Armstrong, N., Bis, J.C. et al. (2015). Genetic contributions to variation in general cognitive function: a meta-analysis of genome-wide association studies in the CHARGE consortium (N=53949). *Mol. Psychiatry* 20: 183–192.

56 Kimberly, W.T., LaVoie, M.J., Ostaszewski, B.L. et al. (2003). Gamma-secretase is a membrane protein complex comprised of presenilin, nicastrin, Aph-1, and Pen-2. *Proc. Natl. Acad. Sci. U.S.A.* 100: 6382–6387.

57 Wakabayashi, T. and De Strooper, B. (2008). Presenilins: members of the gamma-secretase quartets, but part-time soloists too. *Physiology (Bethesda)* 23: 194–204.

58 Crook, R., Verkkoniemi, A., Perez-Tur, J. et al. (1998). A variant of Alzheimer's disease with spastic paraparesis and unusual plaques due to deletion of exon 9 of presenilin 1. *Nat. Med.* 4: 452–455.

59 Rogaeva, E.A., Fafel, K.C., Song, Y.Q. et al. (2001). Screening for PS1 mutations in a referral-based series of AD cases: 21 novel mutations. *Neurology* 57: 621–625.

60 De Jonghe, C., Cruts, M., Rogaeva, E.A. et al. (1999). Aberrant splicing in the presenilin-1 intron 4 mutation causes presenile Alzheimer's disease by increased Abeta42 secretion. *Hum. Mol. Genet.* 8: 1529–1540.

61 Scheuner, D., Eckman, C., Jensen, M. et al. (1996). Secreted amyloid beta-protein similar to that in the senile plaques of Alzheimer's disease is increased in vivo by the presenilin 1 and 2 and APP mutations linked to familial Alzheimer's disease. *Nat. Med.* 2: 864–870.

62 Kuperstein, I., Broersen, K., Benilova, I. et al. (2010). Neurotoxicity of Alzheimer's disease Abeta peptides is induced by small changes in the Abeta42 to Abeta40 ratio. *EMBO J.* 29: 3408–3420.

63 Brooks, W.S., Kwok, J.B., Kril, J.J. et al. (2003). Alzheimer's disease with spastic paraparesis and 'cotton wool' plaques: two pedigrees with PS-1 exon 9 deletions. *Brain* 126: 783–791.

64 Verkkoniemi, A., Kalimo, H., Paetau, A. et al. (2001). Variant Alzheimer disease with spastic paraparesis: neuropathological phenotype. *J. Neuropathol. Exp. Neurol.* 60: 483–492.

65 Jayadev, S., Case, A., Eastman, A.J. et al. (2010). Presenilin 2 is the predominant gamma-secretase in microglia and modulates cytokine release. *PLoS One* 5: e15743.

66 Marchani, E.E., Bird, T.D., Steinbart, E.J. et al. (2010). Evidence for three loci modifying age-at-onset of Alzheimer's disease in early-onset PSEN2 families. *Am. J. Med. Genet. B Neuropsychiatr. Genet.* 153B: 1031–1041.

67 Li, D., Parks, S.B., Kushner, J.D. et al. (2006). Mutations of presenilin genes in dilated cardiomyopathy and heart failure. *Am. J. Hum. Genet.* 79: 1030–1039.

68 Piscopo, P., Marcon, G., Piras, M.R. et al. (2008). A novel PSEN2 mutation associated with a peculiar phenotype. *Neurology* 70: 1549–1554.

69 Wingo, T.S., Lah, J.J., Levey, A.I., and Cutler, D.J. (2012). Autosomal recessive causes likely in early-onset Alzheimer disease. *Arch. Neurol.* 69: 59–64.

70 Bertram, L. (2011). Alzheimer's genetics in the GWAS era: a continuing story of 'replications and refutations. *Curr. Neurol. Neurosci. Rep.* 11: 246–253.

71 Poirier, J. (2003). Apolipoprotein E and cholesterol metabolism in the pathogenesis and treatment of Alzheimer's disease. *Trends Mol. Med.* 9: 94–101.

72 Bekris, L.M., Yu, C.E., Bird, T.D., and Tsuang, D.W. (2010). Genetics of Alzheimer disease. *J. Geriatr. Psychiatry Neurol.* 23: 213–227.

73 Liu, C.C., Kanekiyo, T., Xu, H., and Bu, G. (2013). Apolipoprotein E and Alzheimer disease: risk, mechanisms and therapy. *Nat. Rev. Neurol.* 9: 106–118.

74 Farrer, L.A., Cupples, L.A., Haines, J.L. et al. (1997). Effects of age, sex, and ethnicity on the association between apolipoprotein E genotype and Alzheimer disease: a meta-analysis. APOE and Alzheimer Disease Meta Analysis Consortium. *JAMA* 278: 1349–1356.

75 Strittmatter, W.J., Weisgraber, K.H., Huang, D.Y. et al. (1993). Binding of human apolipoprotein E to synthetic amyloid beta peptide: isoform-specific effects and implications for late-onset Alzheimer disease. *Proc. Natl. Acad. Sci. U.S.A.* 90: 8098–8102.

76 Corder, E.H., Saunders, A.M., Strittmatter, W.J. et al. (1993). Gene dose of apolipoprotein E type 4 allele and the risk of Alzheimer's disease in late onset families. *Science* 261: 921–923.

77 Roses, A.D. (1994). Apolipoprotein E affects the rate of Alzheimer disease expression: beta-amyloid burden is a secondary consequence dependent on APOE genotype and duration of disease. *J. Neuropathol. Exp. Neurol.* 53: 429–437.

78 Corder, E.H., Saunders, A.M., Risch, N.J. et al. (1994). Protective effect of apolipoprotein E type 2 allele for late onset Alzheimer disease. *Nat. Genet.* 7: 180–184.

79 Chen, J., Li, Q., and Wang, J. (2011). Topology of human apolipoprotein E3 uniquely regulates its diverse biological functions. *Proc. Natl. Acad. Sci. U.S.A.* 108: 14813–14818.

80 Frieden, C. and Garai, K. (2012). Structural differences between apoE3 and apoE4 may be useful in developing therapeutic agents for Alzheimer's disease. *Proc. Natl. Acad. Sci. U.S.A.* 109: 8913–8918.

81 Zhong, N. and Weisgraber, K.H. (2009). Understanding the association of apolipoprotein E4 with Alzheimer disease: clues from its structure. *J. Biol. Chem.* 284: 6027–6031.

82 Kim, J., Basak, J.M., and Holtzman, D.M. (2009). The role of apolipoprotein E in Alzheimer's disease. *Neuron* 63: 287–303.

83 Verghese, P.B., Castellano, J.M., Garai, K. et al. (2013). ApoE influences amyloid-beta (Abeta) clearance despite minimal apoE/Abeta association in physiological conditions. *Proc. Natl. Acad. Sci. U.S.A.* 110: E1807–E1816.

84 Castellano, J.M., Kim, J., Stewart, F.R. et al. (2011). Human apoE isoforms differentially regulate brain amyloid-beta peptide clearance. *Sci. Transl. Med.* 3: 89ra57.

85 Bales, K.R., Verina, T., Cummins, D.J. et al. (1999). Apolipoprotein E is essential for amyloid deposition in the APP(V717F) transgenic mouse model of Alzheimer's disease. *Proc. Natl. Acad. Sci. U.S.A.* 96: 15233–15238.

86 Holtzman, D.M., Bales, K.R., Tenkova, T. et al. (2000). Apolipoprotein E isoform-dependent amyloid deposition and neuritic degeneration in a mouse model of Alzheimer's disease. *Proc. Natl. Acad. Sci. U.S.A.* 97: 2892–2897.

87 Morris, J.C., Roe, C.M., Xiong, C. et al. (2010). APOE predicts amyloid-beta but not tau Alzheimer pathology in cognitively normal aging. *Ann. Neurol.* 67: 122–131.

88 Rebeck, G.W., Reiter, J.S., Strickland, D.K., and Hyman, B.T. (1993). Apolipoprotein E in sporadic Alzheimer's disease: allelic variation and receptor interactions. *Neuron* 11: 575–580.

89 Reiman, E.M., Chen, K., Liu, X. et al. (2009). Fibrillar amyloid-beta burden in cognitively normal people at 3 levels of genetic risk for Alzheimer's disease. *Proc. Natl. Acad. Sci. U.S.A.* 106: 6820–6825.

90 Villemagne, V.L., Pike, K.E., Chetelat, G. et al. (2011). Longitudinal assessment of Abeta and cognition in aging and Alzheimer disease. *Ann. Neurol.* 69: 181–192.

91 Huang, Y.A., Zhou, B., Wernig, M., and Sudhof, T.C. (2017). ApoE2, ApoE3, and ApoE4 differentially stimulate APP transcription and Abeta secretion. *Cell* 168 (427–441): e421.

92 Mahley, R.W. (2016). Apolipoprotein E: from cardiovascular disease to neurodegenerative disorders. *J. Mol. Med. (Berl.)* 94: 739–746.

93 Yu, J.T. and Tan, L. (2012). The role of clusterin in Alzheimer's disease: pathways, pathogenesis, and therapy. *Mol. Neurobiol.* 45: 314–326.

94 Jones, S.E. and Jomary, C. (2002). Clusterin. *Int. J. Biochem. Cell Biol.* 34: 427–431.

95 Pasinetti, G.M., Johnson, S.A., Oda, T. et al. (1994). Clusterin (SGP-2): a multifunctional glycoprotein with regional expression in astrocytes and neurons of the adult rat brain. *J. Comp. Neurol.* 339: 387–400.

96 Zwain, I.H., Grima, J., Stahler, M.S. et al. (1993). Regulation of Sertoli cell alpha 2-macroglobulin and clusterin (SGP-2) secretion by peritubular myoid cells. *Biol. Reprod.* 48: 180–187.

97 Saura, J., Petegnief, V., Wu, X. et al. (2003). Microglial apolipoprotein E and astroglial apolipoprotein J expression in vitro: opposite effects of lipopolysaccharide. *J. Neurochem.* 85: 1455–1467.

98 Aronow, B.J., Lund, S.D., Brown, T.L. et al. (1993). Apolipoprotein J expression at fluid-tissue interfaces: potential role in barrier cytoprotection. *Proc. Natl. Acad. Sci. U.S.A.* 90: 725–729.

99 Szymanski, M., Wang, R., Bassett, S.S., and Avramopoulos, D. (2011). Alzheimer's risk variants in the clusterin gene are associated with alternative splicing. *Transl. Psychiatry* 1: e18.

100 Gupta, V.B., Doecke, J.D., Hone, E. et al. (2016). Plasma apolipoprotein J as a potential biomarker for Alzheimer's disease: Australian imaging, biomarkers and lifestyle study of aging. *Alzheimers Dement (Amst.)* 3: 18–26.

101 Kiddle, S.J., Sattlecker, M., Proitsi, P. et al. (2014). Candidate blood proteome markers of Alzheimer's disease onset and progression: a systematic review and replication study. *J. Alzheimers Dis.* 38: 515–531.

102 Schrijvers, E.M., Koudstaal, P.J., Hofman, A., and Breteler, M.M. (2011). Plasma clusterin and the risk of Alzheimer disease. *JAMA* 305: 1322–1326.

103 Thambisetty, M., Simmons, A., Velayudhan, L. et al. (2010). Association of plasma clusterin concentration with severity, pathology, and progression in Alzheimer disease. *Arch. Gen. Psychiatry* 67: 739–748.

104 Schurmann, B., Wiese, B., Bickel, H. et al. (2011). Association of the Alzheimer's disease clusterin risk allele with plasma clusterin concentration. *J. Alzheimers Dis.* 25: 421–424.

105 Xing, Y.Y., Yu, J.T., Cui, W.Z. et al. (2012). Blood clusterin levels, rs9331888 polymorphism, and the risk of Alzheimer's disease. *J. Alzheimers Dis.* 29: 515–519.

106 Du, W., Tan, J., Xu, W. et al. (2016). Association between clusterin gene polymorphism rs11136000 and late-onset Alzheimer's disease susceptibility: A review and meta-analysis of case-control studies. *Exp. Ther. Med.* 12: 2915–2927.

107 Tan, L., Wang, H.F., Tan, M.S. et al., Alzheimer's Disease Neuroimaging I (2016). Effect of CLU genetic variants on cerebrospinal fluid and neuroimaging markers in healthy, mild cognitive impairment and Alzheimer's disease cohorts. *Sci. Rep.* 6: 26027.

108 Qiu, L., He, Y., Tang, H. et al. (2016). Genetically-mediated grey and white matter alteration in normal elderly individuals with the CLU-C allele gene. *Curr. Alzheimer Res.* 13: 1302–1310.

109 Shuai, P., Liu, Y., Lu, W. et al. (2015). Genetic associations of CLU rs9331888 polymorphism with Alzheimer's disease: A meta-analysis. *Neurosci. Lett.* 591: 160–165.

110 May, P.C., Lampert-Etchells, M., Johnson, S.A. et al. (1990). Dynamics of gene expression for a hippocampal glycoprotein elevated in Alzheimer's disease and in response to experimental lesions in rat. *Neuron* 5: 831–839.

111 Calero, M., Rostagno, A., Matsubara, E. et al. (2000). Apolipoprotein J (clusterin) and Alzheimer's disease. *Microsc. Res. Tech.* 50: 305–315.

112 Karch, C.M., Jeng, A.T., Nowotny, P. et al. (2012). Expression of novel Alzheimer's disease risk genes in control and Alzheimer's disease brains. *PLoS One* 7: e50976.

113 Allen, M., Zou, F., Chai, H.S. et al., Alzheimer's Disease Genetics C (2012). Novel late-onset Alzheimer disease loci variants associate with brain gene expression. *Neurology* 79: 221–228.

114 Wu, Z.C., Yu, J.T., Li, Y., and Tan, L. (2012). Clusterin in Alzheimer's disease. *Adv. Clin. Chem.* 56: 155–173.

115 Ghiso, J., Matsubara, E., Koudinov, A. et al. (1993). The cerebrospinal-fluid soluble form of Alzheimer's amyloid beta is complexed to SP-40,40 (apolipoprotein J), an inhibitor of the complement membrane-attack complex. *Biochem. J.* 293 (Pt 1): 27–30.

116 Matsubara, E., Frangione, B., and Ghiso, J. (1995). Characterization of apolipoprotein J-Alzheimer's A beta interaction. *J Biol Chem* 270: 7563–7567.

117 Oda, T., Wals, P., Osterburg, H.H. et al. (1995). Clusterin (apoJ) alters the aggregation of amyloid beta-peptide (A beta 1-42) and forms slowly sedimenting A beta complexes that cause oxidative stress. *Exp. Neurol.* 136: 22–31.

118 Matsubara, E., Soto, C., Governale, S. et al. (1996). Apolipoprotein J and Alzheimer's amyloid beta solubility. *Biochem. J* 316 (Pt 2): 671–679.

119 DeMattos, R.B., O'Dell, M.A., Parsadanian, M. et al. (2002). Clusterin promotes amyloid plaque formation and is critical for neuritic toxicity in a mouse model of Alzheimer's disease. *Proc. Natl. Acad. Sci. U.S.A.* 99: 10843–10848.

120 DeMattos, R.B., Cirrito, J.R., Parsadanian, M. et al. (2004). ApoE and clusterin cooperatively suppress Abeta levels and deposition: evidence that ApoE regulates extracellular Abeta metabolism in vivo. *Neuron* 41: 193–202.

121 Zhang, H., Kim, J.K., Edwards, C.A. et al. (2005). Clusterin inhibits apoptosis by interacting with activated Bax. *Nat. Cell Biol.* 7: 909–915.

122 Baralla, A., Sotgiu, E., Deiana, M. et al. (2015). Plasma clusterin and lipid profile: a link with aging and cardiovascular diseases in a population with a consistent number of centenarians. *PLoS One* 10: e0128029.

123 Voruganti, V.S., Cole, S.A., Ebbesson, S.O. et al. (2010). Genetic variation in APOJ, LPL, and TNFRSF10B affects plasma fatty acid distribution in Alaskan Eskimos. *Am. J. Clin. Nutr.* 91: 1574–1583.

124 Kaminski, W.E., Piehler, A., and Schmitz, G. (2000). Genomic organization of the human cholesterol-responsive ABC transporter ABCA7: tandem linkage with the minor histocompatibility antigen HA-1 gene. *Biochem. Biophys. Res. Commun.* 278: 782–789.

125 Kim, W.S., Li, H., Ruberu, K. et al. (2013). Deletion of Abca7 increases cerebral amyloid-beta accumulation in the J20 mouse model of Alzheimer's disease. *J. Neurosci.* 33: 4387–4394.

126 Ikeda, Y., Abe-Dohmae, S., Munehira, Y. et al. (2003). Posttranscriptional regulation of human ABCA7 and its function for the apoA-I-dependent lipid release. *Biochem. Biophys. Res. Commun.* 311: 313–318.

127 Kim, W.S., Guillemin, G.J., Glaros, E.N. et al. (2006). Quantitation of ATP-binding cassette subfamily-A transporter gene expression in primary human brain cells. *Neuroreport* 17: 891–896.

128 Vasquez, J.B., Simpson, J.F., Harpole, R., and Estus, S. (2017). Alzheimer's disease genetics and ABCA7 splicing. *J. Alzheimers Dis.* 59: 633–641.

129 Vasquez, J.B., Fardo, D.W., and Estus, S. (2013). ABCA7 expression is associated with Alzheimer's disease polymorphism and disease status. *Neurosci. Lett.* 556: 58–62.

130 Jehle, A.W., Gardai, S.J., Li, S. et al. (2006). ATP-binding cassette transporter A7 enhances phagocytosis of apoptotic cells and associated ERK signaling in macrophages. *J. Cell Biol.* 174: 547–556.

131 Tanaka, N., Abe-Dohmae, S., Iwamoto, N. et al. (2011). HMG-CoA reductase inhibitors enhance phagocytosis by upregulating ATP-binding cassette transporter A7. *Atherosclerosis* 217: 407–414.

132 Chan, S.L., Kim, W.S., Kwok, J.B. et al. (2008). ATP-binding cassette transporter A7 regulates processing of amyloid precursor protein in vitro. *J. Neurochem.* 106: 793–804.

133 Cukier, H.N., Kunkle, B.W., Vardarajan, B.N. et al. Alzheimer's Disease Genetics C (2016). ABCA7 frameshift deletion associated with Alzheimer disease in African Americans. *Neurol. Genet.* 2: e79.

134 Allen, M., Lincoln, S.J., Corda, M. et al. (2017). ABCA7 loss-of-function variants, expression, and neurologic disease risk. *Neurol. Genet.* 3: e126.

135 Nuytemans, K., Maldonado, L., Ali, A. et al. (2016). Overlap between Parkinson disease and Alzheimer disease in ABCA7 functional variants. *Neurol. Genet.* 2: e44.

136 Kim, W.S., Fitzgerald, M.L., Kang, K. et al. (2005). Abca7 null mice retain normal macrophage phosphatidylcholine and cholesterol efflux activity despite alterations in adipose mass and serum cholesterol levels. *J. Biol. Chem.* 280: 3989–3995.

137 Kim, W.S., Weickert, C.S., and Garner, B. (2008). Role of ATP-binding cassette transporters in brain lipid transport and neurological disease. *J. Neurochem.* 104: 1145–1166.

138 Crehan, H., Holton, P., Wray, S. et al. (2012). Complement receptor 1 (CR1) and Alzheimer's disease. *Immunobiology* 217: 244–250.

139 Brouwers, N., Van Cauwenberghe, C., Engelborghs, S. et al. (2012). Alzheimer risk associated with a copy number variation in the complement receptor 1 increasing C3b/C4b binding sites. *Mol. Psychiatry* 17: 223–233.

140 Liu, D. and Niu, Z.X. (2009). The structure, genetic polymorphisms, expression and biological functions of complement receptor type 1 (CR1/CD35). *Immunopharmacol. Immunotoxicol.* 31: 524–535.

141 Krych-Goldberg, M., Moulds, J.M., and Atkinson, J.P. (2002). Human complement receptor type 1 (CR1) binds to a major malarial adhesin. *Trends Mol. Med.* 8: 531–537.

142 Khera, R. and Das, N. (2009). Complement receptor 1: disease associations and therapeutic implications. *Mol. Immunol.* 46: 761–772.

143 Schjeide, B.M., Schnack, C., Lambert, J.C. et al. (2011). The role of clusterin, complement receptor 1, and phosphatidylinositol binding clathrin assembly protein in Alzheimer disease risk and cerebrospinal fluid biomarker levels. *Arch. Gen. Psychiatry* 68: 207–213.

144 Biffi, A., Anderson, C.D., Desikan, R.S. et al. Alzheimer's Disease Neuroimaging I (2010). Genetic variation and neuroimaging measures in Alzheimer disease. *Arch. Neurol.* 67: 677–685.

145 Chibnik, L.B., Shulman, J.M., Leurgans, S.E. et al. (2011). CR1 is associated with amyloid plaque burden and age-related cognitive decline. *Ann. Neurol.* 69: 560–569.

146 Barral, S., Bird, T., Goate, A. et al. National Institute on Aging Late-Onset Alzheimer's Disease Genetics S (2012). Genotype patterns at PICALM, CR1, BIN1, CLU, and APOE genes are associated with episodic memory. *Neurology* 78: 1464–1471.

147 Terai, K., Walker, D.G., McGeer, E.G., and McGeer, P.L. (1997). Neurons express proteins of the classical complement pathway in Alzheimer disease. *Brain Res.* 769: 385–390.

148 Gasque, P., Ischenko, A., Legoedec, J. et al. (1993). Expression of the complement classical pathway by human glioma in culture: a model for complement expression by nerve cells. *J. Biol. Chem.* 268: 25068–25074.

149 Hosokawa, M., Klegeris, A., Maguire, J., and McGeer, P.L. (2003). Expression of complement messenger RNAs and proteins by human oligodendroglial cells. *Glia* 42: 417–423.

150 Eikelenboom, P. and Stam, F.C. (1982). Immunoglobulins and complement factors in senile plaques: an immunoperoxidase study. *Acta Neuropathol.* 57: 239–242.

151 McGeer, P.L., Akiyama, H., Itagaki, S., and McGeer, E.G. (1989). Activation of the classical complement pathway in brain tissue of Alzheimer patients. *Neurosci. Lett.* 107: 341–346.

152 Shen, Y., Lue, L., Yang, L. et al. (2001). Complement activation by neurofibrillary tangles in Alzheimer's disease. *Neurosci. Lett.* 305: 165–168.

153 Velazquez, P., Cribbs, D.H., Poulos, T.L., and Tenner, A.J. (1997). Aspartate residue 7 in amyloid beta-protein is critical for classical complement pathway activation: implications for Alzheimer's disease pathogenesis. *Nat. Med.* 3: 77–79.

154 Fonseca, M.I., Chu, S., Pierce, A.L. et al. (2016). Analysis of the putative role of CR1 in Alzheimer's disease: genetic association, expression and function. *PLoS One* 11: e0149792.

155 Mahmoudi, R., Kisserli, A., Novella, J.L. et al. (2015). Alzheimer's disease is associated with low density of the long CR1 isoform. *Neurobiol. Aging* 36 (1766): e1765–e1712.

156 Malik, M., Simpson, J.F., Parikh, I. et al. (2013). CD33 Alzheimer's risk-altering polymorphism, CD33 expression, and exon 2 splicing. *J. Neurosci.* 33: 13320–13325.

157 Griciuc, A., Serrano-Pozo, A., Parrado, A.R. et al. (2013). Alzheimer's disease risk gene CD33 inhibits microglial uptake of amyloid beta. *Neuron* 78: 631–643.

158 Bradshaw, E.M., Chibnik, L.B., Keenan, B.T. et al., Alzheimer Disease Neuroimaging I (2013). CD33 Alzheimer's disease locus: altered monocyte function and amyloid biology. *Nat. Neurosci.* 16: 848–850.

159 Crocker, P.R. (2002). Siglecs: sialic-acid-binding immunoglobulin-like lectins in cell-cell interactions and signalling. *Curr. Opin. Struct. Biol.* 12: 609–615.

160 Crocker, P.R., Hartnell, A., Munday, J., and Nath, D. (1997). The potential role of sialoadhesin as a macrophage recognition molecule in health and disease. *Glycoconjugate J.* 14: 601–609.

161 Raj, T., Ryan, K.J., Replogle, J.M. et al. (2014). CD33: increased inclusion of exon 2 implicates the Ig V-set domain in Alzheimer's disease susceptibility. *Hum. Mol. Genet.* 23: 2729–2736.

162 Tateno, H., Li, H., Schur, M.J. et al. (2007). Distinct endocytic mechanisms of CD22 (Siglec-2) and Siglec-F reflect roles in cell signaling and innate immunity. *Mol. Cell. Biol.* 27: 5699–5710.

163 Linnartz, B. and Neumann, H. (2013). Microglial activatory (immunoreceptor tyrosine-based activation motif)- and inhibitory (immunoreceptor tyrosine-based inhibition motif)-signaling receptors for recognition of the neuronal glycocalyx. *Glia* 61: 37–46.

164 Mhatre, S.D., Tsai, C.A., Rubin, A.J. et al. (2015). Microglial malfunction: the third rail in the development of Alzheimer's disease. *Trends Neurosci.* 38: 621–636.

165 Ishibashi, K., Suzuki, M., Sasaki, S., and Imai, M. (2001). Identification of a new multigene four-transmembrane family (MS4A) related to CD20, HTm4 and beta subunit of the high-affinity IgE receptor. *Gene* 264: 87–93.

166 Howie, D., Nolan, K.F., Daley, S. et al. (2009). MS4A4B is a GITR-associated membrane adapter, expressed by regulatory T cells, which modulates T cell activation. *J. Immunol.* 183: 4197–4204.

167 Zuccolo, J., Bau, J., Childs, S.J. et al. (2010). Phylogenetic analysis of the MS4A and TMEM176 gene families. *PLoS One* 5: e9369.

168 Seshadri, S., Fitzpatrick, A.L., Ikram, M.A. et al. (2010). Genome-wide analysis of genetic loci associated with Alzheimer disease. *JAMA* 303: 1832–1840.

169 Antunez, C., Boada, M., Gonzalez-Perez, A. et al. (2011). The membrane-spanning 4-domains, subfamily A (MS4A) gene cluster contains a common variant associated with Alzheimer's disease. *Genome Med.* 3: 33.

170 Giri, M., Zhang, M., and Lu, Y. (2016). Genes associated with Alzheimer's disease: an overview and current status. *Clin. Interv. Aging* 11: 665–681.

171 Kofler, J., Bissel, S., Wiley, C. et al. (2012). Differential microglial expression of new Alzheimer's disease associated genes MS4A4A and MS4A6A. *Alzheimers Dement* 8: 253.

172 Bianchin, M.M., Capella, H.M., Chaves, D.L. et al. (2004). Nasu-Hakola disease (polycystic lipomembranous osteodysplasia with sclerosing leukoencephalopathy – PLOSL): a dementia associated with bone cystic lesions. From clinical to genetic and molecular aspects. *Cell Mol. Neurobiol.* 24: 1–24.

173 Paloneva, J., Manninen, T., Christman, G. et al. (2002). Mutations in two genes encoding different subunits of a receptor signaling complex result in an identical disease phenotype. *Am. J. Hum. Genet.* 71: 656–662.

174 Bock, V., Botturi, A., Gaviani, P. et al. (2013). Polycystic lipomembranous osteodysplasia with sclerosing leukoencephalopathy (PLOSL): a new report of an Italian woman and review of the literature. *J. Neurol. Sci.* 326: 115–119.

175 Madry, H., Prudlo, J., Grgic, A., and Freyschmidt, J. (2007). Nasu-Hakola disease (PLOSL): report of five cases and review of the literature. *Clin. Orthop. Relat. Res.* 454: 262–269.

176 Neumann, H. and Takahashi, K. (2007). Essential role of the microglial triggering receptor expressed on myeloid cells-2 (TREM2) for central nervous tissue immune homeostasis. *J. Neuroimmunol.* 184: 92–99.

177 Paloneva, J., Autti, T., Hakola, P., and Haltia, M.J. (1993). Polycystic lipomembranous osteodysplasia with sclerosing leukoencephalopathy (PLOSL). In: *GeneReviews(R)* (ed. R.A. Pagon, M.P. Adam, H.H. Ardinger, et al.). Seattle (WA).

178 Benitez, B.A., Cooper, B., Pastor, P. et al. (2013). TREM2 is associated with the risk of Alzheimer's disease in Spanish population. *Neurobiol. Aging* 34: 1711 e1715–1711 e1717.

179 Hooli, B.V., Parrado, A.R., Mullin, K. et al. (2014). The rare TREM2 R47H variant exerts only a modest effect on Alzheimer disease risk. *Neurology* 83: 1353–1358.

180 Pottier, C., Wallon, D., Rousseau, S. et al. (2013). TREM2 R47H variant as a risk factor for early-onset Alzheimer's disease. *J. Alzheimers Dis.* 35: 45–49.

181 Benitez, B.A. and Cruchaga, C., United States-Spain Parkinson's Disease Research G. (2013). TREM2 and neurodegenerative disease. *N. Engl. J. Med.* 369: 1567–1568.

182 Bertram, L., Parrado, A.R., and Tanzi, R.E. (2013). TREM2 and neurodegenerative disease. *N. Engl. J. Med.* 369: 1565.

183 Giraldo, M., Lopera, F., Siniard, A.L. et al. (2013). Variants in triggering receptor expressed on myeloid cells 2 are associated with both behavioral variant frontotemporal lobar degeneration and Alzheimer's disease. *Neurobiol. Aging* 34 (2077): e2011–e2078.

184 Guerreiro, R. and Hardy, J. (2013). TREM2 and neurodegenerative disease. *N. Engl. J. Med.* 369: 1569–1570.

185 Rajagopalan, P., Hibar, D.P., and Thompson, P.M. (2013). TREM2 and neurodegenerative disease. *N. Engl. J. Med.* 369: 1565–1567.

186 Cruchaga, C., Kauwe, J.S., Harari, O. et al. (2013). GWAS of cerebrospinal fluid tau levels identifies risk variants for Alzheimer's disease. *Neuron* 78: 256–268.

187 Guerreiro, R.J., Lohmann, E., Bras, J.M. et al. (2013). Using exome sequencing to reveal mutations in TREM2 presenting as a frontotemporal dementia-like syndrome without bone involvement. *JAMA Neurol.* 70: 78–84.

188 Rayaprolu, S., Mullen, B., Baker, M. et al. (2013). TREM2 in neurodegeneration: evidence for association of the p.R47H variant with frontotemporal dementia and Parkinson's disease. *Mol. Neurodegener.* 8: 19.

189 Cady, J., Koval, E.D., Benitez, B.A. et al. (2014). TREM2 variant p.R47H as a risk factor for sporadic amyotrophic lateral sclerosis. *JAMA Neurol.* 71: 449–453.

190 Rohn, T.T. (2013). The triggering receptor expressed on myeloid cells 2: 'TREM-ming' the inflammatory component associated with Alzheimer's disease. *Oxid. Med. Cell Longev.* 2013: 860959.

191 Golde, T.E., Streit, W.J., and Chakrabarty, P. (2013). Alzheimer's disease risk alleles in TREM2 illuminate innate immunity in Alzheimer's disease. *Alzheimers Res. Ther.* 5: 24.

192 Hickman, S.E. and El Khoury, J. (2014). TREM2 and the neuroimmunology of Alzheimer's disease. *Biochem. Pharmacol.* 88: 495–498.

193 Hsieh, C.L., Koike, M., Spusta, S.C. et al. (2009). A role for TREM2 ligands in the phagocytosis of apoptotic neuronal cells by microglia. *J. Neurochem.* 109: 1144–1156.

194 Zheng, H., Jia, L., Liu, C.C. et al. (2017). TREM2 promotes microglial survival by activating Wnt/beta-catenin pathway. *J. Neurosci.* 37: 1772–1784.

195 Liao, F., Yoon, H., and Kim, J. (2017). Apolipoprotein E metabolism and functions in brain and its role in Alzheimer's disease. *Curr. Opin. Lipidol.* 28: 60–67.

196 Trowsdale, J. and Knight, J.C. (2013). Major histocompatibility complex genomics and human disease. *Annu. Rev. Genomics Hum. Genet.* 14: 301–323.

197 Cree, B.A. (2014). Multiple sclerosis genetics. *Handb. Clin. Neurol.* 122: 193–209.

198 International Multiple Sclerosis Genetics C, Wellcome Trust Case Control C, Sawcer, S. et al. (2011). Genetic risk and a primary role for cell-mediated immune mechanisms in multiple sclerosis. *Nature* 476: 214–219.

199 Hauser, S.L., Chan, J.R., and Oksenberg, J.R. (2013). Multiple sclerosis: prospects and promise. *Ann. Neurol.* 74: 317–327.

200 Ferrari, R., Hernandez, D.G., Nalls, M.A. et al. (2014). Frontotemporal dementia and its subtypes: a genome-wide association study. *Lancet Neurol.* 13: 686–699.

201 Hamza, T.H., Zabetian, C.P., Tenesa, A. et al. (2010). Common genetic variation in the HLA region is associated with late-onset sporadic Parkinson's disease. *Nat. Genet.* 42: 781–785.

202 Ahmed, I., Tamouza, R., Delord, M. et al. (2012). Association between Parkinson's disease and the HLA-DRB1 locus. *Mov. Disord.* 27: 1104–1110.

203 Sun, C., Wei, L., Luo, F. et al. (2012). HLA-DRB1 alleles are associated with the susceptibility to sporadic Parkinson's disease in Chinese Han population. *PLoS One* 7: e48594.

204 Nalls, M.A., Pankratz, N., Lill, C.M. et al. (2014). Large-scale meta-analysis of genome-wide association data identifies six new risk loci for Parkinson's disease. *Nat. Genet.* 46: 989–993.

205 Wissemann, W.T., Hill-Burns, E.M., Zabetian, C.P. et al. (2013). Association of Parkinson disease with structural and regulatory variants in the HLA region. *Am. J. Hum. Genet.* 93: 984–993.

206 Kim, K., Bang, S.Y., Yoo, D.H. et al. (2016). Imputing variants in HLA-DR beta genes reveals that HLA-DRB1 is solely associated with rheumatoid arthritis and systemic lupus erythematosus. *PLoS One* 11: e0150283.

207 Zhao, L.P., Alshiekh, S., Zhao, M. et al., Better Diabetes Diagnosis Study G (2016). Next-Generation Sequencing Reveals That HLA-DRB3, -DRB4, and -DRB5 May Be Associated With Islet Autoantibodies and Risk for Childhood Type 1 Diabetes. *Diabetes* 65: 710–718.

208 Henschke, P.J., Bell, D.A., and Cape, R.D. (1978). Alzheimer's disease and HLA. *Tissue Antigens* 12: 132–135.

209 Mansouri, L., Messalmani, M., Klai, S. et al. (2015). Association of HLA-DR/DQ polymorphism with Alzheimer's disease. *Am. J. Med. Sci.* 349: 334–337.

210 Chauhan, G., Adams, H.H., Bis, J.C. et al. (2015). Association of Alzheimer's disease GWAS loci with MRI markers of brain aging. *Neurobiol. Aging* 36 (1765): e1767–e1716.

211 Yu, L., Chibnik, L.B., Srivastava, G.P. et al. (2015). Association of Brain DNA methylation in SORL1, ABCA7, HLA-DRB5, SLC24A4, and BIN1 with pathological diagnosis of Alzheimer disease. *JAMA Neurol.* 72: 15–24.

212 Ruiz, A., Heilmann, S., Becker, T. et al. (2014). Follow-up of loci from the International Genomics of Alzheimer's Disease Project identifies TRIP4 as a novel susceptibility gene. *Transl. Psychiatry* 4: e358.

213 Metzner, A., Precht, C., Fehse, B. et al. (2009). Reduced proliferation of CD34(+) cells from patients with acute myeloid leukemia after gene transfer of INPP5D. *Gene Ther.* 16: 570–573.

214 Srivastava, N., Sudan, R., and Kerr, W.G. (2013). Role of inositol poly-phosphatases and their targets in T cell biology. *Front Immunol.* 4: 288.

215 Kalesnikoff, J., Lam, V., and Krystal, G. (2002). SHIP represses mast cell activation and reveals that IgE alone triggers signaling pathways which enhance normal mast cell survival. *Mol. Immunol.* 38: 1201–1206.

216 Kalesnikoff, J., Baur, N., Leitges, M. et al. (2002). SHIP negatively regulates IgE + antigen-induced IL-6 production in mast cells by inhibiting NF-kappa B activity. *J. Immunol.* 168: 4737–4746.

217 Kim, C.H., Hangoc, G., Cooper, S. et al. (1999). Altered responsiveness to chemokines due to targeted disruption of SHIP. *J. Clin. Invest.* 104: 1751–1759.

218 Sly, L.M., Rauh, M.J., Kalesnikoff, J. et al. (2003). SHIP, SHIP2, and PTEN activities are regulated in vivo by modulation of their protein levels: SHIP is up-regulated in macrophages and mast cells by lipopolysaccharide. *Exp. Hematol.* 31: 1170–1181.

219 Sly, L.M., Ho, V., Antignano, F. et al. (2007). The role of SHIP in macrophages. *Front Biosci.* 12: 2836–2848.

220 Bao, M., Hanabuchi, S., Facchinetti, V. et al. (2012). CD2AP/SHIP1 complex positively regulates plasmacytoid dendritic cell receptor signaling by inhibiting the E3 ubiquitin ligase Cbl. *J. Immunol.* 189: 786–792.

221 Khiem, D., Cyster, J.G., Schwarz, J.J., and Black, B.L. (2008). A p38 MAPK-MEF2C pathway regulates B-cell proliferation. *Proc. Natl. Acad. Sci. U.S.A.* 105: 17067–17072.

222 Xu, Z., Yoshida, T., Wu, L. et al. (2015). Transcription factor MEF2C suppresses endothelial cell inflammation via regulation of NF-kappaB and KLF2. *J. Cell. Physiol.* 230: 1310–1320.

223 Tang, S.S., Wang, H.F., Zhang, W. et al. (2016). MEF2C rs190982 polymorphism with late-onset Alzheimer's disease in Han Chinese: a replication study and meta-analyses. *Oncotarget* 7: 39136–39142.

224 Janson, C.G., Chen, Y., Li, Y., and Leifer, D. (2001). Functional regulatory regions of human transcription factor MEF2C. *Brain Res. Mol. Brain Res.* 97: 70–82.
225 Potthoff, M.J. and Olson, E.N. (2007). MEF2: a central regulator of diverse developmental programs. *Development* 134: 4131–4140.
226 Akhtar, M.W., Kim, M.S., Adachi, M. et al. (2012). In vivo analysis of MEF2 transcription factors in synapse regulation and neuronal survival. *PLoS One* 7: e34863.
227 Ren, G., Vajjhala, P., Lee, J.S. et al. (2006). The BAR domain proteins: molding membranes in fission, fusion, and phagy. *Microbiol. Mol. Biol. Rev.* 70: 37–120.
228 Tan, M.S., Yu, J.T., and Tan, L. (2013). Bridging integrator 1 (BIN1): form, function, and Alzheimer's disease. *Trends Mol. Med.* 19: 594–603.
229 Taylor, M.J., Perrais, D., and Merrifield, C.J. (2011). A high precision survey of the molecular dynamics of mammalian clathrin-mediated endocytosis. *PLoS Biol.* 9: e1000604.
230 Wigge, P. and McMahon, H.T. (1998). The amphiphysin family of proteins and their role in endocytosis at the synapse. *Trends Neurosci.* 21: 339–344.
231 McMahon, H.T., Wigge, P., and Smith, C. (1997). Clathrin interacts specifically with amphiphysin and is displaced by dynamin. *FEBS Lett.* 413: 319–322.
232 Ramjaun, A.R. and McPherson, P.S. (1998). Multiple amphiphysin II splice variants display differential clathrin binding: identification of two distinct clathrin-binding sites. *J. Neurochem.* 70: 2369–2376.
233 De Rossi, P., Buggia-Prevot, V., Clayton, B.L. et al. (2016). Predominant expression of Alzheimer's disease-associated BIN1 in mature oligodendrocytes and localization to white matter tracts. *Mol. Neurodegener.* 11: 59.
234 Kamboh, M.I., Demirci, F.Y., Wang, X. et al., Alzheimer's Disease Neuroimaging I (2012). Genome-wide association study of Alzheimer's disease. *Transl. Psychiatry* 2: e117.
235 Carrasquillo, M.M., Belbin, O., Hunter, T.A. et al. (2011). Replication of BIN1 association with Alzheimer's disease and evaluation of genetic interactions. *J. Alzheimers Dis.* 24: 751–758.
236 Lambert, J.C., Zelenika, D., Hiltunen, M. et al. (2011). Evidence of the association of BIN1 and PICALM with the AD risk in contrasting European populations. *Neurobiol. Aging* 32 (756): e711–e755.
237 Chapuis, J., Hansmannel, F., Gistelinck, M. et al. (2013). Increased expression of BIN1 mediates Alzheimer genetic risk by modulating tau pathology. *Mol. Psychiatry* 18: 1225–1234.
238 Yang, S., Liu, T., Li, S. et al. (2008). Comparative proteomic analysis of brains of naturally aging mice. *Neuroscience* 154: 1107–1120.
239 Meunier, B., Quaranta, M., Daviet, L. et al. (2009). The membrane-tubulating potential of amphiphysin 2/BIN1 is dependent on the microtubule-binding cytoplasmic linker protein 170 (CLIP-170). *Eur. J. Cell Biol.* 88: 91–102.
240 De Rossi, P., Buggia-Prevot, V., Andrew, R. et al. (2017). BIN1 localization is distinct from tau tangles in Alzheimer's disease. *Matters* https://doi.org/10.19185/matters.201611000018.
241 Di Paolo, G., Sankaranarayanan, S., Wenk, M.R. et al. (2002). Decreased synaptic vesicle recycling efficiency and cognitive deficits in amphiphysin 1 knockout mice. *Neuron* 33: 789–804.

242 Pant, S., Sharma, M., Patel, K. et al. (2009). AMPH-1/Amphiphysin/Bin1 functions with RME-1/Ehd1 in endocytic recycling. *Nat. Cell Biol.* 11: 1399–1410.

243 Leprince, C., Le Scolan, E., Meunier, B. et al. (2003). Sorting nexin 4 and amphiphysin 2, a new partnership between endocytosis and intracellular trafficking. *J. Cell Sci.* 116: 1937–1948.

244 Miyagawa, T., Ebinuma, I., Morohashi, Y. et al. (2016). BIN1 regulates BACE1 intracellular trafficking and amyloid-beta production. *Hum. Mol. Genet.* 25: 2948–2958.

245 Ubelmann, F., Burrinha, T., Salavessa, L. et al. (2017). Bin1 and CD2AP polarise the endocytic generation of beta-amyloid. *EMBO Rep.* 18: 102–122.

246 Calafate, S., Flavin, W., Verstreken, P., and Moechars, D. (2016). Loss of Bin1 promotes the propagation of tau pathology. *Cell Rep.* 17: 931–940.

247 Baig, S., Joseph, S.A., Tayler, H. et al. (2010). Distribution and expression of picalm in Alzheimer disease. *J. Neuropathol. Exp. Neurol.* 69: 1071–1077.

248 Harel, A., Wu, F., Mattson, M.P. et al. (2008). Evidence for CALM in directing VAMP2 trafficking. *Traffic* 9: 417–429.

249 Zhang, B., Koh, Y.H., Beckstead, R.B. et al. (1998). Synaptic vesicle size and number are regulated by a clathrin adaptor protein required for endocytosis. *Neuron* 21: 1465–1475.

250 Wendland, B., Emr, S.D., and Riezman, H. (1998). Protein traffic in the yeast endocytic and vacuolar protein sorting pathways. *Curr. Opin. Cell Biol.* 10: 513–522.

251 Duce, J.A., Tsatsanis, A., Cater, M.A. et al. (2010). Iron-export ferroxidase activity of beta-amyloid precursor protein is inhibited by zinc in Alzheimer's disease. *Cell* 142: 857–867.

252 Xiao, Q., Gil, S.C., Yan, P. et al. (2012). Role of phosphatidylinositol clathrin assembly lymphoid-myeloid leukemia (PICALM) in intracellular amyloid precursor protein (APP) processing and amyloid plaque pathogenesis. *J. Biol. Chem.* 287: 21279–21289.

253 Parikh, I., Fardo, D.W., and Estus, S. (2014). Genetics of PICALM expression and Alzheimer's disease. *PLoS One* 9: e91242.

254 Tian, Y., Chang, J.C., Fan, E.Y. et al. (2013). Adaptor complex AP2/PICALM, through interaction with LC3, targets Alzheimer's APP-CTF for terminal degradation via autophagy. *Proc. Natl. Acad. Sci. U.S.A.* 110: 17071–17076.

255 Moreau, K., Fleming, A., Imarisio, S. et al. (2014). PICALM modulates autophagy activity and tau accumulation. *Nat. Commun.* 5: 4998.

256 Mercer, J.L., Argus, J.P., Crabtree, D.M. et al. (2015). Modulation of PICALM levels perturbs cellular cholesterol homeostasis. *PLoS One* 10: e0129776.

257 Thomas, R.S., Henson, A., Gerrish, A. et al. (2016). Decreasing the expression of PICALM reduces endocytosis and the activity of beta-secretase: implications for Alzheimer's disease. *BMC Neurosci.* 17: 50.

258 Treusch, S., Hamamichi, S., Goodman, J.L. et al. (2011). Functional links between Abeta toxicity, endocytic trafficking, and Alzheimer's disease risk factors in yeast. *Science* 334: 1241–1245.

259 Ponomareva, N.V., Andreeva, T.V., Protasova, M.S. et al. (2017). Quantitative EEG during normal aging: association with the Alzheimer's disease genetic risk variant in PICALM gene. *Neurobiol. Aging* 51: 177 e171–177 e178.

260 Liu, Z., Dai, X., Zhang, J. et al. (2018). The interactive effects of age and PICALM rs541458 polymorphism on cognitive performance, brain structure, and function in non-demented elderly. *Mol. Neurobiol.* .

261 Dustin, M.L., Olszowy, M.W., Holdorf, A.D. et al. (1998). A novel adaptor protein orchestrates receptor patterning and cytoskeletal polarity in T-cell contacts. *Cell* 94: 667–677.

262 Liao, F., Jiang, H., Srivatsan, S. et al. (2015). Effects of CD2-associated protein deficiency on amyloid-beta in neuroblastoma cells and in an APP transgenic mouse model. *Mol. Neurodegener.* 10: 12.

263 Adams, H.H., de Bruijn, R.F., Hofman, A. et al. (2015). Genetic risk of neurodegenerative diseases is associated with mild cognitive impairment and conversion to dementia. *Alzheimers Dement* 11: 1277–1285.

264 Shulman, J.M., Chen, K., Keenan, B.T. et al. (2013). Genetic susceptibility for Alzheimer disease neuritic plaque pathology. *JAMA Neurol.* 70: 1150–1157.

265 Cormont, M., Meton, I., Mari, M. et al. (2003). CD2AP/CMS regulates endosome morphology and traffic to the degradative pathway through its interaction with Rab4 and c-Cbl. *Traffic* 4: 97–112.

266 Lee, J.H., Cheng, R., Honig, L.S. et al. (2008). Association between genetic variants in SORL1 and autopsy-confirmed Alzheimer disease. *Neurology* 70: 887–889.

267 Rogaeva, E., Meng, Y., Lee, J.H. et al. (2007). The neuronal sortilin-related receptor SORL1 is genetically associated with Alzheimer disease. *Nat. Genet.* 39: 168–177.

268 Bettens, K., Brouwers, N., Engelborghs, S. et al. (2008). SORL1 is genetically associated with increased risk for late-onset Alzheimer disease in the Belgian population. *Hum. Mutat.* 29: 769–770.

269 Miyashita, A., Koike, A., Jun, G. et al. (2013). SORL1 is genetically associated with late-onset Alzheimer's disease in Japanese, Koreans and Caucasians. *PLoS One* 8: e58618.

270 Wen, Y., Miyashita, A., Kitamura, N. et al. (2013). SORL1 is genetically associated with neuropathologically characterized late-onset Alzheimer's disease. *J. Alzheimers Dis.* 35: 387–394.

271 Reitz, C., Cheng, R., Rogaeva, E. et al. Genetic, Environmental Risk in Alzheimer Disease C(2011). Meta-analysis of the association between variants in SORL1 and Alzheimer disease. *Arch. Neurol.* 68: 99–106.

272 Vardarajan, B.N., Zhang, Y., Lee, J.H. et al. (2015). Coding mutations in SORL1 and Alzheimer disease. *Ann. Neurol.* 77: 215–227.

273 Taira, K., Bujo, H., Hirayama, S. et al. (2001). LR11, a mosaic LDL receptor family member, mediates the uptake of ApoE-rich lipoproteins in vitro. *Arterioscler Thromb. Vasc. Biol.* 21: 1501–1506.

274 Yamazaki, H., Bujo, H., Kusunoki, J. et al. (1996). Elements of neural adhesion molecules and a yeast vacuolar protein sorting receptor are present in a novel mammalian low density lipoprotein receptor family member. *J. Biol. Chem.* 271: 24761–24768.

275 Schmidt, V., Sporbert, A., Rohe, M. et al. (2007). SorLA/LR11 regulates processing of amyloid precursor protein via interaction with adaptors GGA and PACS-1. *J. Biol. Chem.* 282: 32956–32964.

276 Yin, R.H., Yu, J.T., and Tan, L. (2015). The role of SORL1 in Alzheimer's disease. *Mol. Neurobiol.* 51: 909–918.

277 Dodson, S.E., Andersen, O.M., Karmali, V. et al. (2008). Loss of LR11/SORLA enhances early pathology in a mouse model of amyloidosis: evidence for a proximal role in Alzheimer's disease. *J. Neurosci.* 28: 12877–12886.

278 Sager, K.L., Wuu, J., Leurgans, S.E. et al. (2007). Neuronal LR11/sorLA expression is reduced in mild cognitive impairment. *Ann. Neurol.* 62: 640–647.

279 Louwersheimer, E., Ramirez, A., Cruchaga, C. et al., Alzheimer's Disease Neuroimaging I, Dementia Competence N (2015). Influence of genetic variants in SORL1 gene on the manifestation of Alzheimer's disease. *Neurobiol. Aging* 36 (1605): e1613–e1620.

280 Andersen, O.M., Rudolph, I.M., and Willnow, T.E. (2016). Risk factor SORL1: from genetic association to functional validation in Alzheimer's disease. *Acta Neuropathol.* 132: 653–665.

281 Kajiho, H., Sakurai, K., Minoda, T. et al. (2011). Characterization of RIN3 as a guanine nucleotide exchange factor for the Rab5 subfamily GTPase Rab31. *J. Biol. Chem.* 286: 24364–24373.

282 Kaneko, T., Li, L., and Li, S.S. (2008). The SH3 domain – a family of versatile peptide- and protein-recognition module. *Front Biosci.* 13: 4938–4952.

283 Yoshikawa, M., Kajiho, H., Sakurai, K. et al. (2008). Tyr-phosphorylation signals translocate RIN3, the small GTPase Rab5-GEF, to early endocytic vesicles. *Biochem. Biophys. Res. Commun.* 372: 168–172.

284 Kajiho, H., Saito, K., Tsujita, K. et al. (2003). RIN3: a novel Rab5 GEF interacting with amphiphysin II involved in the early endocytic pathway. *J. Cell Sci.* 116: 4159–4168.

285 Lu, H., Zhu, X.C., Wang, H.F. et al. (2016). Lack of association between SLC24A4 polymorphism and late-onset Alzheimer's disease in Han Chinese. *Curr. Neurovasc. Res.* 13: 239–243.

286 Coulthard, M.G., Lickliter, J.D., Subanesan, N. et al. (2001). Characterization of the Epha1 receptor tyrosine kinase: expression in epithelial tissues. *Growth Factors* 18: 303–317.

287 Wang, X., Lopez, O.L., Sweet, R.A. et al. (2015). Genetic determinants of disease progression in Alzheimer's disease. *J. Alzheimers Dis.* 43: 649–655.

288 Yamazaki, T., Masuda, J., Omori, T. et al. (2009). EphA1 interacts with integrin-linked kinase and regulates cell morphology and motility. *J. Cell Sci.* 122: 243–255.

289 Wilkinson, D.G. (2000). Eph receptors and ephrins: regulators of guidance and assembly. *Int. Rev. Cytol.* 196: 177–244.

290 Zhou, R. (1998). The Eph family receptors and ligands. *Pharmacol. Ther.* 77: 151–181.

291 Lai, K.O. and Ip, N.Y. (2009). Synapse development and plasticity: roles of ephrin/Eph receptor signaling. *Curr. Opin. Neurobiol.* 19: 275–283.

292 Martinez, A., Otal, R., Sieber, B.A. et al. (2005). Disruption of ephrin-A/EphA binding alters synaptogenesis and neural connectivity in the hippocampus. *Neuroscience* 135: 451–461.

293 Sakamoto, A., Sugamoto, Y., Tokunaga, Y. et al. (2011). Expression profiling of the ephrin (EFN) and Eph receptor (EPH) family of genes in atherosclerosis-related human cells. *J. Int. Med. Res.* 39: 522–527.

294 Sharfe, N., Nikolic, M., Cimpeon, L. et al. (2008). EphA and ephrin-A proteins regulate integrin-mediated T lymphocyte interactions. *Mol. Immunol.* 45: 1208–1220.

295 Deuss, M., Reiss, K., and Hartmann, D. (2008). Part-time alpha-secretases: the functional biology of ADAM 9, 10 and 17. *Curr. Alzheimer Res.* 5: 187–201.

296 Janes, P.W., Saha, N., Barton, W.A. et al. (2005). Adam meets Eph: an ADAM substrate recognition module acts as a molecular switch for ephrin cleavage in trans. *Cell* 123: 291–304.

297 Kuhn, P.H., Wang, H., Dislich, B. et al. (2010). ADAM10 is the physiologically relevant, constitutive alpha-secretase of the amyloid precursor protein in primary neurons. *EMBO J.* 29: 3020–3032.

298 Suh, J., Choi, S.H., Romano, D.M. et al. (2013). ADAM10 missense mutations potentiate beta-amyloid accumulation by impairing prodomain chaperone function. *Neuron* 80: 385–401.

299 Yu, M., Liu, Y., Shen, J. et al. (2016). Meta-analysis of BACE1 gene rs638405 polymorphism and the risk of Alzheimer's disease in Caucasion and Asian population. *Neurosci. Lett.* 616: 189–196.

300 Wang, M., Yang, J., and Su, J. (2017). Relationship between the polymorphism in exon 5 of BACE1 gene and Alzheimer's disease. *Aging Clin. Exp. Res.* 29: 105–113.

301 Munck, A., Bohm, C., Seibel, N.M. et al. (2005). Hu-K4 is a ubiquitously expressed type 2 transmembrane protein associated with the endoplasmic reticulum. *FEBS J.* 272: 1718–1726.

302 Heilmann, S., Drichel, D., Clarimon, J. et al. (2015). PLD3 in non-familial Alzheimer's disease. *Nature* 520: E3–E5.

303 van der Lee, S.J., Holstege, H., Wong, T.H. et al. (2015). PLD3 variants in population studies. *Nature* 520: E2–E3.

304 Lambert, J.C., Grenier-Boley, B., Bellenguez, C. et al. (2015). PLD3 and sporadic Alzheimer's disease risk. *Nature* 520: E1.

305 Zhang, D.F., Fan, Y., Wang, D. et al. (2016). PLD3 in Alzheimer's disease: a modest effect as revealed by updated association and expression analyses. *Mol. Neurobiol.* 53: 4034–4045.

306 Rosenthal, S.L., Barmada, M.M., Wang, X. et al. (2014). Connecting the dots: potential of data integration to identify regulatory SNPs in late-onset Alzheimer's disease GWAS findings. *PLoS One* 9: e95152.

307 Beecham, G.W., Hamilton, K., Naj, A.C. et al., Alzheimer's Disease Genetics C (2014). Genome-wide association meta-analysis of neuropathologic features of Alzheimer's disease and related dementias. *PLos Genet.* 10: e1004606.

308 He, F., Umehara, T., Saito, K. et al. (2010). Structural insight into the zinc finger CW domain as a histone modification reader. *Structure* 18: 1127–1139.

309 Stage, E., Duran, T., Risacher, S.L. et al. (2016). The effect of the top 20 Alzheimer disease risk genes on gray-matter density and FDG PET brain metabolism. *Alzheimers Dement (Amst.)* 5: 53–66.

310 Andrews, S.J., Das, D., Anstey, K.J., and Easteal, S. (2017). Late onset Alzheimer's disease risk variants in cognitive decline: the PATH through life study. *J. Alzheimers Dis.* 57: 423–436.

311 Chibnik, L.B., White, C.C., Mukherjee, S. et al. (2017). Susceptibility to neurofibrillary tangles: role of the PTPRD locus and limited pleiotropy with other neuropathologies. *Mol. Psychiatry*.

312 Lev, S., Moreno, H., Martinez, R. et al. (1995). Protein tyrosine kinase PYK2 involved in Ca(2+)-induced regulation of ion channel and MAP kinase functions. *Nature* 376: 737–745.

313 Mitra, S.K., Hanson, D.A., and Schlaepfer, D.D. (2005). Focal adhesion kinase: in command and control of cell motility. *Nat. Rev. Mol. Cell Biol.* 6: 56–68.

314 Sayas, C.L., Ariaens, A., Ponsioen, B., and Moolenaar, W.H. (2006). GSK-3 is activated by the tyrosine kinase Pyk2 during LPA1-mediated neurite retraction. *Mol. Biol. Cell* 17: 1834–1844.

315 Choi, S.H., Kim, Y.H., Hebisch, M. et al. (2014). A three-dimensional human neural cell culture model of Alzheimer's disease. *Nature* 515: 274–278.

316 Dourlen, P., Fernandez-Gomez, F.J., Dupont, C. et al. (2017). Functional screening of Alzheimer risk loci identifies PTK2B as an in vivo modulator and early marker of tau pathology. *Mol. Psychiatry* 22: 874–883.

317 Shulman, J.M., Chipendo, P., Chibnik, L.B. et al. (2011). Functional screening of Alzheimer pathology genome-wide association signals in Drosophila. *Am. J. Hum. Genet.* 88: 232–238.

318 Shulman, J.M., Imboywa, S., Giagtzoglou, N. et al. (2014). Functional screening in Drosophila identifies Alzheimer's disease susceptibility genes and implicates tau-mediated mechanisms. *Hum. Mol. Genet.* 23: 870–877.

319 Tu, Y., Wu, S., Shi, X. et al. (2003). Migfilin and Mig-2 link focal adhesions to filamin and the actin cytoskeleton and function in cell shape modulation. *Cell* 113: 37–47.

320 Chapuis, J., Flaig, A., Grenier-Boley, B. et al. (2017). Genome-wide, high-content siRNA screening identifies the Alzheimer's genetic risk factor FERMT2 as a major modulator of APP metabolism. *Acta Neuropathol.* 133: 955–966.

321 Deming, Y., Li, Z., Kapoor, M. et al., Alzheimer's Disease Neuroimaging I, Alzheimer Disease Genetic C. (2017). Genome-wide association study identifies four novel loci associated with Alzheimer's endophenotypes and disease modifiers. *Acta Neuropathol.* 133: 839–856.

322 Beck, T.N., Nicolas, E., Kopp, M.C., and Golemis, E.A. (2014). Adaptors for disorders of the brain? The cancer signaling proteins NEDD9, CASS4, and PTK2B in Alzheimer's disease. *Oncoscience* 1: 486–503.

323 Singh, M.K., Dadke, D., Nicolas, E. et al. (2008). A novel Cas family member, HEPL, regulates FAK and cell spreading. *Mol. Biol. Cell* 19: 1627–1636.

324 Beisang, D., Reilly, C., and Bohjanen, P.R. (2014). Alternative polyadenylation regulates CELF1/CUGBP1 target transcripts following T cell activation. *Gene* 550: 93–100.

325 Hinney, A., Albayrak, O., Antel, J. et al., Consortium G, Consortium I, Consortium G (2014). Genetic variation at the CELF1 (CUGBP, elav-like family member 1 gene) locus is genome-wide associated with Alzheimer's disease and obesity. *Am. J. Med. Genet. B Neuropsychiatr. Genet.* 165B: 283–293.

326 Kim, S.H., Fountoulakis, M., Cairns, N.J., and Lubec, G. (2002). Human brain nucleoside diphosphate kinase activity is decreased in Alzheimer's disease and Down syndrome. *Biochem. Biophys. Res. Commun.* 296: 970–975.

327 Keim, D., Hailat, N., Melhem, R. et al. (1992). Proliferation-related expression of p19/nm23 nucleoside diphosphate kinase. *J. Clin. Invest.* 89: 919–924.

328 Caligo, M.A., Cipollini, G., Fiore, L. et al. (1995). NM23 gene expression correlates with cell growth rate and S-phase. *Int. J. Cancer* 60: 837–842.

329 Leigh, M.W., Pittman, J.E., Carson, J.L. et al. (2009). Clinical and genetic aspects of primary ciliary dyskinesia/Kartagener syndrome. *Genet. Med.* 11: 473–487.

330 Liu, Y., Yu, J.T., Wang, H.F. et al. (2014). Association between NME8 locus polymorphism and cognitive decline, cerebrospinal fluid and neuroimaging biomarkers in Alzheimer's disease. *PLoS One* 9: e114777.

331 Polymeropoulos, M.H., Lavedan, C., Leroy, E. et al. (1997). Mutation in the alpha-synuclein gene identified in families with Parkinson's disease. *Science* 276: 2045–2047.

332 Spillantini, M.G., Schmidt, M.L., Lee, V.M. et al. (1997). Alpha-synuclein in Lewy bodies. *Nature* 388: 839–840.

333 Singleton, A.B., Farrer, M.J., and Bonifati, V. (2013). The genetics of Parkinson's disease: progress and therapeutic implications. *Mov. Disord.* 28: 14–23.

334 Corti, O., Lesage, S., and Brice, A. (2011). What genetics tells us about the causes and mechanisms of Parkinson's disease. *Physiol. Rev.* 91: 1161–1218.

335 Klein, C. and Westenberger, A. (2012). Genetics of Parkinson's disease. *Cold Spring Harb. Perspect. Med.* 2: a008888.

336 Kim, J.Y., Kim, S.Y., Kim, J.M. et al. (2009). Spinocerebellar ataxia type 17 mutation as a causative and susceptibility gene in parkinsonism. *Neurology* 72: 1385–1389.

337 Houlden, H. and Singleton, A.B. (2012). The genetics and neuropathology of Parkinson's disease. *Acta Neuropathol.* 124: 325–338.

338 Zarranz, J.J., Alegre, J., Gomez-Esteban, J.C. et al. (2004). The new mutation, E46K, of alpha-synuclein causes Parkinson and Lewy body dementia. *Ann. Neurol.* 55: 164–173.

339 Lesage, S., Anheim, M., Letournel, F. et al. (2013). G51D alpha-synuclein mutation causes a novel parkinsonian-pyramidal syndrome. *Ann. Neurol.* 73: 459–471.

340 Appel-Cresswell, S., Vilarino-Guell, C., Encarnacion, M. et al. (2013). Alpha-synuclein p.H50Q, a novel pathogenic mutation for Parkinson's disease. *Mov. Disord.* 28: 811–813.

341 Pasanen, P., Myllykangas, L., Siitonen, M. et al. (2014). Novel alpha-synuclein mutation A53E associated with atypical multiple system atrophy and Parkinson's disease-type pathology. *Neurobiol. Aging* 35 (2180): e2181–e2185.

342 Singleton, A.B., Farrer, M., Johnson, J. et al. (2003). Alpha-Synuclein locus triplication causes Parkinson's disease. *Science* 302: 841.

343 Spira, P.J., Sharpe, D.M., Halliday, G. et al. (2001). Clinical and pathological features of a Parkinsonian syndrome in a family with an Ala53Thr alpha-synuclein mutation. *Ann. Neurol.* 49: 313–319.

344 Kasten, M. and Klein, C. (2013). The many faces of alpha-synuclein mutations. *Mov. Disord.* 28: 697–701.

345 Zimprich, A., Biskup, S., Leitner, P. et al. (2004). Mutations in LRRK2 cause autosomal-dominant parkinsonism with pleomorphic pathology. *Neuron* 44: 601–607.

346 Paisan-Ruiz, C., Jain, S., Evans, E.W. et al. (2004). Cloning of the gene containing mutations that cause PARK8-linked Parkinson's disease. *Neuron* 44: 595–600.

347 Elbaz, A. (2008). LRRK2: bridging the gap between sporadic and hereditary Parkinson's disease. *Lancet Neurol.* 7: 562–564.

348 Huang, Y., Halliday, G.M., Vandebona, H. et al. (2007). Prevalence and clinical features of common LRRK2 mutations in Australians with Parkinson's disease. *Mov. Disord.* 22: 982–989.

349 Greene, I.D., Mastaglia, F., Meloni, B.P. et al. (2014). Evidence that the LRRK2 ROC domain Parkinson's disease-associated mutants A1442P and R1441C exhibit increased intracellular degradation. *J. Neurosci. Res.* 92: 506–516.

350 Ishihara, L., Gibson, R.A., Warren, L. et al. (2007). Screening for Lrrk2 G2019S and clinical comparison of Tunisian and North American Caucasian Parkinson's disease families. *Mov. Disord.* 22: 55–61.

351 Healy, D.G., Falchi, M., O'Sullivan, S.S. et al. (2008). Phenotype, genotype, and worldwide genetic penetrance of LRRK2-associated Parkinson's disease: a case-control study. *Lancet Neurol.* 7: 583–590.

352 Bonifati, V. (2007). LRRK2 low-penetrance mutations (Gly2019Ser) and risk alleles (Gly2385Arg)-linking familial and sporadic Parkinson's disease. *Neurochem. Res.* 32: 1700–1708.

353 Ross, O.A., Wu, Y.R., Lee, M.C. et al. (2008). Analysis of Lrrk2 R1628P as a risk factor for Parkinson's disease. *Ann. Neurol.* 64: 88–92.

354 West, A.B., Moore, D.J., Biskup, S. et al. (2005). Parkinson's disease-associated mutations in leucine-rich repeat kinase 2 augment kinase activity. *Proc. Natl. Acad. Sci. U.S.A.* 102: 16842–16847.

355 Han, K.A., Yoo, L., Sung, J.Y. et al. (2017). Leucine-rich repeat kinase 2 (LRRK2) stimulates IL-1beta-mediated inflammatory signaling through phosphorylation of RCAN1. *Front Cell Neurosci.* 11: 125.

356 Pankratz, N., Nichols, W.C., Uniacke, S.K. et al. (2003). Significant linkage of Parkinson disease to chromosome 2q36-37. *Am. J. Hum. Genet.* 72: 1053–1057.

357 Lautier, C., Goldwurm, S., Durr, A. et al. (2008). Mutations in the GIGYF2 (TNRC15) gene at the PARK11 locus in familial Parkinson disease. *Am. J. Hum. Genet.* 82: 822–833.

358 Bras, J., Simon-Sanchez, J., Federoff, M. et al. (2009). Lack of replication of association between GIGYF2 variants and Parkinson disease. *Hum. Mol. Genet.* 18: 341–346.

359 Guo, Y., Jankovic, J., Zhu, S. et al. (2009). GIGYF2 Asn56Ser and Asn457Thr mutations in Parkinson disease patients. *Neurosci. Lett.* 454: 209–211.

360 Zhang, Y., Sun, Q.Y., Yu, R.H. et al. (2015). The contribution of GIGYF2 to Parkinson's disease: a meta-analysis. *Neurol. Sci.* 36: 2073–2079.

361 Vilarino-Guell, C., Wider, C., Ross, O.A. et al. (2011). VPS35 mutations in Parkinson disease. *Am. J. Hum. Genet.* 89: 162–167.

362 Zimprich, A., Benet-Pages, A., Struhal, W. et al. (2011). A mutation in VPS35, encoding a subunit of the retromer complex, causes late-onset Parkinson disease. *Am. J. Hum. Genet.* 89: 168–175.

363 Lesage, S., Condroyer, C., Klebe, S. et al. (2012). Identification of VPS35 mutations replicated in French families with Parkinson disease. *Neurology* 78: 1449–1450.

364 Deng, H., Gao, K., and Jankovic, J. (2013). The VPS35 gene and Parkinson's disease. *Mov. Disord.* 28: 569–575.

365 Gambardella, S., Biagioni, F., Ferese, R. et al. (2016). Vacuolar protein sorting genes in Parkinson's disease: a re-appraisal of mutations detection rate and neurobiology of disease. *Front Neurosci.* 10: 532.

366 Chartier-Harlin, M.C., Dachsel, J.C., Vilarino-Guell, C. et al. (2011). Translation initiator EIF4G1 mutations in familial Parkinson disease. *Am. J. Hum. Genet.* 89: 398–406.

367 Lesage, S., Condroyer, C., Klebe, S. et al. (2012). EIF4G1 in familial Parkinson's disease: pathogenic mutations or rare benign variants? *Neurobiol. Aging* 33: 2233.e2231–2233.e2235.

368 Nichols, N., Bras, J.M., Hernandez, D.G. et al. (2015). EIF4G1 mutations do not cause Parkinson's disease. *Neurobiol. Aging* 36: 2444.e2441–2444.e2444.

369 Huttenlocher, J., Kruger, R., Capetian, P. et al. (2015). EIF4G1 is neither a strong nor a common risk factor for Parkinson's disease: evidence from large European cohorts. *J. Med. Genet.* 52: 37–41.

370 Lucking, C.B., Durr, A., Bonifati, V. et al. (2000). Association between early-onset Parkinson's disease and mutations in the parkin gene. *N. Engl. J. Med.* 342: 1560–1567.

371 Foroud, T., Uniacke, S.K., Liu, L. et al. (2003). Heterozygosity for a mutation in the parkin gene leads to later onset Parkinson disease. *Neurology* 60: 796–801.

372 Poorkaj, P., Nutt, J.G., James, D. et al. (2004). parkin mutation analysis in clinic patients with early-onset Parkinson [corrected] disease. *Am. J. Med. Genet. A* 129a: 44–50.

373 Wu, R.M., Bounds, R., Lincoln, S. et al. (2005). Parkin mutations and early-onset parkinsonism in a Taiwanese cohort. *Arch. Neurol.* 62: 82–87.

374 Oliveira, S.A., Scott, W.K., Martin, E.R. et al. (2003). Parkin mutations and susceptibility alleles in late-onset Parkinson's disease. *Ann. Neurol.* 53: 624–629.

375 Sun, M., Latourelle, J.C., Wooten, G.F. et al. (2006). Influence of heterozygosity for parkin mutation on onset age in familial Parkinson disease: the GenePD study. *Arch. Neurol.* 63: 826–832.

376 Valente, E.M., Salvi, S., Ialongo, T. et al. (2004). PINK1 mutations are associated with sporadic early-onset parkinsonism. *Ann. Neurol.* 56: 336–341.

377 Hedrich, K., Hagenah, J., Djarmati, A. et al. (2006). Clinical spectrum of homozygous and heterozygous PINK1 mutations in a large German family with Parkinson disease: role of a single hit? *Arch. Neurol.* 63: 833–838.

378 Narendra, D.P., Jin, S.M., Tanaka, A. et al. (2010). PINK1 is selectively stabilized on impaired mitochondria to activate Parkin. *PLoS Biol.* 8: e1000298.

379 Barodia, S.K., Creed, R.B., and Goldberg, M.S. (2016). Parkin and PINK1 functions in oxidative stress and neurodegeneration. *Brain Res. Bull.* 133: 51–59.

380 Scott, L., Dawson, V.L., and Dawson, T.M. (2017). Trumping neurodegeneration: targeting common pathways regulated by autosomal recessive Parkinson's disease genes. *Exp. Neurol.* .

381 Bonifati, V., Rizzu, P., van Baren, M.J. et al. (2003). Mutations in the DJ-1 gene associated with autosomal recessive early-onset parkinsonism. *Science* 299: 256–259.

382 Abou-Sleiman, P.M., Healy, D.G., Quinn, N. et al. (2003). The role of pathogenic DJ-1 mutations in Parkinson's disease. *Ann. Neurol.* 54: 283–286.

383 Alcalay, R.N., Caccappolo, E., Mejia-Santana, H. et al. (2010). Frequency of known mutations in early-onset Parkinson disease: implication for genetic counseling: the consortium on risk for early onset Parkinson disease study. *Arch. Neurol.* 67: 1116–1122.

384 Ottolini, D., Cali, T., Negro, A., and Brini, M. (2013). The Parkinson disease-related protein DJ-1 counteracts mitochondrial impairment induced by the tumour suppressor protein p53 by enhancing endoplasmic reticulum-mitochondria tethering. *Hum. Mol. Genet.* 22: 2152–2168.

385 Xiong, H., Wang, D., Chen, L. et al. (2009). Parkin, PINK1, and DJ-1 form a ubiquitin E3 ligase complex promoting unfolded protein degradation. *J. Clin. Invest.* 119: 650–660.

386 Williams, D.R., Hadeed, A., Al-Din, A.S. et al. (2005). Kufor Rakeb disease: autosomal recessive, levodopa-responsive parkinsonism with pyramidal degeneration, supranuclear gaze palsy, and dementia. *Mov. Disord.* 20: 1264–1271.

387 Ramirez, A., Heimbach, A., Grundemann, J. et al. (2006). Hereditary parkinsonism with dementia is caused by mutations in ATP13A2, encoding a lysosomal type 5 P-type ATPase. *Nat. Genet.* 38: 1184–1191.

388 Park, J.S., Blair, N.F., and Sue, C.M. (2015). The role of ATP13A2 in Parkinson's disease: clinical phenotypes and molecular mechanisms. *Mov. Disord.* 30: 770–779.

389 Djarmati, A., Hagenah, J., Reetz, K. et al. (2009). ATP13A2 variants in early-onset Parkinson's disease patients and controls. *Mov. Disord.* 24: 2104–2111.

390 Paisan-Ruiz, C., Bhatia, K.P., Li, A. et al. (2009). Characterization of PLA2G6 as a locus for dystonia-parkinsonism. *Ann. Neurol.* 65: 19–23.

391 Yoshino, H., Tomiyama, H., Tachibana, N. et al. (2010). Phenotypic spectrum of patients with PLA2G6 mutation and PARK14-linked parkinsonism. *Neurology* 75: 1356–1361.

392 Shi, C.H., Tang, B.S., Wang, L. et al. (2011). PLA2G6 gene mutation in autosomal recessive early-onset parkinsonism in a Chinese cohort. *Neurology* 77: 75–81.

393 Miki, Y., Tanji, K., Mori, F. et al. (2017). PLA2G6 accumulates in Lewy bodies in PARK14 and idiopathic Parkinson's disease. *Neurosci. Lett.* 645: 40–45.

394 Zhou, Q., Yen, A., Rymarczyk, G. et al. (2016). Impairment of PARK14-dependent Ca(2+) signalling is a novel determinant of Parkinson's disease. *Nat. Commun.* 7: 10332.

395 Di Fonzo, A., Dekker, M.C., Montagna, P. et al. (2009). FBXO7 mutations cause autosomal recessive, early-onset parkinsonian-pyramidal syndrome. *Neurology* 72: 240–245.

396 Vingill, S., Brockelt, D., Lancelin, C. et al. (2016). Loss of FBXO7 (PARK15) results in reduced proteasome activity and models a parkinsonism-like phenotype in mice. *EMBO J.* 35: 2008–2025.

397 Consortium IPsDG (2011). A two-stage meta-analysis identifies several new loci for Parkinson's disease. *PLos Genet.* 7: e1002142.

398 Kumar, K.R., Lohmann, K., and Klein, C. (2012). Genetics of Parkinson disease and other movement disorders. *Curr. Opin. Neurol.* 25: 466–474.

399 Lill, C.M., Roehr, J.T., McQueen, M.B. et al. (2012). Comprehensive research synopsis and systematic meta-analyses in Parkinson's disease genetics: the PDGene database. *PLos Genet.* 8: e1002548.

400 Pankratz, N., Beecham, G.W., DeStefano, A.L. et al. (2012). Meta-analysis of Parkinson's disease: identification of a novel locus, RIT2. *Ann. Neurol.* 71: 370–384.

401 Bonifati, V. (2010). Shaking the genome: new studies reveal genetic risk for Parkinson's disease. *Lancet Neurol.* 9: 136–138.

402 Peng, J., Oo, M.L., and Andersen, J.K. (2010). Synergistic effects of environmental risk factors and gene mutations in Parkinson's disease accelerate age-related neurodegeneration. *J. Neurochem.* 115: 1363–1373.

403 Cannon, J.R. and Greenamyre, J.T. (2013). Gene-environment interactions in Parkinson's disease: specific evidence in humans and mammalian models. *Neurobiol. Dis.* 57: 38–46.

404 Farrer, M., Maraganore, D.M., Lockhart, P. et al. (2001). Alpha-synuclein gene haplotypes are associated with Parkinson's disease. *Hum. Mol. Genet.* 10: 1847–1851.

405 Tan, E.K., Chai, A., Teo, Y.Y. et al. (2004). Alpha-synuclein haplotypes implicated in risk of Parkinson's disease. *Neurology* 62: 128–131.

406 Mueller, J.C., Fuchs, J., Hofer, A. et al. (2005). Multiple regions of alpha-synuclein are associated with Parkinson's disease. *Ann. Neurol.* 57: 535–541.

407 Mizuta, I., Satake, W., Nakabayashi, Y. et al. (2006). Multiple candidate gene analysis identifies alpha-synuclein as a susceptibility gene for sporadic Parkinson's disease. *Hum. Mol. Genet.* 15: 1151–1158.

408 Chung, S.J., Armasu, S.M., Biernacka, J.M. et al. (2011). Common variants in PARK loci and related genes and Parkinson's disease. *Mov. Disord.* 26: 280–288.

409 Elbaz, A., Ross, O.A., Ioannidis, J.P. et al. (2011). Independent and joint effects of the MAPT and SNCA genes in Parkinson disease. *Ann. Neurol.* 69: 778–792.

410 Ross, O.A., Soto-Ortolaza, A.I., Heckman, M.G. et al. (2011). Association of LRRK2 exonic variants with susceptibility to Parkinson's disease: a case-control study. *Lancet Neurol.* 10: 898–908.

411 Mata, I.F., Samii, A., Schneer, S.H. et al. (2008). Glucocerebrosidase gene mutations: a risk factor for Lewy body disorders. *Arch. Neurol.* 65: 379–382.

412 De Marco, E.V., Annesi, G., Tarantino, P. et al. (2008). Glucocerebrosidase gene mutations are associated with Parkinson's disease in southern Italy. *Mov. Disord.* 23: 460–463.

413 Neumann, J., Bras, J., Deas, E. et al. (2009). Glucocerebrosidase mutations in clinical and pathologically proven Parkinson's disease. *Brain* 132: 1783–1794.

414 Tan, E.K., Tong, J., Fook-Chong, S. et al. (2007). Glucocerebrosidase mutations and risk of Parkinson disease in Chinese patients. *Arch. Neurol.* 64: 1056–1058.

415 Mitsui, J., Mizuta, I., Toyoda, A. et al. (2009). Mutations for Gaucher disease confer high susceptibility to Parkinson disease. *Arch. Neurol.* 66: 571–576.

416 Choi, J.M., Kim, W.C., Lyoo, C.H. et al. (2012). Association of mutations in the glucocerebrosidase gene with Parkinson disease in a Korean population. *Neurosci. Lett.* 514: 12–15.

417 Gan-Or, Z., Giladi, N., Rozovski, U. et al. (2008). Genotype-phenotype correlations between GBA mutations and Parkinson disease risk and onset. *Neurology* 70: 2277–2283.

418 Sidransky, E., Nalls, M.A., Aasly, J.O. et al. (2009). Multicenter analysis of glucocerebrosidase mutations in Parkinson's disease. *N. Engl. J. Med.* 361: 1651–1661.

419 Kalinderi, K., Bostantjopoulou, S., Paisan-Ruiz, C. et al. (2009). Complete screening for glucocerebrosidase mutations in Parkinson disease patients from Greece. *Neurosci. Lett.* 452: 87–89.

420 Nalls, M.A., Duran, R., Lopez, G. et al. (2013). A multicenter study of glucocerebrosidase mutations in dementia with Lewy bodies. *JAMA Neurol.* 70: 727–735.

421 Cullen, V., Sardi, S.P., Ng, J. et al. (2011). Acid beta-glucosidase mutants linked to Gaucher disease, Parkinson disease, and Lewy body dementia alter alpha-synuclein processing. *Ann. Neurol.* 69: 940–953.

422 Appel, S.H. (2012). Inflammation in Parkinson's disease: cause or consequence? *Mov. Disord.* 27: 1075–1077.

423 Deleidi, M. and Gasser, T. (2013). The role of inflammation in sporadic and familial Parkinson's disease. *Cell. Mol. Life Sci.* 70: 4259–4273.

424 Dzamko, N., Geczy, C.L., and Halliday, G.M. (2014). Inflammation is genetically implicated in Parkinson's disease. *Neuroscience* 302: 89–102.

425 Witoelar, A., Jansen, I.E., Wang, Y. et al. International Parkinson's Disease Genomics Consortium NABEC, United Kingdom Brain Expression Consortium I (2017) Genome-wide pleiotropy between Parkinson disease and autoimmune diseases. *JAMA Neurol.* 74: 780–792.

426 van der Walt, J.M., Nicodemus, K.K., Martin, E.R. et al. (2003). Mitochondrial polymorphisms significantly reduce the risk of Parkinson disease. *Am. J. Hum. Genet.* 72: 804–811.

427 Hudson, G., Nalls, M., Evans, J.R. et al. (2013). Two-stage association study and meta-analysis of mitochondrial DNA variants in Parkinson disease. *Neurology* 80: 2042–2048.

428 Giannoccaro, M.P., La Morgia, C., Rizzo, G., and Carelli, V. (2017). Mitochondrial DNA and primary mitochondrial dysfunction in Parkinson's disease. *Mov. Disord.* 32: 346–363.

Final Thoughts Regarding Alzheimer's Disease, Diet, and Health

Charles S. Brennan[1,2,3,4], *Margaret A. Brennan*[1,2,3], *W.M.A.D. Binosha Fernando*[5,6], *Stephanie J. Fuller*[5] *and Ralph N. Martins*[5,6,7,8,9]

[1] Department of Wine, Food and Molecular Biosciences, Centre for Food Research and Innovation, Lincoln University, PO Box 85084, Lincoln, Christchurch, New Zealand
[2] School of Food Science, South China University of Technology, Guangzhou, China
[3] School of Food Science, Tianjin University of Commerce, Tianjin, China
[4] Riddet Institute, Palmerston North, New Zealand
[5] School of Medical and Health Sciences, Centre of Excellence for Alzheimer's Disease Research and Care, Edith Cowan University, Joondalup, WA, Australia
[6] Australian Alzheimer's Research Foundation, Ralph and Patricia Sarich Neuroscience Research Institute, Nedlands, WA, Australia
[7] Department of Biomedical Sciences, Macquarie University, Sydney, NSW, Australia
[8] School of Psychiatry and Clinical Neurosciences, University of Western Australia, Perth, WA, Australia
[9] KaRa Institute of Neurological Diseases, Sydney, NSW, Australia

We hope the chapters of this book have illustrated to you the complex nature of Alzheimer's disease and some of the other age-associated neurological diseases. The sheer number of scientific papers published that relate to treatments and remedies for neurological diseases, as well as articles which appear in the popular press, together with the attention of the media in general to new discoveries in the field, highlight the fact that these illnesses are of great concern to the public as well as to public health departments. The impending escalation in public health costs due to increases in the number of people around the world with these neurodegenerative conditions, particularly Alzheimer's disease, and the lack of success of Alzheimer's-related drug trials over the past three decades, is driving further research into potential preventative treatments and lifestyle changes.

It remains the wish and aspiration of all of us to ensure that our health is maintained at an optimum level for as long as possible. The onset of a neurodegenerative disease is disturbing to any individual, and sometimes it is hard to establish the difference between symptoms of normal ageing, and symptoms of a neurodegenerative disease. The symptoms, diagnostic methods, and potential causes and risk factors of Alzheimer's disease and neurological dysfunction have been described extensively in the preceding chapters. We have known for many decades that cognitive decline in Alzheimer's disease is associated with neuronal loss, brain atrophy, the formation of neurofibrillary tangles, and the extracellular deposition of amyloid peptide aggregates, as well as microglial infiltration. Importantly, imaging studies and other studies over the last decade have confirmed

---

Neurodegeneration and Alzheimer's Disease: The Role of Diabetes, Genetics, Hormones, and Lifestyle,
First Edition. Edited by Ralph N. Martins, Charles S. Brennan, W.M.A.D. Binosha Fernando, Margaret A. Brennan and Stephanie J. Fuller.
© 2019 John Wiley & Sons Ltd. Published 2019 by John Wiley & Sons Ltd.

what has long been suspected, that these pathological changes start approximately two decades before symptom onset. There are diagnostic methods being researched that are making early pre-clinical diagnosis of Alzheimer's disease in the general population a distinct possibility, and the range of potential early diagnostic tests described in this book give an optimistic outlook that cheap, reliable population screening for Alzheimer's disease will soon be possible. This huge step forward in Alzheimer's disease research will provide a large time-frame for potential prevention or slowing of the disease progress.

The main medications for Alzheimer's disease include several cholinesterase inhibitors and an inhibitor of the N-Methyl-D-aspartate (NMDA) receptor: these can alleviate or stabilise symptoms, but only temporarily. Medication is also available to help alleviate other aspects of Alzheimer's disease (such as depression and anxiety). Current medications do not prevent the continuing neurological degeneration in the disease. There is a proverb that warns us all that 'medicines are not meat to live by'. As a society as a whole, we all-too-often rely on pills and potions as a cure-all for our maladies. We present in this book recent evidence that lifestyle and dietary interventions can be used to prevent disease symptom onset, or at least delay the onset of the disease in individuals at risk, by reducing or slowing the degenerative process.

The links between common midlife conditions and Alzheimer's risk have been described in detail in this book: type 2 diabetes, cardiovascular disease, midlife obesity, insulin resistance, and associated health conditions are all risk factors for Alzheimer's disease. Such disruptions to the healthy state of our physiology are linked to chronic inflammatory responses and increased oxidative stress to our cells. These are detailed in this book, along with the dysregulation of glucose and lipid metabolism which can lead up to the midlife conditions mentioned above. Research now indicates these changes are responsible for the neurotoxicity exhibited during the onset and progression of Alzheimer's disease. As such, oxidative stress could be regarded as a primary marker of the severity of the pathogenic disruptions to normal neuron functionality. The research discussed in the chapter 'Inflammation in Alzheimer's Disease, and Prevention with Antioxidants and Phenolic Compounds' illustrates the effect of oxidative stress and inflammation on Aβ clearance and protein aggregation, for example. Importantly, it also describes evidence that certain antioxidants in our foods can help reduce this oxidative stress and inflammation.

The current knowledge on the influence of genetics on the risk and development of Alzheimer's disease is the subject of another chapter. The chapter demonstrates the vast array of genes and proteins that can impact our risk of Alzheimer's disease, and indicates that a good understanding of a person's genetic make-up will help assess a person's risk of dementia.

In recent years there has been increasing attention placed on the value of certain foods, including herbs and spices, as dietary sources of antioxidants and other health-promoting agents. For example, cinnamon, turmeric, green tea, and extra virgin olive oil have been investigated, with the aim of enhancing or preserving cognitive functionality and reducing the susceptibility to neurological decline. Most of the research which supports the use of these specific foods or diets has been conducted using *in vivo* mice studies. The potency and effectiveness of their utilisation remains to be evidenced using human intervention studies. There has to be a degree of scepticism for some of the health claims attributed to dietary supplements. However, there is a consensus that the polyphenolic components of some foods (green vegetables, berry fruits, herbs and spices, for example) act as protective agents, and that this protection can be attributed to the antioxidant properties of the phenolic compounds. Epidemiological data, for example concerning the Mediterranean diet and Okinawan diet, both long associated with longevity, also provide strong evidence of the importance of antioxidant-rich foods. Studies of these diets and comparisons with the western diet underscore the importance of reducing the omega-6 : omega-3 fatty acid ratio in our diet, as well as reducing intake of saturated fats and sugars. Hopefully the detailed discussions in this book concerning these aspects of diet and their influence on our metabolism have given a good overview of the current understanding of this topic.

Other dietary components have also been shown to exert effects in terms of manipulation of the onset and progression of Alzheimer's disease. The brain–gut axis theory is now becoming better understood, and the utilisation of carbohydrates and proteins through our digestive system and during microbiota fermentation has been shown to influence some of the mechanisms of our cognitive function and brain performance. Elements of this are associated with the relationship between protein digestion and carbohydrate utilisation from our diet, and disruptions of this process lead to metabolic disorders often stemming from poor glycaemic control. It is well-known that disruptions to glucose regulation have been shown to be responsible for the progression of many diseases (cardiovascular disease, obesity, and particularly type 2 diabetes). Evidence presented in this book demonstrates that the selective use of slowly digestible (or indigestible) carbohydrates (mainly non-starch polysaccharides, or more commonly called dietary fibre) can regulate glucose production and absorption, and hence postprandial blood glucose levels. However, glucose regulation is just one mechanism by which these ingredients could exert protective actions against neurodegenerative disease. It is popularly quoted that the number of cells in our body is only a fraction of the number of microbiological cells we have in our gut. The relationship between gut microbiota and the production of short-chain fatty acids (SCFA), thought to provide a protective effect on our brain function, has also been discussed in the chapter 'The Products of Fermentation and Their Effects on Metabolism, Alzheimer's Disease and Other Neurodegenerative Diseases: Role of SCFA'. The old adage of 'we are what we eat' may be true to a point; however, taking into account the considerable influence that the microbial communities in our gut play in the regulation of genetic expression and our physiological pathways, perhaps the saying should be refined to 'we are what our gut microbiota feed on'. There is no doubt that the complexity of what we eat, how it is utilised in our body, and then the way this relates to increased oxidative stress and chronic inflammation, amyloid-complex formation, and other markers/factors of neurological diseases will mean that researchers will increase focus on this topic to determine cause-and-effect relationships.

Finally, we cannot disregard the importance of exercise and activity in both general well-being as well as neurological functionality during ageing. A healthy body will help maintain a healthy mind, and exercise and activity are essential for weight control/loss and good circulation, as well as cognitive function. Regular exercise has a protective effect in terms of stimulating neurological performance in individuals showing signs of neurological ageing diseases. Part of this could be due to the participation of physical activity enhancing oxygen uptake and neurological transmission, and increasing the production of neurotrophic factors, as discussed in the chapter 'The Link Between Exercise and Mediation of Alzheimer's Disease and Neurodegenerative Diseases'.

In addition, the social interactions which occur during many acts of physical activity are crucial for a person's outlook and psychological attitude to life.

We hope that this book has helped in illustrating the interrelationships between food, exercise, and lipid- and glucose-metabolism regulation, which are so important for us in maintaining a healthy mind, body, and outlook on life. There is an old Chinese saying, 食物治療勝過於醫生的治療, which roughly translates as 'Diet cures more than a doctor'. Perhaps we can learn more about future cures or preventions for our diseases if we look to our past and general wisdom passed down through the ages.

List of Abbreviations

24-OH-Chol	24S-hydroxycholesterol
27-OH-Chol	27-hydroxycholesterol
4β-OH	4β-hydroxycholesterol
5-HT1a/5-HT2a	5-hydroxytryptamine receptors/serotonin receptors
α7-nAChR	α7-nicotinic acetylcholine receptor
AA	arachidonic acid (also sometimes abbreviated to ARA)
ABCA1	ATP-binding cassette transporter 1
ABCA7	ATP-binding cassette transporter subfamily A member 7
Aβ	amyloid-β peptide (A-beta), cleavage product of APP, that aggregates to form amyloid
Aβ1-40	Full-length Aβ peptide ending at amino acid 40 of the Aβ peptide sequence
Aβ1-42	Full-length Aβ peptide ending at amino acid 42 of the Aβ peptide sequence
Aβ40	Aβ peptide (or fragments of Aβ) ending at amino acid 40 of the Aβ peptide sequence
Aβ42	Aβ peptide (or fragments of Aβ) ending at amino acid 42 of the Aβ peptide sequence
ACh	acetylcholine
AChEI	acetylcholinesterase inhibitors
AD	Alzheimer's disease
ADAD	autosomal dominant Alzheimer's disease
ADAM10	A disintegrin and metalloprotease 10 (cleaves APP at α-site, also known as α-secretase)
ADAS	Alzheimer's disease assessment scale
ADAS-Cog	Alzheimer's disease assessment scale combination of tests (11 tasks)
ADHD	attention deficit/hyperactivity disorder
ADNI	Alzheimer's disease neuroimaging initiative
ADPD	Autosomal Dominant Parkinson's Disease
AGE	advanced glycation end products
AIBL	Australian Imaging Biomarker and Lifestyle
AICD	amyloid precursor protein intracellular domain

Neurodegeneration and Alzheimer's Disease: The Role of Diabetes, Genetics, Hormones, and Lifestyle,
First Edition. Edited by Ralph N. Martins, Charles S. Brennan, W.M.A.D. Binosha Fernando,
Margaret A. Brennan and Stephanie J. Fuller.
© 2019 John Wiley & Sons Ltd. Published 2019 by John Wiley & Sons Ltd.

ALA	alpha-linoleic acid (essential omega-3 polyunsaturated fatty acid)
ALS	amyotrophic lateral sclerosis
ALS-FTD	amyotrophic lateral sclerosis with frontotemporal lobe dementia
aMCI	amnestic mild cognitive impairment
AMPK	adenosine monophosphate–activated protein kinase
ApoA	apolipoprotein A (protein)
APOE	apolipoprotein E gene
ApoE	apolipoprotein E protein
APP	amyloid-β precursor protein
AR	androgen receptor
ARA	arachidonic acid (also abbreviated to AA)
ATD	acute tryptophan depletion
ATP	adenosine triphosphate – unit of energy used in the body, produced in mitochondria
ATP13A2	probable cation-transporting ATPase 13A2
APP/AβPP	amyloid-β precursor protein
BACE/BACE-1	beta-site APP cleaving enzyme (also known as β-secretase), cleaves APP at N-terminus of Aβ peptide
BBB	blood–brain barrier
BDNF	brain-derived neurotrophic factor
BIN1	bridging integrator 1
BSE	bovine spongiform encephalopathy (mad cow disease)
CAA	cerebral amyloid angiopathy
CAG	the letters stand for 3 bases of DNA that translate to glutamine, CAG repeated in sequence over 36 times can lead to Huntington's disease
CASS4	cas scaffolding protein family member 4
CD2AP	CD2-associated protein
CD33	myeloid cell surface antigen CD33
CDR	clinical dementia rating
CDR–SOB	clinical dementia rating–sum of boxes score
CELF1	CUGBP elav-like family member 1
CERAD	Consortium to Establish a Registry for Alzheimer's Disease
CERAD-nb	Consortium to Establish a Registry for Alzheimer's Disease neuropsychological battery
CETP	cholesteryl ester-transfer protein
ChAT	choline acetyltransferase
CJD	Creutzfeldt–Jakob disease
CLU	clusterin, also known as apolipoprotein J
CNS	central nervous system
COX	cyclooxygenase
CR1	complement receptor 1
CSF	cerebrospinal fluid
CT	computed tomography

CVA	cerebrovascular accident
CVD	cardiovascular disease
DASH	dietary approaches to stop hypertension
DHA	docosahexaenoic acid (an omega-3 polyunsaturated fatty acid)
DHLA	dihydrolipoic acid
DHT	dihydrotestosterone
DJ-1	protein deglycase DJ-1
DLB	dementia with Lewy bodies
DPP-4	dipeptidyl peptidase-4, enzyme that degrades GLP-1 (glucagon-like peptide 1)
DRS	dementia rating scale
EEG	electroencephalography/electroencephalograph
EGCG	epigallocatechin-3-gallate
EIF4G1	eukaryotic translation initiation factor 4 gamma 1
ELISA	enzyme-linked immunosorbent assay – biochemical assay commonly used for testing levels of proteins and peptides
EOAD	early-onset Alzheimer's disease
EOFAD	early-onset AD with strong family history
EOPD	early-onset Parkinson's disease
EPA	eicosapentaenoic acid (an omega-3 polyunsaturated fatty acid)
EPHA1	EPH (erythropoietin-producing hepatocellular carcinoma) receptor A1
ERT	estrogen replacement therapy
FBXO7	F-box protein 7
FDG–PET	^{18}F-deoxyglucose–positron emission tomography
FERMT2	fermitin family member 2
FFAR2	free fatty-acid receptor 2
fMRI	functional magnetic resonance imaging
FSH	follicle stimulating hormone
FTD	frontotemporal (lobe) dementia (also commonly abbreviated to FTLD)
FTLD	frontotemporal lobar degeneration (same as FTD)
FUS	fused-in sarcoma protein
γ-secretase	gamma-secretase, cleaves APP at the C-terminus of the Aβ peptide
GABA	γ-aminobutyric acid (neurotransmitter)
GABA-R	γ-aminobutyric acid receptor
GCS	glucosylceramide synthase
GI	gastrointestinal
GIGYF2	PERQ amino acid rich with GYF domain-containing protein 2
GIP	glucose-dependent insulinotropic polypeptide
GLP1/GLP-1	glucagon-like peptide 1
GLUT1	glucose transporter type 1

GLUT4	glucose transporter type 4
GM-CSF	granulocyte macrophages–colony-stimulating factor
GOT	glutamate oxaloacetate transaminase
GPI	glycosylphosphatidylinositol
GSS	Gerstmann–Straussler–Scheinker syndrome
GSK3-β or GSK-3β or GSK3β	glycogen synthase kinase-3β
GWAS	genome-wide association study
H_2O_2	hydrogen peroxide
hCG	human chorionic gonadotropin (hCG)
HD	Huntington's disease
HDAC	histone deacetylase
HDL	high-density lipoprotein
HLA-DRB1/DRB5	major histocompatibility complex class II DRβ1 and DRβ5
HMG-CoA	3-hydroxy-3-methylglutaryl-CoA
HMPAO-SPECT	SPECT scan using radioactively labelled (99mTC)-hexamethylpropyleneamine oxime
HOMA-IR	homeostatic model assessment of insulin resistance and pancreatic β-cell function
HPG	hypothalamic–pituitary–gonadal
HRT	hormone replacement therapy
HSP	hereditary spastic paraplegia
HTRA2	HtrA serine peptidase 2 (also known as Park13)
IDE	insulin-degrading enzyme
IGF	insulin-like growth factor
IGF1R	insulin-like growth factor 1 receptor
IL	interleukin
IL-1α	interleukin 1α
IL-6	interleukin 6
iNOS	inducible nitric oxide synthase
INPP5D	inositol polyphosphate-5-phosphatase D
iPSC	induced pluripotent stem cell
IR	insulin receptor
IRS-1 or IRS1	insulin receptor substrate 1
JNK	c-Jun N-terminal kinase
JPD	juvenile Parkinson's disease
KO	knock-out, referring to removal or disabling of a particular gene
LB	Lewy bodies
LDL	low-density lipoproteins
LH	luteinising hormone
LOAD	late-onset Alzheimer's disease
LOPD	late-onset Parkinson's disease
LPS	lipopolysaccharide
LRP1	low-density lipoprotein receptor–related protein 1
LRRK2	leucine-rich repeat kinase 2
LTD	long-term depression

LTP	long-term potentiation
MAPK	mitogen-activated protein kinase
MAPT	microtubule-associated protein tau
MCI	mild cognitive impairment
MDRS	Mattis dementia rating scale
MeDi	Mediterranean-style diet
MEF2C	myocyte-specific enhancer factor 2C
miRNA	microRNA, class of small single-stranded non-coding RNA involved in post-transcriptional regulation of gene expression
MIND	Mediterranean-DASH diet intervention for neurodegenerative delay
MIP-1α	macrophage inflammatory protein 1α
MMSE	mini-mental state examination
MND	motor neuron disease
MoCA	Montreal Cognitive Assessment
MRI	magnetic resonance imaging
MS4A	membrane-spanning 4-domains subfamily A
mtDNA	mitochondrial DNA
nAChR	nicotinic acetylcholine receptors
NAD/NADH	nicotinamide adenine dinucleotide, involved in redox reactions, NADH is reduced form
NASH	non-alcoholic steatohepatitis
nDNA	nuclear DNA
NFκβ	nuclear factor kappa beta
NFL	neurofilament light chain
NFT	neurofibrillary tangles
NGS	next-generation sequencing
NHP	non-human primates
NIA–AA	National Institute on Aging–Alzheimer's Association
NMDA	N-methyl-D-aspartate
NMDAR	N-methyl-D-aspartate receptor
NME8	NME/NM23 family member 8
NOS2	nitrogen oxide synthase 2
NSAID	non-steroidal anti-inflammatory drug
p75NTR	p75 neurotrophic receptor
Park1	first gene linked to Parkinson's disease, also known as SNCA, codes for α-synuclein
Park2	second gene linked to Parkinson's disease, also known as Parkin
Park8	eighth gene linked to Parkinson's disease, also known as LRRK2 gene, most frequent cause of early Parkinson's disease
PAS	psychogeriatric assessment scales
PBT1 and PBT2	copper/zinc ionophores related to 8-hydroxyquinoline
PC	phosphatidylcholine
PCD	programmed cell death

PCp	phosphatidylcholine plasmalogen
PCR	polymerase chain reaction
PD	Parkinson's disease
PDE9A	phosphodiesterase 9A
PDGF	platelet-derived growth factor
PDGFRβ	platelet-derived growth factor receptor-β
PE	phosphatidylethanolamine
Pep	phosphatidylethanolamine plasmalogen
PI	phosphatidylinositol
PiB-PET	Pittsburgh compound B positron emission tomography
PiB+ve or PiB−ve	PiB-PET–tested people who have (+ve) or do not have (−ve) significant Aβ plaques in the brain
PICALM	phosphatidylinositol binding clathrin assembly lymphoid myeloid protein
PINK 1	PTEN-induced putative kinase 1
PKC	protein kinase C
PLA2G6	phospholipase A2 group 6
PLD3	phospholipase D3
PLS	primary lateral sclerosis
PLTP	phospholipid transfer protein
PM	prospective memory
PNFA	progressive non-fluent aphasia
PON1	paraoxonase 1
PPA	propionic acid
PPARγ	peroxisome proliferator-activated receptor γ
PRKN	parkin
PrP	prion protein
PS1 and PS2	presenilin-1 and presenilin-2 proteins, respectively
PSC	pluripotent stem cell
PSEN1 and *PSEN2*	presenilin-1 and presenilin-2 genes, respectively
PSP	progressive supranuclear palsy
PTEN	phosphatase and tensin homologue
PTK2B	protein tyrosine kinase 2β
PUFA	polyunsaturated fatty acids
qRT-PCR	quantitative reverse transcriptase-polymerase chain reaction, method to quantitate DNA or RNA fragments
RAGE	receptor for advanced glycation end products
RBD	rapid eye movement sleep behaviour disorder
REM	rapid eye movement
RIN3-SLC24A4	rab interactor 3-solute carrier family 24 sodium/potassium/calcium exchanger member 4 locus
RM	retrospective memory

RNA	ribonucleic acid
RNAi	RNA interference
ROS	reactive oxygen species
SAM	senescence-accelerated mouse
SCD	subjective cognitive decline
SCFA	short-chain fatty acid
SD	semantic dementia
SERM	selective oestrogen receptor modulators
SMA	spinal muscular atrophy
SNCA	alpha-synuclein gene
SOD1	superoxide dismutase 1
SOM	standardised outcome measure
SORL1	sortilin-related receptor 1 (containing LDLR class A repeats)
SPECT	single photon emission computed tomography
SRB1	scavenger receptor class B1
SREBP2	sterol regulatory element binding protein 2
SSRI	selective serotonin reuptake inhibitor
STIM2	stromal interaction molecule 2
STZ	streptozotocin (toxic to pancreatic β-cells)
T2D	type 2 diabetes
TAR	transactive response
TARDP	gene for TDP-43
TCA	tricarboxylic acid cycle
TDP-43	transactive response DNA binding protein-43
TGF-β	transforming growth factor β
THA	tetracosahexaenoic acid
TIA	transient ischaemic attack
TNF-α	tumour necrosis factor α
TREM2	triggering receptor expressed on myeloid cells 2
TSE	transmissible spongiform encephalopathy
TTG	tissue transglutaminase
TZD	thiazolidinedione (insulin sensitisers, such as rosiglitazone and pioglitazone)
UCHL1	ubiquitin carboxy-terminal hydrolase L1
UPS	ubiquitin-proteasome system
VaD	vascular dementia
VEGF	vascular endothelial growth factor
VLDL	very low-density lipoprotein
VPS35	vacuolar protein sorting 35
Wnt/β-catenin	Wnt is a genetics acronym for wingless/integrated; Wnt and its co-activator β-catenin act in signal transduction pathways
WT	wild type
ZCWPW1	zinc finger CW type with PWWP domain 1

Index

a

ABCA1 gene and protein   191, 195
ABCA7 gene and protein   12, 449, 450, 453
ABCC1 transporter   409
Aβ 40 and 42 (same as Aβ1-40 and Aβ-42, respectively)   10, 57–58, 92, 95, 249, 269, 299, 301, 354, 399–400, 402, 407–411, 446–448, 461, 465
Aβ aggregation *see* Aβ and, pathology and aggregation
Abeta *see* Aβ and
Aβ and
  animal models   291–293, 295–302
  anti-Aβ treatments   391–411
  antioxidants   244–253
  apoE   120, 197–201, 203
  brain imaging/diagnosis/biomarker   54–56
  cerebrospinal fluid   54–60, 269
  clearance   63, 95, 120, 122, 168–170, 197–201, 203, 209, 241
  cognitive impairment/decline   54–56, 102, 268–269
  diabetes and insulin resistance   91–103
  diet   118, 122, 126, 130, 249
  exercise and physical activity   377–381
  eye diagnosis   68–69
  genetics   10, 66, 446–456, 459–465
  GPCR (G-protein coupled receptors)   316
  immunotherapy   400–405
  inflammation and oxidative stress   93, 94, 97, 98, 128, 170, 192, 235–241, 243–253
  LRP-1   203
  pathology and aggregation   9, 10, 44, 54–56, 68–69, 132–133, 167–170, 202, 209–210, 241, 248
  plasma biomarker   60–62, 132
  production   6, 10, 44, 131, 167, 241, 340–342, 405–408, 446
  sex hormones   340–342, 345, 347–349, 352–354
  Statins   399–400
AβPP *see* amyloid precursor protein or amyloid-β precursor protein (APP or AβPP)
Acetate   150–151, 312–323
acetylcholine   12, 23, 128, 133, 159–160, 242, 250, 353, 377, 378, 391–396
acetylcholinesterase inhibitors   6, 23, 159, 242–243, 246, 298, 355, 391–396
acetyl-CoA   125, 133, 152, 190, 315, 319, 321, 322
AChEI *see* acetylcholinesterase inhibitors
AD
  brain imaging (*see* imaging diagnostic)
  diagnosis (*see* diagnosis AD (Alzheimer's disease))
  differential diagnosis (*see* differential diagnosis)
  pathology   9, 32, 44–45, 55–58, 64, 95–96, 233, 238, 252
  prevention   13, 121, 154, 233, 243, 302, 350, 353, 378

AD (*contd.*)
  symptoms   10–11, 20, 45–51, 55–56, 242–243, 268–270, 274–276, 292, 297
  treatment   12, 298–302, 350–355, 391–412
ADAM10/ADAM-10 (also α-secretase)   12, 66, 128, 205, 246, 340, 405, 406, 450, 463
ADAM17/ADAM-17   203, 241
ADAS   48, 65, 355, 392, 393, 395, 400
ADAS-COG   48, 65, 355, 392, 393, 395, 400
advanced glycation end-products (AGE)   95, 97, 126, 131, 154, 161, 170–171, 237–239, 241, 292, 408
AGE *see* advanced glycation end products (AGE)
AIBL (Australian Imaging Biomarker and Lifestyle study)   13, 54–55, 61, 63, 64, 92, 340, 347, 352
ALA (alpha-linolenic acid)   121, 207–208
alpha-linolenic acid *see* ALA (alpha-linolenic acid)
alpha-secretase *see* ADAM-10/ADAM-10 (also α-secretase)
alpha-synuclein   18–19, 22–23, 32, 167, 168, 236, 465–467, 470, 472
alpha-tocopherol/α-tocopherol *see* vitamin E/α-tocopherol
ALS *see* amyotrophic lateral sclerosis
Alzheimer's disease *see* AD
AMP-activated protein kinase *see* AMPK
AMPK   236, 320–322
amyloid   15, 16, 18, 57, 91–92, 102, 120, 129, 132, 168, 170, 192, 201–203, 381
amyloid and AD genetics   446, 448, 451, 456, 460–463
  AD treatment   394–396, 398, 401-405, 408–410
  amyloid-β (*see* Aβ and)
  animal models   291–302
  cascade hypothesis   10, 446, 463
  congophilic angiopathy (*see* CAA (cerebral amyloid angiopathy))
  inflammation   235, 238–240, 243, 247, 248, 251

  pathology   9, 10, 43–45, 54–56, 61, 67–69, 95
  sex hormones   340, 342, 347, 348, 352–354
amyloid precursor protein animal models   291–300
amyloid precursor protein or amyloid-β precursor protein (APP or AβPP)   10, 12, 29, 44, 57, 167, 340–341, 347, 378, 405–408, 446
amyotrophic lateral sclerosis   14–15, 27–30, 132, 167, 169, 208, 236, 302, 397, 457, 470
animal models
  in drug development   297–299, 308
  non-human primate   298
  non-transgenic   297
  transgenic mice   291–302
anticholinergic medication   17, 23
antioxidants   4–7, 98, 167, 208, 237, 242, 245–253, 398, 410
antioxidants and apolipoprotein E   201
  diet, vitamins, micronutrient   4–7, 118, 122, 127–131, 153, 208
  polyphenols   245–249, 500–501
  sex steroids   342–344, 352
ApoA or apoA *see* apolipoprotein A
ApoE or apoE *see* apolipoprotein E
apolipoprotein   194–197
apolipoprotein A   192–197, 202
apolipoprotein E   12, 52–53, 95, 120, 153, 191–97, 198–203, 243
  antioxidant   201
  brain   198, 199
  exercise   380, 381
  ε4   12, 59, 101, 120, 154, 189, 197–203, 205, 407–409
  ε4 and AD risk   53, 55, 67, 70, 120, 153, 199
  ε4 and dietary lipids   205, 209, 249
  plasma and CSF levels, biomarker   62–66, 199
  receptors   120, 203, 451
  sex hormones   348, 349, 351
apolipoprotein genetics   67, 153, 197, 199, 448–452, 455, 457, 462, 463
apolipoprotein J (apoJ) *see* clusterin

apolipoprotein mouse models 292
apoptosis 26, 62, 65, 124, 128, 151, 169, 170, 209, 210, 237, 245, 315, 326, 353
apoptosis AD genetics 452–453, 459, 467, 470
APP or AβPP *see* Amyloid β precursor protein (APP or AβPP)
Arterial spin labelling 53
ASL *see* arterial spin labelling
astrocytes 120, 133, 157, 191, 197, 198, 241, 246, 247, 296, 322, 324, 344–345
astrocytes and AD pathology 44, 45
  chronic inflammation 233–236, 239, 241, 251
  Genetics 451, 452, 460
  sex steroids 344–345
atorvastatin 399, 400
ATP-binding cassette subfamily A transporter 7 *see* ABCA7 gene and protein
ATP-binding cassette subfamily C member 1 *see* ABCC1 transporter
ATP-sensitive potassium 154, 160
Australian Imaging Biomarker and Lifestyle *see* AIBL (Australian Imaging Biomarker and Lifestyle study)

b

BACE (also BACE-1, BACE1, β-secretase) 6, 69, 95, 129, 131, 203, 205, 248, 252, 405, 406, 410
  genetics 446, 447, 459–461, 463
  inflammation 241, 248, 252
  mouse models 292, 296
  potential treatments 400, 403–406
  sex hormones 340, 342
BDNF 26, 67, 119, 154, 166, 246, 324, 377-379, 381–382
  genetics 67, 381–382
  reproductive hormones 349, 354, 379
beta-amyloid cleavage enzyme *see* BACE (also BACE-1, BACE1, β-secretase)
beta-secretase *see* BACE (also BACE-1, BACE1, β-secretase)
biomarker 32, 54–71, 92, 206, 237, 238, 270, 372, 400

biomarker CSF 31, 32, 55–60, 71, 400, 406–410, 455, 457, 461, 465
blood biomarkers 32, 60–71, 206, 209, 400
blood brain barrier 6, 60, 91, 124, 157, 190, 238, 247, 248, 297, 398, 406, 460
  hormones 346, 348, 353
  short chain fatty acids (SCFA) 311, 315–317
blood proteins 60–64
blood tests 32, 60–71, 206, 400
bovine spongiform encephalopathy 30
brain derived neurotrophic factor *see* BDNF
brain glucose 15, 52, 53, 56, 91, 92, 159, 203, 252
brain scans 51–56
BSE *see* bovine spongiform encephalopathy
butyrate (dietary) 150, 312–318, 321–325

c

CAA (cerebral amyloid angiopathy) 16, 202, 296
calcium (also Ca^{2+}) cellular 13, 58, 95, 123, 127, 130, 132–133, 234, 237, 239, 246, 296, 353, 396, 402
calcium diet 119, 129, 131, 134
calcium genetics 450, 456, 459, 462, 464, 471
carbohydrates 1–4, 7, 99, 118–119, 122–125, 149–161, 163, 311–314, 318, 501
Cardiovascular disease (CVD) 1, 2, 4, 5, 12, 17, 153, 170, 189, 500–501
Cardiovascular disease (CVD) and AD risk 12, 17, 33, 53, 60, 63, 241, 453
  apolipoprotein E 12, 63, 153, 189–190, 451
  diet and nutrition 117–123, 127, 130, 134, 150, 152, 163, 207, 247, 253, 312, 321
  genetics 451, 453, 473
  inflammation 207, 235, 238, 241, 247
  lipids 190, 204, 205, 207, 312, 321
  physical activity 372–375, 377, 380–381
  sex hormones 346, 350
CD33 67, 450, 455–456
CDR-*see* clinical dementia rating 166

CDR-SOB   48
CERAD   49–51
ceramide   58, 59, 65, 70, 120, 131, 152, 208–209
cerebral amyloid angiopathy *see* CAA (cerebral amyloid angiopathy)
cerebrolysin   17, 393
cerebrospinal fluid *see* CSF
ChAT   250–251
cholesterol   64, 189–210
cholesterol and Aβ production   131, 201, 205, 210, 400
  AD risk   64, 119, 120, 189, 203–204, 399–400
  ApoE   120, 189, 195, 197–210
  biomarkers   58, 60
  brain   90, 190–192, 197, 203, 205
  clusterin (apolipoprotein J)   202
  diet   118–121, 123, 131, 151, 153, 192–194, 205, 247, 248, 297, 317, 320–322
  genetics   12, 445, 449–451, 453
  oxysterols   60, 64, 191–192, 248, 399–400
  statins   17, 120, 204–205, 399–400
  synthesis and metabolism   131, 190–191, 194–196, 210, 399, 449–451, 453, 461
  vascular dementia   16, 449–453
choline acetyl transferase *see* ChAT
cholinergic system   19, 23, 159–160, 242, 391–394, 396, 399
cinnamon/cinnamaldehyde   244–245, 248, 500
citric acid cycle   98, 152, 163, 315
CJD   30–32, 168
clinical dementia rating   47–48, 50, 166, 208
clock drawing   48–51, 56, 59
clusterin   12, 95, 202–203, 452
cobalamin *see* vitamin B12 / cobalamin
cognition   189, 191, 200, 204–205, 210, 267–281, 299, 301
cognition and diet   118–120, 122–123, 126–127, 130–132, 153–158, 248, 249, 252, 324

dietary protein and amino acids   162–171
genetics of neurodegeneration   446, 453, 456, 458, 462, 464, 465, 468–470, 472
glucose control and diabetes type II   89–94, 99–103, 158
glucose, fructose, sucrose   158–162
pathology   44–56, 59, 61, 63–67
physical activity   371–376
sex hormones   338–340, 342, 344, 346–347, 349–352, 354, 355
symptoms and diagnosis   10. 15–26, 31–33
treatments   392–396, 398, 399, 401–404, 407, 409–412
cognitive decline *see* cognition and
complement receptor 1 (CR1)   454–455
complement system and components   58, 234, 238–239, 452–455
copper   125, 131–134, 201, 237, 251
corticosteroids   412
COX-1 or COX1   121, 244, 407, 408, 411
COX-2 or COX2   121, 239, 243–245, 247, 407, 408, 411
Creutzfeldt-Jakob disease *see* CJD
CSF   15, 31, 32, 55–60, 63, 69, 90, 101, 130, 203, 234, 238, 251, 299, 348, 399
  Aβ   55–60, 92, 269, 342, 352, 399–400, 402, 406, 407, 409–410, 455, 461, 465
  insulin   90–91, 93
  lipids and lipoproteins   197–198, 206, 208, 400, 452
  miRNA   68-70
  tau   32, 55–60, 92, 126, 269, 352, 378, 399–400, 457, 462
CT scans   51, 54
curcumin   68, 244, 247–248
cyclooxygenases *see* COX-1 or COX1; COX-2 or COX2
cytokines (including interleukins)   58, 62, 64, 66, 322–323, 345, 403, 407, 411
  diet   128, 150, 152
  genetics   67, 448, 455, 458
  inflammation in AD   234–236, 239–241, 244, 246, 247, 251–252

insulin resistance and diabetes Type II 96, 97, 120–122, 124
probiotics 313

d

DASH (dietary approaches to stop hypertension) diet 118–123
dementia 13, 27–29, 31, 89, 92, 100, 125, 127, 130, 166, 204, 267–281
   exercise or physical activity 372, 375–377, 382
   genetics 446, 447, 456, 466, 470, 472
   and hormones 339, 349–351
   symptoms and diagnosis 9–11, 16, 18–20, 22, 29, 31, 32, 45–52, 55–57, 60, 62–63, 65, 267–281
   treatment 159, 205, 242, 250, 393–400
dementia rating scale (DRS) 49, 50
dementia with Lewy bodies (DLB) or Lewy body disease 18–20, 167, 168, 209, 267, 271, 276–277
   genetics 18, 22, 449, 454, 465, 469, 471, 472
   treatment 393, 395, 397
DHA (docosahexaenoic acid) 121, 122, 128, 206–208, 249–250
diabetes Type II/diabetes/T2D and 2–4, 89–103, 150–152, 159, 235, 236, 346, 372, 380, 408
   Alzheimer's disease risk 12, 33, 63, 89–103, 169–171, 190, 204, 207, 208, 238, 240, 241, 321
   brain function and cognition 89–103
   diet and nutrition 117, 120, 122–124, 134
   dietary fermentation and SCFA 316, 319, 326
   diagnosis
      AD (Alzheimer's disease) 10–11, 15, 16, 20, 32, 43–72, 236, 268–276
      cerebrovascular dementia or vascular dementia (VaD) 11, 16–17, 19, 21, 32–33, 50, 51, 53, 277–279
      DLB (dementia with Lewy bodies) 18–20
      FTD, FTLD (fronto-temporal lobe dementia) 13, 52, 443
      Huntington's disease 10, 24–26, 69, 132, 167, 236
      motor neuron diseases 27–30
      Parkinson's disease 19, 20, 47, 53, 54, 57, 59, 69, 133
diet and 1–5, 13, 17, 91, 99, 117–135, 150, 500–502
   carbohydrate metabolism 122, 150, 153, 312
   lipid and fat metabolism 70, 95–96, 99, 101–103, 119, 134, 151, 153, 161, 192, 194, 205, 207, 209, 245, 252, 319
   Mediterranean or Okinawan 3, 7, 13, 118, 119, 162, 208, 248, 253, 501
differential diagnosis 15, 18–20, 28, 32, 50–52, 57, 68, 269, 276
DLB *see* Dementia with Lewy bodies (DLB) or Lewy body disease
docosahexaenoic acid *see* DHA (docosahexaenoic acid)
donepezil 12, 15, 17, 26, 242, 299, 391–396, 398, 399
DRS *see* dementia rating scale (DRS)
dyslipidaemia/dyslipidemia 17, 33, 53, 70, 117–120, 189, 190, 205, 210, 297, 298, 321

e

EEG 51, 461
EGCG (epigallocatechin-3-gallate) 6, 245–247
eicosapentaenoic acid (EPA) 121, 122, 250
exercise 99, 167, 190, 205, 246, 247, 371–382, 501 *see also* physical activity
eye, diagnosis 68

f

fatal familial insomnia 30
FDG-PET 15, 19, 52–53, 91–92, 159, 410
fermentation (dietary) 6, 311–314, 501
fibre (dietary) 33, 118–119, 123, 135, 150, 153, 158, 312, 313, 315–320, 322, 326, 501
fitness cardiovascular/aerobic 371–375, 381

fMRI (functional MRI)   51, 53, 124, 158–159, 377, 381
folate   117, 125, 127–128
free fatty acid receptors (FFAR)   311, 316–323, 325
fronto-temporal lobe dementia   13–15, 20, 27, 29, 32, 267, 274, 279–280, 295
fructose   122–124, 149, 150, 156, 160–161, 318
FTD or FTLD *see* fronto-temporal lobe dementia

g
GABA (gamma amino butyric acid)   125, 127
GABA receptor   398
galantamine   12, 242, 299, 392, 394–396
gamma-secretase *see* secretases
genetics of
   AD   12, 63, 67, 153, 198, 203, 239, 292, 297, 381, 382, 443–473
   fronto-temporal lobe dementia   14
   Huntington's disease   24
   motor neuron diseases   28–30
   Parkinson's disease   22–23
Gerstmann Straussler Syndrome   30
GLP1/GLP-1   101–102, 317, 318, 320, 321
glucagon-like peptide-1 *see* GLP1/GLP-1 24
glucose   89–91, 93–97, 99–103, 122–126, 149–163, 170, 203, 209, 236, 251, 252, 275, 316, 408
glucose and brain metabolism   15, 52, 53, 56, 91–92, 98, 122, 275, 276, 410, 465
   diet and gut fermentation   312, 317, 319–321
   transporters (GLUT1, GLUT4)   90, 103, 157, 203, 252
GLUT1/GLUT4 *see* glucose, transporters (GLUT1, GLUT4)
glutamate   13, 25, 26, 125, 133, 159, 163, 243, 246, 252, 319, 345, 393, 396–398, 409, 410
glutathione   126, 129, 131, 250–252, 343, 344
glycogen   123, 149–151, 157, 161

glycogen synthase kinase 3β (GSK-3β)   96, 101, 102, 246, 299, 349, 410, 457, 464
GPCR and GPR   207, 311, 316
G-protein coupled receptor *see* GPCR and GPR
green tea polyphenols   6, 245–248, 500 *see also* EGCG (epigallocatechin-3-gallate)
GSS *see* Gerstmann Straussler Syndrome

h
HDL   120, 192–197, 202–204, 321, 352
high density lipoprotein *see* HDL
histone deacetylase (HDAC)   323–324, 409
histones   237, 324
homocysteine   17, 117, 126, 127
hypercholesterolaemia/hypercholesterolemia   90, 120, 123, 192, 399
hyperlipidaemia *see* lipidaemia
hypertension   12, 22, 117, 126, 134, 189, 190, 204, 240, 372, 397

i
IGF *see* insulin-like growth factor
idalopiridine   393, 399
imaging diagnostic   51–56
immunotherapy   299, 400–401
   active   299, 400–401
   passive   299, 400–404
indomethacin   240, 243
inflammation   3, 13, 26, 33, 57, 62, 67, 167, 233–253, 380, 408, 411, 500
   AD animal models   292, 296, 298, 299, 301
   diet and digestion   117, 118, 121–122, 129, 132, 133, 135, 151, 154
   genetics   448, 452, 454, 456–459, 465, 470
   diabetes and insulin resistance   89, 93, 96, 97, 102, 152, 159, 161
   sex steroids   344–346, 355
insulin   89–103, 123, 130, 151–153, 159, 160, 207, 209, 380, 408
   adiponectin deficiency   236
   -degrading enzyme (IDE)   169, 241, 250, 341, 353, 377, 378

diet/digestion   247, 252, 312, 316, 319, 321
-like growth factor (IGF)   101, 124, 131, 152, 166, 234, 377–379, 467
resistance   63, 89–103, 118–120, 123, 124, 151–154, 160, 161, 319, 346
sex hormones   346, 352
signalling   89–103, 130, 151–153, 160, 319, 408
interleukins *see* cytokines
iron   125, 131–134, 237, 246, 251–252, 343–344, 400, 460, 471

k
ketogenic diet   154
ketones   151, 153, 154, 156, 159, 325
ketones 3-beta-hydroxybutyrate   154, 252, 325
kuru   30-31, 168

l
LDL   120–121, 153, 193–196, 202–204, 321, 344, 352, 451, 453
LDL receptor   195–198, 200, 450, 451, 461, 462
leptin   103, 124, 208, 317, 318, 320, 322
Lewy bodies   18
Lewy Body Disease/dementia-*see* DLB
lipidaemia/hyperlipidaemia/dyslipidaemia   12, 17, 33, 53, 70, 90, 117–120, 123, 189, 190, 197, 297–298, 321
lipids   4, 58, 62, 64–66, 90, 97, 119, 121, 122, 129, 133, 167, 170, 189, 190, 192, 194, 208, 210, 237, 326, 451
lipoic acid   250–253
lipoproteins *see* HDL; LDL
liraglutide   102, 410
liver function   103, 121, 126, 128, 149, 151, 160, 163, 190, 191, 193–196, 198, 201, 252, 311–315
Lou Gehring's disease *see* ALS
low density lipoprotein *see* LDL
Low density lipoprotein receptor-related protein 1 *see* LRP-1
LRP-1   95, 192, 195, 196, 198, 200–201, 203

m
mad cow disease *see* CJD
magnesium   119, 125, 129, 131
magnetic resonance imaging *see* MRI; fMRI (functional MRI)
manganese   125, 131, 132
MAPK   244–246, 322, 341, 345
MCI   153, 162, 166, 202–204, 249, 268–275, 297, 377, 381, 464
MCI and diabetes and insulin resistance   90–92, 95, 97–98, 100–101
diagnosis and symptoms   47, 49, 51, 53–71
diet and nutrition   122, 123, 127, 130–133
prospective treatments   393–395, 398, 400, 401, 406, 411
sex hormones   340, 347–348, 351
medication for neurodegeneration   12, 15, 17, 19, 23, 26, 30, 71, 99, 242, 391–412, 500
Mediterranean diet (MeDi)   13, 118–121, 123, 162, 208, 248, 253, 501
memantine   13, 15, 26, 71, 94, 242–243, 298, 299, 393, 395, 396
meningoencephalitis   401
microglia   97, 128, 129, 157, 169, 170, 233–236, 238–240, 243, 245, 251
microglia and animal models   291, 296
current/potential treatments   403–404, 408, 410, 411
genetics   448, 451, 453, 455–458, 472
pathology   43–45
microtubule-associated protein kinase *see* MAPK
mild cognitive impairment *see* MCI and
MIND diet (Mediterranean-DASH diet intervention for neurodegenerative delay)   119, 123
mini-mental state examination *see* MMSE
miRNA   30, 69–71
MMSE   46–51, 56, 59, 64, 161, 166, 249, 342, 395, 400
MND   27–30
MoCA   47, 48
monoamine oxidase   23, 26, 66, 395
monocyte-derived macrophages   169

monocytes 96, 169, 240, 322, 323, 345, 455, 456, 463
Montreal Cognitive Assessment *see* MoCA
motor neuron disease *see* MND
MRI 15, 16, 19, 31, 45, 50–57, 158, 269, 276, 377, 380–381, 410, 455, 470
multi-infarct dementia, *see* VaD

n

neprilysin 58, 95, 169, 205, 241, 316, 341, 354, 377, 378
neurodegeneration 6, 26, 53, 56, 59, 65, 69, 89–91, 96–100, 125, 126, 167, 168, 170, 199, 205, 236, 252, 291, 292, 296–297, 339, 372, 443, 456, 457, 459, 469
neurofibrillary tangles *see* NFT (neurofibrillary tangles); tau
neuroplasticity 349, 372–373, 451
neurotransmission medication 71, 242, 298, 391–399
neurotransmitters 12, 15, 66, 94, 154, 159, 163–165, 205, 209, 316, 372, 377, 378, 464
neurotransmitters diet and micronutrients 117, 125, 127, 128, 131, 133, 134
NFT (neurofibrillary tangles) 9, 43–47, 96, 167, 168, 170, 201, 235, 238, 239, 291 *see also* tau
NFT animal models 291, 295, 297, 301
NFT genetics 456, 464
niacin *see* vitamin, B3/niacin
NMDA 13, 26, 71, 94, 125, 243, 298, 299, 393, 396–397
non-steroidal anti-inflammatory drugs (NSAID) 15, 240, 243–244, 408
NSAID *see* non-steroidal anti-inflammatory drugs (NSAID)

o

obesity 12, 17, 33, 60, 64, 66, 117, 169, 189, 190, 204, 207, 235–236, 451, 465
obesity and diet 95, 120–124, 150–153, 163, 207, 312, 316–319
  inflammation 96, 169, 235, 236, 240, 242, 247
  insulin and diabetes 150–153, 169, 236
  sex hormones 344, 349
oestrogen 130, 297, 335–337, 339–346, 348–354, 379–380
Okinawa diet 3, 7, 118, 123, 162, 253, 501
omega-3 fatty acids or n-3 polyunsaturated fatty acids (PUFA) 3, 118, 119, 121–122, 135, 207–208, 249–-250, 253, 501
omega-6 fatty acids or n-6 polyunsaturated fatty acids (PUFA) 119, 121–122, 207–208, 250, 501
oxidative stress 6, 13, 33, 59, 64, 93, 97–102, 167–168, 170, 233, 236–238, 500
oxidative stress and advanced glycation end products (AGE) 170
  biomarkers 57, 62, 65, 66
  clusterin 452–453
  diet and nutrition 4, 118, 122, 124, 126, 130–133, 245–253
  genetics 452–453, 467, 470
  lipid metabolism 192, 196, 208
  sex steroids 342–344, 353

p

Parkinson's disease (PD) 59, 60, 66, 153, 169, 189, 192, 209, 235–236, 245, 276, 302, 345, 376, 393
  and diet 127, 132, 133, 208
  and tyrosine intake 165
  dementia (PDD) 32
  genetics 443, 454, 457, 465–467, 469, 471
  pathology and diagnosis 18–24, 32, 33, 47, 49, 50, 52–54, 69, 167
PD *see* Parkinson's disease (PD)
PDD *see* Parkinson's disease, dementia (PDD)
PET 15, 19, 32, 51–57, 61–63, 67, 69, 91–92, 157, 159, 200, 340, 348, 352, 371, 377, 381
phosphodiesterase 397
physical activity 5, 17, 33, 117, 161, 247, 371–382, 501–502 *see also* exercise

Pittsburgh compound B PET *see* PiB PET 32, 54–57, 61–63, 67, 69, 91–92, 200, 340, 348, 352, 371, 377, 410
PKC 246, 409
plasma Aβ *see* Aβ plasma
polyphenol antioxidants 245–249, 500
polysaccharides 122, 125, 149–161, 312, 314, 501
positron emission tomography *see* PET
PPARγ (peroxisome proliferator-activated receptor-γ) 150, 236, 297, 243, 320, 344, 411
prebiotics 313
p75 receptor ligand 410
presenilin-1 (*PSEN1* gene, PS1 protein) 10, 65, 291–293, 296, 445–449, 463
presenilin-2 (*PSEN2* gene, PS2 protein) 10, 291–293, 445–449, 463
prion diseases 30–31
probiotics 313
programmed cell death 169 *see also* apoptosis
progressive supranuclear palsy *see* PSP
propionate 128, 150, 312–325
protein kinase C *see* PKC
PrP 30–31, 168
PSP 10, 15, 404, 410
psychogeriatric assessment scales (PAS) 48
pyridoxine see vitamin B6 122, 125, 127

r

RAGE 95, 97, 170–171, 238, 241, 292, 408
receptor for advanced glycation end products *see* RAGE
retinol/retinoic acid see vitamin, A/retinol/retinoic acid
riboflavin *see* vitamin, B2/riboflavin
rivastigmine 12, 23, 71, 242, 392, 394–396
rivastigmine transdermal patches 242, 394
rosiglitazone 94, 100, 393
Rowland Universal Dementia Assessment Scale *see* RUDAS
RUDAS 49

S

SAM *see* senescence accelerated mouse strain (SAM and SAMP8)
SAMP8 *see* senescence accelerated mouse strain (SAM and SAMP8)
SARM *see* selective oestrogen or androgen receptor modulators
SCFA *see* short chain fatty acids (SCFA)
scrapie 30–31
secretases 405–408, 446, 447, 463
secretase alpha-secretase (α-secretase) *see* ADAM10 ADAM-10 (also α-secretase); ADAM17/ADAM-17
secretase beta-secretase (β-secretase) *see* BACE (also BACE-1, β-secretase)
secretase gamma-secretase (γ-secretase) 95, 129, 134, 205, 206, 299, 316, 340, 405–408, 446–448, 463
secretase inhibitors and modulators 405–408
selective oestrogen or androgen receptor modulators 336, 346, 352–354
selenium 125, 131, 132
senescence accelerated mouse strain (SAM and SAMP8) 297
SERM *see* selective oestrogen or androgen receptor modulators
serotonin 15, 23, 26, 66, 127, 164–165, 378, 393, 396–399
seven minute screen 48
short chain fatty acids (SCFA) 6, 123, 150–151, 153, 311–326, 501
simvastatin 205, 399, 400
SMA (spinal muscular atrophy) 27, 30
SNCA gene 22
SOD1 28–30, 167, 168, 292
SPECT 19, 54
spinal muscular atrophy 27
statins 17, 120, 204–205, 399–400
sucrose 122–124, 149, 150, 160–162, 239
sugar 3
sulfatides 59, 209
superoxide dismutase-1 *see* SOD1
synucleinopathy 18, 22

t

tau   15, 29, 32, 56–61, 65, 167, 201, 245, 291, 377–378
   animal models   291, 293–297, 299, 301–302
   cytokines and inflammation   239–240
   diabetes and insulin resistance   92, 94, 96, 99, 102, 103
   diagnosis and phospho-tau   29, 31, 32, 56–61, 68, 269
   diet and nutrition   120, 126, 129, 132, 163
   genetics   291, 449, 450, 457, 459–462, 464–465
   imaging   15
   pathology   10, 14, 29, 31, 167, 168, 170, 235–236, 279, 443, 445
   sex steroids   348–349, 352
TCA cycle   125, 127, 154, 163, 319
TDP-43   14, 29
tea catechins *see* EGCG (epigallocatechin-3-gallate)
testosterone   130, 335–342, 344–354, 379–380
thiamin *see* vitamin B1
transgenic mouse model
   APP23 mice   293, 295, 299–301, 307
   APP/PS1 mice (or APPPS1)   293, 295, 299
   PDAPP mice   299
   Tg2576 mice   294, 295, 298, 299, 307, 309
   5XFAD mice   292, 293, 295, 299, 307
   3XTG mice   293, 295, 299
transient ischaemic attack (TIA)   17
transmissible spongiform encephalopathies (TSE) *see* prion diseases
tricarboxylic acid cycle *see* TCA cycle
tryptophan   65, 117, 125, 127, 164–165
TSE *see* prion diseases
type 2 diabetes mellitus (T2D) *see* diabetes type II/diabetes/T2D and
tyrosine   117, 163–166

v

VaD   16–17, 19–21, 32–33, 50, 51, 53, 277–279
vascular dementia *see* VaD
vascular endothelial growth factor (VEGF)   325, 378, 379
very low density lipoprotein *see* VLDL (very low density lipoprotein)
vitamin
   A/retinol/retinoic acid   125, 128, 129
   B1/thiamin   125, 126
   B2/riboflavin   125, 126
   B3/niacin   125, 127, 165
   B5   125
   B6/pyridoxine   5, 122, 125, 127, 158
   B12/ cobalamin   5, 46, 50, 117, 125, 127
   C   5, 125
   D   125, 129, 130, 134
   E/ α-tocopherol   125, 130, 131, 247
   K   125
VLDL (very low density lipoprotein)   153, 193–196, 201, 202, 451

w

Werdnig Hoffman disease *see* SMA (spinal muscular atrophy)

z

zinc   125, 129, 131–134, 237, 251, 464, 470